Aging 2000: Our Health Care Destiny

Volume I: Biomedical Issues

Aging 2000: Our Health Care Destiny

Volume I: Biomedical Issues

Edited by

Charles M. Gaitz

T. Samorajski

With 71 Figures

Springer-Verlag
New York Berlin Heidelberg Tokyo

Charles M. Gaitz, M.D.
Head, Gerontology Center
Assistant Director
T. Samorajski, Ph.D.
Chief, Neurobiology Section

Texas Department of Mental Health and Mental Retardation
Texas Research Institute of Mental Sciences
Texas Medical Center
Houston, Texas 77030 U.S.A.

Library of Congress Cataloging in Publication Data
Main entry under title:
Aging 2000.
Edited proceedings of a symposium held Oct. 23–26, 1983 in Houston, Tex.; sponsored by the Texas Research Institute of Mental Sciences.
Bibliography: v. 1, p.
Includes index.
Contents: v.1. Biomedical issues.
1. Aged—Medical care—Congresses. 2. Aging—Congresses. 3. Geriatrics—Congresses. 4. Geriatric psychiatry—Congresses. 5. Health—Congresses. I. Gaitz, Charles M. II. Samorajski, T. (Thaddeus), (date). III. Texas Research Institute of Mental Sciences. [DNLM: 1. Geriatrics—congresses. 2. Health Services for the Aged—trends—congresses. 3. Geriatrics—trends—congresses. W3 TE77 17th 1983a / WT 30 A2689 1983]
RA777.6.A37 1985 362.1′0880565 84-22196

ISBN-13: 978-1-4612-9544-0 e-ISBN-13: 978-1-4612-5058-6
DOI: 10.1007/978-1-4612-5058-6
1985 $0.00 + .20
Typeset by Ampersand, Inc., Rutland, Vermont.

9 8 7 6 5 4 3 2 1

Preface

The seventeenth annual symposium sponsored by the Texas Research Institute of Mental Sciences was held October 23–26, 1983, in Houston, Texas. The theme was *Aging 2000: Our Health Care Destiny*. This volume on biomedical aspects and a companion volume on psychosocial aspects include edited versions of the presentations by about 80 speakers.

Their papers were directed at practitioners, researchers, and medical educators who will be active and productive in the year 2000, and we focused on those who would influence the evolution of care of elderly persons during the next 17 years. We chose topics that would be of particular interest to teachers and current planners in the disciplines concerned with delivery of health and social services. We believe that having a core of more qualified and better trained practitioners will help the population of aged persons achieve a higher level of physical and mental health, life satisfaction and happiness, to find better coping techniques and control of environmental stresses, and to attain personal and social goals.

Our Goals

While preparing for the symposium we knew that the status of the art in 1983 obviously would be the base from which we would work, but we asked our speakers to give priority to future planning and directions. A compilation of background material and reviews of data relevant to the symposium topics was distributed before the meeting to each participant so that the material could be studied; speakers were thus confronted by an informed audience able to address issues with a future-oriented view. Readers of these volumes, then, should not expect them to replace textbooks of geriatric medicine or psychiatry.

To clarify research needs, we asked our speakers to raise questions based on current status and to suggest solutions based on current knowledge. Problems of individuals, families, and society were discussed and we explored ways of dealing more effectively with social and health problems. We inquired into what is known about prevention and normal aging, asked how services could be organized for more efficient delivery, and how we might pay for such services. Much attention was given to application of present knowledge, and practitioners were informed of creative new programs already in operation. Obstacles to delivery of services were defined and techniques for more effective application of present knowledge were discussed.

In attempting to delineate needed research, we did this knowing that resources for both services and research will be limited in the next 17 years, and so we emphasized a practical approach. We gave priority to the relevance of research and its potential for finding solutions that will contribute to the general welfare of aged persons. It became clear that alternatives for the delivery of service, the roles of practitioners, and quality-of-life issues all need further investigation, but so does the biological science approach to clinical problems that are currently not understood but offer hope of being resolved.

Throughout the conference, we emphasized the relationship of researchers and practitioners, not as antagonists but as partners—as representatives of the society to which they belong. Better communication between these groups will lead to a clearer definition of the problems and issues, especially of those that only scientific advances can solve. Moral and ethical aspects, political and social implications of the questions and proposals were highlighted, as were the more typical problems of disease prevention and the care and treatment of patients.

Format

Approximately half the meeting time was devoted to plenary sessions and the rest to smaller concurrent group meetings to discuss specific problems. The approach enabled each participant to get a broad overview and, at the same time, to follow a track that gave a more intensive review of issues interesting to specific health care disciplines or researchers in a particular field. Our broad approach ranged from such diverse areas as basic mechanisms of biologic aging to often neglected patient groups like those with mental retardation. Discussion of treatment for depression ranged from very recent progress in psychopharmacology to social services, such as supportive and intensive psychotherapy.

The diversity of topics and approaches is reflected in the chapters of these two publications. Decision-makers, researchers, and practitioners must, in the future, collaborate with colleagues in other disciplines and use many methods of solving problems. We attempted to highlight as many relevant issues as possible within the constraints of a three-day meeting. Understandably, some topics were given minimal attention and others omitted entirely.

Training and Education Aspects

We hope that participation in a symposium, and now reading these two books, will be a stimulating educational experience. From the first planning stage, we sought ways to disseminate the substance of the conference. These volumes are one approach. A home study course, with some additional material, is also being prepared. An intense effort has been made to assure that this conference will have an impact beyond the ordinary publication of proceedings that collect dust on bookshelves.

The symposium planners were ambitious. We wanted to address social, psychological, health, economic, and cultural issues of particular interest to psychiatrists and other physicians, psychologists, social workers, nurses, and other health professionals. The need for more trained practitioners was known, so the publications contain many implications for students, faculty members, and educational institutions. Throughout the conference, we emphasized the application of current knowledge and encouraged a dialogue with scientists about issues and conditions for which there is no present solution.

We hope that our readers will recall the intent and format of the symposium and will integrate its concepts and ideas into their work as practitioners, researchers, and teachers. We cannot provide all the answers, but we do offer a concise presentation of many important issues. Applying the knowledge we have now and searching for more will lead to a healthier, more satisfying life for our aged population in the years to come.

Charles M. Gaitz, M.D.
T. Samorajski, Ph.D.

Contents for Volume I

Contents for Volume II

Part VII. Delivery of Care for the Aged in a State Mental Health and Mental Retardation System

Part VIII. Rehabilitation with the Future Aged

Part IX. Long-Term-Care System for Future Elders

Part X. Future Financing of Health Care

Part XI. Legal and Ethical Concerns in Care of the Aged

Part XII. Concluding Visions

Acknowledgments

It is impossible to express formal thanks to everyone who contributed to the implementation and success of the symposium on *Aging 2000: Our Health Care Destiny*. The comprehensiveness of the program, the quality of presentations by our speakers, and the persistent interest and enthusiasm of our audience justified the many hours of planning and the heavy investment of energy and money.

A large grant by Sandoz was the vehicle that made it possible, but the material contributions, while necessary and useful, were less significant than the assistance provided by Bill Connelly, Bob Essner, and Krystyna Belendiuk, who gave us much support and help in planning the conference and attracting an internationally known group of speakers and participants.

The program was organized collaboratively by several staff members of the Texas Research Institute of Mental Sciences. Dr. George Niederehe, Dr. Roy Varner, and Ms. Nancy Wilson participated as representatives of their professional disciplines, and offered a multidisciplinary approach. Dr. Jary Lesser joined us after he came on staff early in 1983. Howard Rabinowitz did an extraordinary job of facilitating and coordinating everyone's efforts, and his attention to details in his usual affable manner averted serious crises. Dr. Linda Webb and other members of the training division staff, Peter Baer and his associates in the audiovisual section, and Lore Feldman and Kathleen Kimball-Baker of the publications staff were all extremely co-operative, efficient, and conscientious in helping us. We also are grateful for the remarkable and consistent support of our secretaries, Gerry

Meeker, Susan Samson, and Mildred Beaman, who were always available and performed at a superior level.

Finally, we express our appreciation to Dr. Joseph Schoolar, Director of TRIMS, and his staff for their encouragement and assistance in bringing our aspirations to fulfillment with the publication of these two volumes.

Contributors

Kenneth Z. Altshuler, M.D., Stanton Sharp Professor and Chairman, Department of Psychiatry, University of Texas Health Science Center, Dallas, Texas, USA.

Stanley H. Appel, M.D., Professor and Chairman, Department of Neurology, Baylor College of Medicine, Houston, Texas, USA.

Richard W. Besdine, M.D., Assistant Professor of Medicine, Division on Aging, Harvard Medical School, Boston, Massachusetts; Director, Geriatric Education Center and Geriatric Fellowship Training, Harvard Medical School, Cambridge, Massachusetts, USA.

Robert H. Binstock, Ph.D., Henry R. Luce Professor of Aging, Health, and Society, Case Western Reserve University, Cleveland, Ohio, USA.

James E. Birren, Ph.D., Dean, Gerontology Center, Professor of Psychology, University of Southern California, Los Angeles, California, USA.

William Bondareff, Ph.D., M.D., Professor of Psychiatry and Gerontology, Della Martin Professor of Medical Research in Psychiatry, University of Southern California School of Medicine and Andrus Gerontology Center, Los Angeles, California, USA.

R. Nick Bryan, M.D., Ph.D., Professor of Radiology, Department of Radiology, Baylor College of Medicine, Houston, Texas, USA.

Roger J. Bulger, M.D., Professor of Medicine and Professor of Public Health and President of the University of Texas Health Science Center at Houston, Texas, USA.

Ewald W. Busse, M.D., Sc.D., Associate Provost and Dean Emeritus, Duke University Medical Center; J.P. Gibbons Professor of Psychiatry, Duke University School of Medicine, Durham, North Carolina, USA.

Arvid Carlsson, M.D., Professor of Pharmacology, Institute of Pharmacology, University of Gothenberg, Gothenberg, Sweden.

Arthur Cherkin, Ph.D., Research Biochemist, Departments of Medicine and Psychiatry and Biobehavioral Sciences, University of California School of Medicine, Los Angeles, California, USA.

S. Chierichetti, M.D., B.Sc., Medical Director, Sandoz Ptooloti Farmaceutici S.P.A., Milano, Italy.

Gene D. Cohen, M.D., Ph.D., Director, Program on Aging, National Institute of Mental Health, Rockville, Maryland, USA.

John Copeland, M.A., M.D., F.R.C.P., F.R.C. Psych., D.P.M., Professor of Psychiatry, University Department of Psychiatry, Royal Liverpool Hospital, Liverpool, England.

Joseph T. Coyle, M.D., Professor of Psychiatry, Neuroscience, Pharmacology, and Pediatrics, The Johns Hopkins University, Baltimore, Maryland, USA.

D. Cucinotta, M.D., Postgraduate School of Geriatrics and Gerontology, University of Parma, Parma, Italy.

Mony J. de Leon, Ed.D., Research Assistant Professor of Psychiatry, New York University Medical Center, New York, New York, USA.

Gunnar Dybwad, Ph.D., Professor Emeritus of Human Development, Florence Heller Graduate School for Advanced Studies in Social Welfare, Brandeis University, Waltham, Massachusetts, USA.

Fumio Eto, M.D., Associate, Department of Geriatrics, Faculty of Medicine, University of Tokyo, Tokyo, Japan.

William E. Fann, M.D., Professor of Psychiatry, Associate Professor of Pharmacology, Baylor College of Medicine; Chief, Psychiatry Service, Veterans Administration Medical Center, Houston, Texas, USA.

Steven H. Ferris, Ph.D., Associate Professor of Psychiatry, New York University Medical Center, New York, New York, USA.

Caleb E. Finch, Ph.D., Professor of Biological Sciences and Gerontology, University of Southern California, Los Angeles, California, USA.

James F. Flood, Ph.D., Research Psychopharmacologist, Department of Psychiatry and Biobehavioral Sciences, University of California, Los Angeles, California, USA.

Marshal F. Folstein, M.D., Eugene Meyer Professor of Psychiatry and Medicine, Departments of Psychiatry and Medicine, Johns Hopkins Institute, Baltimore, Maryland, USA.

Kjell Fuxe, Ph.D., Department of Histology, Karolinska Institute, Stockholm, Sweden.

Ajax E. George, M.D., Professor of Radiology, New York University School of Medicine, New York, New York, USA.

Menek Goldstein, Ph.D., Professor of Neurochemistry, New York University School of Medicine, Department of Psychiatry, New York, New York, USA.

Carl G. Gottfries, M.D., Ph.D., Professor of Psychiatry, Department of Psychiatry and Neurochemistry, St. Jörgen's Hospital, University of Göteborg, Hisings Backa, Sweden.

Barry J. Gurland, F.R.C. Psych., M.R.C.P., Professor of Clinical Psychiatry, Department of Psychiatry, Columbia University, New York, New York, USA.

Herman B. Hamot, M.A., Sandoz Research Institute, East Hanover, New Jersey, USA.

Leonard Hayflick, Ph.D., Professor and Director, Center for Gerontological Studies, University of Florida, Gainesville, Florida, USA.

Leo E. Hollister, M.D., Professor of Medicine, Psychiatry, and Pharmacology, Stanford University School of Medicine, Palo Alto, California, USA.

Fritz Huber, M.D., Medical Director and Head of the First Geriatric Clinic, Felix Pfeller Hospital, Basel, Switzerland.

John M. Kane, M.D., Associate Professor of Psychiatry, School of Medicine, Health Sciences Center, State University of New York at Stony Brook, Stony Brook, New York, USA.

Wolfgang Kehr, M.D., Research Laboratory of Schering AG, Berlin (West) and Bergkamen, Federal Republic of Germany.

Susan Köberle, M.D., Scientific Collaborator, Clinical Research, Sandoz Ltd., Basel, Switzerland.

Karin Kurth, Research Laboratories of Schering AG, Berlin (West) and Bergkamen, Federal Republic of Germany.

Jow Y. Lew, Ph.D., Neurochemistry Research Laboratories, New York University Medical Center, New York, New York, USA.

Abraham Lieberman, M.D., Department of Neurology, New York University Medical Center, New York, New York, USA.

Mary Jane Lucas, R.N., Johns Hopkins Medical Center, Baltimore, Maryland, USA.

Rudolf Markstein, Ph.D., Preclinical Research, Sandoz Ltd., Basel, Switzerland.

Edward J. Masoro, Ph.D., Professor and Chairman, Department of Physiology, University of Texas Health Science Center at San Antonio, San Antonio, Texas, USA.

William Meier-Ruge, M.D., Associate Professor of Neuropathology, Laboratory of Gerontological Brain Research, Department of Neuropathology, Institute of Pathology, University of Basel, Basel, Switzerland.

George S. Merz, Ph.D., Head, Tissue Culture Laboratory, Department of Pathological Neurobiology, New York State Institute for Basic Research in Developmental Disabilities, Staten Island, New York, USA.

Kosei Ojika, M.D., Assistant Professor, Department of Neurology, Baylor College of Medicine, Houston, Texas, USA.

John R. Patin, Sandoz Research Institute, East Hanover, New Jersey, USA.

Eric Pfeiffer, M.D., Professor of Psychiatry, University of South Florida College of Medicine; Director, Suncoast Gerontology Center, University of South Florida Medical Center, Tampa, Florida, USA.

Bruce W. Richman, M.D., Department of Psychiatry, Baylor College of Medicine, Houston, Texas, USA.

Martin N. Rossor, M.A., M.R.C.P., Senior Registrar, Department of Neurology, Kings College Hospital, London, England.

John W. Rowe, M.D., Associate Professor of Medicine, Director, Division on Aging, Harvard Medical School, Boston, Massachusetts; Deputy Director, Division on Health Policy Research and Education, Harvard University, Cambridge, Massachusetts, USA.

Harvey L. Ruben, M.D., M.P.H., Associate Clinical Professor of Psychiatry, Department of Psychiatry, Yale University School of Medicine, New Haven, Connecticut, USA.

T. Samorajski, Ph.D., Neurobiology Section, Texas Research Institute of Mental Sciences, Houston, Texas, USA.

V. Santini, M.D., Sandoz Ptooloti Farmaceutici S.P.A., Milan, Italy.

Charles A. Shamoian, M.D., Ph.D., Associate Professor of Clinical Psychiatry and Pharmacology, Cornell Medical College, New York, New York, USA.

Yukito Shinohara, M.D., Professor and Chairman of Department of Neurology, Tokai University School of Medicine, Isehara, Japan.

Jack M. Singer, M.D., Medical Director, Sandoz Research Institute, East Hanover, New Jersey; Clinical Assistant Professor of Psychiatry, Rutgers Medical School, University of Medicine and Dentistry of New Jersey, Piscataway, New Jersey, USA.

René Spiegel, Ph.D., Lecturer at the University of Basel, Department of Psychology, Basel, Switzerland; Scientific Collaborator, Clinical Research, Sandoz Ltd., Basel, Switzerland.

Helmut Wachtel, M.D., Research Laboratories of Schering AG, Berlin (West) and Bergkamen, Federal Republic of Germany.

Kenneth M. Weiss, Ph.D., Professor of Genetics, Center for Demographic and Population Genetics, University of Texas Graduate School of Biomedical Sciences, Houston, Texas, USA.

Leslie A. Widrow, B.A., Department of Psychiatry and Behavioral Sciences, Stanford University School of Medicine, Stanford, California, USA.

David E. Wilder, Ph.D., Adjunct Professor of Sociology and Education, Teachers College, Columbia University, New York, New York, USA.

Henryk M. Wisniewski, M.D., Ph.D., Director, New York State Institute for Basic Research in Developmental Disabilities, Staten Island, New York, USA.

Jerome A. Yesavage, M.D., Assistant Professor of Psychiatry, Department of Psychiatry and Behavioral Sciences, Stanford University School of Medicine, Stanford, California, USA.

Masaki Yoshikawa, M.D., Professor Emeritus, University of Tokyo, Tokyo, Japan.

Part I

Overview

Chapter 1

Health Care of the Aging: Trends, Dilemmas, and Prospects for the Year 2000

Robert H. Binstock

Summary

Improvements in mortality are not being accompanied by comparable improvements in morbidity among older persons. Consequently, increased longevity is sharply exacerbating a number of trends—in public policy, social structure, and particularly the costs of health care—that make it highly probable that the financing, delivery mechanisms, and use of health care resources in the United States will be drastically altered by the year 2000. As these alterations in the health care system unfold, old age is highly likely to be a focal point for a number of moral, financial, and social dilemmas. These dilemmas and their societal implications are explored in this chapter.

During the past few years the media dramatically focused public concern on the so-called crisis in Social Security. Our attention was drawn to both short-term and longer-term issues. We were confronted with the immediate fact that the Social Security payroll tax was not yielding enough revenue to pay the Old Age and Survivors Insurance (OASI) benefits that were due during 1983. At the same time the public began to appreciate some of the possible implications of the "graying of America"—the demographic trends through which our population will have increasingly larger absolute numbers and higher proportions of older persons in the years ahead. In particular, these demographic projections generated anxieties about our societal capacity to sustain Social Security retirement benefits in the 21st century when the "dependency ratio"—the proportion of workers to retired persons—is expected to fall sharply.

The Social Security Amendments that Congress enacted in March of 1983 and the President signed in April may alleviate the sense of crisis regarding this issue for some time. But even if they do, our attention will very quickly be absorbed by a somewhat different crisis in public policy toward aging.

It will soon become apparent to most Americans that the recently resolved crisis in Social Security was negligible compared to the crises emerging in the arena of health care and aging. The most serious implications of a graying America—I would argue—lie in the financing, organization, and utilization of health care resources.

Many policy analysts, journalists, and other observers have looked at the demographic trends of a graying America, and at the fact that we are currently spending 27% of our annual federal budget, $218 billion in Fiscal Year 1983 (U.S. Senate Special Committee on Aging, 1983), on benefits to the aged. They have extended these observations to forecast, for instance, that shortly after the year 2000, federal expenditures on the aged will have more than tripled in real dollars, and will constitute 40% of the federal budget (Califano, 1978). On the basis of such dramatic projections, they have questioned sharply whether our society can afford the costs of an aging population (e.g., Samuelson, 1978). But in doing so, they are not framing the issue in an appropriate context.

Numbers that express the percentages of governmental expenditures devoted to a single function such as "benefits to the aged" or "defense" may be dramatic political symbols. But they do not necessarily represent unsustainable economic burdens. The pertinent question to ask is: What kinds of public benefits to the aged, if any, are unsustainable—either through current taxing policies or, more broadly, through the Gross National Product (GNP), the total annual output of goods and services in the nation? When this issue is confronted, the answer becomes readily apparent. What appears to be unsustainable are the rapidly inflating costs of health care for the aging, and of health care in general.

This conclusion can be reached easily, either in the narrower content of specific governmental programs or in the broader context of the total economy. In the governmental context we can look, for instance, at the Medicare program through which all persons over the age of 64 are eligible to have certain health care expenses reimbursed by the national government. This Medicare program currently costs $55 billion per year (U.S. Senate Special Committee on Aging, 1983). The funds for paying Medicare benefits, financed by Social Security payroll taxes, will be exhausted before the end of this decade unless drastic changes are made in the methods for financing them and/or in the benefits for which they pay (Demkovich, 1983; U.S. Senate Special Committee on Aging, 1983).

In a broader framework, economists Robert Clark and John Menefee (1981) have taken account of the fact that health care costs have inflated at a much greater rate in recent years than the general rate of inflation, as measured by the Consumer Price Index (CPI). Consequently, they have projected that health care costs for older persons will primarily account for a doubling—a 100% increase—in the proportion of GNP expended on total public benefits to the aged over the next 40 years. In contrast, they have also projected that *if* health care costs could be contained at the general level of inflation for other goods, services, and cost-of-living adjustments, the proportion of GNP expended on public benefits to the aged would drop 28% by the year 2000, and remain that low through the year 2025. It is important to note that both projections take account of the millions of additional older persons who will become eligible for government benefits in the years ahead.

By looking at these and other forecasts based on projections of current trends and existing policies (Davis, 1983), it is reasonably safe to predict that the financing, organization, and utilization of health care resources in the U.S. will undergo drastic changes by the year 2000, if not before. In the remainder of this discussion, I will consider some of the elements that will be involved as these consequences of increased longevity unfold. First, I will briefly consider the capacity of older persons to pay for a larger burden of health care costs. Second, I will touch upon some trends in the need for long-term care of older persons, and in public financing and family participation for providing home care alternatives to institutionalization of aged persons. Finally, I will discuss some of the major possibilities that may emerge as the financing, organization, and use of health care resources undergo change.

The Capacity of Older Persons to Pay for Health Care

Expenditures on health care for older persons account for 33% of total health care expenditures in the United States, even though the aged account for only 11% of the population. In 1981, the latest year for which figures are available, the total bill for the health care of the elderly—persons over the age of 64—was more than $83 billion; the average cost of health care for an elderly individual was about $3200 per year (U.S. Senate Special Committee on Aging, 1983).

While government pays for over two-thirds of these health care expenditures for the elderly, the proportion and amounts paid by older persons out-of-pocket are hardly insignificant. Older persons pay an average of about 30% of their health expenditures out-of-pocket. This distribution will clearly be undergoing a change in the years immediately ahead, as governmental insurance programs are "capped," and patients are required to pay more "coinsurance" out-of-pocket.

As health care costs continue to rise, and as the proportion of government reimbursements for those costs are limited through various mechanisms, what capacity will older persons have to pay additional amounts out of their pockets for health care? There are many approaches to measuring the income adequacy and income sources of older persons. And each of these approaches and their specific measures can yield a result that is substantially different from the others. Without engaging in an extensive and technical discussion of these techniques, it is possible to make several summary observations that are substantiated elsewhere (Binstock, 1983; Schulz, 1984) about the capacity of older persons to pay for their health care.

At present, it is very difficult for about two-thirds of the older persons in the U.S. to contribute significantly to further financing of their health care. In the years immediately ahead, the capacity of older Americans to pay for their health care will become even more limited. The Social Security Amendments of 1983 have cut back on the generosity of the formulas that will be used in the future to provide annual cost-of-living adjustments for Social Security retirement benefits. A new provision that subjects some Social Security benefits to taxation will cut down the financial capacity of moderate-income older persons. Increases in the amount of coinsurance payments under Medicare (i.e. the proportions of health care changes that the government will not reimburse to health care providers) are having an impact on both low- and moderate-income persons. And private pensions from industry, and public pensions for state and local government employees, are only adjusted for inflation on an ad hoc basis; even then such adjustments do not come close to matching increases in the Consumer Price Index, let alone the substantially higher rate of inflation in health care prices.

To date, very little has been documented regarding the impact of intrafamily transfers, the income that older persons may receive from their children and other kin, or vice versa. Available data indicate that relatively large transfers may flow both ways, with perhaps slightly more aged families receiving assistance than assisting younger children (Moon, 1977).

The equity that many older persons have in their homes represents a potential source of additional income for them. But converting this asset into a liquid stream of income, through such instruments as Reverse Annuity Mortgages, is not as simple as it would seem. Substantial changes would be needed in financial and marketing practices, and in statutory law, in order to "unlock" home equity in the U.S.A.; such changes may take many years to take effect in a responsible and widespread fashion. The potential of unlocking home equity is a good idea, but a great deal will need to be done to bring it to fruition in the U.S.A., in a manner that will substantially help older persons (Scholen and Chen, 1980).

At this time, therefore, neither home equity nor intrafamily transfers seem likely to be panaceas for the stresses on older persons to increase their out-of-pocket payments for health care. It is possible, of course, that government might require families to pay for an older person's health care expenses before an older person can become eligible for government health insurance benefits that are available to low-income persons of all ages under Medicaid.

Long-Term Care and the Family Situations of Older Persons

Although improvements in mortality rates have been notable in this century, such improvements are not accompanied by equivalent improvements in morbidity. Unfortunately, the optimistic argument presented by Fries (1980), predicting the compression of morbidity in old age, has been responsibly and effectively demolished (Schneider and Brody, 1983). Ironically, an unintended consequence of improvements in longevity has been extension of the life span into the pathways of long-term, chronic, disabling conditions that rob life of its quality. The age-specific prevalence of long-term chronic diseases and other disabling conditions, particularly organic brain syndromes such as Alzheimer's disease, rises exponentially in the last decades of life, particularly in the late 70s and 80s (Gruenberg, 1977). Yet, for instance, we are spending less than $20 million a year (in the U.S.A.) on research to understand the causes of these brain diseases so that they might be prevented or detected early enough to reverse, even though we have had good clues on some of the key issues regarding brain syndromes, particularly Alzheimer's disease, for some time (Butler, 1978). This compares with over $1 billion annually spent for research on heart disease, cancer, and strokes.

The number of Americans in their late 70s and 80s will increase substantially in the decades ahead. By the year 2000, half of the people over 65 years of age in the U.S.A. will be over 75 years of age, and about 15% will be over 85 years old (U.S. Senate Special Committee on Aging, 1983). To the extent that further progress is made against heart disease, cancer, and strokes, even more people will reach this age category. On the basis of current age-specific rates, it can be estimated that the incidence of organic brain syndromes will rise sharply during the decades ahead. For instance, Schneider and Brody (1983) report that the prevalence of Alzheimer's disease is above 15% in persons over 80 years old.

There has been a great deal of talk in recent years about reducing the financial costs of long-term care, and avoiding the dehumanizing aspects of institutionalization by providing "home care alternatives" to nursing homes and other extended care facilities. These home care alternatives have been perceived as part of a "continuum of care" that can enable many persons to remain relatively independent in their own homes, and able to avoid unnecessary institutionalization. Among other things, this continuum includes such elements as companionship services, homemaker services, chore services, shopping assistance, meal-preparation assistance, transportation, periodic monitoring, adult day care, and respite programs. But as much as these services and the concept of home care alternatives have been talked about, they are not funded sufficiently to be implemented on a substantial scale. Medicare and Medicaid, the government health-insurance programs, do not reimburse a patient for most elements of the continuum of care, but only for the most "medicalized" components of the continuum (U.S. Comptroller General, 1979). As a consequence, one suspects that the marginal decision to institutionalize oneself—or one's parent, in-law, spouse, or sibling—may often be influenced by the existing reimbursement possibilities. Talk about home care alternatives is nice. But if one cannot obtain them or afford them, and if institutionalization is financially viable because of government reimbursement programs, the odds favor a decision to institutionalize.

As an alternative to public reimbursement for the full range of home care components, many have looked to the family as a source for supportive care (Cantor and Little, in press). Elaine Brody (1981) has estimated that some 75–80% of the various elements of the continuum of care necessary for living in the community is provided by family members on a voluntary basis. In most cases this means that care is provided by middle-aged daughters and daughters-in-law—persons whom Brody has termed "women in the middle." But if we consider the labor-force participation pattern of women in this age bracket, we cannot rely on a continuation of this level of support from the family, as much as the family may wish to provide it. In the last 40 years, there has been more than a fivefold increase in the labor-force participation of women who are 45–54 years of age—from 11% to a current rate of 60%. An occasional quarterly report from the federal government indicates a short-term drop in this upward trend of women's trends in labor-force participation; but the long-term trend has been steadily upward. What this may imply, of course, is that many family members who may wish to provide many of the elements of the continuum of care at home for their elderly relatives may find it impossible to provide all of those components if they are also working.

Related elements that may be weakening family ties and propensities to provide supportive care are high rates of divorce, single-parent families, remarriages, and unmarried couples living together for extended periods. In contemporary American society, it is not always easy to know whose mother-in-law is whose. As British historian Peter Laslett has pointed out, patterns of family support seem to weaken with the aging of populations, and particularly in relation to such cultural variables as rates of divorce, rates of remarriage, adoption, and so on (Laslett, 1981).

In short, neither trends in public financial support, nor trends in family life suggest that the dilemmas of financing health care of the aging and/or providing it in a humane, community context will be easily resolved. Meanwhile, the potential for continued improvement in mortality rates may not bode well for the aggregate health status or morbidity rates of the older population, its need for health care, and the costs of that care.

Emergent Health Policy Developments

What policies are likely to emerge out of this situation? In the immediate to longer-term future, national health insurance or some variant of it is very unlikely. There has been no formal Congressional action on national health insurance since 1974. Bills have been introduced for that purpose but there have been no hearings or committee action. Perhaps there will be a reemergence of such proposals in the late 1980s because of three factors: first, a lack of universal protection against large health care expenses; second, unequal access to health care; and third, the uncontrolled rate of cost increases in health care, which we have discussed earlier.

But even if we see something in the form of national health insurance enacted by the end of the decade, it is unlikely that it will be a totally governmental approach—all government financed and administered. Since the prime impetus for health care reform is likely to be cost control for the decades ahead, the most likely approach is a mixed government and private-market system. There will be enough federal control to make the delivery system respond. But there will not be a total governmental approach, because the financial burdens for public spending will be seen as too enormous.

How will this be likely to play out with particular reference to health policies affecting the aging? As suggested earlier, the problem of who will pay the health care costs of the aging is one of the most explosive issues of domestic social policy that lies ahead of us. The short term is bringing us some incremental measures: caps are being put on Medicare and Medicaid; small changes are continuously being made in coinsurance or "cost sharing." Marginal mechanisms of various kinds are being launched to cut down on health care costs through prospective-payment devices such as special Health Maintenance Organizations (HMOs) for Medicare-eligible clients, Medicare vouchers, and reimbursements determined on the basis of Diagonistically Related Groups (DRGs). One of the newer proposals for health-cost containment is in legislation currently being considered by the Congress. It would prevent doctors who treat Medicare patients in hospitals from billing for any charges beyond what Medicare reimburses

(Pear, 1983). But I suspect that the real battle will be fought out in parameters defined by broader economic, political, and social factors.

Health care expenditures in the United States are now approaching 11% of the Gross National Product (Stevens, 1982). In the face of continuing exponential increases in the costs of health care, the federal government has been attempting to hold down public expenditures while appropriately insisting that equal quality of care be provided to patients whose expenses are reimbursed by the government. At the same time, hospitals have not been fully reimbursed by Medicare and Medicaid at the customary rates which they have established for specific services and facilities. To compensate for less-than-full rates of governmental reimbursement, hospitals have been redistributing the unreimbursed portion of such costs by building them into their overall structure of charges or, in other words, "cost shifting" to patients whose bills are paid out-of-pocket and/or through private insurance. The Hospital Insurance Association of America recently estimated that cost shifting to insurance companies has reached an annual level of more than $8 billion.

Insurance companies, apparently, are not going to passively accept this cost shifting and its consequences for them. Their customers are resisting higher premiums, and the companies are facing ever-increasing expenditures. In Massachusetts, and in several other states, statutes have been recently enacted at the behest of insurance companies and corporations to curb hospital costs and cost shifting (Kinzer, 1983). Under Chapter 372 of the Commonwealth of Massachusetts, for example, all hospitals will have to live within budgets determined in advance by taking 1981 costs and adding an inflation factor, with allowances for certain "costs beyond control" of the institution, and some increment reflecting increases in services (Caper and Blumenthal, 1983). Such increases, however, are limited by formulas reflecting changes in either numbers of patients or numbers of services per patient—in other words, geared to increases in productivity.

It is highly likely that most states will soon adopt some such hospital cost-containment legislation. The issue will be: Where will hospitals turn in order to contain their costs? It seems to me that there are four immediate possibilities: (1) reductions in physician fees; (2) reductions in the costs of plant, facilities, and nonphysician personnel; (3) less purchase and use of high-cost technology and procedures; and (4) the practice of two-class medicine, brought about by restraints upon cost shifting from patients who rely upon Medicare and Medicaid (see also Platt, 1983). In the context of the power held by physicians in the institutions that provide health care (Starr, 1983), and the relatively low wages and unionization of other health personnel, it would seem that the third and fourth possibilities are most likely. But both of these options—the rationing of high-cost technology and procedures, and the evolution of two-class health care—raise ominous prospects for the elderly. Such developments will begin to make manifest the latent ethical issues concerning the value of one life compared with another (see Hilfiker, 1983).

Rationing issues are customarily framed with a bias against older persons. Especially when the underlying issue is so-called "cost-effectiveness," the policy analysis is customarily framed to weight the answer in favor of those who can be presumed to have a longer potential life span.

The issue of rationing health care on the basis of old-age criteria has already been raised in prominent American public forums. Last April, speaking to the annual meeting of the Health Insurance Association of America—obviously, a receptive audience—economist Alan Greenspan pointed out the facts that 30% of the annual Medicare budget is expended on older patients who die within the year, and that those patients represent only 5–6% of the total number of patients covered by Medicare. Greenspan explicitly asked "whether it is worth it to spend large amounts of money" on such patients (Schulte, 1983). It is worth noting that this proposition was put forward by a highly centrist figure in American politics. Greenspan, after all, was recently the chairman of the Bipartisan Commission on Social Security Reform that resolved the so-called crisis in Social Security. He was chosen as the chairman because he was acceptable to Democrats, Republicans, business, labor, and all other major factions involved in recommending a resolution to the Social Security crisis of 1983.

The prospect of official rationing of health care on the basis of chronological old age is hardly farfetched. It is already done in other nations. Up to now, in the United States, we have had the luxury of pretending that all physicians and their associates have been doing everything they can for everyone. Unofficially, of course, health care rationing has taken place on demographic and socioeconomic bases in many different ways. But before the year 2000, I suspect that such rationing will take place officially, and we will no longer have the luxury of pretending that it does not occur. Moreover, I suspect that old age is highly likely to be one of the prime criteria used in such rationing. The moral and ethical dilemmas raised by such policies require widespread public discussion and consideration before they become official, are firmly entrenched, and we find ourselves overtaken by them.

The same can be said, of course, with respect to two-class health care, in which extraordinary and high-cost procedures are not available to those whose care is financed by public and private insurance, but only to those who can pay for them from their own accumulated private resources. As indicated by my earlier discussion of the capacity of older persons to pay for their health care, about two-thirds of the elderly in the United States will not be able to pay for the more costly health care procedures out of their own pockets. The moral and ethical implications of unequal health care on the basis of income status pose issues that are applicable, of course, to all age groups in society.

In the context of this chapter, I will not dwell on these prospects, their implications, or the moral and ethical arguments that can be mobilized. Rather, let us turn briefly to consider some more optimistic prospects.

A major possibility is that the demands of adult children—particularly middle-income children—will bring about some new developments. Many adult children—faced with the choices of expending $21,000 per year for high-quality (guilt-free) institutional care, or institutionalizing a parent in a Medicaid (guilt-exacerbating) warehouse, the Space Age version of the British Elizabethan Poorhouse, or absorbing the economic, psychological, social, and other costs of maintaining a chronically ill older person in their own home—may push strongly for new alternatives.

One arena in which this demand could be expressed is the private-sector market. Many adult children may be only too happy and able to pay for selected components of the continuum of care that can make community or home-based alternatives to institutions truly viable. This may turn into a significant market for private enterprise.

Another way in which such a demand could be expressed is through collective bargaining efforts aimed at extending corporate employee benefits. Many corporations now allow their employees to maintain their group medical and dental benefits in retirement. If labor unions regain their strength in the context of a more vital American economy, new collective bargaining efforts may well focus on (1) extending most employee medical benefits past the point of retirement; (2) broadening group medical benefit coverage (both in working years and in retirement) to the nonmedical components of the long-term continuum of care; and (3) even providing workers with insurance against the possibility of having to pay long-term care bills for their parents. To be sure, the actuarial parameters of such forms of insurance are highly uncertain at the present time. But the potential market is tremendous. I will be very surprised if insurance companies do not soon begin to take the risks of underwriting broad coverage for long-term care, because they will find it hard to resist the lure of the dollar volume that would be generated by premiums for such policies. Analyses of the economics of artifically structured "life care" communities, through which older persons pay entry sums and other fees for residence and any subsequent care they may need, suggest that the financial risks are predictable and manageable (Winklevoss and Powell, 1984). A very recent analysis, by Jacobs and Weissert (1983), suggests that viable insurance parameters can also be extended to long-term-care costs in natural community settings and in long-term-care institutions.

Still another arena in which the demand for long-term care may be expressed is national politics. A distinct possibility is a compulsory national insurance program for long-term care, similar to the compulsory program of Old Age and Survivors Insurance. Indeed, if the demand for long-term care and for a viable means of financing it becomes strong enough, it may be considered as an option to replace Social Security old-age benefits. We may, as a nation, come to consider it more important to insure against the financial catastrophes of long-term care in old age, than against reduced income in retirement.

Finally, another way in which the demand for adequate long-term-care supportive services may find expression is through the development of locally felt senses of crises, and local government financing for such services. Such crises provide powerful incentives to those who undertake to solve them, namely the people who directly feel the impact of them. If we view the history of the United States we will find that fully developed services (beyond the token or symbolic level) have not developed from national initiatives, but from local crises. It was the extreme impact of sudden and large waves of immigrants from Europe in the latter half of the 19th century that led to the development of professional police services, fire-protection services, and public health services. Similarly, I believe that the best prospects for developing the community services that will be needed for an ever-growing, chronically disabled older population will be in the crises that will be felt in the lives of individuals and which are felt and expressed profoundly in local communities. Even when resources are scarce, the identification of *essential* services is a dynamic process that continually brings about different answers, in the form of resource allocation, at the community level. Cohesion in values is always easier to achieve at the community level than at the level of a mass society of 240 million persons.

Conclusion

The picture just presented of our health-care destiny is not especially uplifting. I have tried to place the trends, dilemmas, and prospects for the health care of the aging in their proper perspective. I hope that I have made clear that the crises emerging in the arena of health care and aging are far more serious than other implications of increased longevity. Our current approaches to the financing, organization, and use of health care resources for older persons, and for all of us, are unlikely to survive this century.

The longer-term emergent policy and societal trends and the alternatives I have outlined may not be agreeable. Indeed, they may not be accurate visions. But I do hope that I have helped you to share my fundamental view that we need to restructure our issues and priorities if we are to resolve the profound contemporary and future dilemmas of health care for older persons.

References

Binstock, R.H.: The aged as scapegoat. *The Gerontologist 23*, 136–143 (1983).

Brody, E.M.: Health and its social implications. In A.J.J. Gilmore, A. Svanberg, M. Marois, W.M. Beattie, and J. Piotrowski (Eds.): Aging: A Challenge to Science and Social Policy, Vol. II, Medicine and Social Science, pp. 189–201. London: Oxford University Press, 1981.

Butler, R.N.: Advances in aging research. In Symposium on the Care of the Elderly, pp. 85–88. Worcester, Mass.: University of Massachusetts Medical Center, 1978.

Califano, J.A., Jr.: U.S. policy for the aging—a commitment to ourselves. *Nat. Journ. 10*, 1576 (1978).

Cantor, M., and Little, V.: Aging and social care. In R.H. Binstock and E. Shanas (Eds.): Handbook of Aging and the Social Sciences, Chapter 26. New York: Van Nostrand Reinhold, in press.

Caper, P., and Blumenthal, D.: What price cost control?—Massachusetts' new hospital payment law. *New Eng. J. Med. 308*, 542–543 (1983).

Clark, R.L., and Menefee, J.A.: Federal expenditures for the elderly: past and future. *The Gerontologist 21*, 132–137 (1981).

Davis, K.: Health implications of aging in America. Proceedings of Conference on the Impact of Technology on Aging, Feb. 16–18, 1983. Washington, D.C.: Office of Technology Assessment, U.S. Congress, in press.

Demkovich, L.E.: Medicare on the critical list—can Congress plug a $200 billion gap? *Nat. Journ. 15*, 1580–1585 (1983).

Fries, J.F.: Aging, natural death, and the compression of morbidity. *New Eng. J. Med. 303*, 130–135 (1980).

Gruenberg, E.M.: The failures of success. *Milbank Mem. Fund Quart., 55*, pp. 3–24. Winter, 1977.

Hilfiker, D.: Allowing the debilitated to die: facing our ethical choices. *New Eng. J. Med. 308*, 716–719 (1983).

Jacobs, B., and Weissert, W.: Home equity financing of long-term care. Unpublished presentation at the Fifth Annual Conference of the Association for Public Policy Analysis and Management, Philadelphia, Pa., Oct. 21, 1983.

Kinzer, D.M.: Massachusetts and California—two kinds of hospital cost control. *New Eng. J. Med. 308*, 838–841 (1983).

Laslett, P.: The comparative history of aging and the aged: with particular reference to the household position of aged persons. In A.J.J. Gilmore, A. Svanberg, M. Marois, W.M. Beattie, and J. Piotrowski (Eds.): Aging: A Challenge to Science and Social Policy, Vol. III, Medicine and Social Science. London: Oxford University Press, 1981.

Moon, M.: The Measurement of Economic Welfare—Its Application to the Aged Poor. New York: Academic Press, 1977.

Pear, R.: House unit would bar additions to Medicare bills. New York Times, p. 1 (Oct. 20, 1983).

Platt, R.: Cost containment—another view. *New Eng. J. Med. 309*, 726–730 (1983).

Samuelson, R.J.: Aging America—who will shoulder the growing burden? *Nat. Journ. 10*, 1712–1717 (1978).

Schneider, E.L., and Brody, J.A.: Aging, natural death, and the compression of morbidity. *New Eng. J. Med. 309*, 854–855 (1983).

Scholen, K., and Chen, Y-P.: Unlocking Home Equity for the Elderly. Cambridge, Mass.: Ballinger Publishing Company, 1980.

Schulte, J.: Terminal patients deplete Medicare, Greenspan says. Dallas Morning News (April 26, 1983).

Schulz, J.: The Economics of Aging, 3rd edition. Belmont, Calif.: Wadsworth Publishing Co., 1984.

Starr, P.: The Social Transformation of American Medicine. New York: Basic Books, 1983.

Stevens, W.K.: High medical costs under attack as drain on the nation's economy. New York Times (March 28, 1982).

U.S. Comptroller General: Entering a Nursing Home—Costly Implications for Medicaid and the Elderly. Washington, D.C.: U.S. General Accounting Office, 1979.

U.S. Senate Special Committee on Aging: Developments in Aging, 1982, Vol. I. Washington, D.C.: U.S. Government Printing Office, 1983.

Winklevoss, H.E., and Powell, A.V.: Continuing Care Retirement Communities—an Empirical, Financial and Legal Analysis. Homewood, Ill.: Richard O. Irvin, Inc., 1984.

Chapter 2

The Next Twenty Years: Medical Science and the Practice of Geriatrics

Ewald W. Busse

Summary

For the next 20 years, geriatrics will require and receive increased attention. The treatment, prevention, health promotion, and research related to aging and the aged will be influenced by socioeconomic factors and by the status and trends of the health and disability characteristics of the elderly population. The increase in longevity has not been accompanied by a significant change in the onset of disability, namely, the compression of infirmity. New and existing diseases should be anticipated. Hence flexibility is needed to respond to changes associated with diagnosis, treatment, and long-term care. Rapidly emerging scientific knowledge and technological advances will greatly alter medical practice. Innovative models of patient care must be initiated with careful cost-effectiveness and cost/benefit evaluations. The allocation of limited resources will be a serious problem for the medical profession and will be a major political issue.

Introduction

The focus of this presentation is upon the future of geriatrics—the treatment, prevention, health promotion, and the emerging advances in biomedical and behavioral sciences associated with aging and the diseases and disabilities of late life. Social, political, and economic factors associated with chronic disability, long-term care, and allocation of limited resources are discussed in Chapter 1. Often determinants, as discussed in that chapter, seem obscure or are apparently unrelated, but it is a fact that numerous determinants have serious impact upon the practice of geriatrics and the advancement of science.

The World Population

Life expectancy at birth is a prediction based upon assumptions, such as no major changes in the organization of medical care or preventive public health measures, no catastrophic change such as war or an epidemic, and no substantial change in environmental, social, or economic conditions. Life expectancy at birth in the U.S.A. in 1982 was 70.8 years for males and 78.2 for females. A white male 65 years of age can expect to live 14.4 years, a female 18.8 years. The prediction for the life expectancy in the year 2000 is 73.42 years for men and 81.05 for women. These changes in life expectancy are important for our planning but are likely to result in an overwhelming problem for the developing nations of the world.

As of 1980 the United States population was 227,658,000 (Myers, 1983) and the total world population was estimated at 4.4 billion (4,432,100,000). Of this world population, 375,800,000 are 60 years of age and over. Forty-five point four percent (45.4%) are living in more developed nations, and 54.6% in less-developed nations. By the year 2000 there will be a remarkable change. Only 39% of older persons will be living in developed regions and 61% in less developed regions. There will be an increase of over 200,000,000 old people in slightly less than 20 years. Of this increased number, 155,000,000 will be living in the less-developed regions. The increased burden of caring for so many old people may well be a significant deterent to improving the social and economic conditions of many nations and regions.

Chronic Disease and Disability (NIA, 1983)

Eighty-six percent (86%) of older people have some form of chronic disease. The most frequently recorded chronic conditions are arthritis, heart problems, hypertension, diabetes, brain impairment, and vision and hearing defects. However, only 5% of those not in institutions are housebound, and only 1% bedridden. The over-65 age group averages 16 days per year confined to bed. Most confinements in the older group are attributed to chronic conditions rather than to acute illnesses. Mental disturbances are common affecting approximately 10% of the population over 65 and 20% of those over 80. Of those in nursing homes, one-half suffer from some degree of intellectual impairment. In addition to organic brain disease, the most frequently reported mental conditions are chronic depression and anxiety.

To care for these increasing and disabling health problems, older people make more frequent use of medical services both as inpatients and outpatients. They account for 15% of all doctors' visits, 25% of all prescriptions, and 34% of all days in short-stay hospitals. It is evident that older persons do suffer from acute disorders as well as exacerbations of chronic disorders, and this does require hospital attention. They are hospitalized for much longer periods of time than are young people, and surgical procedures have increased more among people over 65 than in any other age group.

Longevity and Disability

A national survey of the aged (1983) was conducted in 1962 and repeated in 1975. Medicare became effective in 1966; therefore, this report provided an opportunity to determine whether Medicare affected (1) how old people function, (2) how old people feel about their health, and (3) whether Medicare and other social programs of health services have made a difference in the provision of direct services to the elderly sick. There is increasing evidence that the extension of the life span has not been paralleled by a delayed onset of chronic disease and disability.

The elderly who are defined as restricted in mobility include the bedfast, the housebound, and those who can go outdoors only with difficulty. Of this group, there was no major change between 1962 and 1975. In 1962, about 11 of every 100 persons had restrictions on their mobility in contrast to 14 of 100 in 1975. More women than men reported such restrictions since there is a higher percentage of elderly women in older populations. The institutionalized population of elderly at any one time was estimated in 1962 at 4%, while it was 5% in 1975.

In this study an index of incapacity was developed. The old person was asked specifically: Can you go outdoors? Can you walk up and down stairs? Can you get about the house? Can you wash and bathe yourself? Can you dress and put on shoes? Can you cut your own toenails? The answers to these questions were scored on the basis of (1) without difficulty, (2) with minor difficulty, or (3) with the help of another person. In both 1962 and 1975 the proportion of those with no incapacities remained the same; 7 of every 10 were able to perform all of the tasks. However, there was a difference in that incapacitated elderly people were more likely to have seen a doctor in 1975 than in 1962. Six of every 10 had seen a doctor during the preceding month in 1975, 5 of every 10 in 1962. According to the 1982 National Plan for Research on Aging, "There is no substantial evidence that the elderly of today have better or worse health than the elderly of yesterday." Thus, the influence of Medicare is negligible.

Nursing Homes

Between 1974 and 1978, the number of nursing home residents increased by more than 21%. Some 20% of the aging will enter a nursing home before dying. It is projected that nursing home residents will increase 54% by the year 2000. For persons 65 years of age and over, the median age in nursing homes was 81 in 1977. Forty percent of the elderly nursing home residents were 85 years of age and over. The ratio of women to men was approximately 3 to 1, and approximately 93.2% were white. Nursing home use rates are nine times higher among unmarried than among married elderly persons (National Research on Aging Planning Panel, 1982).

Health Promotion and Prevention

The prevention of disease and disability is not health promotion. A health promotion program is one that seeks to facilitate community and individual measures which can foster the development of life-styles to maintain and enhance health and well-being. These programs deal with enhancing the effectiveness of known information such as stopping smoking, eliminating the misuse of alcohol and drugs, improving diet and nutrition, managing stress and exercise, adhering to medical regimes for certain illnesses such as diabetes and hypertension, and making appropriate use of education and services that reduce the risk of illness and premature death (Office of Disease Prevention and Health Promotion, 1982).

Between 1950 and 1978 there has been a substantial shift in the rankings of the leading causes of death among those 65 years of age and over. Although heart disease has declined, it remains the predominant cause of death. The disease listed as the cause of death may not contribute to long-term care as much as some other conditions, such as arthritis and organic brain disease.

There are two indicators which are often used to determine quality of life. These are the number of days of restricted activity and the number of "bed-disability days." Some surveys utilize a questionable approach to defining restricted-activity days. These surveys count those days in which the individual is unable to engage in his or her customary activity. The problem is that customary activity is not defined and this may shift not only between individuals, but between cohorts as well. Bed-disability days may be a more accurate way of measuring the health status of individuals.

Alternatives to institutionalization programs may not be as effective as imagined. Three evaluative studies have been done on two psychogeriatric day hospitals in and near Edinburgh, Scotland. Approximately 40% of the patients suffer from organic brain disease and the remainder from a variety of mental disorders. The study concluded that psychogeriatric day care does not provide any clear-cut support for daycare being either an alternative to institutionalization care or means of significantly delaying entry of the elderly mentally infirm into such institutional care. It does appear that this program permits a type of short-term support until long-term beds become available rather than altering admission to hospitals. Patients' relatives did receive a definite benefit as they were relieved of certain burdens of care. Apparently the question remains whether the cost of this type of care is proportionate to its benefits (*Psychiatric News*, 1983).

Sex Differences in Longevity

Since 1900, the percentage of the U.S.A. population aged 65 and over has more than doubled. The actual number of aged persons has increased seven- to eight-fold from 3 million to over 25.7 million people (in 1980). In the last 80 years, there has been a clear reversal in life expectancy trends for men and women. In 1900 in the U.S.A., there were 98 old women to every 100 old men, but since that date, an important trend has developed. During the period 1900–1902 life expectancy for white females below age 20 was lower than for males of a like age, but slightly higher for females through the adult years. By 1964 the longevity of the young female had improved remarkably and had considerably surpassed that of the young male. Apparently this was not the result of selected immigration, that is, more men than women coming into the country, but a shift in health as related to sex.

As previously noted, life expectancy in the U.S.A. is now approximately 70 years for men and over 78 years for women. This difference in mortality rates has resulted in women now outnumbering men by 4.5 million. Sixty percent of those aged 65 years of age and over are women. By the year 2000 the ratio of women to men 65 and over will be 150 to 100. For those over 75 years of age by the year 2000, there will be 185 women to 100 men. Most older men are married and living with their wives, while most older women are widows. Older men are seven times more likely to be married than older women.

There are sex differences in the morbidity and mortality ratios in the three major cardiovascular diseases. These are coronary heart disease, hypertension, and vascular lesions of the central nervous system, that is, stroke. In the U.S.A. coronary heart disease is the cause of death in twice as many men as women. Stroke is somewhat higher in men than in women, but hypertension is essentially the same for both sexes. These differences suggest that although there may be some causative factors in common between these three disorders, they are far from identical. One factor that may result in a woman's lower risk of coronary heart disease may be the protective effect of female sex hormones. The mechanism of the effective estrogen is far from understood. Women given estrogen prior to a natural or surgical menopause have an increased risk of coronary heart disease. In contrast, estrogen when given to postmenopausal women appears to reduce the risk of coronary disease.

In the United States the high mortality of males compared to females appears to be a complex interaction between genetically determined physiological differences, socioeconomic factors and cultural values, and expectations and environmental conditions that may be more dangerous to the man than to the woman.

Research on Aging

The goal of research on aging is not merely to extend the life span, but to extend the vigorous and productive years of life. This goal includes the reduction of the pain and disability that accompanies illnesses and disorders now common in late life. The improvement of the health and quality of life not only is affected by modifying the aging processes and diseases of late life, but also by society's attitudes toward aging and the older population. Aging research includes achieving a better understanding of the biological processes of aging, the diseases common to late life, social and behavioral factors, and improved methods of meeting the needs of the elderly.

Recent advances in biomedical research have been spectacular and new doors have been opened to the study of aging in basic molecular genetics and the opportunity to combine chemical analysis with sophisticated biophysical, morphological, and functional assessment of cells. The diseases of late life also are under exciting investigation. The appearance of numerous pharmacologic agents that have some value will undoubtedly be expanded and their effectiveness improved. A few of the disorders that need immediate attention include cardiovascular diseases and stroke, organic brain syndrome including Alzheimer's disease, osteoporosis, osteomalacia and osteoarthritis, cancer, benign prostatic hyperplasia, diabetes, mental disorders, and perceptual defects (NIA, 1983).

Biomedical research is increasingly influenced by declining financial resources, by political intervention, and by the influence of the news media that emphasize the sensational and are responsible to press groups with limited objectives. This unfortunate situation forces the scientific investigator to shift to current favorite subjects rather than to direct the limited resources of medical science to those chronic diseases and disabilities that are and will have an increasing impact on the health and well-being of all people.

Early this year, a report (NIA, 1983) was transmitted to Secretary Heckler of the Department of Health and Human Services. (Fortunately

Secretary Heckler is very cognizant of the serious health problems associated with aging. As a member of the House of Representatives, she played a major role in establishing and expanding the efforts of the Veterans Administration in dealing with the problems of aging and has recently put in place a task force which will address the area of dementia of the Alzheimer's type and associated disorders.) This report was based upon an in-depth review of past and current aging research, an assessment of current knowledge, and a careful look at needs, opportunities, and future directions for research on aging. This background material was prepared by a panel of experts from a wide range of disciplines. Four subpanels were put in place including one panel devoted to basic mechanisms of aging, a second to clinical manifestations of aging, a third to interactions between older people and society, and the fourth to increasing productivity among older people. This carefully developed and comprehensive report is directly relevant to my presentation today. I shall present a few representative excerpts from the report.

1. Research on aging requires more scholars who can bridge the gaps between the biomedical sciences and psychology, sociology, economics, history, and anthropology, and who can apply sophisticated research methods in a multidisiplinary framework appropriate to life-span perspective (p. 8).
2. The major need in the neurosciences is the development of adequate laboratory models of many of the basic aging processes and of major age-related diseases as they occur in man. For example, neurofibillary tangles, the ultrastructural hallmark of senile dementias of the Alzheimer's type, has never been observed among aging rodents (p. 8).
3. A vital aspect of geriatric research relates to the health-care strategy employed to diagnose, treat, and prevent major diseases. There is a great need to build a health-care system that can better respond to the unique needs of the elderly (p. 10).
4. As to Alzheimer's disease, "A major effort needs to be directed towards identifying etiological factors. In some familial cases, there is an apparent genetic component; the application of new techniques for identifying the gene(s) responsible should be considered a priority area. Identifying nongenetic risk factors will require extensive epidemiologic studies" (p. 12).
5. Pharmacology. "Special problems exist with the use of drugs in treatment of the elderly as a result both of the presence of multiple illnesses and, hence, multiple drugs (polypharmacy), and because of increased adverse reactions in older patients" (p. 13).

5a. Continued investigation of active metabolites, or drug–drug interactions, and of the increased sensitivity of older subjects to certain drugs is needed (p. 13).

6. Nutrition. "Methodological problems in assessing nutrition of elderly populations need to be addressed" (p. 13).
7. "Investigate the behavioral, cultural, social, and psychological factors that may influence the onset, course, and recovery from major illnesses affecting the elderly, and that may also influence the support network, especially the family" (p. 15).

An Emerging Ethical Issue

A number of articles have appeared recounting the early work involving brain grafting in certain types of disorders in Europe. In actuality to date only one experiment has been conducted and this involved two patients with Parkinson disease (Kolata, 1983).

Parkinson disease is to a large degree due to a lack of dopamine. Therefore, cells taken from the patient's own adrenal glands were moved to the brain. There they continued to produce dopamine and did partially eliminate the patient's need for supplementation of L-dopa. Alzheimer's is another disease that is apparently related to a deficiency of a neurotransmitter, particularly acetylcholine. There is a problem in that there is no other organ in the human body that has the cells that could produce acetylcholine. Consequently, there cannot be any autotransplant. The only known source would be cells from the brains of human fetuses. Obviously, this could produce an ethical problem. However, it is conceivable that cell colonies could be established utilizing as a source a single fetus. It would be possible to develop a cell line utilizing cell-sorting techniques to get the cells as pure as possible before grafting and to establish banks of these cells so that donors and recipients could be matched as closely as possible. Considerable work has been done on rats and it does appear that by brain cell transplants, certain skills can be improved such as maintaining balance in a precarious situation, and correcting memory impairments. It is obvious that many problems need to be resolved, but eventually an attempt will be made to treat Alzheimer's disease utilizing a brain grafting technique.

Training in Geriatrics

A training program in geriatric psychiatry has existed at Duke University Medical Center since 1965. As of 1974, a single program in the U.S.A. existed for training in geriatrics for specialists in internal medicine. In 1978 the Institute of Medicine of the National Academy of Sciences made an extensive report "Aging and Medical Education." This recommended the expansion of geriatric training at all levels of the medical education process. It did not recommend the creation of a medical specialty in geriatrics. The report indicated that there were an adequate number of physicians who would provide care for the elderly patients, but many required additional training to properly function as geriatricians. In the last few years federal and state agencies have provided financial support for training in geriatrics in the medical fields of internal medicine, family practice, psychiatry and neurology. While the American Board of Medical Specialties has discouraged the formation of separate subspecialty boards and new boards, it does favor certification in subspecialties by existing specialty boards.

Some people today advocate developing a specialty of geriatrics pointing to Great Britain where a more or less distinct hospital-based specialty of geriatrics has emerged. Although there have admittedly been some gains in Britain, there have also been some losses, particularly because the specialty is hospital based. Moreover, the emergence of a geriatrics specialty in the United Kingdom has spanned a period of 25 years and is tied to a system of health insurance and social assistance that has not been acceptable in the U.S.A.

Summary

Geriatrics has clearly been established as a special area of expanding medical knowledge and that knowledge is considerably beyond that of caring for the young and middle-aged adult. The teaching of geriatrics is rapidly becoming integrated into the medical school curriculum and into postgraduate training. It is probable that the physician who has been established in an existing medical specialty will seek further recognition of clinical competence in geriatrics. Currently this appears not to be a possibility for the diplomate of the American Board of Family Practice. However, some accommodation and recognition of the skills of the family practitioner will have to be made. It is my opinion that the family physician will carry a major portion of the task of caring for the elderly.

Models of long-term care must be tested and evaluated not only for their cost effectiveness, but also for their cost benefit. I doubt if we will ever develop an ideal system, but certainly we will improve on the continuity of care for the elderly person. This will involve improved communication beween physicians, and other members of the health profession as well.

In recent years, there is no doubt that medical science has advanced rapidly, but I believe that this will be accelerated and there will be numerous new affective pharmacologic agents and diagnostic procedures. A version of the PDR will become part of the computer capability in the practitioner's office. This will also include evaluations of diagnostic procedures, reviewing both the sensitivity and the specificity of the diagnostic tests.

Numerous ethical problems will emerge; one is already with us—the use and limitations of the "living" will. Within the very near future the ethics of brain transplants, especially those utilizing human fetal cell transplant into an aging brain, will surface.

The failure to recognize that the prolongation of life expectancy has not been paralleled by an equivalent delay in the onset of chronic disabilities is producing some serious defects in planning for the year 2000. It is possible that in the early part of the next century many chronic disabilities will be delayed, reduced, or eliminated. But that will require extensive research and clinical trials.

In the U.S.A., I feel confident that an adequate level of care will be available to all of our citizens; however, I am equally certain that there will be small groups of individuals who will get superior care just as they do today.

The male/female differences which are appearing, particularly in late life, do produce an interesting dilemma. Should we devote biological research to a better understanding of the causes of the male's early demise so that an equal balance can be attained? Is an equal balance really desirable or is there some other solution that will be just as useful to society in the year 2000?

Many aspirations for the elderly will not take place unless medical research is directed toward the incapacitating, chronic diseases. Until many of these are dealt with, it is very unlikely that the latter part of our life span will truly be the golden years.

References

Kolata, G.: Brain grafting work shows promise. *Science 221*, 1277–1278 (1983).

Myers, G.C.: Reading from material of the 1980 Bureau of the Census. Personal communication, 1983.

National Institute on Aging: Report of the National Advisory Council on Aging: For a National Plan on Research on Aging, 1983.

National Research on Aging Planning Panel: Toward an Independent Old Age: A National Plan for Research on Aging. U.S. Department of Health and Human Services (NIH) Publication No. 82-2453, 1982.

Office of Disease Prevention and Health Promotion: Prevention '82. Department of Health and Human Services (PHS) Publication No. 82-50157, 1982.

Psychiatric News XVIII(16), 1983.

Shanas, E. (preparer): National Survey of the Aged. U.S. Department and Human Services (OHDS) Publication No. 83-20425, 1983.

Part II

Basic Mechanisms of Biologic Aging

Chapter 3

The Biology of Aging and the Quality of Later Life

Kenneth M. Weiss

Summary

In biomedical terms, the quality of later life is related to the processes of physiological change with age. The timing of these changes is determined by the basic nature of human biology, and is similar for a wide variety of different physiological systems as well as for the onset pattern of the major degenerative diseases. Efforts to modify the aging pattern will have consequences in terms of the quality of later life which are not independent of the biological constraints on the aging process. In particular, extension of the lifespan by the curing or prevention of specific diseases is likely to diminish the quality, or contribute to the "dysquality," of later life in ways which can be quantified. Even the extension of the lifespan by slowing down the overall aging process would probably have the consequence of a less, not a more, square survivorship curve and an increase, not a decrease, in the amount of dysquality the average individual would experience. Since there thus does not appear to be a single optimal way to extend life and minimize dysquality simultaneously, the role of the individual is as important as that of science in determining the quality of later life in the years to come.

Introduction: The Flight of Time

As one might expect, poets have written much about time and life. Often, they have used aeronautical metaphors; Herrick admonished the virgins to

> Gather ye rosebuds while ye may,
> Old time is still a-flying,
> And this same flower that smiles today,
> Tomorrow will be dying.
>
> *To the Virgins,*
> *to Make Much of Time*

In his paean to drink, Omar Khayyam wrote

> Come, fill the Cup and in the Fire of Spring
> The Winter Garment of Repentence fling:
> The Bird of Time has but a little way
> To fly—and Lo! the Bird is on the Wing.
>
> *Rubiyat*

I, too, think that time and life can aptly be described in aeronautical terms, but I think we may find more relevance in the words of Longfellow, who

> . . . shot an arrow into the air,
> It fell to earth I know not where
>
> *The Arrow and the Song*

and who elsewhere said,

> If you would hit the mark, you must aim above it;
> Every arrow that flies feels the attraction of the earth.
>
> *Elegaic Verse*

Biomedical issues concerning the quality of later life may have more to do with ballistics than with birds on the wing. While it is true that each bird, like each arrow, must come to rest on the earth, the arrow's path, unlike that of the bird, can be predicted: with the greatest respect to Longfellow, an arrow was useful precisely because it fell to earth we do know (more or less) where. Given its initial acceleration and angle of trajectory, it will follow a reasonably nice parabola.

The determinants of the quality of life at any stage are many, but above all they are sociocultural. However, my topic concerns biomedical, and not sociocultural, aspects of the aging process, so I will touch upon social issues only briefly, though we should not underrate them. From the biomedical point of view, the quality of later life has to do with the nature and amount of physical and physiologic decline, with disease, and with death. Because we are biological organisms, formed over many millions of years of selection and evolution, these factors obey laws just as compulsory as do arrows, and if we are serious about understanding what can be done to alter the quality of later life, we must consider the problem in terms of its natural laws.

The Clockworks: Regularity in Biological Aging Processes

Though we might think from everyday experience that much of what determines the length as well as the quality of later life is the accumulating result of the chance and happenstance of our individual life histories, the fact is that nonetheless most of the aging processes which we can measure follow regular patterns. In studies of a wide variety of physiologic functions, in terms of the percent of function present at age 30 which has been lost by subsequent ages, it has been found that these functions accumulate loss in a roughly linear way with age. The rates of change—the slopes—vary, but the form of the change, a straight line, remains roughly the same for many systems (Shock, 1960, 1961, 1972; Strehler and Mildvan, 1960; Strehler, 1977; Kohn, 1971).

A similar phenomenon occurs for the age patterns of onset of disease or of death, a fact noted at least as early as 1825 by Benjamin Gompertz and followed closely, we may be sure, by insurance carriers ever since. Typically, the risk of disease increases after age 30 in a way which is exponential, or very curved, if we plot it on natural scales of risk and age. But if we plot the age-onset data on paper logarithmic in both scales the pattern becomes notably more linear after age 30 or 40. Again, the form of the curve is very similar for many different kinds of diseases in different organ systems, though the slope may differ. The data are by no means perfectly linear even on this scale, but the considerable similarity in shape is not something one would necessarily predict a priori, and the systems they involve, and the nature of the pathologies, are diverse in the extreme.

We do not know the ultimate cause for heart disease, diabetes, or kidney failure, nor why such diseases follow these observed risk curves. However, we do know a considerable amount about one family of diseases which follows a very similar age relationship quite closely, namely, the adult-onset cancers. These arise as the result of a series of mutational steps in stem cells. Mutations are probably random occurrences, which might be expected to lead to irregular age-onset patterns, but the number of at-risk stem cells is so large that, as Figure 3-1 shows, the actual resulting cancer patterns follow a log–log linear age pattern very closely (Whittemore, 1978; Weiss et al., in prep.).

Many of these sites are epithelial tissues. Female breast cancer stops increasing much in risk after the age of the menopause, showing that indeed certain deterministic aging processes do regulate the age-rate of risk increase. On the other hand, male prostate cancer is very rare in younger men, but once its risk starts increasing it accelerates very rapidly. The other epithelial tissues are somewhat intermediate. Leukemias and certain other nonepithelial tissues have much lower absolute rates but surprisingly similar onset patterns (for the adult forms of the disease).

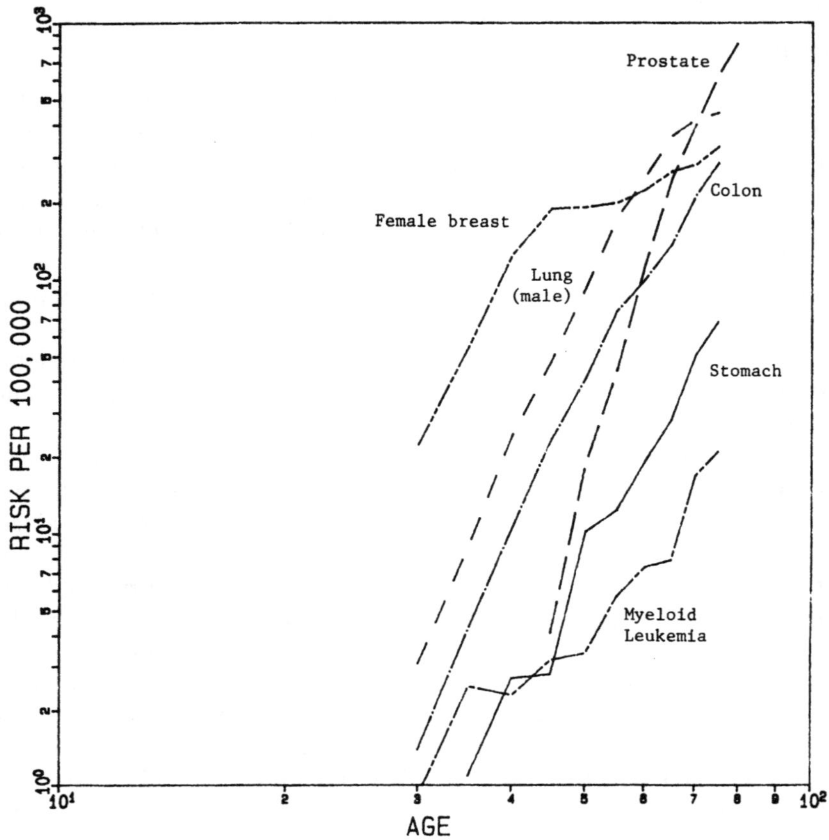

Figure 3-1. Typical age-onset patterns of adult cancers. (Source: Connecticut, 1970 data from Waterhouse et al., 1976.)

The leukemia curve is irregular because of sampling errors, not, I think, because the process is irregular.

It might seem contradictory that physiologic functions deteriorate linearly with age but disease frequency rises exponentially. These facts can probably be reconciled. First of all, we should note that the linear decline in function relates to the amount of function lost per year, not to the rate of its loss. The rate of loss, which is equal to the amount lost divided by the amount remaining at any age, changes exponentially—roughly as the square—of age. Note also that physiologic measures are measures of capacity, whereas diseases are discrete categories. The process leading up to categories such as cancer or heart disease may have effects which appear gradually as lost functional capacity over time—for example, the number of stem cells in a tissue having suffered a mutational change, or the number of arterial plaques in the circulatory system.

However, the clinical entity of disease may have to do with avoiding a specific condition, such as multiple mutations in a single stem cell, or the closing of any single coronary artery. An intestine is free of cancer until some single cell has been affected by all the required mutations, and as long as there are open anastamotic pathways, the blockage of an artery or vein, while it may affect functional efficiency, is not generally lethal. A slow increase in the rate of functional decline can lead to a much more exponential path of acceleration in the rate at which diseases arise, although the latter will be much less in absolute amount. For a review of other methods of reconciling the decline and mortality patterns, one may consult Strehler (1977) or Kohn (1971).

In the case of cancers, we are fairly sure that environmental factors affect the rate at which tissue damage such as mutations accumulate, and this is probably the way in which smoking or dietary components act to produce disease. If we examine the age-onset patterns of one tumor, say, colon cancer, across the world's range of national population risk levels, we can see, as shown in Figure 3-2, that the pattern has the same shape. However, as we move from Thailand to the Switzerland the risk factors—whatever they are—act to produce a different slope for the resulting age-pattern of risk. Note that while we discussed physiologic function in terms of the life of an individual, these curves represent the *risks* an individual must pass through; however, because an individual can contract colon cancer at most once (as a rule), these data really are of a populational rather than an individual nature, a point to which we will return later.

To recall our arrow analogy, this set of colon cancer age curves is like tracing the parabolic flights of arrows released at different angles of trajectory. Most of the adult-onset tumors follow this kind of a pattern to a reasonable degree, often for all adult ages for which data are reliable.

This pattern regularity is even deeper than so far shown. A straight line is defined by two parameters, the intercept and the slope. If we separately fit a multistage risk model to data on a single tumor, for a large number of the world's populations, we will obtain estimates of the pair of parameters characterizing the risk line in each such population, and can plot these points on a single graph to summarize the nature of worldwide variation in tumor patterns. Actually, I do not fit a linear model to the data, but instead a slightly different version of the multistage model which fits the data very well and also, like a straight line, has two parameters (Weiss et al., in prep; Appendix A). Colon cancer would illustrate this nicely, but in Figure 3-3 we present values of parameters fitted to lung cancer data from populations around the world. Not only does the age curve fit the model very closely within most populations, but across the range of human exposure levels the fitted parameters themselves have a linear pattern. This strongly suggests that although an environmental agent affects the particular slope of the age-onset curve, changes in the exposure level are

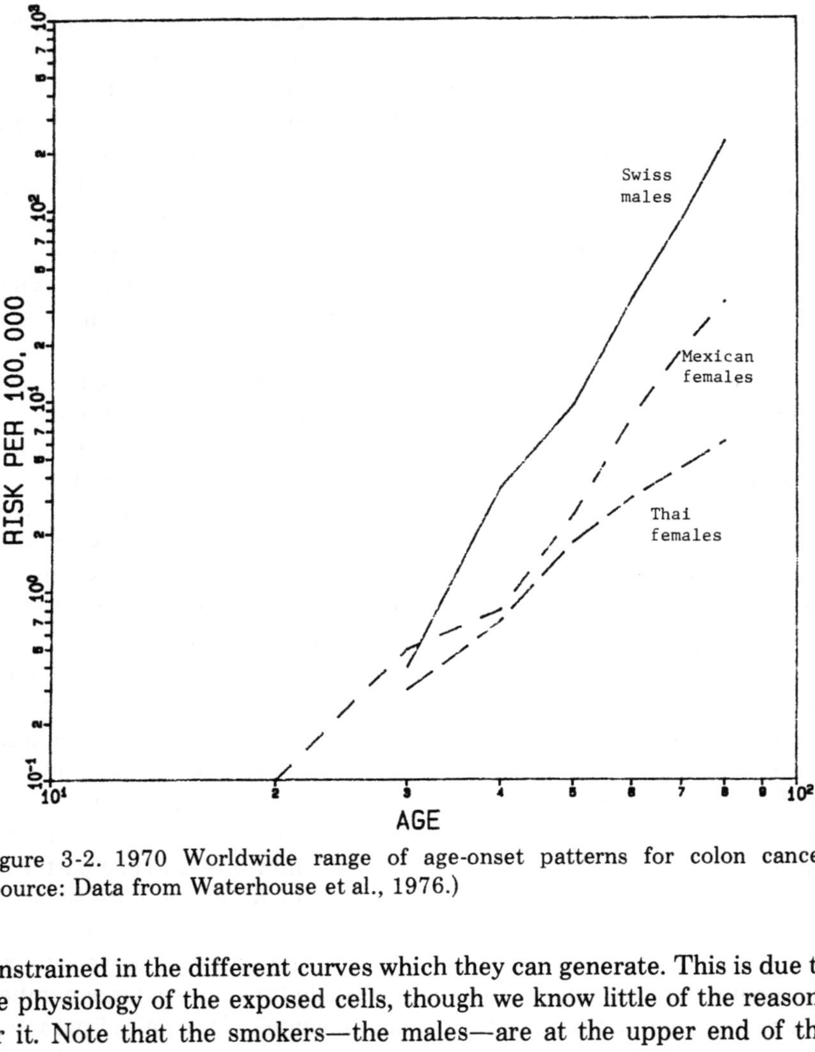

Figure 3-2. 1970 Worldwide range of age-onset patterns for colon cancer. (Source: Data from Waterhouse et al., 1976.)

constrained in the different curves which they can generate. This is due to the physiology of the exposed cells, though we know little of the reasons for it. Note that the smokers—the males—are at the upper end of the line.

It is unexpected from any theoretical consideration, and quite fascinating to find that a very similar pattern-among-patterns also obtains for other tumors, and indeed that very nearly the same parameter line can be found for tumors occurring in quite different organs. This is shown in Figure 3-4 in which the parameter-pairs obtained from fitting stomach and colon cancer are plotted on the same graph. Clearly there is an almost complete overlap, though there are many differences between stomachs and colons and the things they are exposed to. Nonetheless, there is an exposure level such that almost the entire age-specific risk schedule could be found for stomach cancer as well as for colon cancer at some corresponding exposure level. Indeed this pattern applies even more

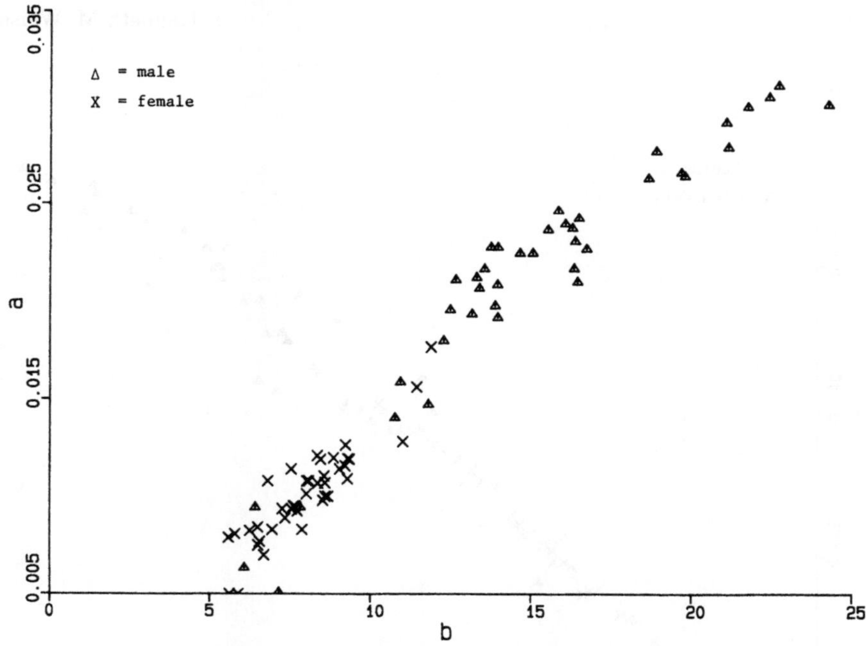

Figure 3-3. Multistage parameters fitted to lung cancer data from 1970 worldwide data. (Source: Data from Waterhouse et al., 1976. Parameters as fitted to equation (3), Appendix A. Data were a sample of tumor registries from different nations, and sexes were treated separately in each.)

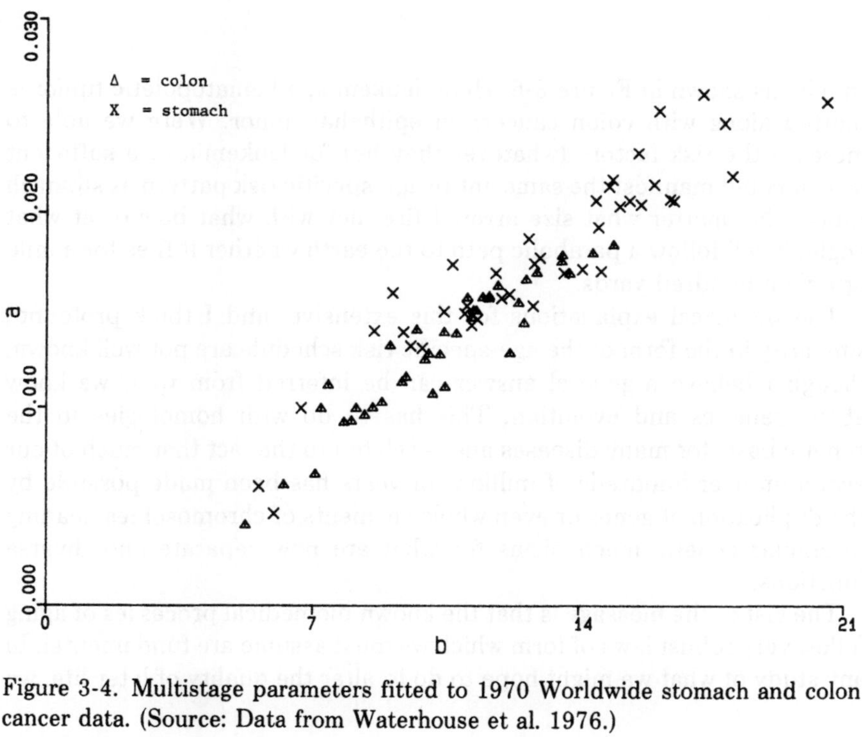

Figure 3-4. Multistage parameters fitted to 1970 Worldwide stomach and colon cancer data. (Source: Data from Waterhouse et al. 1976.)

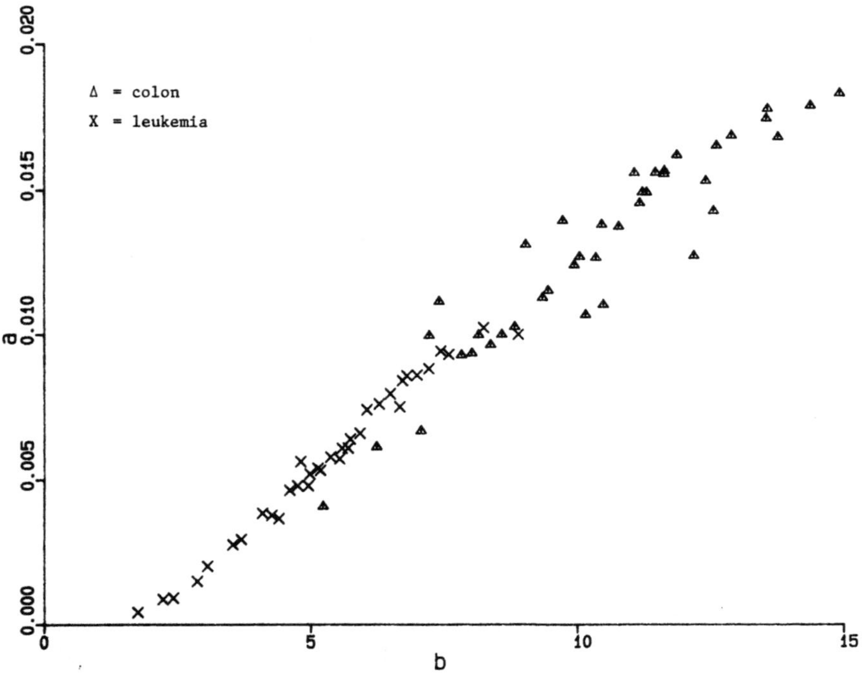

Figure 3-5. Multistage parameters fitted to 1970 Worldwide colon cancer and leukemia data. (Source: Data from Waterhouse et al., 1976.)

widely, as shown in Figure 3-5. Here, leukemia, a hematopoietic tumor is plotted along with colon cancer, an epithelial tumor. Were we able to increase the risk factors (whatever they be) for leukemia to a sufficient level it could manifest the same entire age-specific risk pattern as stomach cancer. No matter what size arrow I fire, nor with what bow or at what angle, it will follow a parabolic path to the earth whether it flies for a mile or only a hundred yards.

The biological explanations for this extensive, and I think profound, similarity in the form of the age-specific risk schedule are not well known, though I believe a general answer can be inferred from what we know about genetics and evolution. This has to do with homologies in the genetic basis for many diseases and is related to the fact that much of our evolution over hundreds of millions of years has been made possible by the duplication of genes or even whole segments of chromosomes, leading to similar genetic mechanisms for what are now separate and diverse functions.

The gist of the message is that the known biomedical processes of aging follow very robust laws of form which we must assume are fundamental. In any study of what we might hope to do to alter the quality of later life, we must accept the probability that there will be nontrivial constraints in the manner in which we can alter the age patterns of physiologic change.

The Dysquality Index and Its Dynamics

The assessment of the quality of later life is subjective and is determined by the integrated experience of all of our physiologic systems. However, we can gain some understanding by looking at the pattern of age changes in its component parts, like muscle strength, joint flexibility, sight, or hearing. We have seen that these generally deteriorate linearly with age. We can assume for simplicity that the quality of life is diminished as physiologic function declines, and that the amount of such loss in quality, which we can here term "dysquality," is proportional to the amount of decline which has occurred. Let us then attempt to measure the total amount of such dysquality an individual has had to bear up to his or her current age. This will be proportional to the area under the line of physiologic decline. Since physiologic decline of any measurable amount begins at about age 30, we can measure all ages as the number of years since age 30 rather than since birth. This is illustrated by Figure 3-6, in which the inner solid-line triangle to age 80 is the area of interest. We may call this area the Dysquality Index at age x, $DI\ (x)$. It is very simple to compute this area. It is equal to half the slope of the line times the square of the age above 30 years (Appendix B). If we use the life expectancy as the age of interest the value of the Dysquality Index will be the amount of dysquality experienced, from the specified physiologic system, by the average person in the population who has lived at least to age 30, until the end of his or her life.

The length of life itself is determined by the multiplicity of causes of death and death is a complex phenomenon. It results from our failure to prevent or cure some particular cause, that is, by our failure to avoid Hamlet's "slings and arrows of misfortune." The general approach of medical science is perforce to stop disease once it has occurred, and prevention, especially in regard to chronic diseases caused by the effects of ordinary habits of life, is relegated to second place. This is probably as it must be, since the acute condition and its treatment already occupy more than our current research resources and the chronic problem is generally of very poorly understood etiology. That prevention can effectively be applied by public policy, however, can easily be seen by the examples of hygiene, antisepsis, and seat belts. Let us assume that by improved curative therapy we could shield ourselves from the penetration of the slings and arrows of disease for some years and that the life expectancy were thus extended. What would this do to the total amount of dysquality experienced by the average person in the population? Figure 3-7 shows this for increases in life expectancy at age 30 up to a doubling of

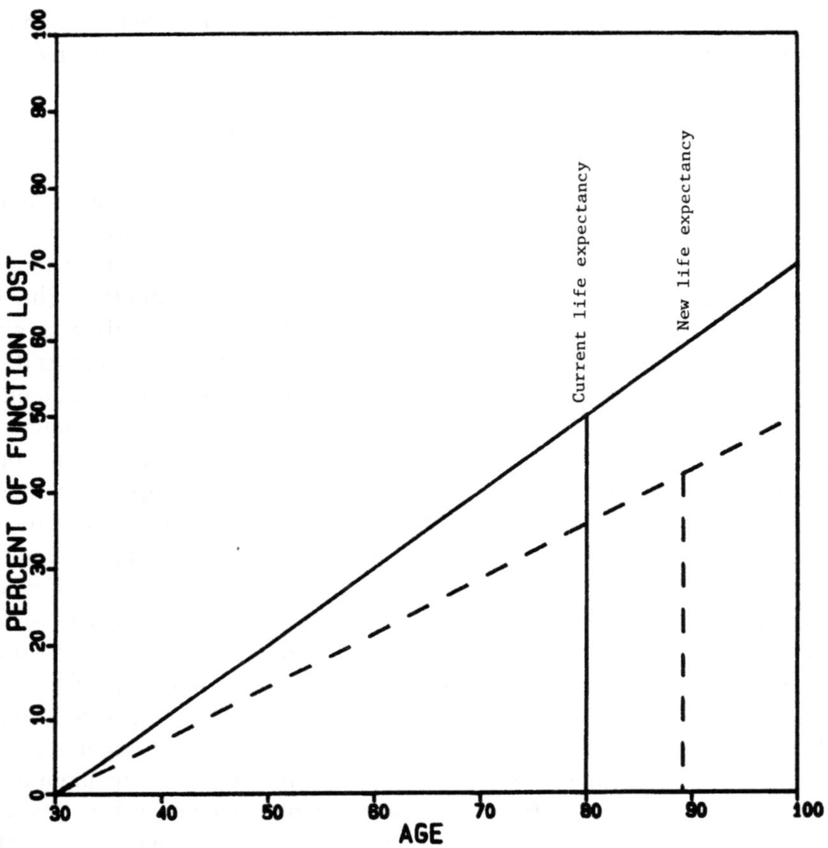

Figure 3-6. Relationship between longevity and dysquality, and definition of the dysquality index.

it. The Dysquality Index increases by the square of the factor by which life expectancy is increased.

Clearly, what we want is not simply to extend life if we do nothing substantial to alter the rate of decline in physiologic functions. All we would accomplish would be to decrease the quality of our later lives, by trading the addition of quantity for an increase in dysquality. Indeed, there may be a threshold of dysquality which is basically intolerable and to which many of us would be condemned by such unidimensional life extension. Perhaps this level is already experienced by many of today's elderly individuals.

What must be done is to alter the rate of decline in function, not merely the length of life. To do this, we must not dream that we would alter the basic shape of the decline function, to the extent that this is bound in natural law, but rather of altering its slope. If we could lower the slope of functional decline by some factor, by how much could we increase life

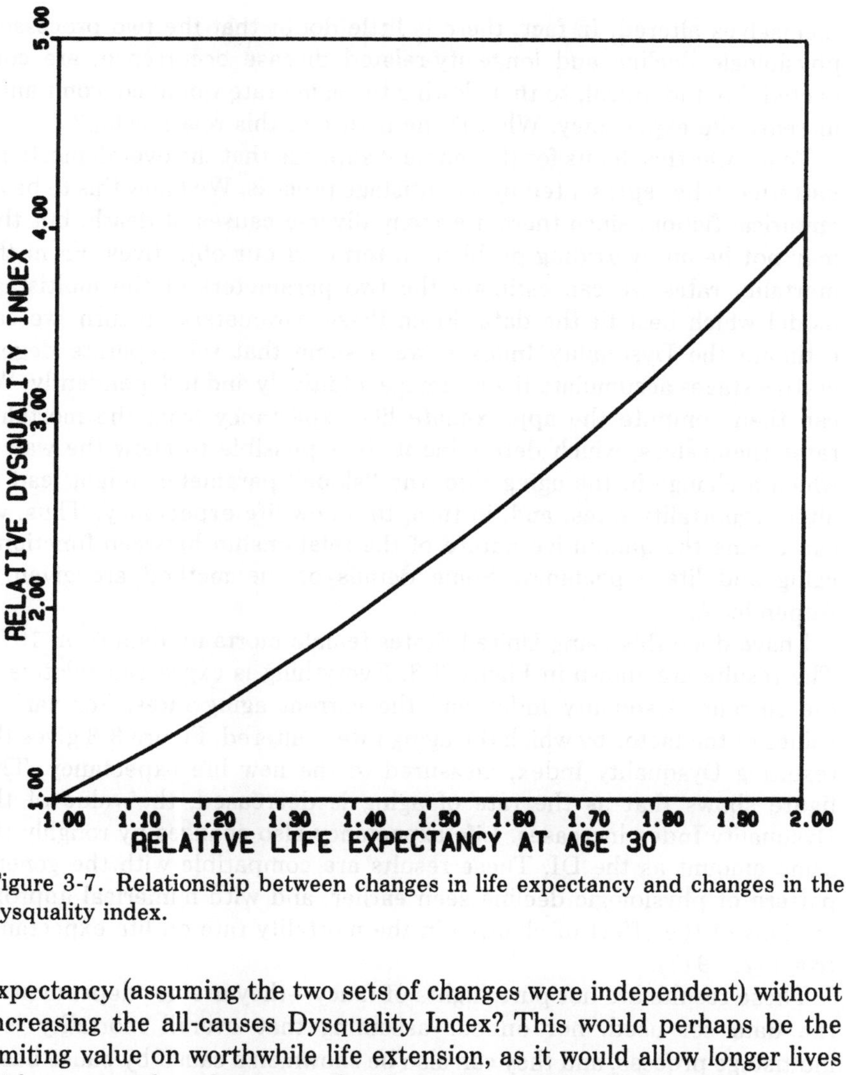

Figure 3-7. Relationship between changes in life expectancy and changes in the dysquality index.

expectancy (assuming the two sets of changes were independent) without increasing the all-causes Dysquality Index? This would perhaps be the limiting value on worthwhile life extension, as it would allow longer lives with no more than the current burdens of dysquality. This is shown as the inner dotted-line triangle in Figure 3-6. By lowering the aging rate, we could increase life expectancy to the point shown without increasing the total dysquality. Obviously, the new life expectancy value is dependent on the aging rate of the system in question, and would therefore be different for each system as well as for different degrees of alteration in the aging rates.

Relationship Between Length and Quality

We have just seen that by itself curing disease would lead to an increase in the Dysquality Index unless the processes leading to disease were themselves altered. In fact, there is little doubt that the two processes, physiologic decline and longevity-related disease occurrence, are connected if not identical, so that slowing the aging rate would concomitantly increase life expectancy. What is the nature of this relationship?

To answer this, let us for the moment suppose that the overall mortality pattern can be represented by a multistage process. We know this to be an empirical fiction, since there are many diverse causes of death, but this may not be an overriding problem in terms of our objectives. From the mortality rates we can estimate the two parameters of the multistage model which best fit the data. From these parameters, in turn, we can estimate the Dysquality Index if we assume that the separate degenerative stages accumulate their damage additively and independently. We can then compute the approximate life expectancy from the mortality rates themselves, which determine it. It is possible to show the way in which a change in the aging rate, the "slope" parameter, might lead to altered mortality rates, and, in turn, to a new life expectancy. Thus, we can exaine the qualitative nature of the relationship between functional aging and life expectancy. Some details of the method are given in Appendix A.

I have done this using United States female mortality data from 1976. The results are shown in Figure 3-8. Everything is expressed relative to the current Dysquality Index and the current aging rates. For various values of the factor by which the aging rate is altered, Figure 3-8 gives the resulting Dysquality Index, measured to the new life expectancy. This figure shows that as the rate of aging is decreased, the value of the Dysquality Index increases. Life expectancy also changes by roughly the same amount as the DI. These results are compatible with the general pattern of physiologic decline seen earlier, and with numerical approximations of the effect of changes in the mortality rate on life expectancy (Keyfitz, 1977).

These results are not pure flights of fancy—they are not dependent on the data set used, nor on our assuming that overall mortality is a multistage process, and they can also be shown on a cause-by-cause basis. They derive from the fact that considerable functional loss can accumulate before a life-terminating event results, so that if aging is slowed, more "dysquality" will be experienced by the average person, even though he or she lives longer. Aging and longevity are not independent phenomena.

The Marksman versus the Fusillade: The Competing Objectives of Individual and Population

So far we have dealt only with patterns of decline as they are experienced along the lifetime of a single, average, person. But nearly none of us are average. First of all, we are genetically diverse, and for many—if not

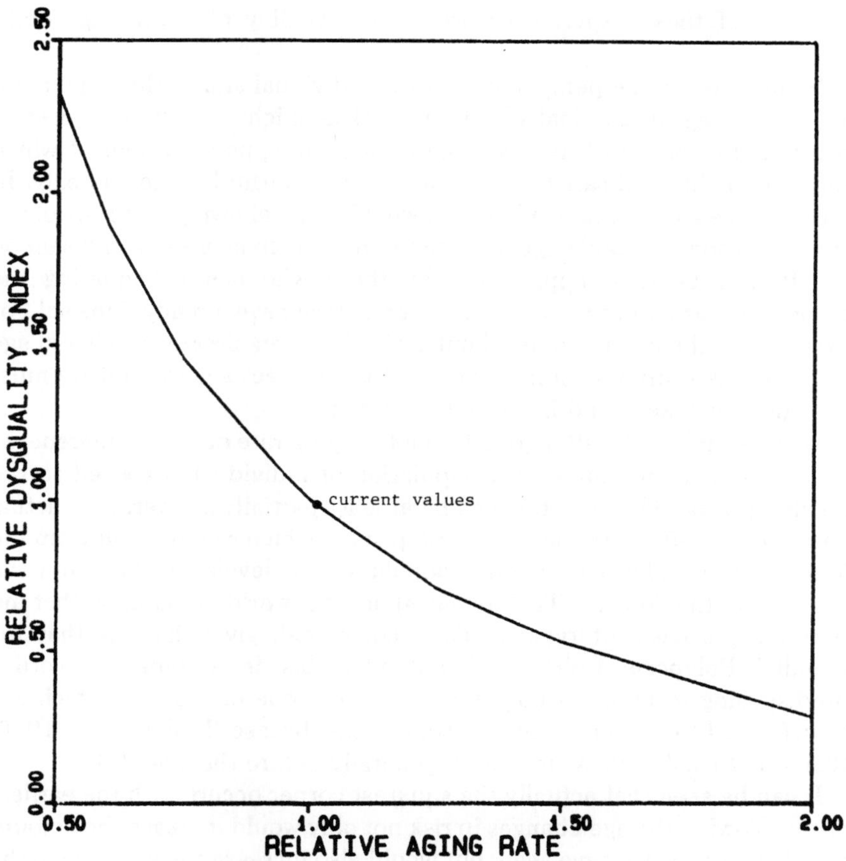

Figure 3-8. Relationship between changes in the aging rate and changes in the dysquality index.

most—the genes we carry make us very different in terms of risk and of what would have to be done to improve our life-quality. The sickle-cell or PKU infant are clear, dramatic cases, but what of the person susceptible to colon cancer or diabetes? Our individual genes and life experiences are so varied that it is difficult to conceive simple medical or environmental changes we might make which could provide a commensurate benefit to every recipient.

The extent of this variability can easily be seen in relationship simply to the end of life. In 1967, there were about 1,733,000 girls born in the U.S.A. Their life expectancy was 74.22 years, or 74 years 80 days (data from Keyfitz and Flieger, 1971). Of these girls, only about 106 will die on their appointed day. The life expectancy only applies exactly to .006% of the cohort, but not to the remaining 99.994%. To each individual his or her own experience is what counts, but to the population the mean and variance of these experiences are more revealing of prevailing conditions.

In many ways, the perspectives of the individual and of the population are competing. In an ideal world, many of us might prefer the causes of death and disease to leave us alone until some appointed hour at which time we might, well satisfied from a full and fruitful life, go willingly. In terms of the survivorship curve, this would mean allowing more people to survive to some suitable age and then to die, much as insects and salmon do. It may be underappreciated by those who desire "squaring the corner" in this manner that to a great extent we have already done so! For example, in the Netherlands, about 80% of women already survive to age 70. There is some way still to go to get the perfect square, but we must consider what we would have to do attain it.

What would be the effect of altering the aging rate on the "squareness" of the survivorship curve of a population of individuals exposed to the resulting risks? This question can be at least partially answered by actual data. Figure 3-9 shows the survivorship curve which would result from the imposition of colon cancer on a population, at levels ranging from the highest to the lowest (Thai females) in the world, assuming that no competing causes intervened. The highest risk given here is that for Familial Polyposis Coli (FPC) patients; this is a genetic disorder predisposing to multiple polyps in the colon, one or more of which are transformed to cancer in most victims of the disease (Lipkin et al., 1980; Weiss and Chakraborty, in press), generally before the age of 60.

It can be seen that actually the squarest corner occurs with the earliest onset. Slowing the age-changes in risk not only would increase the amount of dysquality, as we have seen, but would also increase the variance in the age at which the disease struck, that is, would "unsquare" the survivorship pattern. Note that to experience these effects we would have to live much longer than currently, even centuries longer; this may simply not be practicable with all of the nonaging (e.g., accident) risks we must also survive. The point is that as the aging rate declines, if life is thereby extended, the variance in age at death increases.

An exactly analogous situation would occur for all causes combined. Figure 3-10 shows the survivorship curve which would result from the alterations in the overall aging rate used earlier to relate dysquality to that rate. Clearly, though the effect is more compressed in time than we just saw for the hypothetical case of colon-cancer risk only, slowing aging means a more dispersed distribution of age at death. This would be true even if disease rates did not continue to increase throughout an extended lifespan (Schneider and Brody, 1983). Whether it is a fair trade to increase our probability of surviving to a much older age, for the increased sense of inequity which those unlucky enough to be affected much earlier would feel, is an individual judgment. However, it is in this way that the perspectives of the individual, who must gamble personal experience

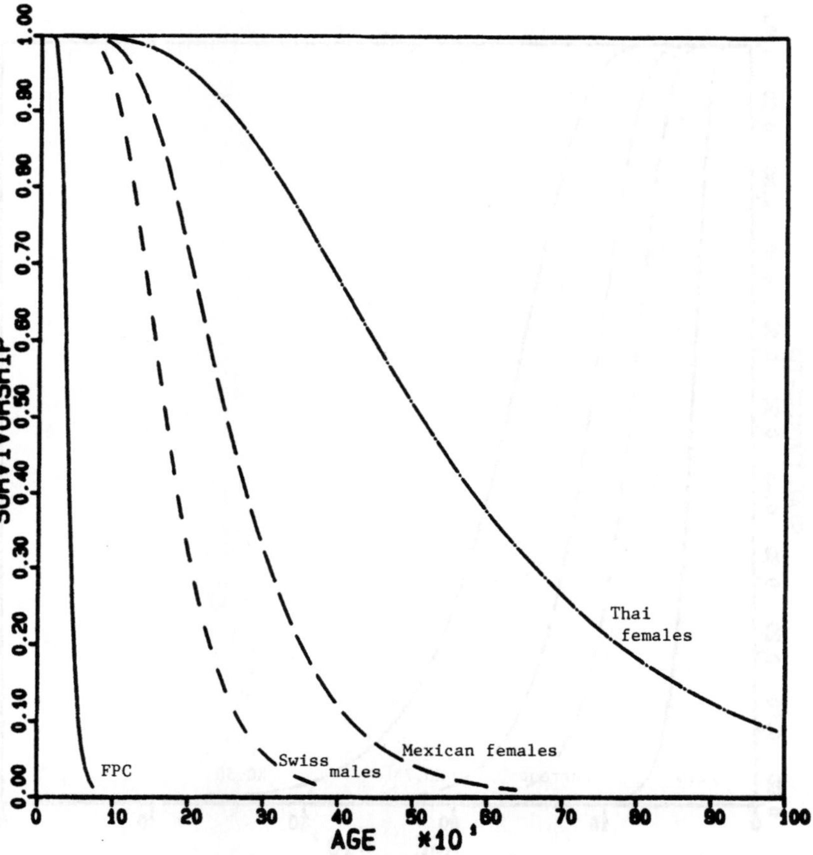

Figure 3-9. Survivorship schedules for colon cancer at extremes of worldwide risk assuming no other causes of death occur.

against the prevailing odds, and the population, which can be characterized by its collective experience, are at odds with each other.

We are now living in the time in which the variance in age at death is less than ever before, i.e., history's fairest and most equitable society in the face of death (Weiss, 1980), although there is empirical evidence that the variance is increasing again, as we forestall the fatal effects of degenerative diseases by a few years (Schneider and Brody, 1983). Today's squared corner in overall survivorship pattern is due to the elimination of early causes of death, however, and not to any substantial alteration of the onset pattern of degenerative disease, nor to any extension of our biological longevity potential, whatever that may be. Our survivorship pattern is now dominated by the multiplicity of degenerative causes all increasing in risk exponentially with adult ages. No single cause could, by

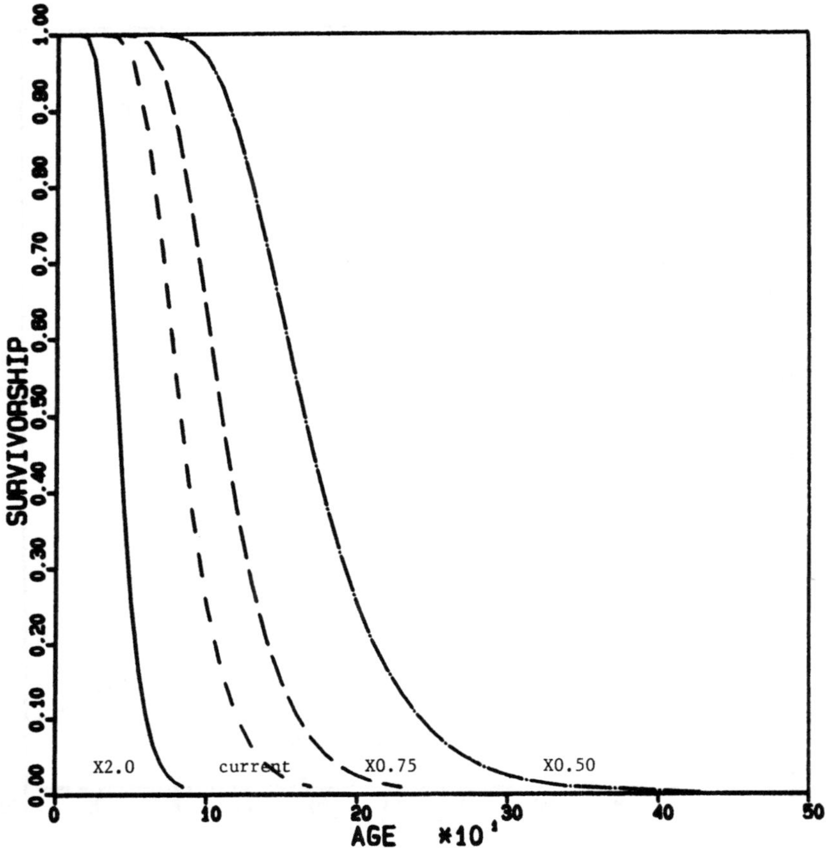

Figure 3-10. Survivorship schedules resulting from changes in overall aging rate. (Source: *Vital Statistics of the United States, 1966, Vol. II–Mortality*. U.S. National Center for Health Statistics, Washington, D.C., 1968.)

being removed, produce much increase in survivorship; indeed, as shown in Figure 3-9 single causes by themselves have a life expectancy of hundreds of years if other causes did not intervene. In that sense, on a cause-by-cause basis there is no justification for the statement that we have a programmed maximum lifespan potential calibrated by a deterministic clock, as are the timing of parturition, puberty, and menopause. However, this is a somewhat controversial point, being largely a matter of how one interprets or extrapolates from the available data which, of course, come only from those who only live to age 100 or so at most. For different views, see Fries (1980), Kohn (1982), Hayflick (1982), Schneider and Brody (1983), and Weiss (1983). The multiplicity of independent causes, by itself, suffices to reduce our probability of survival beyond a century or so virtually to zero. Slowing the aging rate would not square the corner of survivorship at 100, but would extend our maximum survival beyond 100 and reduce the squaring of the curve. Even if there is a cytological limit to survival, slowing of the aging process would probably also slow the processes leading to that limit, hence deferring the age of cytological decline; this seems to be shown by the results of Masoro (this volume) and other dietary life-extension experiments. Much of our idea about squaring the curve comes from comparison of our experience to that in other less-developed countries and to animals; but there the unsquared aspects of the curve have to do with early mortality, not with a different time calibration of degenerative processes.

Conclusion

Nothing in what I have presented depends on the particular mathematical forms of physiologic decline or disease-rate increase. The examples given only illustrate the nature of the relationships between the phenomena of aging, longevity, and "quality." However, I believe that the conclusions reached would be essentially the same were I to use much more extensive and detailed data.

It seems very likely that any combination of research or behavioral/environmental change can alter the basic aging processes themselves, which are determined by the nature of cells, genes, and their reactions to the outside world. It might be possible, within limits, to alter the rate at which these changes take place by controls placed on various kinds of exposure. In some cases we might alter this rate effectively to zero, that is, by preventing certain diseases. However, as we have seen, any slowing of the aging rate actually acts to raise the dysquality produced by causes not cured or prevented.

For these reasons, there seems to be no single point at which longevity is maximized and dysquality minimized. Hence, within the constraints of biology, we ourselves must determine goals we might choose to attain by scientific research. Palliation of existing disease and dysquality is obviously one area in which great strides can be expected. But we cannot expect science to deliver a specified optimal change in the quality of later life as this is determined by the aging process. Science does not work that predictably. Furthermore, where such an optimum may lie is an issue still up in the air, and is a social, not a biomedical, issue. It will probably change with the times, and judgments on the level of balance between longevity and quality will remain personal ones.

We leave where we came in, acknowledging the importance of social factors in the question of the quality of later life. Our current policy is to reduce exposures to disease-causing agents, or at least to inform people before they choose to become exposed to them, and to educate the public about the disease consequences of various aspects of behavior. This will probably remain the best policy in the foreseeable future. It will allow us to make an informed choice as to those life-ways, among the ones available at any given time, whose probable consequences most suit us. It will allow each of us to live our lives as individual trajectories, more or less independently of the fusillade of which, by being members of a population, we are a part. The hit pattern of that fusillade may be of small interest to the individual. Under these conditions, though still following the natural migratory laws, the bird of spring may be free to choose a peaceful, even enjoyable, course by which to fly south for the winter.

Acknowledgments

This paper was written with the partial support of grant CA-19311 from the U.S. National Cancer Institute. This is Demographic Epidemiology of Aging and Disease, Paper Number 19.

Mathematical Appendices

The various figures in the text were derived from the following mathematical equations and relationships.

Appendix A: Multistage Risk Models for Degenerative Disease

Frequently, a log-log linear equation of risk with age has been fitted to data. Such an equation has been show empirically to fit the data closely, and also has been derived from probability processes thought appropriate for diseases like cancer. The log-log linear equation is

$$\log(\text{risk}) = a + b\log(\text{age}) \tag{1}$$

and the parameters a and b are estimated from data.

This has often been interpreted as a multistage process leading to disease risk, although such an interpretation is not necessary and the equation can be used purely empirically. In treating disease as a multistage process, one can use any of a number of formulations of the process. Here, a specific model is used, though not interpreted as a biological model but because it fits the data well. The probability that an individual has the disease at some time at or before age t is given in this model by

$$P(t) = (1 - e^{-at})^b. \tag{2}$$

Many degenerative diseases fit this model very closely. From equation (2) we can derive the age-specific risk, or hazard, function as

$$h(t) = \frac{P'(t)}{1 - P(t)}$$
$$= \frac{abe^{-at}(1 - e^{-at})^{b-1}}{1 - (1 - e^{-at})^b}. \quad (3)$$

In deriving this, $1 - P(t)$ is the survivorship at age t, or the population at risk, and $P'(t)/[1 - P(t)]$ is the usual way to compute a rate, or hazard function.

To derive a life expectancy for a given set of age-specific risks, $h(t)$, we follow the definition of life expectancy. First, call survivorship at age t, $l(t)$. This is defined in terms of the age-specific hazard as

$$l(t) = \exp\left(\int_0^t h(x)dx\right) \quad (4)$$

and the life expectancy at age t is the sum of survivorship from age t onward:

$$E(t) = \int_t^\infty l(x)dx. \quad (5)$$

In this paper, we have looked at the effect of changes in aging rates, represented by the rate a in equation (2), on life expectancy from equation (5). This was done by determining the age-specific death rates from equation (3). Hence, by changing the value of a, the aging rate, the effect on life expectancy can be determined. For the U.S.A., mortality fitted in the text, equation (3) was used to estimate the parameters a and b for all causes. No biological interpretation is implied.

Appendix B: Computations Regarding the Dysquality Index

We assume maximum physiologic function at age 30, and define dysquality to be the amount of lost function. Assuming a linear accumulation of lost function by an amount A per year, the dysquality at age t, $d(t)$, is

$$d(t) = A(t - 30). \quad (6)$$

The Dysquality Index at age t, $DI(t)$, is defined as the sum of dysquality from age 30 to age t. This is computed from $d(t)$ as follows:

$$\mathrm{DI}(t) = \int_{30}^t d(x)dx$$
$$= \int_{30}^t a(x - 30)dx$$
$$= \frac{a}{2}(t - 30)^2. \quad (7)$$

If life expectancy is changed from age t to t', we could keep the Disquality Index (to the new life expectancy) unchanged by altering the aging rate by an amount given as follows: Let $T = t - 30$ and $T' = t' - 30$, and let a be the original aging rate and a' be the new rate. We want the value of $DI(t) = DI'(t')$ after the change in the aging rate, or

$$(a/2)T^2 = (a'/2)T'^2$$

or

$$t' = \sqrt{(a/a')}\,(t - 30) + 30. \tag{8}$$

References

Fries, J.: Aging, natural death, and the compression of morbidity. *New Eng. J. Med. 303*, 130–135 (1980).

Gompertz, B.: On the nature of the function expressive of the law of human mortality and on a new mode of determining life contingencies. *Phil. Trans. R. Soc. Lond. Ser. A 115*, 513–585 (1825).

Hayflick, L.: Biological aspects of aging. In Preston, SH (Ed.), Biological and Social Aspects of Mortality and the Length of Life. Liege: Ordina Editions, pp. 223–256, 1982.

Keyfitz, N.: Applied Mathematical Demography. New York: Wiley, 1977.

Keyfitz, and Flieger, W.: Population: Facts and Methods of Demography. San Francisco: Freeman, 1971.

Kohn, R.R.: Principles of Mammalian Aging. Englewood Cliffs, NJ: Prentice-Hall, 1971.

Kohn, R.R.: Cause of death in very old people. *J. Am. Med. Assoc. 247*, 2793–1797 (1982).

Lipkin, M., Sherlock, P., and DeCosse, J.: Risk factors and preventive measures in the control of cancer of the large intestine. In Current Problems in Cancer, Vol. IV, No. 10. Chicago: Yearbook Medical, 1980.

Schneider, E.L., and Brody, J.A.: Aging, natural death,and the compression of morbidity: another view. *New Eng. J. Med. 309*, 854–856 (1983).

Shock, N.W.: Biology of Aging. Washington, DC: American Institute of Biological Sciences, 1960.

Shock, N.W.: Physiological aspects of aging in man. *Ann. Rev. Physiol. 23*, 97–122 (1961).

Shock, N.W.: Energy metabolism, calorie intake and physical activity of the aging. In Carlston, L.A. (Ed.), Nutrition in Old Age. X Symposium of the Swedish Nutrition Foundation. Uppsala: Almqvistand Wiksell, 1972.

Strehler, B.L.: Time, Cells, and Aging. 2d Ed. New York: Academic Press, 1977.

Strehler, B.L., and Mildvan, A.S.: General theory of mortality and aging. *Science 132*, 14–21 (1960).

Waterhouse, J., Muir, C., Correa, P., and Powell, J.: Cancer Incidence in Five Continents, Vol. III. Lyon: International Agency for Research on Cancer, 1976.

Weiss, K.M.: Evolutionary perspectives on human aging. In Amoss, P., and Harrell, S. (Eds.), Other Ways of Growing Old. Stanford: Stanford University Press, pp. 25–52 (1980).

Weiss, K.M.: Aging *J. Am. Med. Assoc 249*, 2328–2329 (1983).

Weiss, K.M., Chakraborty, R., Ward, R.H., and Yucel, M.: Estimating the parameters which determine the age pattern of cancer. In prep.

Weiss, K.M., Chakraborty, R.: Multistage risk models and the age pattern of familial polyposis coli. Cancer Investigation, in press.

Whittemore, A.S.: Quantitative theories of oncogenesis. *Adv. Cancer Res. 27*, 55–88 (1978).

World Health Organization 1970 Mortality Data (supplied as Computer Tapes, also published as WHO Demographic Yearbook, 1971).

Chapter 4

Extending the Mammalian Life Span

Edward J. Masoro

Summary

That food restriction increases the length of life of laboratory rodents has long been known. Recent data indicate that in addition to increasing life span, food restriction also retards age-related physiological deterioration and age-related disease processes. Food restriction started in adult life is as effective as food restriction started in early life in regard to these effects. Restriction of protein but not calories did increase the median length of life but did not affect life span. The sum of these data strongly suggest that food restriction slows the aging process. The hypotheses that have been proposed as mechanisms by which food restriction retards the aging process are reviewed and each has been found to be wanting. A general metabolic hypothesis is proposed in which a specific metabolic event or events couple food restriction to the slowing of the aging process. Future research should focus on defining the specific nature of this metabolic couple.

Introduction

Recently there has been a proliferation of claims that dietary and/or pharmacologic interventions can slow the aging process and increase the life span. These claims include complex dietary programs involving periods of fasting and the inclusion of certain foods with the exclusion of others, the fortifying of diets with antioxidants (e.g., Vitamin E), the addition of the neurotransmitter, dopamine, to the diet, the use of dehydroepiandrosterone, and many others. Thus, it is surprising that only one experimental intervention, that of food restriction, has been consistently shown to increase the life span of a mammalian species (Sacher, 1977).

It was in 1935 that McCay and his colleagues (McCay et al., 1935) first clearly showed that restricting the food intake of rats increased longevity. This finding has been often repeated and it has also been shown to occur in mice and other rodent species (Barrows and Kokkonen, 1977). Moreover, recent studies have established that in addition to increasing life span, food restriction also delays and, in part, prevents age-related physiologic deterioration and age-related disease (Masoro et al., 1980). Thus, it seems highly probable that food restriction slows the basic aging process or processes.

If food restriction does indeed slow basic aging processes as seems likely, it should provide a powerful tool for the experimental exploration of these processes. Moreover, such explorations are likely to provide clues to interventions that may modulate aging in humans. It is for this reason that we and many other investigators have been intensively studying food restriction. The findings have been exciting and strongly indicate that further experimental work in this area should be a primary focus of experimental gerontology for at least the next 20 years. This chapter will review these recent findings with primary focus on the work of the author's laboratory.

Experimental Design

Since the research from our laboratory will be the primary focus, a brief description of the design of our studies is in order. Male Fischer 344 rats were used. They were purchased as weanlings (4 weeks of age) from the Charles River Laboratories and were specific pathogen-free. The animals were housed throughout life in a barrier facility to maintain the specific pathogen-free status. They were fed a semisynthetic diet with a caloric composition of 21% protein, 57% carbohydrate, 22% fat unless otherwise noted.

The first of our studies which was completed 4 years ago was comprised of two groups. The rats in Group A were allowed to eat *ad libitum* throughout life and the rats in Group R were fed 60% of the mean food intake of the Group A rats from 6 weeks of age on.

The second study which has just been completed involved five dietary groups. Group 1 was a repeat of Group A of the first study and Group 2 was a repeat of Group R. The rats in Group 3 were restricted to 60% of the food intake of Group 1 rats from 6 weeks of age to 6 months of age, but at all other ages were fed *ad libitum*. The rats in Group 4 were restricted to

60% of the food intake of Group 1 rats starting at 6 months of age. The rats in Group 5 were fed *ad libitum* from 6 weeks of age on a diet with the following caloric composition: 12.6% protein, 65.4% carbohydrate, and 22% fat. Thus, the second study involved (a) dietary restriction limited to early life, (b) dietary restriction started in adult life, and (c) restriction of protein but not calories as well as the dietary regimens of the first study.

Longevity Findings

Data from the longevity component of our first study (Yu et al., 1982) are presented in the form of survival curves in Figure 4-1. The survival curve for the rats of Group A ($n = 115$) is quite rectangular which is to be expected for a genetically homogeneous rat population maintained under specific pathogen-free conditions in a controlled environment and a constant-composition diet. The survival curve for the Group R rats is less rectangular but shifted to the right with a marked increase in both the median length of life and the life span. The fact that the curve is less rectangular, however, is somewhat surprising since technology and medicine has rectangularized the human survival curve during the past 2000 years; however, technology and medicine have not influenced human life span since a few citizens of Ancient Rome (median length of life of 21 years) lived 100 years and the same is true of the life span of the 20th

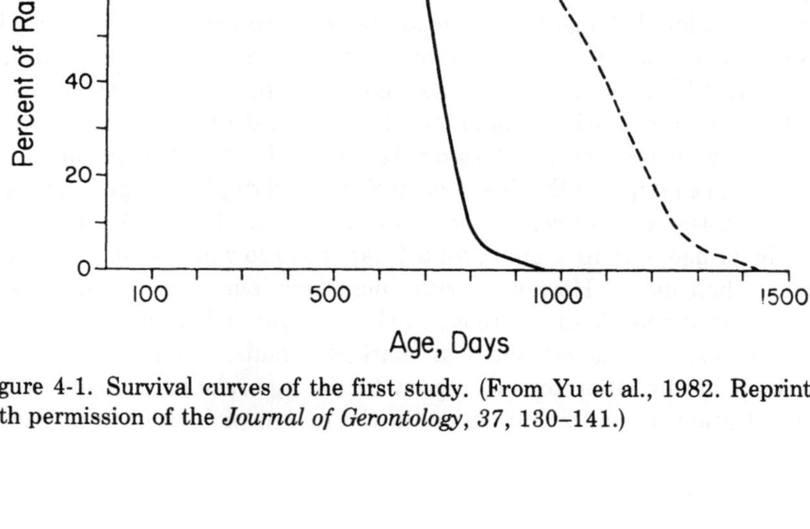

Figure 4-1. Survival curves of the first study. (From Yu et al., 1982. Reprinted with permission of the *Journal of Gerontology*, *37*, 130–141.)

century United States, even though the median length of life is now in excess of 70 years.

Although longevity data are important to obtain, it is expensive to do so using 115 rats per group. Because of the highly standardized living conditions of our studies, it seemed possible to decrease the *n* and still obtain accurate longevity data. Thus, in the second study, we used 40 rats per group. The survival curve for Group 1 rats which were treated the same as the Group A rats but some four years later was almost identical to that of Group A and the survival curve of Group 2 was also similar to that of Group R rats. Thus, an *n* of 40 proved to be quite adequate for highly reproducible survival curves between studies carried out years apart.

The survival curve of Group 3 rats indicates that this dietary regimen resulted in small but significantly greater median length of life and life span than is the case for the rats in Group 1. However, these increases were much less than what was obtained with Group 2 or R rats. Thus, food restriction limited to early life was not very effective in promoting longevity.

In contrast, the survival curve of the Group 4 rats shows that this dietary regimen markedly extended median length of life and life span. In regard to the latter, it was as effective as the dietary regimen of the Group 2 rats. Thus, food restriction started in early adult life is very effective in promoting longevity.

The survival curve of the Group 5 rats shows that this dietary regimen results in a small but significant increase in median length of life with little effect on life span. Thus, protein restriction in the absence of caloric restriction does not influence longevity markedly.

Physiologic Deterioration

Physiologic changes occur with aging and the nature of these changes, for the most part, are detrimental to the organism. The general pattern of these age-related changes in *ad libitum* fed and food-restricted rats can be described as follows: During early adult life, there is little difference between *ad libitum* fed and food restricted rats, but with increasing age, a marked and progressive change occurs in the *ad libitum* fed rats while such change is delayed and less marked in the food restricted rats.

A typical example of this is shown in Figure 4-2 depicting age changes in serum cholesterol concentrations (Masoro et al., 1983). At 6 and 12 months of age, Group 1 and Group 2 rats have low and similar levels of serum cholesterol. However, with increasing age, serum cholesterol concentrations markedly increase in Group 1 rats while in Group 2 rats this increase is delayed and less marked. Similar findings have been obtained in our laboratory in regard to the age-related changes in the concentration of serum hormones, in the action of hormones on target

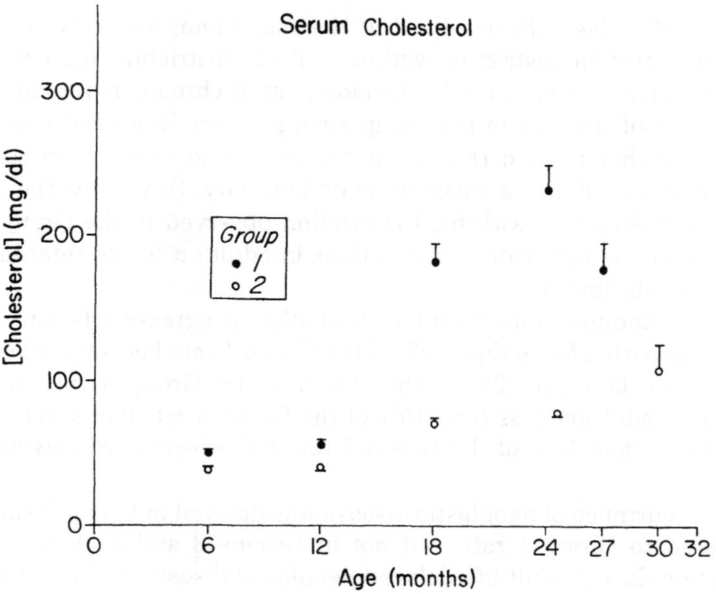

Figure 4-2. Serum cholesterol concentrations from the second study. (Modified from Masoro et al., 1983. Reprinted with permission of the American Institute of Nutrition.)

cells, on the loss of muscle mass, on the loss of muscle function, and on the loss of bone mass (Masoro et al., 1980). Other laboratories have reported similar results. For instance, Levin et al. (1981) found that the age-related loss of dopamine receptors in the corpus striatum of the rat is markedly retarded by food restriction. Moreover, extensive studies (Weindruch et al., 1979; Fernandes et al., 1978) have been carried out on the immune system of mice and food restriction was found to retard the age-related loss of immune competence and the age-related development of autoimmunity.

Age-Related Disease

In rats, chronic nephropathy in many respects is similar to atherosclerosis in humans. It is found in almost all individuals and progresses in severity with increasing age. In many but not all individuals, the disease process becomes clinically manifest at advanced ages. Food restriction started at 6 weeks of age (Group 2) or 6 months of age (Group 4) markedly retarded the progression of these kidney lesions with age. At death, more than 50% of the Group 1 rats have a severity of lesion associated with clinical renal failure while less than 5% of the Group 2 or Group 4 rats had lesions of this severity. Restricting food from 6 weeks to 6 months of age (Group 3) was less effective with one-third of the rats having very severe lesions. However, protein restriction without caloric restriction (Group 5) was quite effective in retarding the development of chronic nephropathy with about 10% of the rats in the group having severe lesions at death. It is interesting that protein restriction, which was so effective in retarding renal lesions, had only a small effect on longevity. Obviously, the marked increase in longevity with food restriction observed in the Group 2 and Group 4 rats results from other actions in addition to the retardation of chronic nephropathy.

Similar findings were found with another progressive lesion, that of cardiomyopathy. More than 20% of the Group 1 rats had severe lesions at death while less than 2% of the Group 2 and Group 4 rats had such lesions. In addition, less than 10% of the Group 5 rats had severe lesions while more than 10% of the Group 3 rats had severe cardiomyopathy at death.

The occurrence of neoplastic disease was delayed in Group 2 and 4 rats compared to Group 1 rats, but not in Groups 3 and 5. Although food restriction during adult life delayed neoplastic disease, it did not prevent its occurrence. Indeed, a greater percentage of the Group 2 and 4 rats at death had neoplastic disease than the rats in the other groups. However, it must be kept in mind that the rats in Groups 2 and 4 died at much older ages than the rats in the other groups.

Mechanisms of Action

The mechanism(s) by which food restriction slows the aging process is not known. McCay originally proposed that food restriction acts by retarding maturation. Indeed, he hypothesized that aging was a postmaturational event and that if maturation were prevented, aging would not occur. He used food restriction in an attempt to prevent maturation and thus test his hypothesis. He interpreted his findings as support for this hypothesis in that food restriction did not prevent but it did delay maturation and, in so doing, he believed it increased longevity presumeably because it had retarded the aging processes. Our findings with the Group 4 rats make it most unlikely that food restriction acts by delaying maturation since maturation should have been completed before 6 months of age when food restriction was initiated.

A related hypothesis was the proposal that food restriction slows the aging process by decreasing the rate of growth and prolonging its duration. This concept was based on the view that aging does not start until growth has been completed. Indeed, there are data showing that the length of life correlates inversely with the rate of growth and directly with the duration of growth (Goodrick, 1980). However, our findings with the Group 4 rats make it unlikely that this is an important component of the action of food restriction on the aging process since growth is nearly complete in the 6-month-old male Fischer 344 rat.

Another view that has been widely held is that food restriction acts by maintaining the rats lean. Indeed, the food-restricted rats do have a lower fat content than the *ad libitum* fed rats. However, data reported from our laboratory (Bertrand et al., 1980) make it unlikely that food restriction retards the aging process by reducing body fat. Within the Group A population, there was no correlation between the length of life and the body fat and within the Group R population (the lean food-restricted rats), there was a positive correlation, i.e., the fatter the rat the longer it lived.

In 1977, Sacher (Sacher, 1977) proposed that food restriction slowed the rate of aging by reducing the metabolic rate per gram of body mass. This view has been rather widely embraced. He based his hypothesis on studies of Ross (Ross, 1969) in which a spectrum of diets were used which caused markedly different life spans. He found that the number of kilocalories used by the rats per gram body weight per lifetime was almost the same for all rat groups. Thus, he felt the reason the rats on restricted diets lived longer was that their metabolic rate was lower, therefore requiring a longer period of time before this limiting lifetime caloric expenditure was reached. This view was in accord with the findings of Rubner at the turn of the Century that a variety of domestic animals had the same lifetime caloric expenditure if expressed in terms of kilocalories per kilogram body weight. It also is in accord with the rate of living theory of aging proposed by Pearl in 1928 (Pearl, 1928).

However, it was clear that, in using the limited amount of data in the published paper of Ross, Sacher had to make assumptions in generating his calculations. Moreover a different choice of assumptions would have led to a different conclusion. We, therefore, decided to make the calculations from the raw data of our first study, thus circumventing the need for any assumptions. We found that Group R rats did not consume less calories per gram body weight per day than Group A rats, but rather consumed more (Masoro et al., 1982). However, if lean body mass were used as the basis, Group A and Group R rats consumed the same number of kilocalories per day per gram lean body mass. Moreover, the mean lifetime caloric consumption per gram body mass was 92 kcal for Group A rats and 134 kcal for Group R rats; thus, Group R rats lived longer and consumed significantly more kilocalories per gram body weight during their lifetime than Group A rats. These findings do not support the hypothesis that food restriction prolongs life by reducing the metabolic rate per unit body mass.

If all seriously proposed hypotheses appear to be incorrect, what other possibilities are there for the mechanism by which food restriction prolongs life and slows the aging process? My colleague, Dr. B. P. Yu, and I have developed a framework which we call the General Metabolic

Hypothesis. We feel this framework will be useful in guiding future research aimed at exploring this question. This hypothesis is schematically presented in Figure 4-3 (Masoro, in press). The central point of this hypothesis is that food restriction modulates a specific metabolic process(es) and that it is the change in this metabolic process(es) that slows the basic aging process. The slowing of the aging results in the retardation of physiologic deterioration, immune deterioration, and age-related disease processes, all of which are viewed as being secondary to the modulation of one or more basic aging processes. The increase in longevity is viewed to be a result of the retardation of these secondary events. Future research should focus on learning the nature of these specific metabolic alterations that couple food restriction to the slowing of the aging process. Metabolic processes that generate or degrade free radicals appear to be a particularly fertile area to explore in this regard at this time.

Relevance to Humans

The question always arises as to whether food restriction would have similar actions in humans as those just described for laboratory rodents. Hard data on this are not available nor are they likely to be in the near future. Although our major reason for studying food restriction in rodents is to use it as a tool to explore the basic aging processes, it is our feeling that our findings may also provide a basis for interventions in human aging. On theoretical grounds, it seems likely that a regimen that so markedly influences aging in rodents will similarly influence all mammals. However, this should not be interpreted to mean that food restriction in humans would increase the human life span above 100–115 years.

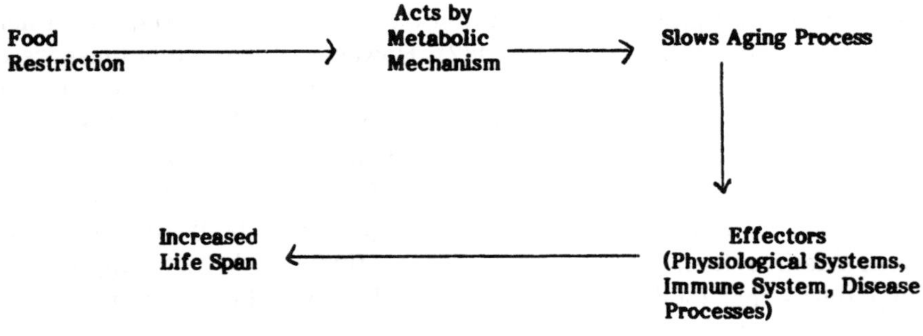

Figure 4-3. General metabolic hypothesis. (From Masoro, 1984. Reprinted with permission of the *Journal of the American Geriatric Society*, *32*, 296–300.)

Laboratory rats and other rodents have been maintained nutritionally in a rather unique way; they have been allowed to eat *ad libitum* and their diet has been very high in protein. This was done because the primary aim was to have a high rate of reproduction and a high rate of growth in order to supply the needs of investigators for experimental animals. Although some in the human population have a dietary history similar to the *ad libitum* fed rats, it is almost certain that a fraction of the billions of people for which longevity data are available have had dietary histories similar to that restricted rats. Since 115 years is the longest length of human life that can be documented, it is doubtful that food restriction or anything we learn from food restriction research will cause the human life span to exceed 115 years. Rather, what the application of our knowledge of food restriction is likely to achieve is an increase in the percent of people who live to 95 years or more.

References

Barrows, G.H., and Kokkonen, G.C.: Relationship between nutrition and aging. *Adv. Nutr. Res. 1*, 253–298, 1977.

Bertrand, H.A., Lynd, F.T., Masoro, E.J., and Yu, B.P.: Changes in adipose mass and cellularity through the adult life of rats fed ad libitum or a life prolonging restricted diet. *J. Geront. 35*, 827–835, 1980.

Fernandes, G., Friend, P., Yunis, E.J., and Good, R.A.: Influence of dietary restriction on immunologic function and renal disease in (NZB × NZW) F_1 mice. *Proc. Natl. Acad. Sci. USA 75*, 1500–1504, 1978.

Goodrick, C.L.: Effects of long-term voluntary wheel exercise on male and female Wistar rats. I. Longevity. *Gerontology 26*, 22–33, 1980.

Levin, P., Janda, J.K., Joseph, J.A., Ingram, D.K., and Roth, G.S.: Dietary restriction retards the age-associated loss of rat striatal dopaminergic receptors. *Science 214*, 561–562, 1981.

Masoro, E.J.: Food restriction and the aging process. *J. Am. Geriat. Soc. 32*, 296–300, 1984.

Masoro, E.J., Compton, C., Yu, B.P., and Bertrand, H.: Temporal and compositional dietary restrictions modulate age-related changes in serum lipids. *J. Nutr. 113*, 880–892, 1983.

Masoro, E.J., Yu, B.P., and Bertrand, H.A.: Action of food restriction in delaying the aging process. *Proc. Natl. Acad. Sci. USA 79*, 4239–4241, 1982.

Masoro, E.J., Yu, B.P., Bertrand, H.A., and Lynd, F.T.: Nutritional probe of the aging process. *Fed. Proc. 39*, 3178–3182, 1980.

McCay, C.M., Crowell, M.F., and Maynard, L.A.: The effect of retarded growth upon the length of life span and upon the ultimate body size. *J. Nutr. 10*, 63–79, 1935.

Pearl, R.: The Rate of Living. New York: Alfred Knopf, 1928.

Ross, M.H.: Aging, nutrition and hepatic enzyme patterns in the rat. *J. Nutr. 97, Suppl. 1, Part II*, 563–602, 1969.

Sacher, G.A.: Life table modification and life prolongation. In Finch, C. and Hayflick, L. (Eds.): Handbook of Biology of Aging, pp. 582–638. New York: Van Nostrand Reinhold, 1977.

Weindruch, R., Kristie, J.A., Cheney, K.E., and Walford, R.L.: Influence of controlled dietary restriction on immunologic function and aging. *Fed. Proc. 38*, 1007–1016, 1979.

Yu, B.P., Masoro, E.J., Murata, I., Bertrand, H.A., and Lynd, F.T.: Life span study of SPF Fischer 344 male rats: Longevity, growth, lean body mass and disease. *J. Geront. 37*, 130–141, 1982.

Chapter 5

Aging Humans and Aging Cells

Leonard Hayflick

Summary

After reaching sexual maturity, individual members of a species accumulate physiologic decrements that lead to an increase in their likelihood of dying. This decline in function is called aging. For humans, the likelihood of dieing doubles every 7 years beyond the age of 30.

The triumphs of modern medicine have not lengthened the human lifespan. Medical successes merely have permitted more people to reach what appears to be a fixed upper age limit. Life expectation has increased but life span has not. In many developed countries, one can now reasonably expect to become old, which is a very new phenomenon.

If the two leading causes of death in developed countries were to be eliminated (cardiovascular diseases and cancer), about 14 years of additional life expectation would occur for all age groups. Resolving all other causes of death would add an additional 2 years of life expectation. Thus if all causes of premature death were to be eliminated, all humans would live to be about 100 years of age. They would then die as the result of normal losses in physiologic function which previously increased their vulnerability to an earlier death caused by disease or accidents. The diseases of old age are simply superimposed on the normal physiologic decrements that occur after sexual maturation.

Studies on isolated human cells grown in laboratory cultures indicate that normal cells have a limited capacity to divide and to function. They have a chronometer that limits their replicative and functional capacity. Cells grown in culture from older donors have a reduced capacity to divide and function when compared to cells grown from younger donors. Before cells die in culture they reveal several hundred changes, many of which are similar to those changes that occur in the intact older human.

Current evidence leads to the belief that age changes are substantially due to changes that occur in the genetic machinery of individual cells. The changes apparently are induced by the same genetic program that operates throughout the life of the individual.

Introduction

Of all the conflicting views on the causes of biological aging, few gerontologists disagree with the axiom that after reaching sexual maturity and cessation of growth, animals accumulate physiologic decrements that lead to an increase in their likelihood of dying. In fact, for humans, the data, first analyzed by the English actuary Gompertz in 1825, reveal that the force of mortality doubles every 7 years after the age of 30. That is, after maturity, the rate and probability of dying are exponential with increasing age. A variety of human physiologic functions, although subject to some individual variation, show a slow, nearly linear decline from 30 years of age. The rate constants for this linear loss seem to occur at about 0.8–0.9% loss per year of the functional capacity present at the age of 30 (Strehler and Mildvan, 1960).

The common impression that the triumphs of modern medicine have lengthened the human life span is not supported by either vital statistics or biological evidence. The fact is that in the developed countries, the prevention and treatment of ills which occur in the early years has improved, permitting more people to reach what appears to be an immutable, upper age limit. Thus life expectation has increased (Fig. 5-1), but the human life span has remained virtually unchanged for many hundreds of thousands of years.

Medical achievements have simply allowed more people to reach the limit of that fixed life span. Deaths in the early years are becoming increasingly less frequent in the developed countries, resulting in life tables that are simply becoming more rectangular, as indicated by the direction of the arrow in Figure 5-2. In many privileged countries, one can now expect to become reasonably old, which is a relatively new phenomenon.

Effects of the Resolution of Diseases

If cardiovascular diseases, which are the leading cause of death in the United States, are prevented, approximately 12 years of additional life can be expected (Table 5-1). If the second greatest cause of death—cancer—is eliminated, about 2 years of additional life expectation will result. The net increase in life expectancy at birth achieved in the United

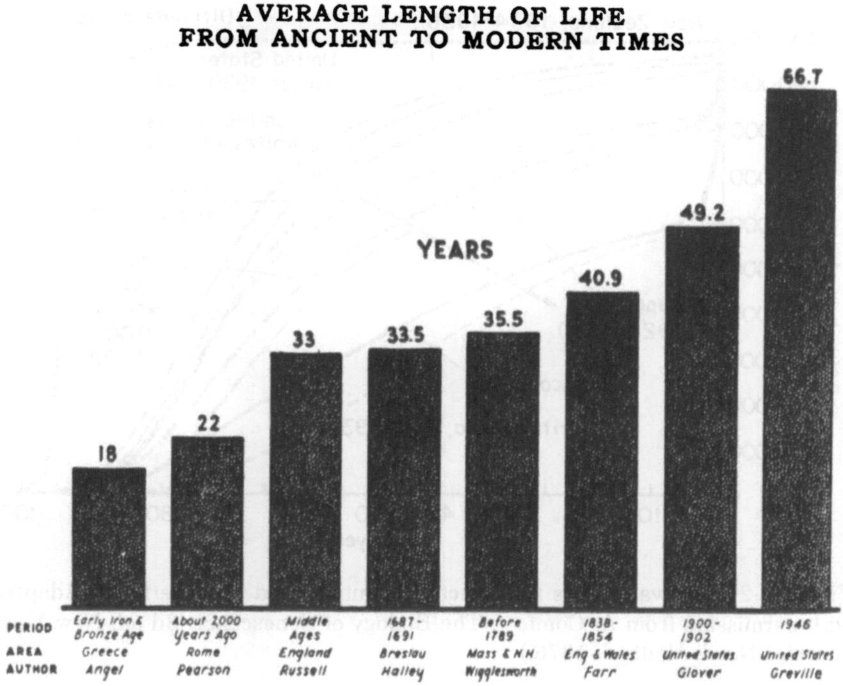

Figure 5-1. Average length of life at birth in various eras. (From L.I. Dublin, A.J. Lotka, and M. Spiegelman, Length of Life. New York: Ronald Press, 1949. Reprinted with permission of John Wiley and Sons.)

States from 1900 to 1950 was almost 20 years. This increase resulted from the decrease in the large number of deaths that occurred before the age of 65. However, the gain in life expectancy at 65 and 75 years of age from 1900 to 1969 was, respectively, only 2.9 and 2.2 years.

What would be the effect on human longevity and the human life span in a world in which all causes of death resulting from disease and accidents were totally eliminated (Table 5-1)? The effect on human longevity would be to realize the ultimate rectangular curve (Figure 5-2) in which citizens would live out their lives free of the fear of premature death, but with the certain knowledge that their normal physiologic decrements would result in death on about their 100th birthday.

These concepts have forced gerontologists to the conclusion that the disease-oriented approach to medical research might increase life expectation but will have little impact on increasing the human life span. If such an increase is desirable (and there is considerable doubt that it is), one must first separate the disease-related causes of death from the age-dependent normal physiologic decrements that give rise to the manifestations of old age. The diseases of old age are simply superimposed on these normal physiologic decrements but must be separately regarded to consider ways of increasing the human life span. Although age-associated

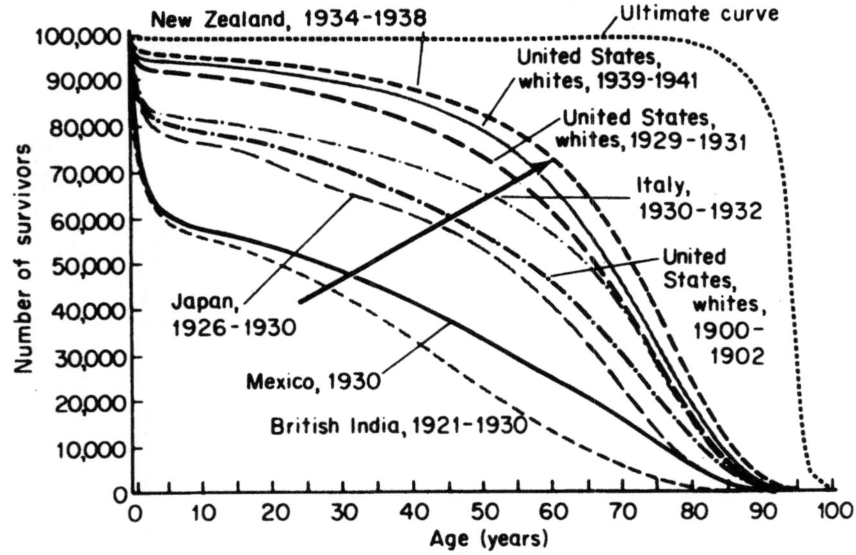

Figure 5-2. Survival curves for selected countries and time periods. (Adapted with permission from A. Comfort, The Biology of Senescence, 3d ed. New York: Elsevier-North Holland, 1976.)

Table 5-1. Gain in expectation of life at birth and at age 65 due to elimination of various causes of death, 1969–71

Cause of Death	Gain (yr) in Expectation of Life if Cause was Eliminated: At Birth	At Age of 65
Major cardiovascular-renal diseases	11.8	11.4
Diseases of the heart	5.9	5.1
Cerebrovascular diseases	1.2	1.2
Malignant neoplasms*	2.5	1.4
Motor vehicle accidents	0.7	0.1
All accidents excluding motor vehicles	0.6	0.1
Influenza and pneumonia	0.5	0.2
Diabetes mellitus	0.2	0.2
Infectious and parasitic diseases	0.2	0.1
Tuberculosis	Less than 0.05	

*Including neoplasms of lymphatic and hematopoietic tissues.

Source: U.S. Public Health Service, National Center for Health Statistics, U.S. Life Tables by Causes of Death: 1969–71, by T.N.E. Greville, *U.S. Decennial Life Tables for 1969–71, 1*, 5, 1976.

physiologic decrements surely increase vulnerability to disease, the fundamental causes of death are not diseases (or many kinds of accidents) but the physiologic decrements that make their occurrence more likely.

Biomedical research has directed its efforts almost exclusively on the disease-associated causes of death. Scant attention has been paid to the underlying cause of biologic aging that are not disease-associated, but which, in clocklike fashion, dictate for each species a specific maximum life span. To be sure, the physiologic decrements that occur in advancing years increase vulnerability to disease, but unless more attention is paid to the fundamental non-disease-related biological causes of aging, the fate of each person will be death on about his or her 100th birthday.

Prospects for Increasing Human Longevity

As stated, there are two ways in which the efforts of biomedical research can be expected to extend human longevity in the next 25 years. The first is to reduce or eliminate the major causes of death. For most developed countries, this would mean eliminating cardiovascular diseases and cancer. In the developing countries, life expectancy can be extended by the simple expedient of motivating the political and economic infrastructure to provide citizens with the necessary food, hygienic conditions, and medical care that are commonplace in developed countries. The results of reducing the role of minor diseases in developed countries will be minimal. For example, in the United States, if tuberculosis were completely eliminated, the gain in life expectation at birth would be less than 0.05 year (Table 5-1). Thus it could be argued that if an increase in life expectation becomes the main goal of biomedical research in the developed countries, all such research should be directed toward the elimination of the two major causes of death. This position, although less than humane and not likely to attract many adherents, is nonetheless the most logical conclusion to be drawn from life-table studies and the projections dealt with in Table 5-1.

The second way in which biomedical research can deal with human longevity is to address itself specifically to the underlying non-disease-related fundamental causes of age changes. These are not diseases but are the basic biological changes that result in the physiologic decrements characteristic of normal aging. On these changes is superimposed an increasing vulnerability to disease. Such an approach, then, does not directly concern itself with efforts to increase human life expectation but rather to extend what appears to be a fixed life span.

As a measure of the current effort put forth toward these two approaches, funds spent in the United States on cardiovascular disease and cancer research are about 20 times greater than the funds spent in gerontology. It is also probable that the number of researchers, and consequently the amount of effort, in both these areas also differs 20-fold. Consequently, the likelihood that any significant increase in human longevity will occur in the next 15 years depends on (1) significantly better cure rates for cardiovascular diseases or cancer or both, and (2) significant advances in our understanding and ability to manipulate the biologial clocks that set a maximum life span for each species.

Demographic Projections

That the proportion of persons in developed countries over the age of 65 has been steadily increasing is well known. In the last 100 years, their proportion of the total population in the United States has increased from 3.4 to 11.6% (Fig. 5-3).

Within 50 years, those over 65 are expected to number nearly 40 million in the United States. This prediction does not take into account any major resolution within 50 years of the two leading causes of death (cardiovascular disease and cancer). If some significant cure rate were to occur, however, the United States might have as many persons over 65 as under 15 in the year 2025.

Aging at the Cellular Level

The notion that aging occurs in animals that reach a fixed size after maturity is beyond dispute. But is the inevitability of the aging and death of individual cells composing that organism predetermined? A superficial

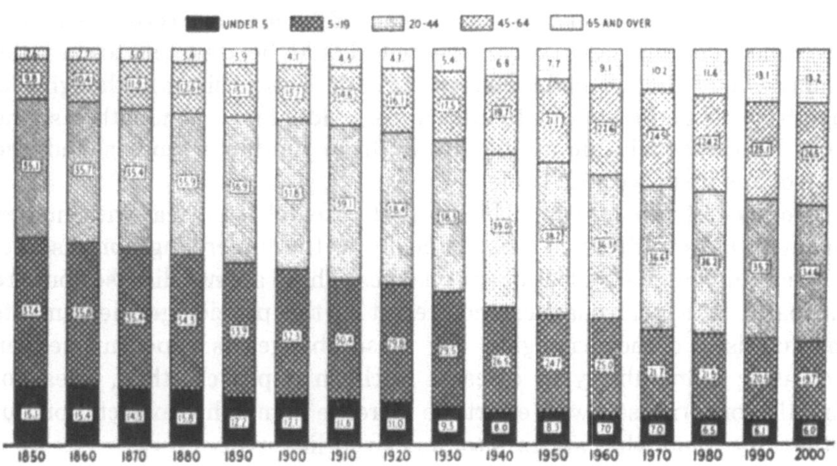

Figure 5-3. Proportion of persons in various age groups as a function of various decades in the United States. (From L.I. Dublin, A.J. Lotka, and M. Spiegelman, Length of Life. New York: Ronald Press, 1949. Reprinted with permission of John Wiley and Sons.)

consideration of this thought may provoke some incredulity since it is intuitively obvious that a dead or aging organism must consist of dead or aging cells. Nevertheless, whatever causes age changes and death in the whole organism undoubtedly does not produce similar changes, and at the same rate, in each cell composing that organism. If the rates of aging vary among organs, tissues, and their constituent cells, then the root causes of aging may occur as a consequence of decrements in some few cell types where the rate is fastest and the effects greatest. Let us explore the notion that normal somatic cells are predestined to undergo irreversible functional decrements that lead to aging in the whole organism.

There are at least two ways in which this question has been put to the test. First, vertebrate cells have been serially cultured in laboratory glassware, and second, similar cells, containing specific markers allowing them to be distinguished from host cells, have been serially transplanted in isogenic laboratory animals. The goals of such studies, as they pertain to the science of gerontology, have been directed toward answering this fundamental question: Can vertebrate cells, functioning and replicating under ideal conditions, escape from the inevitability of aging and death that is universally characteristic of the whole animals from which they were derived?

In respect to studies undertaken in cell culture, one investigation stood out as the classic response to this intriguing question. In the early part of this century, Alexis Carrel, a noted cell culturist, described experiments purporting to show that the fibroblasts derived from chick heart tissue could be cultured seriatim indefinitely. The culture was voluntarily terminated after 34 years. This experiment is important to gerontologists because it implied that if cells released from in vivo control could divide and function normally for a period in excess of the life span of a species, then either the types of cells cultured play no role in the aging phenomenon or aging is the result of changes occurring at the supracellular level; that is, aging would be the result of decrements that occur only in organized tissue or whole organs as a result of the physiologic interactions between those organized cell hierarchies. The inference would be that aging per se is not the result of events occurring at the cell level.

In the years that followed Carrel's observations, support for his experimental results seemed to be forthcoming from the many laboratories in which it was observed that cultured cell populations, derived from many tissues of a variety of animal species and from humans, had the striking ability to replicate apparently indefinitely. These cell populations number in the hundreds and are best known by the prototype cell lines HeLa (derived from a human cervical carcinoma in 1952) and L cells (derived from mouse mesenchyme in 1943). They continue to flourish even to this day in cell-culture laboratories throughout the world. They arise by some unknown spontaneous process, or they can be purposely provoked by the introduction of chemical carcinogens or certain oncogenic viruses into cultures of normal cells. Nevertheless, what seemed to be incontrovertible evidence for the potential immortality of vertebrate cells soon fell to new insights and a preponderance of opposing evidence.

Aging Under Glass

Of central importance to the question is whether the cell populations studied in vitro are composed of normal or abnormal cells. Clearly the aging of animals occurs in normal cell populations. If we are to equate the behavior of normal cells in vivo with that of similar cells in vitro, then the latter must be shown to be normal as well. For this reason the "immortal" cell lines described earlier, of which the HeLa and L cell populations are prototypes, must be excluded from consideration because they are composed of cells that are abnormal in one or more important properties. For example, all immortal cell lines vary in their chromosomal constitution; they do not reveal either the exact number or the precise morphology of chromosomes characteristic of the cells composing the tissue of origin. The widespread use of these cell lines for a variety of research purposes in laboratories throughout the world is subject to the criticism that in most cases they are not characteristic of any cell type found in human or animal tissue. Much experimental data generated from the use of such cell populations cannot be extrapolated to apply to cells that characterize the animal species from which they originally descended. Consequently, the use of cell lines is questionable because such cells undoubtedly represent laboratory artifacts whose behavior may be unrelated to cells found in vivo.

This fundamental flaw in interpreting normal cell behavior in vitro can, in fact, be circumvented. Cell populations entirely typical of normal cells found in vivo can be cultured, and with respect to gerontologic inquiry, the findings are profoundly different from the behavior of abnormal cell lines.

Twenty-three years ago, Paul Moorhead and I found that cultured normal human embryonic fibroblasts underwent a finite number of serial subcultivations or population doublings and then they died (Hayflick and Moorhead, 1961). We demonstrated that when such cells were grown under the most favorable conditions, death was inevitable after about 50 population doublings (the Phase III Phenomenon). We also showed that the death of the normal cells was not due to some trivial explanation involving medium components or cultural conditions, but that the death of cultured normal cells was an inherent property of the cells themselves. That observation has now been confirmed in hundreds of laboratories in which variations in medium components and cultural conditions have been as numerous as the laboratories themselves (Hayflick and Moorhead, 1961; Hayflick, 1965).

Since normal diploid cell strains have a limited doubling potential in vitro, studies on any single strain would be severely curtailed were it not possible to preserve these cells at subzero temperatures for apparently indefinite periods of time. The reconstitution of frozen human fetal diploid cell strains has revealed that regardless of the doubling level reached by the population at the time it is preserved, the total number of doublings that can be expected is about 50 when those made before and after preservation are combined. Storage of human diploid cell strains merely arrests the cells at a particular population doubling level but does not influence the total number of expected doublings (Hayflick and Moorhead, 1961; Hayflick, 1965).

We have reconstituted about 130 ampules of our human fetal diploid cell strain WI-38, which was placed in liquid nitrogen storage 22 years ago. All have yielded cell populations that have undergone 50 ± 10 cumulative population doublings. This represents the longest period of time that viable normal human cells have been arrested at subzero temperatures.

Since normal human embryo fibroblasts are able to undergo only a fixed number of reproductive cycles in vitro, we postulated that this observation might be interpreted as aging at the cell level. Although we and others were skeptical of this interpretation at first, subsequent experimental data have tended to support the validity of this notion. I have named the burgeoning field of cellular aging *cytogerontology*. However, before considering the newer developments in this field, it is necessary to reconsider Carrel's experiment, in which a presumptive normal chicken cell population was cultured for 34 years and then voluntarily terminated. The cells cultured by Carrel are presumed to have been normal simply because abnormal immortal cell lines have never been reported to arise from chick tissue. In the years following Carrel's observation, and even in very recent times when more sophisticated cell-culture techniques have been used, no one has been able to culture chick fibroblasts serially in a state of continuous, rapid proliferation beyond 1 year. Thus there is serious doubt that the original interpretation of Carrel's work can be accepted because it has never been confirmed. I have proposed one explanation for Carrel's findings that was subsequently supported by personal communications from one of his laboratory technicians. The method of preparation of chick embryo extract, used as a source of nutrients for his cultures and prepared daily under conditions of low-speed centrifugation, allowed for the survival and introduction of new, viable fibroblasts into the so-called immortal culture at each feeding (Hayflick, 1970, 1972).

Donor Age Versus Cell Doubling Potential

Because cultured normal human cells derived from embryonic tissue have a finite proliferative capacity of about 50 population doublings and because this may represent cellular aging, it is important to determine the proliferative capacity of normal cells derived from human adults of varying ages. Our first report of such studies did indeed show a diminished proliferative capacity for cultured normal human adult fibroblasts in which 14–29 doublings occurred in cells derived from 8 adult donors (Hayflick, 1965). This compared with a range of 35–63 doublings found in cells cultured from 13 human embryos.

Subsequent to these studies a report by Martin, Sprague, and Epstein (1970) not only confirmed the principle we observed but extended it significantly. These investigators cultured fibroblasts derived from biopsies taken from the upper arm of human donors ranging from fetal to 90 years of age. They found the regression coefficient, from the first to the ninth decade, to be −0.20 population doublings per year of life with a standard deviation of 0.05 and a correlation coefficient of −0.50.

In the past 14 years, several additional studies on human tissue have been reported. LeGuilly, Simon, Lenoir, and Bourel (1973) used human liver tissue; Schneider and Mitsui (1976), Goldstein, Moerman, Soeldner, Gleason, and Barnett (1978), and Vracko and McFarland (1980) studied fibroblasts from skin biopsies; Bierman (1978) examined arterial smooth-muscle cells; and Walford, Jarwaid, and Naeim (1981) and Walford (1982) used T-lymphocytes. All of these studies tend to support our original contention that the number of population doublings achievable by cultured normal human cells is inversely proportional to donor age (Hayflick, 1965). Nevertheless, these findings must be tempered with observations that the relationship may be clouded when different tissue sites are compared (Schneider, Mitsui, Aw, and Schorr, 1977) or where the physiologic state of the donor is abnormal. For example, strains derived from diabetics have been found to undergo fewer doublings in vitro than their normal, age-matched counterparts (Goldstein, Moerman, Soeldner, Gleason, and Barnett, 1978).

Direct Proportionality Between Maximum Species Life Span and Population Doubling Potential

Several years ago I suggested that the population doubling potential of cultured fibroblasts from several animal species revealed a surprisingly good direct correlation with maximum species life span (Hayflick, 1976). In the years that followed several other reports have appeared that have substantiated this idea, especially that of Rohme (1981). One report in which several marsupial species were studied does not support this finding; however, the authors did not determine population doublings by conventional means nor is the maximum life spans of the species they studied known (Stanley, Pye, and MacGregor, 1975). Figure 5-4 shows the direct proportionality between different species' maximum life spans and the population doubling potential of their cultured fibroblasts. Embryonic fibroblasts were used in the ten species studied except that of the Galapagos tortoise, where cells from a juvenile were used.

If this relationship is extended and confirmed it suggests the presence of a chronometer or pacemaker within all normal cells that is characteristic for each species and that dictates maximum cell doubling or functional capacity with an apparent evolutionary basis. The postulated chronometer may or may not be the same one that we postulate controls the inverse relationship between donor age and population doubling potential.

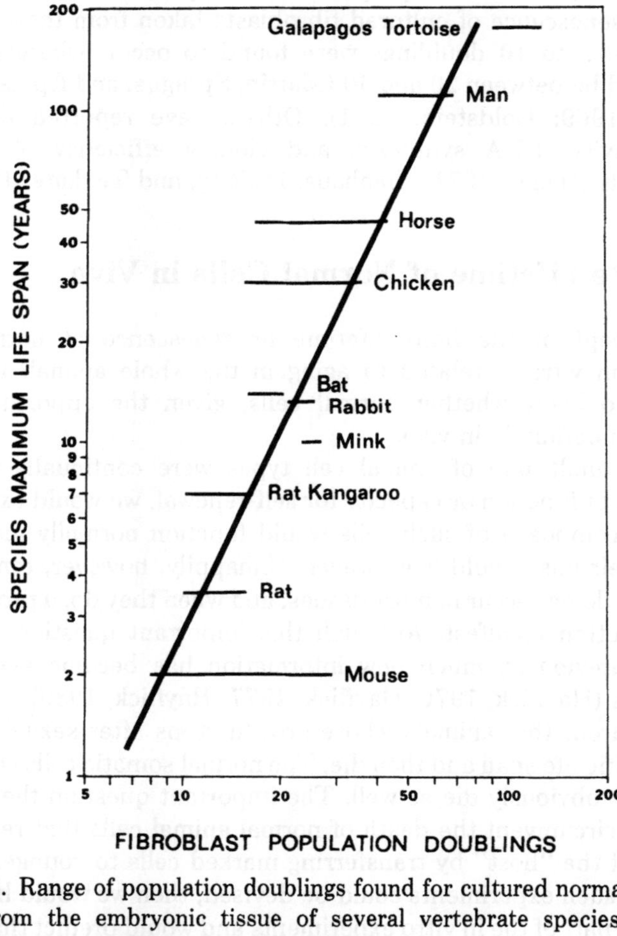

Figure 5-4. Range of population doublings found for cultured normal fibroblasts derived from the embryonic tissue of several vertebrate species. Galapagos tortoise tissue was obtained from a juvenile animal.

Progeria and Werner's Syndrome

Progeria (Hutchinson-Guilford syndrome) is a human condition leading to a severe deceleration of growth in patients as young as 9 years of age (Reichel, Garcia-Bunuel, and Dilallo, 1971). A very rare disease, it is thought by many to represent a model for precocious aging in which individuals, at the end of the first decade of life, manifest the physical signs of aging typical of their normal counterparts in the seventh decade of life. Werner's syndrome is similar to progeria in many ways, although its salient manifestations occur in later years. The full clinical picture shows early graying and loss of hair, short stature, juvenile cataracts, proneness to diabetes, atherosclerosis and calcification of the blood vessels, osteoporosis, and high incidence of malignancy (Epstein, Martin, Schultz, and Motulsky, 1966).

If Werner's syndrome and progeria are examples of accelerated aging, when does senescence of cultured fibroblasts taken from these patients occur? From 2 to 10 doublings were found to occur, whereas normal values would be between 20 and 40 (Martin, Sprague, and Epstein, 1970; Goldstein, 1969; Goldstein, 1971). Others have reported decreased mitotic activity, DNA synthesis, and cloning efficiency of cultured progeria cells (Danes, 1971; Nienhaus, DeJong, and Tenkate, 1971).

The Finite Lifetime of Normal Cells in Vivo

If the concept of the finite lifetime or senescence of normal cells replicating in vitro is related to aging in the whole animal, then it is important to know whether normal cells, given the opportunity, can proliferate indefinitely in vivo.

If all the multitude of animal cell types were continually renewed, without loss of function or capacity for self-renewal, we would expect that the organs composed of such cells would function normally indefinitely and that their host would live forever. Unhappily, however, renewal cell populations do not occur in most tissues, and when they do, a proliferative finitude is often manifest. Although this important question has been discussed previously, much new information has become available in recent years (Hayflick, 1970; Hayflick, 1977; Hayflick, 1980).

It is apparent that animals whose growth stops after sexual maturity have a specific life span and then die. The normal somatic cells composing their tissues obviously die as well. The important question then is: Is it possible to circumvent the death of normal animal cells that result from the death of the "host" by transferring marked cells to younger animals seriatim? If such experiments could be devised, then we would have an in vivo counterpart of the in vitro experiments and would predict that normal cells transplanted serially to proper inbred hosts would, like their in vitro counterparts, age. Such experiments would largely rule out those objections to in vitro findings that are based on the artificiality of in vitro cell cultures. The question could be answered by serial orthotopic transplantation of normal somatic tissue to new, young, inbred hosts each time the recipient approaches old age.

Data from seven different laboratories in which mammary tissue (Daniel, deOme, Young, Blair and Faulkin, 1968; Young, Medina, deOme and Daniel, 1971), skin (Krohn, 1962), and hematopoietic cells (Ford, Micklem, and Gray, 1959; Cudkowicz, Upton, Shearer, and Hughes, 1964; Siminovitch, Till, and McCulloch, 1964; Harrison, 1973; Harrison, 1975; Hellman, Botnick, Hannon, and Vigneulle, 1978) were employed indicate that normal cells serially transplanted to inbred hosts do not survive indefinitely. Furthermore, the trauma of transplantation does not appear to influence the results (Krohn, 1962). And finally, in heterochronic transplants, survival time is related to the age of the grafted tissue (Krohn, 1962). It is well known that under similar conditions of tissue transplantation, cancer cell populations can be serially passed indefinitely (Stewart, Snell, Dunham, and Schylen, 1959; Daniel, Aidells, Medina, and Faulkin, 1975; Till, McCulloch, and Siminovitch, 1964). The implications of this may be that acquisition of potential for unlimited cell division or escape from senescent changes by mammalian cells in vitro or in vivo can only be achieved by somatic cells that have acquired some or all of the properties of cancer cells.

Paradoxically, this leads to the conclusion that in order for mammalian somatic cells to become biologically "immortal," they first must be induced to an abnormal or neoplastic state either in vivo or in vitro, at which time they can be subcultivated or transplanted indefinitely. Krohn (1962) found some transplants capable of surviving several years beyond the maximum life span of the mouse, but they were ultimately lost. It is important to note that long survival time is not equivalent to proliferation time or rounds of division; hence these long-surviving grafts consist of cells having a very slow rate of reproductive turnover. This is analogous to holding cell cultures at room temperature, which also extends calendar time for cell survival but does not result in an increase in population doublings.

A series of experiments has been reported that clearly shows that the birth rate of mouse mammary epithelium declines during in vivo serial transplantation (Daniel, deOme, Young, Blair, and Faulkin, 1968; Daniel and Young, 1971; Daniel, 1973). Mouse mammary epithelium was propagated in isogenic female hosts by periodic transplantation of tissue samples into the mammary fat pads from which the host gland was surgically removed. These workers repeatedly observed that unlike cancerous and precancerous mammary tissue, normal mammary epithelium displays a characteristic decline in proliferative capacity with repeated transplantation (Daniel, deOme, Young, Blair, and Faulkin,

1968). It also has been found that when transplants that are allowed to proliferate continuously are compared with transplants in which growth is restricted, the decline in cell proliferation is related to the number of population doublings undergone rather than to the passage of metabolic time (Daniel and Young, 1971). This represents the first in vivo confirmation of our in vitro data (Hayflick and Moorhead, 1961; Hayflick, 1965). At that time, we suggested that somatic cells have an intrinsic, predetermined capacity for division under the most favorable environmental conditions. Others (Hay and Strehler, 1967; McHale, Moulton, and McHale, 1971), however, have invoked the passage of "metabolic time" as the determinant of in vitro senescence. That metabolic time is not the governing factor, but that population doublings are, has been demonstrated beyond doubt (Dell'Orco, Mertens, and Kruse, 1974; Harley and Goldstein, 1978). The in vivo finding that population doublings dictate cell senescence and not "metabolic time" (Daniel and Young, 1971) is especially significant because it results from studies on cells grown entirely in situ and thus circumvents arguments leveled at similar data obtained from the alleged "artificial" conditions of in vitro cell culture. These investigators conclude that "the ability of grafts from old donors to proliferate rapidly in young hosts suggests that the life span of mammary glands is influenced primarily by the number of cell divisions rather than by the passage of chronological or metabolic time" (Young, Medina, deOme, and Daniel, 1971).

The study of single antibody-forming cell clones in vivo has shown that these cells are also capable of only a limited capacity to replicate after serial transfer in vivo (Williamson and Askonas, 1972; Williamson, 1972). Harrison (1972) and Harrison (1973) report that when marrow cell transplants from young and old normal donors are made to a genetically anemic recipient mouse strain, the anemia is cured. He further reports that such transplants to anemic mice ultimately expire, exhibiting once again the finitude of normal cell proliferation in vivo (Harrison, 1975).

In connection with findings that bear on the proliferative capacity of cells in vivo as a function of age, several other intriguing reports should be mentioned here. The most informative of such studies are those bearing on the major cell renewal system: the hematopoietic cells of the bone marrow, the epidermis, the lymphatic cells of the thymus, the spleen and lymph nodes, the sperm cells in the seminiferous tubules of the testes, and the epithelial cells lining the small intestine. It has been found, for example, in the latter system in the mouse that cell generation time increases with age (Lesher, Fry, and Kohn, 1961a,b; Thrasher and Greulich, 1965). The increase in generation time, however, is not a linear increase from early youth to extreme old age (Lesher and Sacher, 1968).

Thus we can see a wide variety of examples of in vivo constraints on the proliferative capacity of replicating cell cohorts. It is likely that different proliferative cell systems may display variations on this general theme. Based on our in vitro data, the fibroblasts may represent the upper limit of proliferative potential, although one should not exclude a higher limit being placed on such cell removal systems as hematopoietic cells or skin epithelium, neither of which have been shown to proliferate in vitro for long periods of time and still retain normal characteristics and functional capacities.

Decrements Occurring in Cultured Normal Human Cells

The probability that animals age because one or more important cell populations lose their proliferative capacity is unlikely. It is more probable that, as we have shown, normal cells have a finite capacity for replication and that this finite limit is rarely, if ever, reached by cells in vivo but is, of course, demonstrable in vitro. We would therefore suggest that other functional losses that occur in cells prior to the cessation of division capacity produce physiologic decrements in animals much before their normal cells have reached their maximum proliferative capacity. Indeed, we are now becoming aware of many functional changes that take place in normal human cells grown in vitro and expressed well before they lose their capacity to replicate (Hayflick, 1980). Over 125 functional changes occur in cultured normal human cells as they age. These changes occur in such things as DNA, RNA, enzymes, cell cycle, karyology, lipids, carbohydrates, morphology, and protein synthesis. It is more likely that these changes, which herald the approaching loss of division capacity, play the central role in the expression of aging and result in the death of the individual animal well before its cells fail to divide (Hayflick, 1976).

To be sure, those several classes of cells which are incapable of division in mature animals, such as neurons and muscle cells, may play a greater role in the expression of age changes than those cell classes in which division commonly occurs. It is important, therefore, to indicate that the cessation of mitotic activity is only one functional decrement whose genetic basis may be similar to those functional decrements known to occur in nondividing cells. It is suggested, therefore, that the same kind of gene action resulting in physiologic decrements in aging nondividing cells also occurs in aging cells that can divide. It is not our contention, therefore, that age changes result necessarily from losses in cell-division capacity, but simply in loss of function in any class of cells. That function might be measured as reduced division capacity or any number of the myriad functional decrements characteristic of aging cells. The genetic changes leading to these decrements is postulated to be the common denominator, so that the measurement of loss of population doubling potential in vitro may have the same basis as the loss of other cell functions characteristic of nondividing cells. It follows, therefore, that an understanding of the mechanism by which cultured normal cells lose their capacity to replicate could provide insights into the causes of decrements in other functional properties that are characteristic of such nondividing cells as neurons. These decrements may be even more direct causes of biological aging.

This chapter is dedicated to the memory of Dr. Henry S. Kaplan, Professor of Radiology, Stanford University School of Medicine; scholar, physician, teacher, friend, and champion of just causes.

References

Bierman, E.L.: The effect of donor age on the in vitro lifespan of cultured human arterial smooth-muscle cells. *In Vitro 14*, 951–955 (1978).

Cudkowicz, G., Upton, A.C., Shearer, G.M., and Hughes, W.L.: Lymphocyte content and proliferative capacity of serially transplanted mouse bone marrow. *Nature 201*, 165–167 (1964).

Danes, B.S.: Progeria: A cell culture study on aging. *J. Clin. Invest. 50*, 2000–2003 (1971).

Daniel, C.W., deOme, K.B., Young, J.T., Blair, P.B., and Faulkin, L.J., Jr.: The in vivo lifespan of normal and preneoplastic mouse mammary glands: A serial transplantation study. *Proc. Nat. Acad. Sci. U.S.A. 61*, 53–60 (1968).

Daniel, C.W., and Young, L.J.T.: Influence of cell division on an aging process. *Exp. Cell Res. 65*, 27–32 (1971).

Daniel, C.W.: Finite growth span of mouse mammary gland serially propagated in vivo. *Experientia* (Basel) *29*, 1422–1424 (1973).

Daniel, C.W., Aidells, B.D., Medina, B., and Faulkin, L.J., Jr.: Unlimited division potential of precancerous mouse mammary cells after spontaneous or carcinogen-induced transformation. *Fed. Proc. 34*, 64–67 (1975).

Dell'Orco, R.T., Mertens, J.G., and Kruse, P.F., Jr.: Doubling potential, calendar time, and donor age of human diploid cells in culture. *Exp. Cell Res. 84*, 363–366 (1974).

Epstein, C.J., Martin, G.M., Schultz, A.L., and Motulsky, A.G.: Werner's syndrome: A review of its symptomatology, natural history, pathologic features, genetics and relationship to the natural aging process. *Medicine* (Baltimore) *45*, 177–221 (1966).

Ford, C.E., Micklem, H.S., and Gray, S.M.: Evidence of selective proliferation of reticular cell-clones in heavily irradiated mice. *Brit. J. Radiol. 32*, 280 (1959).

Goldstein, S.: Lifespan of cultured cells in progeria. *Lancet 1*, 424 (1969).

Goldstein, S.: The biology of aging. *New Engl. J. Med. 285*, 1120–1129 (1971).

Goldstein, S., Moerman, E.J., Soeldner, J.S., Gleason, R.E., and Barnett, D.M.: Chronologic and physiologic age effect replicative lifespan of fibroblasts from diabetics, prediabetics, and normal donors. *Science 199*, 781–782 (1978).

Harley, C.B., and Goldstein, S.: Cultured human fibroblasts: Distribution of cell generations and a critical limit. *J. Cell Physiol. 97*, 509–516 (1978).

Harrision, D.E.: Normal function of transplanted mouse erythrocyte precursors for 21 months beyond donor lifespans. *Nature New Biol. 237*, 220–222 (1972).

Harrison, D.E.: Normal Production of erythrocytes by mouse marrow continuous for 73 months. *Proc. Nat. Acad. Sci. U.S.A. 70*, 3184–3188 (1973).

Harrision, D.E.: Normal function of transplanted marrow cell lines from aged mice. *J. Gerontol. 30*, 279–285 (1975).

Hay, R.J., and Strehler, B.L.: The limited growth span of cell strains isolated from the chick embryo. *Exp. Gerontol. 2*, 123–135 (1967).

Hayflick, L., and Moorhead, P.S.: The serial cultivation of human diploid cell strains. *Exp. Cell Res. 25*, 585–621 (1961).

Hayflick, L.: The limited in vitro lifetime of human diploid cell strains. *Exp. Cell Res. 37*, 614–636 (1965).

Hayflick, L.: Aging under glass. *Exp. Gerontol. 5*, 291–303 (1970).

Hayflick, L.: Cell senescence and cell differentation in vitro. Band 4, 1–15. In H. Bredt and J.W. Rohen (Eds.), Aging and Development. Stuttgart: F.K. Schattauer Verlag, 1972.

Hayflick, L.: The biology of human aging. *Am. J. Med. Sci. 265*, 433–445 (1973).

Hayflick, L.: The cell biology of human aging. *New Engl. J. Med. 295*, 1302–1308 (1976).

Hayflick, L.: The cellular basis for biological aging. In C. Finch and L. Hayflick (Eds.), Handbook of the Biology of Aging, pp. 159–186. New York: Van Nostrand Reinhold, 1977.

Hayflick, L.: Cell aging. In C. Eisdorfer (Ed.), Annual Review of Gerontology and Geriatrics, pp. 26–67. New York: Springer, 1980.

Hellman, S., Botnick, L.E., Hannon, E.C., and Vigneulle, R.M.: Proliferative capacity of murine hematopoietic stem cells. *Proc. Nat. Acad. Sci. U.S.A. 75*, 490–494 (1978).

Krohn, P.L.: Review lectures on senescence. II: Heterochronic transplantation in the study of aging. *Proc. Roy. Soc. Lond.* [Biol.] *157*, 128–147 (1962).

LeGuilly, Y., Simon, M., Lenoir, P., and Bourel, M.: Long-term culture of human adult liver cells: Morphological changes related to in vitro senescence and effect of donor's age on growth potential. *Gerontologia 19*, 303–313 (1973).

Lesher, S., Fry, R.J.M., and Kohn, H.I.: Age and the generation time of the mouse duodenal epithelial cell. *Exp. Cell Res. 24*, 334–343 (1961a).

Lesher, S., Fry, R.J.M., and Kohn, H.I.: Age and the generation cycle of intestinal epithelial cells in the mouse. *Gerontologia* (Basel) 5, 176–181 (1961b).

Lesher, S., and Sacher, G.A.: Effects of age on cell proliferation in mouse duodenal crypts. *Exp. Gerontol. 3*, 211–217 (1968).

Martin, G.M., Sprague, C.A., and Epstein, C.J.: Replicative lifespan of cultivated human cells. Effects of donor's age, tissue, and genotype. *Lab. Invest. 23*, 86–92 (1970).

McHale, J.S., Moulton, M.L., and McHale, J.T.: Limited culture lifespan of human diploid cells as a function of metabolic time instead of division potential. *Exp. Gerontol 6*, 89–93 (1971).

Nienhaus, A.J., DeJong, B., and Tenkate, L.P.: Fibroblast culture in Werner's syndrome. *Humangenetik 13*, 244–246 (1971).

Reichel, W., Garcia-Bunuel, R., and Dilallo, J.: Progeria and Werner's syndrome as models for the study of normal human aging. *J. Am. Geriatr. Soc. 19*, 369–375 (1971).

Rohme, D.: Evidence for a relationship between longevity of mammalian species and lifespans of normal fibroblasts in vitro and erythrocytes in vivo. *Proc. Nat. Acad. Sci. U.S.A. 78*, 5009–5013 (1981).

Schneider, E.L., and Mitsui, Y.: The relationship between in vitro cellular aging and in vivo human age. *Proc. Nat. Acad. Sci. U.S.A. 73*, 3584–3588 (1976).

Schneider, E.L., Mitsui, Y., Aw, K.S., and Shorr, S.: Tissue-specific differences in cultured human diploid fibroblasts. *Exp. Cell Res. 108*, 1–6 (1977).

Siminovich, L., Till, J.E., and McCulloch, E.A.: Decline in colony-forming ability of marrow cells subjected to serial transplantation into irradiated mice. *J. Cell Comp. Physiol. 64*, 23–31 (1964).

Stanley, J.F., Pye, D., and MacGregor, A.: Comparison of doubling numbers attained by cultured animal cells with the life span of species. *Nature 255*, 158–159 (1975).

Stewart, H.L., Snell, K.C., Dunham, L.J., and Schylen, S.M.: Transplantable and transmissible tumors of animals. Washington, D.C., Armed Forces Institute of Pathology (1959).

Strehler, B.L., and Mildvan, A.S.: General theory of mortality and aging. *Science 132*, 14–21 (1960).

Thrasher, J.D., and Greulich, R.C.: The duodenal progenitor population. I: Age related increase in the duration of the cryptal progenitor cycle. *J. Exp. Zool. 159*, 39–46 (1965).

Till, J.E., McCulloch, E.A., and Siminovitch, L.: Isolation of variant cell lines during serial transplantation of hematopoietic cells derived from fetal liver. *J. Nat. Cancer Inst. 33*, 707–720 (1964).

Vracko, R., and McFarland, B.M: Lifespan of diabetic and non-diabetic fibroblasts in vitro. *Exp. Cell Res. 129*, 345–350 (1980).

Walford, R.L., Jawaid, S.Q., and Naeim, F.: Evidence for *in vitro* senescence of T-lymphocytes cultured from normal human peripheral blood. *Age 4*, 67–70 (1981).

Walford, R.L.: Studies on immunogerontology. *J. Am. Geriat. Soc. 30*, 617–625 (1982).

Williamson, A.R., and Askonas, B.A.: Senescence of an antibody-forming cell clone. *Nature 238*, 337–339 (1972).

Williamson, A.R.: Extent and control of antibody diversity. *Biochem. J. 130*, 325–333 (1972).

Young, L.J.T., Medina, D., deOme, K.B., and Daniel, C.W.: The influence of host and tissue age on the lifespan and growth rate of serially transplanted mouse mammary gland. *Exp. Gerontol. 6*, 49–56 (1971).

Chapter 6

A Progress Report on Neurochemical and Neuroendocrine Regulation in Normal and Pathologic Aging

Caleb E. Finch

Summary

Recent findings from this lab include the progressive decrease during normal human aging of caudate D_2 receptors and cortical S_2 receptors. Also, the ovary-dependent neuroendocrine aging syndrome of female rodents is described.

Introduction

Aging in the central nervous system, as elsewhere in the mammalian organism, appears to involve a series of highly regulated, selective changes. Some age-correlated changes are interrelated and can be described as a cascade of interactions which involve hormones, neurotransmitters, and other physiologic factors (Finch, 1976; Finch et al., 1980*). Such cascades suggest a great potential to intervene and experimentally manipulate events of aging.

According to the familiar view derived from the two centuries of Western physiology, the body is an hierarchically organized community of cells that has interactions across both time and space. Many changes in

---

*This article was prepared from a transcript of my lecture in this symposium and does not contain a complete bibliography or discussion of many basic issues. It is best considered as a progress report with restricted referencing. Some of the articles I cite will do more justice to the work of many other laboratories also studying these complex problems than this curtailed presentation.

regulatory factors during aging have been documented as occurring relatively early in the life span, as well as in middle age and in the later years. For a review of this aspect, see "*Biological Markers of Aging*," edited by M.E. Reff and E.L. Schneider, NIH publ. 82-2221 (1982). Some changes that can be traced into pre-midlife may represent a progressive set of cascading and causally related events. In some cases, the events of aging may be traceable back to early development.

Studies on Brain Monoamine Receptors

My laboratory at the University of Southern California has recently analyzed receptor changes in the human brain from studies done collaboratively with colleagues in several parts of the world, particularly in Sweden with Drs. Bengt Winblad, Jan Marcusson, and Carl-Gerhart Gottfries. These colleagues provided postmortem brain specimens with a well-documented health status, which for specimens from elderly persons is essential to defining any changes as normal aging and not consequences of neurologic diseases or drug treatment. Figure 6-1 shows the results of assays for what neuropharmacologists call the D_2 dopaminergic receptor, which we measured in human caudates of several normal age groups of differing age. Other data (not shown) evaluated the same individuals whose brain tissue was analyzed with a 7-point Scatchard binding isotherm using spiperone or fluphenazine as a binding ligand and appropriate competitors, to eliminate other classes of dopaminergic binding. Both ligands detected a progressive change across the human life span; there is a reassuring correlation found between the B_{max} values observed with the two ligands (Morgan and Finch, unpubl.). These results suggest a class of changes that arise before midlife and that progress during the entire lifespan. This progressive decrease of D_2 sites in the caudate is very similar to that found in the aging mouse striatum (Severson and Finch, 1980).

Further studies are being made to characterize age effects on receptor subtypes. With fluphenazine as the binding ligand in the same assay using appropriate concentrations of spiroperidol and apomorphine as competitors to distinguish D_1 and D_2, we find that a D_1-type binding component in the caudate increases during the human lifespan (Morgan and Finch, unpubl.). Thus, the ratio of D_1 to D_2 shifts progressively in favor of the D_1-type; this shift may have neuropharmacologic and neurologic consequences. It seems important that not everything decreases during aging. The increase of some brain parameters during the normal aging process suggests possible interrelationships between the D_1 and D_2 dopaminergic loci. We hypothesize the increase of D_1 is a postdenervation supersensitivity phenomenon consequent to a loss of nigro-striatal cells during normal aging (McGeer et al., 1977), whereas the

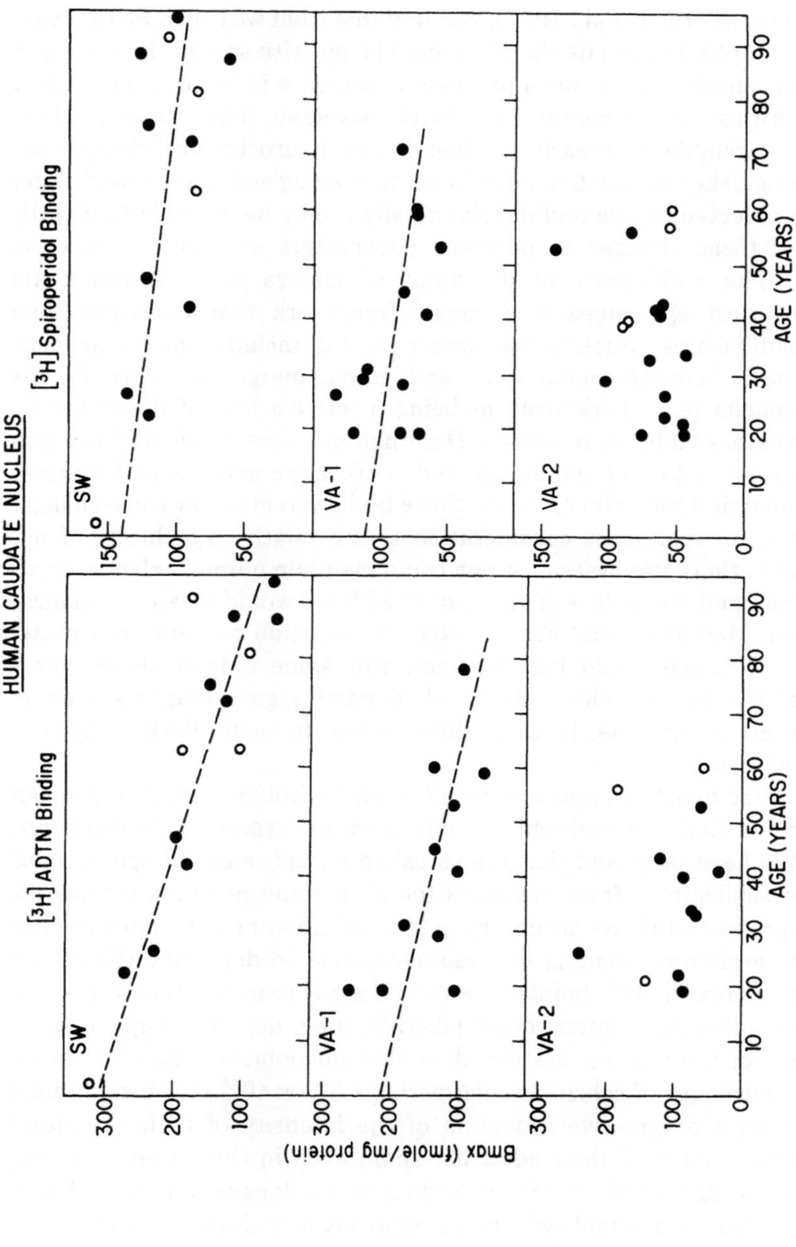

Figure 6-1. Age-related changes in D_2 binding sites of normal human caudate. Each point represents the B_{max} as determined by Scatchard analysis of binding isotherms. (From Severson et al., 1982.)

decrease of D_2 is associated with loss of striatal cells (Bugiani et al., 1978).

We have also examined effects of age on serotonergic sites. Figure 6-2 shows the S_2 site in the human cortex, which progressively declines with adult age. We have subfractionated the S_2 site by competition with ketanserin (Morgan et al., 1984), and find that what we called S_2b above is really an alpha-1-type site that does not change with age. In the same sets of brain samples, there was a progressive increase in imipramine binding sites with age in the cerebral cortex (J. Severson, pers. comm.). These findings strengthen our early conclusions that neurochemical changes can be distinguished during the normal course of aging and that some changes can be detected before midlife. Eventually it may be possible to identify some of these changes as potential pacemakers or primary causes of others. The multiplicity of directions of change in neurotransmitter systems with age suggests a causal framework that describes their interrelationships. Such a framework would include the antagonism postulated between cholinergic and dopaminergic systems in the basal ganglia (e.g., Parkinsonism being a relative loss of dopaminergic tone, whereas motor symptoms in Huntingtonism are considered to result from a relative loss of cholinergic and GABAergic neurons and a excess dopaminergic tone; Finch, 1980). Since both systems show some changes with age, an important consideration is the relative synchrony of age changes in these two systems which could maintain normal balance, or, on the other hand, faster loss of one system with age would create imbalances (Morgan, Marcusson and Finch, 1984). Information on neurotransmitter balance with age would help us know why some individuals are more susceptable to the side effects of dopaminergic antagonists or to cholinergic antagonists, leading, alternatively, to senile Parkinsonism or senile chorea.

The same questions apply to cognitive and affective functions. A major view holds that schizophrenia results from an excess of dopaminergic tone. We have proposed that the so-called paraphrenias of aging, which are the schizophrenifrom disorders found in some people after age 65, may represent a relative asychrony in favor of greater cholinergic loss than dopaminergic tone, leading to a relative excess in dopamine (Finch and Morgan, in press). This point of view could apply to many other interacting systems, some interactions being positive, some negative, depending on the state of the nervous system. A related phenomenon may be the so-called "burnout" of schizophrenia; perhaps 30 or 40% of schizophrenics experience a progressive reduction of the intensity of their symptoms during the course of their adult life span, even in the absence of drug therapy (Bridges et al., 1978). According to the dopamine-excess view of schizophrenia, individuals who had a relatively high dopamine tone would then, because of the loss of dopaminergic functions, return toward normal domain (Finch and Morgan, in press). In normal individuals, however, such

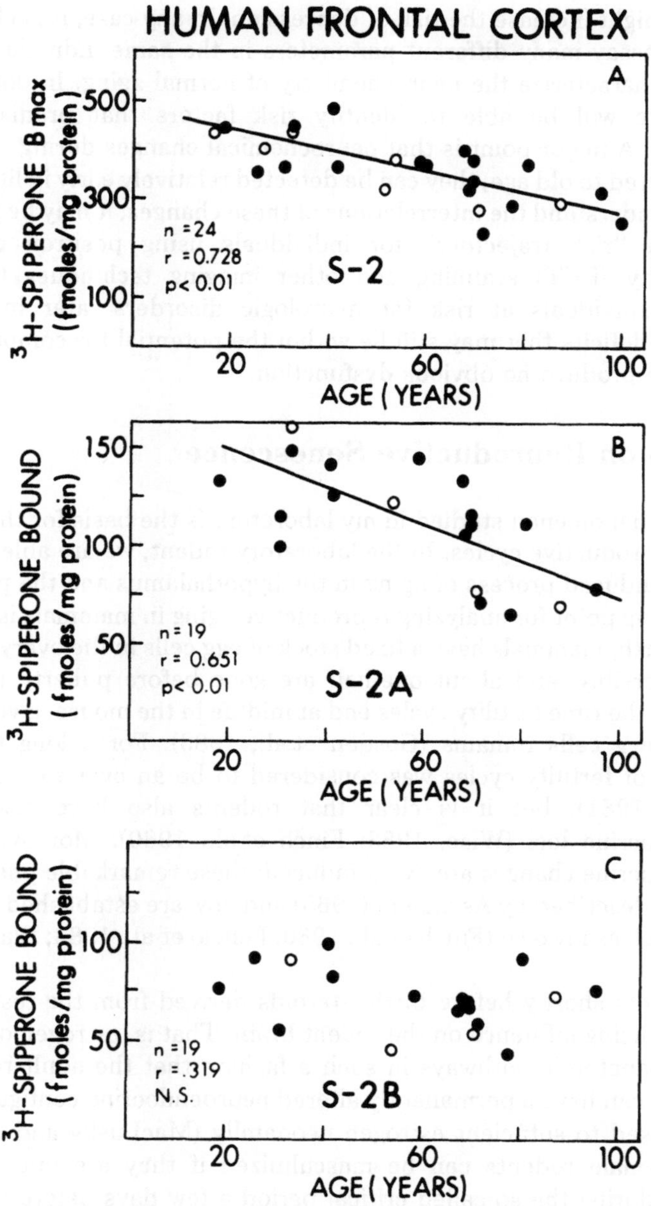

Figure 6-2. Age-related changes in S-2 binding sites of human frontal cortex. Each point represents the B_{max} determined by Scatchard analysis. Total S-2 (panel A) is binding of (3H)spiperone with competition by 0.5 micromolar ketanserine. S-2A and S-2B (panels B and C) determined from competition of (3H)spiperone with methysergide; the S-2B site was recently shown to be an alpha-1 adrenergic component (Morgan et al., 1984). The females are open circles. (From Marcussen et al., in press.)

changes might increase the risk of depression. In any case, it is clear that we must assay many different parameters in the same individual specimens to characterize the neurochemistry of normal aging. In doing so, I believe we will be able to identify risk factors that predispose to pathology. A major point is that neurochemical changes during aging are not restricted to old age; they can be detected relatively early in life. As we begin to understand the interrelations of these changes, it may be possible to plot a "risk trajectory" for individuals using positron emission tomography (PET) scanning and other imaging techniques that will identify individuals at risk for neurologic disorders later in life by emergent deficits that may still lie within the potential for compensation and hence produce no obvious dysfunction.

Studies on Reproductive Senescence

Another phenomenon studied in my laboratory is the basis for the loss of female reproductive cycles. In the laboratory rodent, we are able to show an ovary-induced process of aging in the hypothalamus and the pituitary. The starting point for analyzing reproductive aging in mammals is the fact that, at birth, mammals have a fixed stock of egg cells in the ovary that are lost irreversibly, and about one-half are gone before puberty (Talbert, 1977). By the time fertility cycles end at midlife in the mouse, a very small stock of egg cells remains (Gosden et al., 1983). For a long time the cessation of fertility cycles was considered to be an ovarian exhaustion (Guyton, 1981), but it is clear that rodents also have changes in neuroendocrine loci (Wise, 1983; Finch et al., 1980). Moreover, some neuroendocrine changes are ovary induced; these remarkable phenomena were first described by Aschheim (1965) and now are established by other labs, as well as my own (Finch et al., 1980; Felicio et al., 1983; Blake et al., 1983).

In rodents shortly before birth, steroids derived from the testes have a masculinizing influence on the rodent brain. That is, estrogen organizes the neuroanatomic pathways in such a fashion that the adult rodent of either sex can have a permanently altered neuroendocrine configuration if it is exposed to sufficient estrogen neonatally (MacLusky and Naftolin, 1981). Female rodents can be masculinized if they are injected with estrogen during the so-called critical period a few days before and after birth. Subtle phenomena have recently been discovered in which the sex of the fetal neighbor in the uterus modulates the extent of masculinization of the brain (vom Saal and Bronson, 1978). Females flanked by males in utero are very different behaviorally and physiologically from females flanked by other females. The female embryos flanked by males have higher plasma estrogen prenatally and have more masculine behavior as adults.

The animal model we study is an inbred mouse strain, the C57BL/6J mouse. We chose mice because the finely detailed genetic maps that are emerging through recombinant DNA technology (e.g., Blatt et al., 1983) will eventually enable us to build biochemical genetic models of the aging process.

Table 6-1 lists a series of markers for reproductive aging in the mouse strain. Each event shown in Table 6-1 has now been opened to experimental manipulation. We can retard or accelerate its age of onset and intensity, depending on the animal's steroid exposure or history. This gives us a context for looking for stages in an aging process which involves changes in the brain and the pituitary in which the ovary has a major directing role. A major age change in neuroendocrine functions is the impaired surge in luteinizing hormone (LH), an episodic output from the

Table 6-1. Manipulations of reproductive aging; the ovary-induced neuroendocrine aging syndrome of rodents

Markers of Reproductive Aging	Chronic Ovariectomy Delays	Chronic-E2 Accelerates
1. Ovarian cycles lost	Refs. 1, 2	Refs. 3, 4, 5
2. Smaller postovariectomy LH rise	Refs. 6, 7	Ref. 4
3. Decreased negative feedback sensitivity	Ref. 8	Not known
4. Glial hyperactivity in arcuate nucleus	Ref. 9	Ref. 3
5. Lactotrophe adenomas (a late effect)	Refs. 10, 11	Refs. 12, 13
6. Increased pituitary G6PDH and dopamine	Ref. 14	Not known

See Finch et al. (1984), *Endocrine Rev.* for recent details.
[1]Aschheim, P. (1965).
[2]Felicio et al. (1983).
[3]Brawer et al. (1978).
[4]Mobbs et al. (1984a)
[5]Kawashima, S. (1960).
[6]Gee et al. (1983).
[7]Blake et al. (1983).
[8]Mobbs, C., and Finch, C. (unpubl.).
[9]Schipper et al. (1981).
[10]Nelson et al. (1980).
[11]Mobbs et al. (1984b).
[12]Brawer et al. (1975).
[13]Casaneuva et al. (1982).
[14]Gordon, M., Telford, N., and Finch, C. (unpubl.)

pituitary that causes the ovary to ovulate and also prepares for continuing reproductive cycles. The LH surge is induced by an interaction of ovarian steroids with the brain and pituitary over the normal sequence of a 4-day cycle. Progressively during aging, as rodents approach the loss of cyclicity, their ability to produce the LH surge diminishes; by the time cycles have stopped, the estradiol-induced LH surge has disappeared (Finch et al, 1980; Mobbs et al., 1984a).

My colleagues and I have found that by removing the ovaries of young animals and allowing them to age in the absence of the ovary, the LH surge is largely maintained into the age at which it normally would have disappeared (Felicio et al., 1983; Mobbs et al., 1984a). This striking result is part of the evidence for an ovary-dependent neuroendocrine aging process. Removal of the ovary arrests specific aspects of neuroendocrine aging, including pituitary tumors which are prevalent in older animals (Felicio et al., 1980; Nelson et al, 1980; Mobbs et al., 1984a). Using some biochemical markers, we can show that aging changes in the pituitary are also arrested by early ovariectomy: Levels of dopamine in the pituitary normally increase two- or threefold with age; glucose-6-phosphate dehydrogenase increases also, but more modestly. However, these increases are arrested if mice were ovariectomized when young and allowed to age in the absence of the ovary (M. Gordon, N. Telford, and C. Finch, unpublished). We believe here that the increased dopamine reflects a pretumorogenic change in the control of the pituitary, and may imply estrogen-induced disturbances in the arcuate dopaminergic neurons (Casanueva et al., 1982). Another marker of reproductive aging (Table 6-1) is the glial hyperactivity in the dopamine-rich arcuate nucleus of the hypothalamus which suggests the possibility that neurons or neuronal processes are deteriorating under ovarian influences. At present, there are more than ten distinct parameters which are delayed or arrested by early ovariectomy. When rodents age in the absence of the ovary, these changes do not happen, or are greatly attenuated.

These manipulations led us to think that steroids might have a cumulative impact on neuroendocrine loci during successive cycles, perhaps a sort of "estrogen staircase." One would predict, then, that with each progressive cycle a progressive increment would be registered in neuroendocrine functions in terms of physiologic time, rather than absolute time (Finch et al., 1980). According to this hypothesis, it should be possible to arrest the accumulation of estradiol by ovariectomy at a young age. It should then be possible to reactivate the process by replacing ovaries in animals at midlife. This result was demonstrated by an ovarian transplant experiment in which young ovaries were implanted in mice of differing ages. The decline of cycling in the young-to-young transplant is virtually superimposed upon the normal changes in the intact animal. Young ovaries implanted in an old animal, which was intact at the time its cycles had ceased, resulted in only limited reactivation of cycles.

Young ovaries, given to animals which had been aging without an ovary, i.e. ovariectomized between the ages of 6 and 16 months caused the animals to have almost as many cycles (80%) as normal controls (Felicio et al., 1983). We found, therefore, that some neuroendocrine aging processes can be arrested by ovariectomy and then much later can be reactivated by replacing the ovaries.

Thus, we postulate that specific ovarian steroids induce changes in neuroendocrine systems. Estrogen is a major candidate for the process, as was demonstrated by giving young adult mice an intense exposure to estrogen, which causes a long-lasting, irreversible effect on neuroendocrine functions (Mobbs et al., 1984b). Mice were given a depot injection of estradiol valerate. Eight months later, the extent of their LH surge was examined; even after ovariectomy for 4 months, which should have eliminated circulating estrogen completely, the mice had residual, major impairments in their LH surge. This demonstrates the phenomenon that the adult neuroendocrine system has a susceptibility to long-lasting, steroidal memories as a consequence of exposure to estrogen and perhaps other steroids.

Some of the same markers of reproductive aging, which are retarded or delayed by chronic ovariectomy, are correspondingly accelerated in young animals by exposure to estrogen (Table 6-1). In these experiments, we were able to not only stop the syndrome, but to start and speed it up by administering estradiol to young mice. These results give an intriguing experimental system for studying neuroendocrine aging under the control of peripheral hormones; this paradigm is also pertinent in designing experiments for other aspects of aging processes that may involve sympathetic and endocrine influences on the brain.

Returning to the developmental side, I mentioned the remarkable phenomenon that the sex of the fetal neighbor influences a mammal's adult behavioral physiology; moreover, that female fetuses flanked by males in utero have different reproductive aging patterns than females flanked by females. Recently, the male-flanked fetuses were found to have a several-month-earlier loss of fertility (vom Saal and Moyer, in press). Thus, the process of reproductive neuroendocrine aging may be considered as a developmental continuum, in which fetal and developmental influences form the substrate for subsequent neuroendocrine aging changes induced by the ovary. It seems plausible then that perinatal developmental exposure to steroids sets specific extraovarian limits on the number of estrous cycles, and this raises a major question. Does postpubertal exposure to steroids act on the same locus as it does in the perinate? We hope to investigate this question in depth, using recombinant DNA techniques to see which genes are affected by estrogen at various stages of development and aging.

These estrogen-induced aging phenomena lead us to consider that an important factor in the ovary-dependent neuroendocrine age mechanisms

Table 6-2. Cell damage and death results from unremitting receptor stimulation

Agent	Effects
1. E2	Reduced dopamine in arcuate n; impaired control of LH[1]
	Glial hyperactivity, arcuate n[2]
2. Neuroleptics	Irreversible tardive dyskinesia[3,4]
3. Kainic acid (excitotoxins)	Death of cholinergic and GABAergic neurons[5,6]
4. Noise	Damage to hair cells of inner ear[7,8]

[1]Casaneuva et al. (1982).
[2]Brawer et al. (1978).
[3]Smith and Baldessarini (1980).
[4]Seide and Müller (1967).
[5]Mason and Fibiger (1979).
[6]Coyle and Schwarcz (1976).
[7]Rosen et al. (1962).
[8]Kryter, K. (1970).

is unremitting receptor stimulation. There is good evidence that continual receptor occupancy leads to neurologic damage in some other conditions (Table 6-2). These studies are ongoing and much more work needs to be done. As we learn more about the molecular basis for cell damage that results from receptor occupancy, it may be possible to propose a general unifying hypothesis related to many aspects of the nervous system including the neurological diseases of aging.

Acknowledgments

These studies were supported by NIA grants AG-00446, AG-00117, and AG-03272 to CEF. I am indebted to Lane Kannegieter for compassionate and capable assistance in preparing this manuscript.

References

Aschheim, P.: Resultats fournis per la greffe hererochrone des ovarie dans l' etude de la regulation hypothalamus-hypophyso-ovariene de la ratte senile. *Gerontologia 10*, 65–67 (1965).

Blake, C.A., Elias, K.A., and Hoffman, L.J.: Ovariectomy of young adult rats has a sparing effect on the suppressed ability of aged rats to release luteinizing hormone. *Biol. Repro. 28*, 575–585 (1983).

Blatt, C., Mileham, K., Haas, M., Nesbitt, M.N., Harper, M.E., and Simon, M.I.: Chromosome mapping of the mink cell focus-inducing and xenotropic env gene family in the mouse. *Proc. Nat. Acad. Sci. 80*, 6298–6302 (1983).

Brawer, J.R., Naftolin, R., Martin, J., and Sonnenschein, C.: Effects of a single injection of estradiol valerate on the hypothalamic arcuate nucleus and on reproductive function in the female rat. *Endocrinology 103*, 510–512 (1978).

Brawer, J.R., and Sonnenschein, C.: Cytopathological effects of estradiol on the arcuate nucleus of the female rat. A possible mechanism for pituitary tumorigenesis. *Am. J. Anat. 144*, 157–187 (1975).

Bridges, T.P., Cannon, H.E., and Wyatt, R.J.: Burned-out schizophrenia: evidence for age effects in schizophrenia symptomatology. *J. Gerontology 33*, 835–839 (1978).

Bugiani, C., Salvariani, S., Perdelli, F., Mancardi, G.L., and Leonardi, A.: Nerve cell loss with aging in the putamen. *Eur. Neurol. 17*, 286–291 (1978).

Casanueva, F., Cocchi, D., Locatelli, V., Flauto, C., Zambotti, F., Bestetti, G., Rossi, G.L., and Muller, E.: Defective central nervous system dopaminergic function in rats with estrogen-induced pituitary tumors, as assessed by plasma prolactin concentrations. *Endocrinology 110*, 590–599 (1982).

Coyle, J.T., and Schwarcz, R.: Lesion of striatal neurons with kainic acid provides a model for Huntington's chorea. *Nature 263*, 244–246 (1976).

Felicio, L.S., Nelson, J.F., Gosden, R.G., and Finch, C.E.: Restoration of ovulatory cycles by young ovarian grafts in aging mice: potentiation by long-term ovariectomy decreases with age. *Proc. Nat. Acad. Sci. 80*, 6076–6080 (1983).

Finch, C.E.: Relationships of aging changes in the basal ganglia to manifestations of Huntington's chorea. *Ann. Neurol. 7*, 406–411 (1980).

Finch, C.E., Felicio, L.S., Flurkey, K., Gee, D.M., Mobbs, C., Nelson, J.F., and Osterburg, H.H.: Studies in ovarian–hypothalamic–pituitary interactions during reproductive aging in C57BL/6J mice. *Peptides, 1, Suppl. 1*, 163–176 (1980).

Finch, C.E., and Morgan, D.G.: Aging and schizophrenia: a hypothesis relating asynchrony in neural aging processes to manifestations of schizophrenia and other neurologic diseases with age. In Miller, N.E. and Cohen, G.N. (Eds.), Schizophrenia, Paranoia, and Schizophreniform Disorders of Later Life. New York: Guilford, in press.

Finch, C.E., and Mobbs, C.V.: Hormonal influences on hypothalamic sensitivity during aging in female rodents. In Meites, J. (Ed.), Neuroendocrinology of Aging, pp. 143–171. New York: Plenum, 1983.

Gee, D.M., Flurkey, K., and Finch, C.E.: Aging and the regulation of luteinizing hormone in C57BL/6J mice: Impaired elevations after ovariectomy and spontaneous elevations at advanced ages. *Biol. Repro. 28*, 598–607 (1983).

Gee, D.M., Flurkey, K., and Finch, C.E.: The regulation of the LH surge by estradiol in ovariectomized C57BL/6J mice. Effects of estradiol implant size, postovariectomy duration and aging. *Endocrinology 114*, 685–693 (1984).

Gosden, R.G., Liang, S.C., Felicio, L.S, Nelson, J.F., and Finch, C.E.: Imminent oocyte exhaustion and reduced follicular recruitment mark the climacteric in aging mice. *Biol. Repro. 28*, 255–260 (1983).

Guyton, A.C.: Textbook of Medical Physiology, 6th ed, p. 1016. Philadelphia: Saunders, 1981.

Kawashima, S.: Influence of continued injections of sex steroids on the estrous cycle in the adult rat. *Annot. Zool. Japan 33*, 226–232 (1960).

Kryter, K.: The effects of noise on man. New York: Academic, 1970.

MacLusky, N.J., and Naftolin, F.: Sexual differentiation of the central nervous system. *Science 211*, 1294–1303 (1981).

Marcussen, J.O., Morgan, D.G., Winblad, B., and Finch, C.E.: Serotonin-2 binding sites in human frontal cortex and hippocampus. Selective loss of S-2A sites with age. *Brain Res.*, in press (1984).

Mason, S.T., and Fibiger, H.C.: Kainic acid lesions of the striatum in rats mimic the spontaneous motor abnormalities of Huntington's disease. *Neuropharmacology 18*, 403–407 (1979).

McGeer, P.L., McGeer, E.G., and Suzuki, J.S.: Aging and extrapyramidal function. *Arch. Neurol.* (Chicago) *34*, 33–35 (1977).

Mobbs, C.V., Flurkey, K., Gee, D.M., Yamamoto, K., Sinha, Y.N., and Finch, C.E.: Estradiol-induced anovulatory syndrome in female C57BL/6J mice: age-like neuroendocrine, but not ovarian impairments. *Biol. Repro. 30*, 556–563 (1984a).

Mobbs, C.V., Gee, D.M., and Finch, C.E.: Reproductive senescence in female C57BL/6J mice: ovarian impairments and neuroendocrine impairments that are partially reversible and delayable by ovariectomy. *Endocrinology*, in press (1984b).

Morgan, D.M., Marcusson, J.O., and Finch, C.E.: Contamination of serotonin-2 binding sites by an alpha-1 adrenergic component in assays with (3H)spiperone. *Life Sci. 34*, 2507–2514 (1984).

Nelson, J.F., Felicio, L.S., Sinha, Y.N., and Finch, C.E.: An ovarian role in the spontaneous pituitary tumorigenesis and hyperprolactinemia of aging female mice. *The Gerontologist 20 Part II* (Abstract), 171 (1980).

Rosen, S., Bergman, M., Plester, D., El-Mofty, A., and Satti, M.H.: Presbycusis study of a relatively noise-free population in the Sudan. *Ann. Otol. Rhinol. Laryngol. 71*, 727–743 (1962).

Schipper, H., Brawer, J.R., Nelson, J.F., Felicio, L.S., and Finch, C.E.: The role of the gonads in the histologic aging of the hypothalamic arcuate nucleus. *Biol. Repro. 25*, 413–419 (1981).

Seide, H., and Müller, H.: Choreiform movements as side effects of phenothiazine medication in geriatric patients. *J. Am. Ger. Soc. 15*, 517–522 (1977).

Severson, J.A., and Finch, C.E.: Reduced dopaminergic binding with aging in the rodent striatum. *Brain Res. 192*, 147–162 (1980).

Smith, J.M., and Baldessarini, R.J.: Changes in prevalence, severity and recovery in tardive dyskinesia with age. *Arch. Gen. Psychiat. 37*, 1368–1373 (1980).

Talbert, G.: Aging of the female reproductive system. In Finch, C.E., Hayflick, L. (Eds.), Handbook of the Biology of Aging, pp. 318–356. New York: Van Nostrand, 1977.

vom Saal, F.S., and Bronson, F.H.: In utero proximity of female mouse fetuses to males: effect on reproductive performance during later life. *Biol. Repro. 19*, 842–853 (1978).

vom Saal, F.S., and Moyer, C.L. Prenatal effects on reproductive capacity during aging in female mice. *Biol. Rev.*, in press.

Wise, P.M.: Aging of the female reproductive system. *Rev. Biol. Res. Aging 1*, 195–222 (1983).

Chapter 7

New Approaches to Alzheimer's Disease: Neurotrophic Factors

Stanley H. Appel and Kosei Ojika

Summary

The etiology of Alzheimer's disease (AD) is unknown. Furthermore, specific therapy for this condition is almost totally lacking. Our own thesis is that Alzheimer's disease is due to the failure of a neurotrophic hormone normally elaborated or stored in cortical or hippocampal tissue and exerting its effect in a retrograde fashion on cortical or hippocampal projections originating in nucleus basalis or medial septal regions. Depletion of such hormone or interference with its action on basalis or septal neurons may result from many different processes and lead to gradual neuronal failure and the progressive impairment of memory as well as cognitive and emotional function characteristic of Alzheimer's disease.

Introduction

Recent advances in developmental neurobiology have documented the importance of target-cell trophic factors for the survival, growth, and differentiation of innervating neurons. This principle is most convincingly documented in the peripheral autonomic nervous system where nerve growth factor (NGF) can be demonstrated to influence neuronal viability and maturation in vivo and in vitro (Bradshaw, 1978). Further evidence supporting the potential role of neurotrophic factors acting in a retrograde fashion is provided by the phenomenon of retrograde transneuronal degeneration (Torch, Hirano, and Solomon, 1977). Such retrograde transneuronal degeneration has been noted in the limbic system; that is, in the medial mamillary nucleus of the ventral tegmental nucleus following lesions in the limbic cortex or cerebral cortex (Cowan, 1970). It has also been demonstrated in pyramidal cells of precentral cortex following limb amputation or in the inferior olivary nucleus following cerebral or Purkinje cell damage. Lesions of the occipital visual cortex have been noted to give rise to changes in retinal ganglion cells, optic nerve, and lateral geniculate body presumably secondary to retrograde transneuronal degeneration. This process may take from several weeks to several months and may even take up to several years. Thus, it is reasonable to suggest that neurotrophic factors, synthesized or perhaps stored in the postsynaptic cell, may have long-term retrograde effects on innervating neurons. Different neurotrophic factors may exist for different specific networks, and impairment of neurotrophic function may contribute to certain degenerative diseases of man.

Diseases of Aging: ALS, Parkinsonism, and Alzheimer's Disease

Amyotrophic lateral sclerosis, parkinsonism, and Alzheimer's disease represent three of the most common and most devastating diseases of the nervous system. Each of these conditions is presently considered to be a degenerative disease of unknown origin. In each, multiple etiologies including viral or immunologic causes have been implicated, but never proven. In all three the changes in the disease state resemble alterations known to occur in older individuals. Thus, all three disorders may represent accelerated aging of specific neuronal pathways.

Our thesis is that each of these disorders results from the lack of a neurotrophic hormone elaborated or stored in the synaptic target of the affected neurons and exerting a specific retrograde effect (Appel, 1981). Any process which depletes neurotrophic hormones, or interferes with their retrograde action on presynaptic receptors, may result in gradual neuronal failure. This failure could be considered the result of premature aging which in turn results from many different etiologic factors. The common denominator would be a diminution in retrograde trophic effects.

In our own laboratory, we have documented the existence of neurotrophic proteins from rat, calf, and human skeletal muscle which can promote neuron survival, neuritic outgrowth, and enhance acetylcholine synthesis in cultured ventral spinal cord (Smith and Appel, 1983). The relevant protein is not nerve growth factor since neither nerve growth factor nor antibody to nerve growth factor had significant effects on dissociated ventral cord cultures in the presence or absence of muscle extract. We have been able to separate a morphologic and cholinergic activity by charge and by molecular weight. The factors responsible for neurite elongation represent a glycoprotein of approximately 33–37,000 daltons. The cholinergic activities reside in proteins of different sizes: a high-molecular-weight species of 55,000 daltons, a lower-molecular-weight species of approximately 17,000 daltons, as well as a peptide of under 1500 daltons. Our success in identifying such factors from the motor system has prompted a similar investigation in the pathways relevant to Alzheimer's disease.

Alzheimer's Disease

Alzheimer's disease is a disorder characterized clinically by diffuse deterioration of mental function primarily in thought and memory and secondarily in feeling and conduct. It is a disorder of the later decades of life which is diagnosed primarily by exclusion. Secondary causes of loss of memory and impaired cognitive function by multiple infarcts, intracranial mass lesions, infections, or toxic and metabolic disorders must be ruled out.

The etiology of Alzheimer's disease is unknown. Although viral and immunologic causes have been suggested, no convincing reproducible data support the presence of an infectious agent or a cell-mediated or humoral immune factor. However, despite the paucity of data regarding the etiology, there has been substantial clarification of the pathology of this syndrome. The most striking changes include the loss of neurons in the nucleus basalis of Meynert (Whitehouse et al., 1982). These cells are known to convey cholinergic input to cortical tissues, in the same way that medial septal projections provide cholinergic input to the hippocampus (Johnston, McKinney, and Coyle, 1979). Accompanying such a loss is a consistent biochemical abnormality, namely the loss of an enzyme unique to cholinergic neurons (Davies and Maloney, 1976), choline acetyltransferase. Thus, a good correlation is known to exist between the presence of senile plaques, the depletion of cells in nucleus basalis and the depletion of cholinergic activity.

In this framework, Alzheimer's disease becomes a much more specific and limited network structural defect analogous to Parkinson's disease and ALS rather than a widespread diffuse cortical destructive process. Within this new framework, one can postulate a lack of a specific neurotrophic hormone elaborated or released from hippocampus and cortical cells which would result in impairment of medial septal and nucleus basalis neurons respectively. It is important to keep in mind that in rapidly progressive cases of Alzheimer's disease in younger individuals, impairment of noradrenergic projections from locus ceruleus has also been noted (Bondareff, Mountjoy, and Roth, 1982), and that several neuropeptides, most especially somatostatin, have been noted to be decreased in Alzheimer's disease (Davies, Katzman, and Terry, 1980). The former finding might reflect the lack of retrograde neurotrophic effects within the noradrenergic system in selected patients, although the latter finding has no such simple explanation.

ALS, Parkinson's Disease, Alzheimer's Disease, and Normal Aging

All three of these diseases appear to represent disorders of specific neural networks in which the presynaptic neuronal input is altered with secondary alterations of the target tissue. All three occur as sporadic diseases later in life and have an increased incidence with advancing age. A familial form of each of the diseases is present in 5–10% of patients. Furthermore, in all three heavy-metal intoxication has been implicated as the secondary cause of the syndrome: lead in ALS, manganese in Parkinsonism, and aluminum in Alzheimer's disease, although the evidence favoring aluminum is at best extremely tenuous. In all three diseases, the respective abnormalities are reflected in presynaptic neuronal systems known to deteriorate normally with age. For example, rat motor neurons demonstrate less sprouting following injury in older animals (Pestronk, Drachman, and Griffin, 1980). An age-related decrease in dopamine as well as in tyrosine hydroxylase occurs in mammalian striatum (Finch, 1973), and there is an age-related diminution in CAT activity in brain (Davies, 1978). With age the gradual appearance of muscle wasting, bradykinesia, and impaired memory may suggest that ALS, Parkinson's disease, and Alzheimer's disease respectively are merely accentuations or accelerations of the normal aging processes within the nervous system. It is an accepted finding that older individuals experience some degree of slowing of intellectual processes, mild forgetfulness and inability to find the correct word or recall details of a recent event. When present to a limited extent these are considered characteristic of normal aging. From a pathological point of view, senile plaques and neurofibrillary tangles do occur during normal aging. By the ninth decade, 90% of all brains may have neurofibrillary tangles in the hippocampus. However, the number of plaques in the neocortex and the number of neurofibrillary tangles in the hippocampus are markedly increased in the brains of patients with Alzheimer's disease as opposed to age-matched individuals without dementia. Furthermore, neurofibrillary tangles in the neocortex occur almost exclusively in patients with dementia (Terry, 1983).

Our hypothesis, suggesting an impairment of neurotrophic hormone function, suggests that the premature aging is not an intrinsic process of the neurons undergoing degeneration, but rather an impairment of extrinsic factors which normally influence the maintenance and survival of neurons. In Alzheimer's disease, trauma, viruses, infections, and vascular disease may attack the relevant neuronal population by interfering with the function of the neurotrophic factors elaborated by the cortex and hippocampus, thereby impairing the viability of nucleus basalis and medial septal neurons. Such degeneration may occur either by interfering with the synthesis or release of the neurotrophic hormone from cortex and hippocampus, by blocking or inactivating trophic hormone prior to its interaction with the presynaptic neuron, or by blocking trophic receptors of the presynaptic cells. Thus, immunologic processes, for example, may well be directed against the neurotrophic hormones and prevent such hormones from acting on nucleus basalis and septal presynaptic terminals. This situation would be analogous to diseases of the endocrine system such as juvenile diabetes in which antibodies directed either against insulin or against insulin receptors may be responsible for the disease symptomatology.

Neurotrophic Effects in the Septal-Hippocampal System

In order to determine whether such neurotrophic factors do exist and whether hippocampal factors can influence medial septal neuron function, we have employed tissue culture systems. Medial septal tissues are obtained from the brains of 16-day embryonic albino Sprague-Dawley rats and are grown in Sato's media (Bottenstein and Sato, 1979). The addition of hippocampal extract at three days in vitro results in a gradual increase in the length and density of fiber outgrowth compared to control cultures. These effects begin within 1–2 days and can be monitored for the next several days in culture.

As an assay for cholinergic neurons, acetylcholine synthesis is monitored over the same 6-day period. After application of the hippocampal extract at day 3 in vitro, acetylcholine synthesis increases significantly and by day 6 is more than twice control value. Other tissues such as cortex, striatum, cerebellum, spinal cord, muscle, liver, and kidney do not give the same effect. Several of these tissues do give some enhancement over control, but this increase is related to the fact that explants are being cultured in defined media. In addition, there is some effect on survival, since in the absence of hippocampal extract, there is a diminution of acetylcholine synthesis between days 6 and 8. Thus, the effects of the extract from day 3 to day 8 are a combination of increased survival as well as enhancement of acetylcholine synthesis independent of survival.

Nerve growth factor (NGF) has been reported to enhance cortical cholinergic activity, but there is no evidence that it is responsible for our observed neurotrophic effects on morphology or acetylcholine synthesis. NGF produces no morphologic nor cholinergic effects in our cultured septal tissue, whereas it has a quite marked effect on rat dorsal root ganglion cells and superior cervical ganglion cells grown in our laboratory. Furthermore, antibodies to NGF have no effect on the enhancement noted in the presence of hippocampal extract or medial septal nucleus morphology and acetylcholine synthesis. The neurotrophic effect of hippocampal tissue is present both in soluble and particulate components. The particulate activity is not specific for the hippocampus, but is found in liver and kidney. Within the hippocampus, it is present not only in the synaptic membranes, but as well in myelin and microsomal fractions. It is absent in mitochondrial fractions. The supernatant activity, however, is specific for the hippocampus, and resides in a peptide fraction with a molecular weight less than 2000 daltons.

Discussion

Our tissue culture experiments have established the fact that neurotrophic factors do exist, and that the most potent activity resides in peptides smaller than 2000 daltons. Our present efforts are in purifying such components to homogeneity, and in preparing antibodies to determine whether these neurotrophic peptides perform similar functions in vivo as they do in vitro. Purification of these peptides, and the production of antibodies against them, will enable us to devise a radioimmunoassay which can test their relevance to the pathophysiology of Alzheimer's disease. It is important to note that both somatostatin or vasoactive intestinal peptides, which have been implicated in the process of memory, have no neurotrophic effects in our culture systems. Thus, our peptides probably represent a novel constitutent not heretofore described. It remains to be determined whether these neurotrophic hormones are applicable to the problem of Alzheimer's disease. Purification of these peptides and clarification of their mechanism of action may not only shed light on long-term cell–cell interaction, but it may also provide a basis for understanding the pathophysiology of Alzheimer's disease.

Acknowledgments

We are grateful to the John A. Hartford Foundation and the Robert J. Kleberg, Jr. and Helen C. Kleberg Foundation for their support of these investigations.

References

Appel, S.H.: A unifying hypothesis for the cause of amyotrophic lateral sclerosis, parkinsonism and Alzheimer's disease. *Ann. Neurol. 10*, 499 (1981).

Bondareff, W., Mountjoy, C.Q., and Roth, M.: Loss of neurons of origin of the adrenergic projection to cerebral cortex (nucleus locus ceruleus) in senile dementia. *Neurology 32*, 164 (1982).

Bottenstein, J.E., and Sato, G.H.: Growth of a rat neuroblastoma cell line in serum-free supplemented medium. *Proc. Natl. Acad. Sci. USA 76*, 514–517 (1979).

Bradshaw, R.A.: Nerve growth factor. *Ann. Rev. Biochem. 47*, 191 (1978).

Cowan, W.M.: Anterograde and retrograde transneuronal degeneration in the central and peripheral nervous system. In Nahta, W.J., and Ebbson, S.D. (Eds.), Contemporary Research Methods in Neuroanatomy, p. 217. New York: Springer, 1970.

Davies, P., and Maloney, A.J.F.: Selective loss of central cholinergic neurons in Alzheimer's disease. *Lancet 2*, 1403 (1976).

Davies, P.: Loss of choline acetyltransferase activity in normal aging and in senile dementia. *Adv. Exp. Med. Biol. 113*, 251 (1978).

Davies, P., Katzman, R., and Terry, R.D.: Reduced somatostatin-like immunoreactivity in cerebral cortex from cases of Alzheimer's disease and Alzheimer's senile dementia. *Nature 288*, 279 (1980).

Finch, C.E.: Catecholamine metabolism in the brains of aging male mice. *Brain Res. 52*, 261 (1973).

Johnston, M.V., McKinney, M., and Coyle, J.T.: Evidence for a cholinergic projection to neocortex from neurons in basal forebrain. *Proc. Natl. Acad. Sci. USA 76*, 5392 (1979).

Pestronk, A., Drachman, D.B., and Griffin, J.W.: Effects of aging on nerve sprouting and regeneration. *Exp. Neurol. 70*, 65 (1980).

Smith, R.G., and Appel, S.H.: Extracts of skeletal muscle increase neurite outgrowth and cholinergic activity of fetal rat spinal motor neurons. *Science 219*, 1079 (1983).

Terry, R.: Cortical norphometry in Alzheimer's disease. In Katzman, R. (Ed.), Banbury Report, Biological Aspects of Alzheimer's Disease, p. 95. New York: Cold Spring Harbor, 1983.

Torch, W.C., Hirano, A., and Solomon, S.: Anterograde transneuronal degeneration in the limbic system: Clinical–anatomic correlation. *Neurology 27*, 1157 (1977).

Whitehouse, P.J., Price, D.L., Clark, A.W., Coyle, J.T., and DeLong, M.R.: Alzheimer's disease and senile dementia: Loss of neurons in the basal forebrain. *Science 215*, 1237 (1982).

Part III

Neurochemistry of Aging and Age-Related Diseases

Chapter 8

Neurochemistry of the Aging Brain and Senile Dementia

William Meier-Ruge

Summary

Neurochemical investigations demonstrate that normal brain aging is characterized by a moderate decrease in glycolytic turnover capacity. There is an age-dependent increase in soluble hexokinase activity and a significant decrease in activity of the key glycolytic enzyme phosphofructokinase. This decrease in the glycolytic turnover capacity lowers acetyl coenzyme A, necessary for the biosynthesis of acetylcholine. Therefore normal aging of the brain is additionally characterized by a moderate decline of the cholinergic activity. The monaminergic neurotransmitters also decrease, which results in a neurotransmitter imbalance.

In normal aging the brain stays within the limits of the functional reserve capacity. This reserve capacity can be exhausted by ischemic, traumatic, or toxic brain lesions, shifting the normal aging brain into a psychoorganic defect syndrome or a senile dementia.

In Alzheimer's disease and in senile dementia of Alzheimer's type, in addition to a decrease of mitochondrial hexokinase and phosphofructokinase activity, there is a significant decrease in aldolase, triosephosphate isomerase, phosphoglucose isomerase, and phosphogylceromutase activity. The functional consequence of this decrease in glycolytic energy supply is a massive impairment of acetylcholine synthesis, which is accompanied by a massive decline in choline acetyltransferase. Senile dementia can be defined as a cholinergic insufficiency of the brain. A drug treatment which improves the glycolytic turnover may be an etiological therapy concept enhancing cholinergic brain activity by increasing acetyl coenzyme A and choline acetyltransferase activity.

Introduction

During the last decades, aging has become a matter of special concern. A steady increase in the number of people over 65 contrasts with a declining working population. In Northern Europe the ratio between the birth rate and the retirement rate is already 1 to 1, and this trend is foreseen in the future, even in countries which today still have an excess of births (Selby and Schechter, 1982). The tendency of human populations to grow older and to reach their physiologic limits of life, as a consequence of better medical treatment of infectious diseases, heart and circulatory diseases, etc., leads to a paradoxical increase in social costs because more and more people reach an age advanced enough for them to experience mental impairment and cognitive dysfunction (Katzman and Karasu, 1975; Selby and Schechter, 1982). In this connection long-term institutional care becomes a source of considerably increased social costs (Butler, 1978a,b). With these facts in mind, the fundamental importance of therapeutic principles to help the elderly to stay mentally healthy and independent as long as possible, becomes clear.

In view of these facts, the relationship between gerontology and pharmacology has therefore become increasingly important in recent years. Insight into the pathogenesis of the aging process and senile dementia, therefore, is a fundamental prerequisite of a more effective and confident use of drugs in geriatric therapy.

This chapter will present neurochemical studies in normal brain aging and in senile dementia. The aim of these investigations was to obtain insights into the pathogenesis of mental impairment in old age.

Neurochemical Investigations of the Normal Aging Brain

In order to investigate the metabolic performance of the normal aging brain neurochemical investigations were started. In contrast to work reported in the literature on neurotransmitter enzymes and neurotransmitter metabolites (Samorajski, 1977; Carlsson et al., 1980; McGeer and McGeer, 1980, 1982), we studied enzymes of the glycolytic pathway, since it is well known that glucose turnover is the main energy source of the brain.

It was found that most of the 13 enzymes of the glycolytic pathway remain practically unchanged during aging. However, aldolase and phosphoglycerate mutase and the two key glycolytic enzymes hexokinase

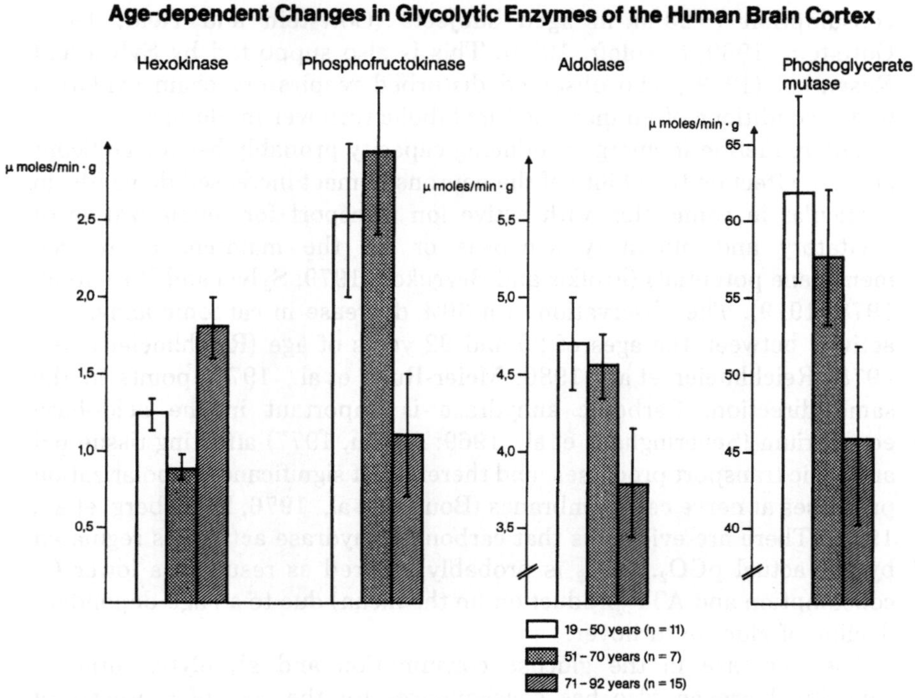

Figure 8-1. Age-related changes in the activity of the key glycolytic enzymes hexokinase and phosphofructokinase, and the glycolytic enzymes aldolase and phosphoglycerate mutase.

and phosphofructokinase are changed (Meier-Ruge et al., 1978; Iwangoff et al., 1978; Iwangoff et al., 1979, Meier-Ruge 1982).

The activity of soluble hexokinase increases and the activity of phosphofructokinase, aldolase, and phosphogylcerate mutase decrease significantly with age (Fig. 8-1). For normal functioning, hexokinase is bound to the mitochondrial membrane. The release of hexokinase leading to a corresponding increase in soluble hexokinase represents a loss of functionally active hexokinase. Therefore, the increase in soluble hexokinase is identical with a decrease in mitochondrial hexokinase activity. Even more important from a functional point of view is the decrease of the key enzyme phosphofructokinase, which results in a decline of the glucose turnover.

Despite the fact that we are unable to explain the etiology of this finding, it demonstrates that the aging brain has a limited capability of increasing the turnover rate of glucose, which is necessary to synthesize a sufficient amount of acetyl coenzyme A and the energy carrier ATP. These observations appear to be consistent with the reduced glucose consumption (−23%) in aged subjects (Gottstein and Held, 1969; Gottstein, 1980; Sokoloff, 1975). This is also supported by Sylvia and Rosenthal (1979), who observed disturbed respiratory chain oxidation under conditions of an increased metabolic turnover in old age.

The reduction in energy-producing capacity probably has a significant adverse effect on the ability of the neurons to meet increased demands, in particular in connection with active ion transport for repolarization of excitatory and inhibitory synapses or for the maintenance of cell membrane potentials (Frolkis and Bezrukov, 1979; Sylvia and Rosenthal, 1978, 1979). The observation of a 30% decrease in carbonic anhydrase activity between the ages of 20 and 92 years of age (Reichlmeier et al., 1978; Reichlmeier et al., 1980; Meier-Ruge et al., 1978) points in the same direction. Carbonic anhydrase is important in the acid–base equilibrium (Severinghaus et al., 1969; Annau, 1977) affecting tissue pH and ionic transport processes, and therefore of significance in polarization processes at nerve cell membranes (Bourke et al., 1976; Kimelberg, et al., 1978). There are evidences that carbonic anhydrase activity is regulated by the actual pCO_2. pCO_2 is probably lowered as result of a lower O_2 consumption and ATP production (in the mean) due to an age-dependent decline of glucose turnover.

The decrease in the glucose consumption and glycolytic turnover capacity, however, also has consequences for the rate of synthesis of acetylcholine: The decline in the glycolytic turnover decreases the level of acetyl coenzyme A (Fig. 8-2), which is the key substrate for the acetylation of choline to acetylcholine, resulting in a lower cholinergic activity of the brain (Gibson and Blass, 1976; Blass et al., 1980; Siesjö and Rehncrona, 1980). In fact, neurotransmitter studies have revealed that cholinergic activity and choline acetyltransferase (ChAT) are significantly reduced with increasing age (Perry et al., 1978; Perry, 1980; McGeer and McGeer, 1982).

Catecholaminergic neurotransmitter concentrations are also diminished in old age (McGeer and McGeer, 1980; Carlsson, 1978).

In summary, neurochemistry of the normal aging brain can be characterized by (1) a decline in glycolytic turnover capacity; (2) a slight decrease in cholinergic activity; and (3) a slight neurotransmitter imbalance. The clinical consequences of these findings in aging individuals were shown by Obrist and Busse (1965), Roubicek (1977), Busse (1978), Busse and Wang (1979), and others. They demonstrated, as a functional consequence of these age-related changes in brain metabolism, a decrease in the dominant α-EEG frequency. In chronospectographic EEG investigations a corresponding rapid loss of vigilance in old age was observed, characterized by a high theta frequency and a low alpha frequency. Perry et al. (1978) demonstrated a relationship between choline actyltransferase activity and mental test score rates. High mental test scores are linked

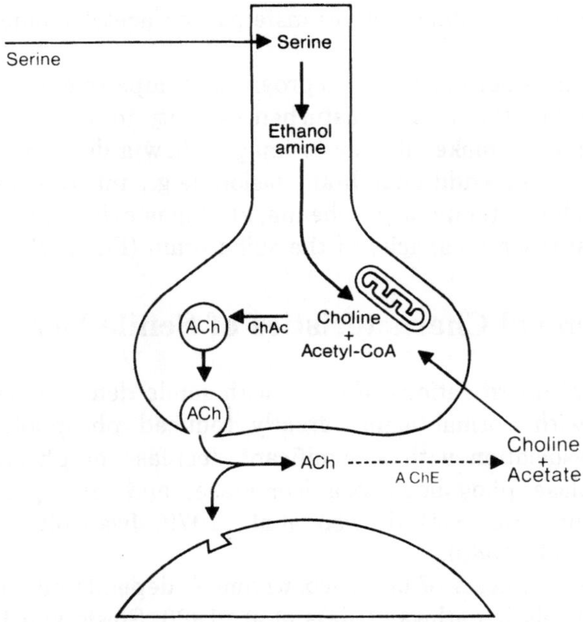

Figure 8-2. Metabolic cycle of the neurotransmitter acetylcholine (ACH = acetylcholine; AChE = acetylcholine esterase; ChAc = choline acetyltransferase; Acetyl-CoA = acetyl coenzyme A).

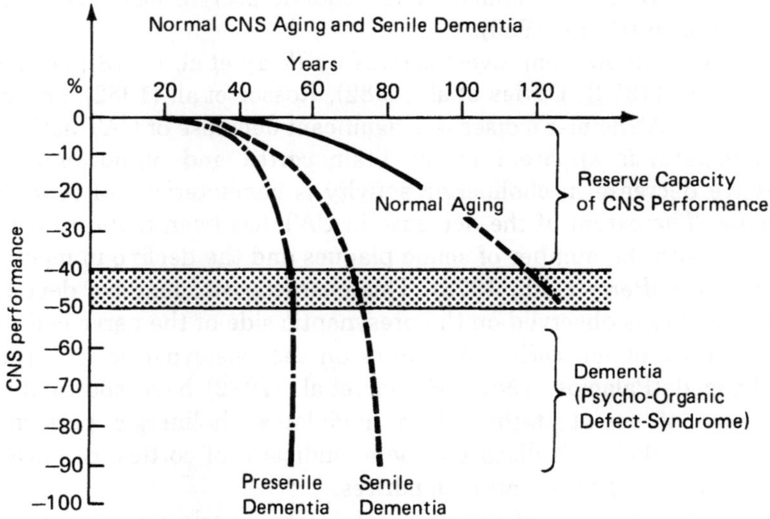

Figure 8-3. Schematic representation of the functional and metabolic differences of normal brain-aging and senile dementia. In normal aging, metabolism and brain function stays within the range of the functional reserve capacity of the brain. In senile dementia the functional reserve and metabolic turnover rates are progressively exhausted.

with high rates of choline acetyltransferase or acetylcholine, and vice versa.

In general terms normal aging is a progressive impairment of adaptation to environmental stimuli. The disturbed capacity to adapt to increased metabolic demands makes it easy to imagine how a dementia syndrome may develop if an additional brain lesion (e.g., intoxication, trauma, hypovolemic shock, temporary ischemia, etc.) may exhaust the metabolic and functional reserve capacity of the aging brain (Fig. 8-3).

Neurochemical Characteristics of Senile Dementia

Neurochemical investigations of cases with senile dementia revealed, in comparison with normal aging, greatly reduced phosphofructokinase activity in association with a significant decrease of phospholycerate mutase, aldolase phosphoglucose isomerase, and triosephospate isomerase activity (Fig. 8-4) (Bowen et al., 1979; Iwangoff et al., 1980; Meier-Ruge et al., 1980).

The rate of synthesis of acetyl-coenzyme A depends on the turnover rate of the glycolytic pathway (Blass et al., 1980; Siesjö and Rehncrona, 1980).

The functional consequences of the pronounced decrease in the glycolytic turnover, therefore, is a marked lowering of the acetyl coenzyme A level in the presynaptic compartment (Fig. 8-2), which results in a lower rate of acetylation of choline by the choline acetyltransferase (CAT) to acetylcholine (Perry, 1980).

Today we know from investigations by Perry et al. (1978), Davies and Yamamura (1978), Davies et al. (1982), Rossor et al. (1982), and others that also in Alzheimer's disease a significant decrease of CAT activity and somatostatin is apparent in the brain cortex and hippocampus. The massive decrease in cholinergic activity is characteristic of Alzheimer's disease. The extent of the decrease in CAT has been found to correlate directly with the number of senile plaques and the decline in mental test score rates (Perry et al., 1978). This characteristic massive decrease in CAT activity is observed on the presynaptic side of the nerve cells, while the number of muscarinic receptors on the postsynaptic side remains unchanged (Palacios, 1982). Rossor et al. (1982) have shown that the decrease of somatostatin, which modulates cholinergic performance, seems in Alzheimer's disease to be an indicator of cortical cell loss or at least of a loss of presynaptic dendrites.

With the discovery of the decrease in cholinergic activity we became aware that the key pathogenetic mechanism in senile dementia is the disturbance of the cholinergic system. Findings by Gibson and Blass (1976), Gibson et al. (1978), and Siesjö and Rehncrona (1980) have

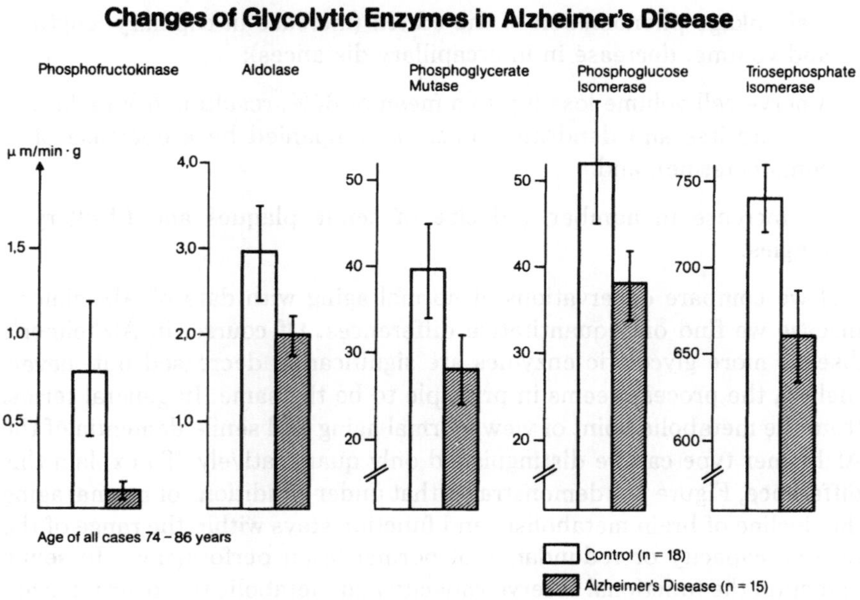

Figure 8-4. Senile dementia of Alzheimer's type is characterized by a marked decrease in phosphofructokinase, aldolase, phosphoglycerate mutase, phosphoglucose isomerase, and triosephosphate isomerase in comparison to age-matched controls.

provided further indications in this direction. These authors have shown that the cholinergic system is highly dependent on energy formation which remains intact. Recovery of acetylcholine synthesis after energy deprivation is much slower than the recovery of energy-rich phosphates or catecholamines. Damage to the cholinergic system has massive effects on memory and learning, which is understandable if one remembers that, generally speaking, the brain is cholinergically innervated but catecholaminergically modulated.

The most important pathogenetic steps in the development of cognitive dysfunction and senile dementia are accordingly

disturbed glycolytic energy supply,

a decrease of acetyl coenzyme A,

a decrease in CAT activity, and

a decrease in acetylcholine synthesis.

As a consequence of these metabolic disturbances a series of morphological alterations occur:

a shrinkage phenomenon of the cortex (increase in capillary length and volume, decrease in intercapillary distances);

a nerve cell volume loss (up to a mean of 65%, resulting from a loss of dendrites and dendritic spines, accompanied by a decrease of somatostatine); and

an increase in number and size of senile plaques and fibrillary tangles.

If we compare observations of normal aging with data of Alzheimer's disease we find only quantitative differences. Of course, in Alzheimer's disease more glycolytic enzymes are significantly decreased but, nevertheless, the process seems in principle to be the same. In general terms, from the metabolic point of view, normal aging and senile dementia of the Alzheimer type can be distinguished only quantitatively. To explain this difference, Figure 8-3 demonstrates that under conditions of normal aging the decline of brain metabolism and function stays within the range of the reserve capacity or redundancy of normal brain performance. In senile dementia the functional reserve capacity and metabolic turnover rates are progressively exhausted (Fig. 8-3).

It seems necessary to distinguish between Alzheimer's disease or presenile dementia in its narrow sense, which normally is a disease developing in the fifth to sixth decade, and senile dementia in old age. The latter is often induced by a hypoxic, toxic, or traumatic exhaustion of the functional reserve capacity of the normal aging brain.

In contrast to senile dementia in old age (>70 years) Alzheimer's disease (Olson and Shaw, 1969; Nordenson et al., 1980; Whalley et al. 1982; Heston 1982; Whalley, 1982) seems to have some common links with Down's Syndrome (Heston, 1982; Whalley, 1982).

Insights into the pathogenesis of dementing brain disease in old age offer a basis for a rational neuropharmacologic concept of treatment. The following pharmacological approaches are presently under investigation.

Approaches in Experimental Pharmacology of Senile Dementia

Pathogenetical-Oriented Concept

1. transmitter substitution (choline, lecithine)
2. favoring of cholinergic mechanisms by AChE inhibition (physostigmine, etc.)
3. cholinergic stimulation (arecoline, etc.)
4. improvement of transmitter response (ergot alkaloids, e.g., codergocrine, bromokriptine, etc.; polypeptides, etc.)

Etiological-Oriented Concept

Improvement of energy formation by boosting glycolysis which causally increases cholinergic activity (e.g., codergocrine).

The improvement of disturbed glucose utilization in the aging brain may have a corrective action on neurotransmitter imbalance and cholinergic activity. As a consequence an improvement in cognitive function may be expected.

References

Annau, Z.: The effect of carbonic anhydrase inhibition on electrical self-stimulation of the brain during hypoxia. *Life Sci. 20*, 1043–1050 (1977).

Blass, J.P., Gibson, G.E., Shimada, M., Kihara, T., Watanabe M., and Kurinioto, K.: Brain carbohydrate metabolism and dementias. In Roberts, P.J. (Ed.), Biochemistry of Dementia, pp. 121–134. London, England: John Wiley & Sons, 1980.

Bourke, R.S., Kimelberg, H.K., and Nelson, L.R.: The effects of temperature and inhibitors on HCO_3-stimulated swelling and ion uptake of monkey cerebral cortex. *Brain Res. 105*, 309–323 (1976).

Bowen, D.M., White, P., Spillane, J.A., Goodhardt, M.J., Curzon, G., Iwangoff, P., Meier-Ruge, W., and Davison, A.N.: Accelerated aging or selective neuronal loss as an important cause of dementia? *Lancet I*, 11–14 (1979).

Busse, E.W.: Duke longitudinal study. I: Senescence and senility. In Katzman, R., Terry, R.D., Bick, K.L. (Eds.), Alzheimer's Disease: Senile Dementia and Related Disorders (Aging Vol. 7), pp. 59–68. New York: Raven, 1978.

Busse, E.W., and Wang, H.S.: The electroencephalographic changes in late life: A longitudinal study. *J. Clin. Exp. Geront. 1*, 145–158 (1979).

Butler, R.N.: Pharmacological interventions of the aging process. In Pharmacological Intervention in the Aging Process. Roberts, J., Adelman, R.C., and Cristofalo, V.J. (Eds.), New York, Plenum Press (1978).

Butler, R.N.: Alzheimer's disease—senile dementia and related disorders: The role of NIA. In Alzheimer's disease: Senile dementia and related disorders, pp. 5–9. Katzman, R., Terry, R.D., and Blick, K.L. (Eds.), Aging, Vol. 7, New York: Raven, 1978b.

Carlsson, A.: Age-dependent changes in central dopaminergic and other monoaminergic systems. *Adv. Exp. Med. Biol. 113*, 1–13 (1978).

Carlsson, A., Adolfsson, R., Aquilonius, S.-M., Gottfries, C.-G., Oreland, L., Svennerholm, L., and Winblad, B.: Biogenic amines in human brain in normal aging, senile dementia and chronic alcoholism. In Goldstein, M., Calne, D.G., Lieberman, A., and Thorner, M.O. (Eds.): Ergot Compounds and Brain Function. Advances in Biochemical Psychopharmacology, Vol. 23, pp. 295–304. New York: Raven, 1980.

Davies, P., Katz, D.A., and Crystal, H.A.: Choline acetyltransferase, somatostatin and substance P in selected cases of Alzheimer's disease. In Corkin, S. et al. (Eds.), Alzheimer's Disease: A Report of Progress, pp. 9–14. New York: Raven, 1982.

Davis, K.L., and Yamamura, H.I.: Cholinergic underactivity in human memory disorders. *Life Sci. 23*, 1729–1734 (1978).

Frolkis, V.V., and Bezrukov, V.V.: Aging of the central nervous system. *Interdiscipl. Topics Geront.* (Karger, Basel) *16*, 1–131 (1979).

Gibson, G.E., and Blass, J.P.: Impaired synthesis of acetylcholine in brain accompanying mild hypoxia and hypoglycemia. *J. Neurochem. 27*, 37–42 (1976).

Gibson, G.E., Schimada, M., and Blass, J.P.: Alterations in acetylcholine synthesis and cyclic nucleotides in mild cerebral hypoxia. *J. Neurochem. 31*, 757–760 (1978).

Gottstein, U.: Risk factors and cerebral blood flow and metabolism. *Proc. Int. Cerebrovascular Diseases SIR* 219–238.

Gottstein, U., and Held, K.: Effekt der Haemodilution nach intravenöser Infusion von niedermolekularen Dextranen auf die Hirnzirkulation des Menschen. *Dtsch. Med. Wschr. 94*, 522–526 (1969).

Heston, L.L.: Alzheimer's dementia and Down's Syndrome: Genetic evidence suggesting an association. *Ann. N.Y. Acad. Sci. 396*, 29–37 (1982).

Iwangoff, P., Armbruster, R., Enz, A., Meier-Ruge, W., and Sandoz, P.: Glycolytic enzymes from human autoptic brain cortex: Normally aged and demented cases. In Roberts, P.J. (Ed.), Biochemistry of Dementia, pp. 258–262. London: John Wiley & Sons, 1980.

Iwangoff, P., Enz, A., and Meier-Ruge, W.: Incorporation, after single and repeated application of radioactive labelled DH-ergot alkaloids in different organs of the cat, with special reference to the brain. *Gerontology*, Suppl. 1, *24*, 126–138 (1978).

Iwangoff, P., Reichlmeier, K., Enz, A., and Meier-Ruge, W.: Neurochemical findings in physiological aging of the brain. *Interdiscipl. Topics Gerontol.* (Karger, Basel) *15*, 13–33 (1979).

Katzman, R., and Karasu, T.: Differential diagnosis of dementia. In Field, W.S. (Ed.), Neurological and Sensory Disorders in the Elderly, pp. 103–104. New York: Stratton Intercont. Med. Book Corp., 1975.

Kimelberg, H.K., Biddlecome, S., Narumi, S., and Bourke, R.S.: ATPase and carbonic anhydrase activities of bulk-isolated neuron, glia and synaptosome fractions from rat brain. *Brain Res. 141*, 305–323 (1978).

McGeer, G., and McGeer, P.L.: Aging and neurotransmitter systems. In Goldstein, M., Calne, D.B., Lieberman, A., and Thorner, M.O. (Eds.), Ergot Compounds and Brain Function, Series Advances in Biochemical Psychopharmacology, Vol. 23., pp. 305–314. New York: Raven, 1980.

McGeer, E.G., and McGeer, P.L: Neurotransmitters in normal aging. In D. Platt (Ed.), Geriatrics, Vol. 1, pp. 263–282. New York: Springer-Verlag, 1982.

Meier-Ruge, W.: Neurochemistry of the aging brain. In Platt, D. (Ed.), Geriatrics, Vol. 1, pp. 241–256. New York: Springer-Verlag, 1982.

Meier-Ruge, W., Emmenegger, H., Enz, A., Gygax, P., Iwangoff, P., and Wiernsperger, N.: Pharmacological aspects of dihydrogenated ergot alkaloids in experimental brain research. *Pharmacology 16, Suppl. 1*,45–62 (1978).

Meier-Ruge, W., Hunziker, O., Iwangoff, P., Reichlmeier, K., and Sandoz, P.: Alterations of morphological and neurochemical parameters of the brain due to normal aging. In Nandy, K. (Ed.), Senile Dementia: A Biomedical Approach, Developmental Neuroscience Vol. 3., pp. 33–44. New York: Elsevier/North-Holland, 1978.

Meier-Ruge, W., Iwangoff, P., Reichlmeier, K., and Sandoz, P.: Neurochemical findings in the aging brain. In Goldstein, M. et al. (Eds.), Ergot Compounds and Brain Function: Neuroendocrine and Neuropsychiatric Aspects, Advances in Biomedical Psychopharmacology Vol. 23, pp. 323–338. New York: Raven, 1980.

Nordenson, I., Adolfsson, R., Beckman, G., Bucht, G., and Winblad, B.: Chromosomal abnormality in dementia of the Alzheimer type. *Lancet 1*, 481–482 (1980).

Obrist, W.D., and Busse, E.W.: The electroencephalogram in old age. In Wilson, W.P. (Ed.), Applications of Electroencephalography in Psychiatry, pp. 185–205. Durham: Duke University, 1965.

Olson, M.I., and Shaw, C.M.: Presenile dementia and Alzheimer's disease in mongolism. *Brain 92*, 147–156 (1969).

Palacios, J.M.: Autoradiographic localization of muscarinic cholinergic receptors in the hippocampus of patients with senile dementia. *Brain Res. 243*, 173–175 (1982).

Perry, E.K.: The cholinergic system in old age and Alzheimer's disease. *Age and Ageing* (England) *9*, 1–8 (1980).

Perry, E.K., Tomlinson, B.E., Blessed, G., Bergmann, K., Gibson, P.H., and Perry, R.H.: Correlation of cholinergic abnormalities with senile plaques and mental test scores in senile dementia. *Brit. Med. J. II*, 1457–1459 (1978).

Reichlmeier, K., Enz, A., Iwangoff, P., and Meier-Ruge, W.: Age-related changes in human brain enzyme activities: A basis for pharmacological intervention. In Roberts, J., Adelman, R.C., and Cristofalo, V.J., Pharmacological Intervention in the Aging Process, Adv. Exper. Med. Biol., Vol. 97, pp. 251–252. New York: Plenum, 1978.

Reichlmeier, K., Iwangoff, P., Enz, A.: Enzymatic changes in the aging brain and some aspects of its pharmacological intervention with ergot compounds. In Eisdorfer, C., and Fann, W.E. (Eds.), Psychopharmacology of Aging, Chapter 2, pp. 13–46. New York: Spectrum, 1980.

Rossor, M.N., Emson, P.C., Iversen, L.L., Mountjoy, C.Q., Roth, M., Fahrenkrug, J., and Rehfeld, J.F.: Neuropeptides and neurotransmitters in cerebral cortex in Alzheimer's disease. In Corkin, G. et al. (Eds.), Alzheimer's Disease: A Report of Progress, Aging, Vol. 19, pp. 15–24. New York: Raven, 1982.

Roubicek, J.: The electroencephalogram in the middle-aged and the elderly. *J. Am. Geriatr. Soc. 25*, 145–152 (1977).

Samorajski, T.: Central neurotransmitter substances and aging: a review. *J. Am. Geriatr. Soc. 25*, 337–348 (1977).

Selby, Ph., and Schechter, M.: Aging 2000: A Challenge for Society. MTP Lancaster: MTP Press 1982.

Severinghaus, J.W., Hamilton, F.N., and Coter, S.: Carbonic acid production and the role of carbonic anhydrase in decarboxylation in brain. *Biochem. J. 114*, 703–705 (1969).

Siesjö, B.K., and Rehncrona, S.: Adverse factors affecting neuronal metabolism: Relevance to the dementias. In Roberts, P.J. (Ed.), Biochemistry of Dementia, pp. 91–120. London: John Wiley & Sons, 1980.

Sokoloff, L.: Cerebral circulation and metabolism in the aged. In Gershon, A., and Raskin, A. (Eds.), Genesis and Treatment of Psychologic Disorders in the Elderly, Aging, Vol. 2, pp. 45–54. New York: Raven, 1975.

Sylvia, A.L., and Rosenthal, M.: The effect of age and lung pathology on cytochrome a,a_3 redox levels in rat cerebral cortex. *Brain Res. 146*, 109–122 (1978).

Sylvia, A.L., and Rosenthal, M.: Effects of age on brain oxidative metabolism in vivo. *Brain Res. 165*, 235–248 (1979).

Whalley, L.J.: The dementia of Down's Syndrome and its relevance to aetiological studies of Alzheimer's disease. *Ann. N.Y. Acad. Sci., 386*, 39–53 (1982).

Whalley, L.J., Carothers, A.D., Collyer, S., DeMey, R., and Frackiewicz, A.: A study of familial factors in Alzheimer's disease. *Brit. J. Psychiatr. 140*, 249–256 (1982).

Chapter 9

Brain Neurotransmitters in Normal Aging

Arvid Carlsson

Summary

Neuronal decay in aging is not a random phenomenon but indicates a selective vulnerability of certain brain regions and certain types of neuron. Susceptibility to the aging process may be at least in part related to a general vulnerability to disturbances in energy supply, etc. Catecholaminergic neurons appear to be especially susceptible to aging. This is possibly due to the formation of cytotoxic quinonoid oxidation products formed from the catecholamines by a nonenzymatic reaction with neuromelanin as the end product.

Substitution therapy of age-induced neurotransmitter deficiency, analogous to the use of L-dopa in Parkinson's disease, will probably have to await more precise identification and mapping of the major age-related neurotransmitter deficiencies, as well as the advent of an arsenal of receptor agonists suitable for drug therapy. In a longer perspective prophylactic measures may be considered (e.g., the possibility of interfering with the formation of hypothetical, cytotoxic oxidation products responsible for degenerative processes in the aging brain).

Introduction

Twenty years ago neurologists did not believe much in drug therapy in degenerative brain disorders. With the advent of L-dopa therapy in Parkinson's disease this attitude has changed. We now know that even the severe loss of neurons of a certain type, perhaps of the order of 80–90%, or even more, can be compensated by substituting for the loss of their specific chemical product(s), namely, their neurotransmitter(s). In Parkinson's disease this can be done by giving the dopamine precursor L-dopa or a directly acting dopamine receptor agonist, such as bromocriptine or lisuride. The direct agonists tried so far have not done as well as L-dopa, but more specific and efficacious agonists may in the not-too-distant future prove equal or even superior to L-dopa. Can the same strategy be applied to other cases of nerve cell degeneration, as occurs, for example, in aging?

Aging is essentially a degenerative process. Aging neurons undergo a loss of mass with a reduction of dendritic spines, etc. (Scheibel, 1978). Finally entire cells are lost. At least in the mammalian brain loss of neurons is not replaced to any detectable extent. Future grafting techniques may possibly make replacement feasible, though probably only to a very limited extent in cases of strictly localized cell loss.

Needless to say, substitution therapy like that applied in Parkinson's disease would appear the more promising, the more selective the damage. The aging process does not affect all brain regions equally, and within a given brain region different types of nerve cells may show marked differences in age dependency. For example, the cerebral cortex is more affected than the brain stem, and within the brain stem some nuclei are affected by the aging process, whereas others are remarkably resistant (Brody, 1975; McGeer, 1978).

Nevertheless, in comparison with Parkinson's disease, where the cell loss is mainly restricted to dopaminergic neurons, the aging process attacks the nerve cells of the brain rather broadly. This means that in all probability more than one neurotransmitter will have to be replaced in order to compensate for the various age-induced losses of brain function.

Our knowledge of the brain neurotransmitters is still very incomplete, and this is even more true of their age dependence. This chapter will focus on those rather few neurotransmitters where at least some knowledge is available. Peptides will not be discussed here, since they are dealt with in Chapter 10 in this volume.

Selectivity of Neuronal Aging

Several lines of evidence indicate that catecholamine-producing neurons are especially susceptible to aging. There is even morphologic evidence to support this contention. As mentioned, brain stem nuclei in general appear to be remarkably resistant to aging. There are two notable exceptions, however: locus ceruleus and substantia nigra, i.e., sites of noradrenaline-and dopamine-producing neurons, respectively. Thus,

Brody (1975) reported that whereas several nuclei of the human brain stem appeared to have constant cell counts throughout life, the cell count of locus ceruleus dropped considerably during senescence. McGeer (1978) found a similar decrease in the cell count of the pigmented cells in substantia nigra.

Biochemical evidence indicating a relatively pronounced age dependence of catecholamine-producing neurons is also available. Thus, McGeer (1978) reported that the activity of the first enzyme in the synthesis of catecholamines (tyrosine hydroxylase) decreases with age in the human striatum. Much less striking age-related changes were observed in two other enzymes in the same structure, namely, glutamic acid decarboxylase and choline acetyltransferase, involved in the synthesis of GABA and acetylcholine, respectively.

In our own studies, where the levels of monoamines and several of their metabolites were measured in various human brain regions, an age-dependent decrease in dopamine was observed in the caudate nucleus, in the putamen and in the mesencephalon, while noradrenaline decreased in the hippocampus. 5-HT showed an age-dependent decrease in the gyrus cinguli (see Carlsson et al, 1980).

Only a few investigators have been unable to confirm the age dependence of human catecholamine neurons (for review, see Loew and Singer, 1983). Observations in rhesus monkeys also show age-related reductions in brain catecholamines (Goldman-Rakic and Brown, 1981). For similar studies on the role of aging in rodent brains, see Chapter 11 in this volume.

The age dependence of neurotransmitters shows regional differences reminiscent of those observed morphologically. For example, the cerebral hemispheres appear to be more susceptible than the brain stem. In our own study, all the statistically significant negative correlations of monoamine levels to age were found in the cerebral hemispheres, except in the case already mentioned, dopamine in the mesencephalon. Remarkably enough, the 5-HT level in the medulla oblongata was positively correlated to age.

An interesting example of regional differences in neurotransmitter susceptibility to aging is given by comparing the caudate nucleus with the putamen (two nuclei of the cerebral hemispheres with almost identical histological appearance and very similar biochemistry). Nevertheless, the former nucleus is clearly more susceptible to aging than the latter. Thus, whereas both nuclei show decreased levels of dopamine with increasing age, the ratio of dopamine in the putamen to that in the caudate nucleus increases significantly with age (see Carlsson, 1981a). Similarly, the dopamine receptor density, measured by means of binding techniques in vitro, shows a significant decrease with age in the caudate nucleus, but not in the putamen (Severson et al., 1982). It should be noted that these receptors are largely located on nondopaminergic neurons and may be looked upon as markers of postsynaptic neurons receiving a dopaminergic nerve supply. This is in contrast to the level of dopamine which occurs in nerve terminals whose cell bodies are located in a brain stem nucleus, namely the pars compacta of the substantia nigra. Finally, in the study of McGeer (1978), choline acetyltransferase activity was found to be negatively correlated to age in the caudate nucleus, whereas no such correlation was found in the putamen.

These observations suggest that regional differences in age dependence exist, which comprise neurons of many different types. The possibility should thus be considered that a local age-related factor exists, which has a general, unspecific influence on nerve cells and which may influence cell bodies and nerve terminals alike. What could be the nature of this factor?

Several decades ago, the progressive loss of brain function in senescence was largely attributed to "arteriosclerosis." Later this view was abandoned, since no correlation between these symptoms and arteriosclerotic changes in the brain could be detected. Nevertheless, it is tempting to suggest that the factor hypothesized above might reside in the blood vessels; possibly the small vessels may undergo changes which are not so readily detected with the microscope but may still interfere with the blood supply to the tissue.

Another, very interesting possible explanation of regional differences might be the existence of trophic factor(s), as discussed in Chapter 7 of this volume. Among possible trophic factors, neurotransmitters may also be considered. If neurotransmitters with general trophic functions do indeed exist, they may play a key role in age-related degenerative processes.

Turnover of Neurotransmitters

In the study referred to above little or no age dependence of the monoamine metabolites was found. For example, the reduction of 5-HT levels with age in the gyrus cinguli was not accompanied by any decrease in the metabolite 5-hydroxyindoleacetic acid. This acid actually showed an insignificant upward trend. Likewise, the age-related decrease in noradrenaline in the hippocampus was accompanied by an insignificant upward trend of its metabolite (3-methoxy-4-hydroxyphenylglycol). These observations suggest that the reduction of neurotransmitter levels is not necessarily accompanied by a corresponding decrease in neurotransmitter turnover. A similar discrepancy has previously been described in Parkinson's disease, where the decrease in striatal dopamine is generally more pronounced than the decrease in its metabolite homovanillic acid (Hornykiewicz, 1966). A plausible explanation of these phenomena is provided by the feedback control of monoaminergic neurons, which has been so amply documented in animal experiments. When a number of neurons within a nucleus such as the pars compacta of substantia nigra start to deteriorate and finally die, the remaining neurons are stimulated by means of feedback mechanisms to increase their synthesis and release of neurotransmitter. This may further reduce the transmitter level but will raise the level of transmitter metabolites.

In Carlsson et al. (1980), which incidentally was a joint effort of several different Swedish research laboratories, the monoamine oxidase activity was also measured. It was found that the B enzyme, but not the A enzyme, was strikingly age dependent; however, it was positively correlated with age. In fact, the activity of monoamine oxidase B shows a more striking age dependence than any other biochemical measure performed on brain tissue to date. The significance of this observation is not clear. The B enzyme, in contrast to the A enzyme, does not seem to be heavily involved in the metabolism of monoamine neurotransmitters. It primarily acts on substrates of doubtful physiologic significance, such as phenethylamine. Experimental data suggest that the B enzyme preferentially resides in glial cells (Student and Edwards, 1977) and that a selective increase in the B enzyme can be induced by nerve degeneration (Oreland et al., 1980; Fowler et al., 1979). The age dependence of the B enzyme may thus tentatively be interpreted as a sign of glial proliferation in response to nerve cell degeneration. Nevertheless, these observations may prove relevant for the possible therapeutic use of monoamine oxidase inhibitors in neurogeriatric cases.

Possible Mechanisms Underlying Selectivity

Nerve-cell death in senescence is obviously not a random phenomenon. Why are some nerve cells more susceptible to aging than others?

It has been proposed that those nerve cells which show a strong age dependence are vulnerable in a more general sense. For example, they are liable to damage in acute conditions affecting the energy metabolism of the brain, such as ischemia, hypoxia, hypoglycemia, and epileptic seizures (Siesjö, 1979). It has been suggested that anoxia as such is not an immediate causal factor, since cell damage following anoxia and ischemia may not occur until oxygen is again supplied. Oxidative reactions, leading for example to peroxidation of intracellular membranes by free radicals, have been suggested to be common denominators of nerve cell damage. This in turn may be induced by failure of protective mechanisms, serving to quench free radicals enzymatically, such as superoxide dismutase, catalase, and glutathione peroxidase, or capable of preventing oxidation or scavenging free radicals, by means of vitamins E and C and glutathione, for example.

According to this line of thinking, the selective vulnerability of certain nerve cells could be related to the intensity and nature of the intraneuronal metabolic processes. Aging may be hypothesized to come into the picture in various ways. Vascular damage may be one factor involved, lipofuscin granules ("age pigment") another—these granules have been reported to contain peroxidized lipid (for references, see Siesjö, 1979).

The apparently selective age-related vulnerability of catecholamine neurons may provide a special case. It has been shown that catecholamines can be cytotoxic, and actually mutagenic, under special conditions. A prerequisite for such activity has been shown to be the formation of semiquinones and quinones, which are the compounds mainly responsible for the toxic effects. These compounds are capable of forming covalent bonds with DNA, protein, and so forth. If the formation of these compounds, which incidentally occurs largely or entirely nonenzymatically, is prevented by means of an antioxidant, the toxic action is likewise prevented. The toxicity of the quinonoid compounds is further enhanced by the simultaneous formation of toxic oxygen species such as the superoxide anion (see Moldéus et al., 1983).

Since the various antioxidants present in body fluids are very efficient in preventing the formation of the quinonoid conversion products of the catecholamines, it may be questioned, as did Moldéus at al. (1983), whether these products are at all formed in the tissues. One argument strongly favors the view, however, that these compounds are indeed formed in certain sites, especially in nerve cells containing neuromelanin: the quinonoids are generally considered to be intermediates in neuromelanin formation. This provides some basis for the postulate that neuromelanin-containing nerve cells are committing suicide slowly over the years by manufacturing cytotoxic material. This may explain the selective age dependence of the neuromelanin-containing catecholaminergic neurons in the locus ceruleus and substantia nigra.

6-Hydroxydopamine is an interesting example of catecholamine toxicity. This compound is even more than dopamine subject to nonenzymatic oxidation ending up in melanin. When injected systemically it causes degeneration of adrenergic nerves. While the formation of toxic oxidation products should result in general cytotoxicity, the selective degeneration of adrenergic nerves is a consequence of a carrier-mediated uptake mechanism, by means of which catecholamines, including 6-hydroxydopamine, are concentrated in these particular nerves. When injected into the central nervous system, where it cannot reach otherwise, it is taken up by noradrenergic as well as dopaminergic neurons and causes them to degenerate (see Jonsson et al., 1975).

The higher cytotoxicity of 6-hydroxydopamine, when compared to the physiologic catecholamines, could be due to its remarkable liability to form oxidation products of quinonoid nature, making the various physiologic oxidation-preventive mechanisms insufficient. Theoretically, the cytotoxicity of dopamine could result from conversion of this compound into 6-hydroxydopamine. Although this reaction has been proposed to occur in vivo, resulting in cell damage, this remains to be demonstrated. Besides, it does not seem necessary to postulate this reaction to account for the cytotoxicity of dopamine. Nevertheless, the fact that 6-hydroxydopamine is overtly and selectively neurotoxic also in vivo lends some credibility to the above speculations on a corresponding, though much less severe, neurotoxicity of dopamine and noradrenaline.

Oxidative damage as the cause of the selective vulnerability of catecholamines neurons in relation to aging has also been recently proposed by Timiras et al. (1983), although these authors emphasized the role of toxic oxygen species rather than quinonoid compounds for the toxic reaction.

Further work is needed to decide whether oxidative reactions are indeed relevant for age-related nerve-cell degeneration and, if so, to what extent this will open up new possibilities for prevention, for example, by strengthening the protective mechanisms referred to above.

Functional Aspects

Despite our limited knowledge of the functional role of the various neurotransmitters, it would not be difficult to envisage a relationship between reduced neurotransmitter availability and age-related loss of brain function. For example, a decrease in dopamine function might well contribute to the loss of initiative and psychic energy as well as reduced motor capacity often seen in the aged. Likewise, the lowered mood frequently observed in the elderly could be at least partly due to diminished function of all the three major monoamines. Memory loss is often associated with a reduction of cholinergic function, which does indeed occur to some extent during normal aging, according to several studies, although it is less prominent than in dementia of the Alzheimer type, especially its presenile form. However, the monoamines are important regulators of wakefulness, which is a prerequisite for normal memory function, and may thus play a role also in this context.

It must not be forgotten that the aging brain may function quite well, at least under optimal conditions. This may be due to the remarkable ability of the nerve cells to compensate for neuronal loss, for example, by increasing the activity of the remaining neurons. As long as this compensation operates satisfactorily, the only consequence of nerve cell loss will be a reduction of reserve capacity, which may show up, for example, as the well-known age-related liability to delirium under stressful conditions. However, when the nerve-cell loss has reached a certain degree, the compensatory mechanisms do not suffice any more, and overt insufficiency develops. Epidemiologic studies indicate that the occurrence of severe dementia increases progressively above the age of 70 and may approach the 50% level at the age of 90–100 years (Adolfsson et al., 1981). Thus, provided that we live long enough, we will probably all end up in a demented state.

The demarcation between normal aging and various pathologic states, such as dementia, depression, and Parkinsonism, is not sharp. Are these conditions just exaggerations of the changes occurring in normal aging? This question cannot be answered as yet. Certainly many features of the senile brain disorders are reminiscent of normal aging. On the other hand, qualitative differences may exist. For example, whereas decay of cholinergic neurons is not a prominent feature in normal aging, it shows up as an important aspect of Alzheimer's disease. Likewise, the biochemical profile of Parkinson's disease differs from normal aging, for example, with respect to the general vulnerability of the basal ganglia: in Parkinson's disease the putamen is more affected than the caudate nucleus (Lloyd et al., 1975), whereas the reverse is true in normal aging. Therefore, Parkinson's disease may not simply be due to accelerated aging of dopaminergic neurons.

Given the apparently very efficient compensatory mechanisms referred to above, it is reasonable to assume that the degenerative age-related processes have proceeded over several years, perhaps even decades, before manifest symptoms arise. This implies that in the "normal" aged population a certain, probably rather high, percentage of individuals have ongoing changes which a number of years later will lead to manifest symptoms. In other words, the study of apparently normal aged individuals may give important information of the early changes that will ultimately result in manifest symptoms. This should apply especially to dementia, considering its high prevalence in the later decades of life. It therefore seems logical to suggest that the degenerative changes in catecholamine neurons, which appear to be so prominent in aging, may be looked upon as early signs, foreboding the changes in cholinergic and serotoninergic neurons, for example, that characteristically occur in cases of overt dementia.

How much neuronal loss can be tolerated without manifest symptoms? In the case of Parkinson's disease it has to be quite substantial, maybe some 80%, before symptoms arise. In the normal aged population the level of dopamine in the caudate nucleus starts to decrease at an elevated rate around the age of 65, and is reduced by 40–50% at the age of 90 years (Carlsson, 1981b). It should be noted that the presence or absence of symptoms may be due to the balance between different systems rather than the absolute strength of each system. Moreover, losses may be functionally additive. For example, the age-related loss of dopamine is accompanied by a reduction of postsynaptic dopamine receptors in the caudate nucleus. In that case symptoms may show up at less severe transmitter deficiencies.

Prophylaxis and Treatment of Age-Related Disorders

A rational approach to senile brain disorders will have to await a more precise mapping of the age-related losses of neurons and neurotransmitters. In theory, substitution therapy would appear possible, provided that the biochemical deficiency can be localized and identified, and that suitable agonists substituting for the missing neurotransmitters are available.

Even more intriguing is the prospect of prophylaxis. As indicated above, the selective vulnerability of certain neurons to aging may be due to mechanisms which are not necessarily inherent in the aging per se but rather may be superimposed on this process. If these mechanisms can be manipulated, the aging may occur with less imbalance between different neuronal systems. For example, if oxidative damage will indeed prove relevant for selective vulnerability, as discussed above, measures to increase the levels of physiologic antioxidants in the body fluids, or to otherwise support the protective mechanisms, should have a beneficial influence.

Hopefully some progress towards this end will have been made by the year 2000.

References

Adolfsson, R., Gottfries, C.-G., Nyström, L., and Winblad, B.: Prevalence of dementia in institutionalized Swedish old people. *Acta Psychiat. Scand. 63*, 225–244 (1981).

Brody, H.: Cell counts in cerebral cortex and brainstem. In Katzman, R., Terry, R.D., and Bick, K.L. (Eds.), Alzheimer's Disease: Senile Dementia and Related Disorders, Aging, Vol. 7, pp. 345–352. New York: Raven, 1975.

Carlsson, A.: Aging and brain neurotransmitters. In Crook, Th., and Gershon, S. (Eds.), Strategies for the Development of an Effective Treatment for Senile Dementia, pp. 93–106. New Canaan: Mark Powley, 1981.

Carlsson, A.: Aging and brain neurotransmitters. In Platt, D. (Ed.), Funktionsstörungen des Gehirns im Alter, pp. 67–81. Stuttgart–New York: F.K. Schattauer Verlag, 1981b.

Carlsson, A., Adolfsson, R., Aquilonius, S.-M., Gottfries, C.-G., Oreland, L., Svennerholm, L., and Winblad, B.: Biogenic amines in human brain in normal aging, senile dementia, and chronic alcoholism. In Goldstein, M., Calne, D.B., Lieberman, A., and Thorner, M.O. (Eds.), Ergot Compounds and Brain Function, Adv. in Biochem. Psychopharm., Vol. 23, pp. 295–304. New York: Raven, 1980.

Fowler, C.J., Oreland, L., Wiberg, Å., Carlsson, A., and Magnusson, T.: The inhibition of rat brain monoamine oxidase-B by J-508 (N-methyl-N-propargyl-(1-indanyl)-ammonium hydrochloride) and its use for the titration of this enzyme form. *Med. Biol.* 57, 406–411 (1979).

Goldman-Rakic, P.S., and Brown, R.M.: Regional changes of monoamines in cerebral cortex and subcortical structures of aging Rhesus monkeys. *Neuroscience 6*, 177–187 (1981).

Hornykiewicz, O.: Metabolism of brain dopamine in human Parkinsonism: Neurochemical and clinical aspects. In Costa, E., Coté, L.J., and Yahr, M.D. (Eds.), Biochemistry and Pharmacology of the Basal Ganglia, pp. 171–181. New York: Raven, 1966.

Jonsson, G., Malmfors, T., and Sachs, C. (Eds.): Chemical Tools in Catecholamine Research. I. 6-Hydroxydopamine as a Denervation Tool in Catecholamine Research, pp. 1–372. Amsterdam: North Holland, 1975.

Lloyd, K.G., Davidson, L., and Hornykiewicz, O.: The neurochemistry of Parkinson's disease: Effect of L-dopa therapy. *J. Pharmacol. Exp. Ther. 195*, 453–464 (1975).

Loew, D., and Singer, J.M.: Stimulants and senility. In Creese, J. (Ed.), Stimulants: Neurochemical, Behavioral, and Clinical Perspectives, pp. 237–268. New York: Raven, 1983.

McGeer, E.G.: Aging and neurotransmitter metabolism in the human brain. In Katzman, R., Terry, R.D., and Bick, K.L. (Eds.), Alzheimer's Disease: Senile Dementia and Related Disorders, pp. 427–440. New York: Raven, 1978.

Moldéus, P., Nordenskjöld, M., Bolcsfoldi, G., Eiche, A., Haglund, U., and Lambert, B.: Genetic toxicity of dopamine. *Mutation Res. 124*, 9–24 (1983).

Oreland, L., Fowler, C.J., Carlsson, A., and Magnusson, T.: Monoamine oxidase-A and -B activity in the rat brain after hemitransection. *Life Sci. 26*, 139–146 (1980).

Scheibel, A.B.: Structural aspects of the aging brain. In Katzman, R., Terry, R.D., and Bick, K.L. (Eds.), Alzheimer's Disease: Senile Dementia and Related Disorders, pp. 353–374. New York: Raven, 1978.

Severson, J.A., Marcusson, J., Winblad, B., and Finch, C.E.: Age-correlated loss of dopaminergic binding sites in human basal ganglia. *J. Neurochem. 39*, 1623–1631 (1982).

Siesjö, B.: Mechanisms of cellular damage in the brain. In Hoffmeister, F. and Müller, C. (Eds.), Bayer Symposium VII. Brain Function in Old Age, pp. 381–384. Berlin: Springer-Verlag, 1979.

Student, A.K., and Edwards, D.J.: Subcellular localization of types A and B monoamine oxidase in rat brain. *Biochem. Pharmacol. 26*, 2337–2342 (1977).

Timiras, P.S., Cole, G., Croteau, M., Hudson, D.B., Miller, C., and Segall, P.E.: Changes in brain serotonin with aging and modification through precursor availability. In Agnoli, A., Crepaldi, G., Spano, P.F., and Trabucchi, M. (Eds.), Aging, Vol. 23, pp. 23–26. New York: Raven, 1983.

Chapter 10

Neuropeptides in Human Aging and Dementia

Martin M. Rossor

Summary

Large numbers of neuronally localized peptides have been discovered which act as neurotransmitters or neuromodulators. Many are stable postmortem and can be measured in routine autopsy samples. Minor decreases in neuropeptide concentrations may be seen with age but they have not been studied in detail. A somatostatin deficit is the most consistent peptide abnormality in dementia and is found in the cerebral cortex of patients with Alzheimer's disease and of those with Parkinson's disease with a coexistent dementia. Since somatostatin is found within cerebral cortical neurons, the deficit may reflect selectivity of cortical neuronal damage in these diseases.

Introduction

The last decade has seen the dramatic discovery of neuronally localized peptides which appear to act as neurotransmitters or neuromodulators. More than 40 neuropeptides have now been described in mammalian brain and the total number is likely to be well in excess of that figure (Snyder, 1980). Many peptides can be released by depolarizing stimuli, and can be demonstrated to have potent postsynaptic effects and interactions with specific receptor sites consistent with a neurotransmitter role. (For review see Snyder, 1980; Krieger and Martin, 1981; Iversen, 1982).

Neuropeptides have characteristic anatomical distributions within the central nervous system established both by regional dissection and radioimmunoassay, and by immunohistochemistry, although many peptides coexist with other peptides and with classical neurotransmitters. The anatomy of peptides systems has, for obvious reasons, been determined largely in animals, but peptides can be measured by radioimmunoassay in routine postmortem tissue and the majority have now also been demonstrated in human brain. The remarkable postmortem stability of peptides in brain contrasts with the liability in plasma which may relate to the localization within synaptic vesicles (Emson et al., 1980). Similarly, for many peptides immunostaining can be performed on routine fresh autopsy material and formalin-fixed tissue. In both animal and human studies the use of immunological techniques introduces the problem of specificity and the nature of immunoreactivity should be confirmed by alternative physicochemical techniques. In strict usage the term peptide-like immunoreactivity should be used, but for the sake of clarity this has been omitted from this text.

Some peptides have been related to particular functions such as substance P and enkephalins in pain transmission in the spinal cord, but in general the physiologic functions of peptides are obscure. However, although changes in peptides cannot be readily related to abnormal function, the regional specificity and neuronal localization make peptides useful cellular markers. Both normal aging and degenerative disease are characterized histologically by selectivity of neuronal loss and this specificity can be explored further by measuring neurotransmitter and peptide systems.

Neuropeptides in the Aging Brain

Aging may be defined as the decline in function from maturity to senescence and a feature of this in the nervous system is the progressive loss of neurons. However, the loss of neurons is selective since cerebral cortical neurons (Henderson et al., 1980) and cerebellar Purkinje cells (Hall et al., 1975) decline in number but neuron counts in the trochlear nuclei (Vijayashankar and Brody, 1973) and certain other brain stem nuclei remain stable throughout life. The selectivity of neuronal loss may not necessarily have a neurotransmitter correlate, although changes in the dopaminergic (McGeer et al., 1977) and cholinergic systems (Bartus et al., 1982) have been related to motor and cognitive declines with aging. At the present time there are no obvious peptide correlates of neuronal loss or functional decline with aging, although there have been a few studies which have specifically addressed this question. Some studies of the normal distribution of peptides or of comparisons of control groups with disease groups have also analyzed the peptide data as a function of the

Table 10-1. Summary of changes in peptide immunoreactivities in normal aging

	SRIF	CCK	VIP	ENK	SP	NT
Cerebral cortex	NS[1,2,3]	NS[4,5]	NS[4,5]	NS[6]	NS[2]	NS[2]
Striatum	NS[1,2]	NS[4]	NS[5]	NS[7]	NS[2,7,8]	NS[2]

NS = no statistically significant ($p > 0.05$) change; SRIF = somatostatin; CCK = cholecystokinin; VIP = vasoactive intestinal polypeptide; ENK = (met) enkephalin; SP = substance P; NT = neurotensin.

[1]Rossor et al. (1980b).

[2]Cooper et al. (1981).

[3]Davies and Terry (1981).

[4]Rossor et al. (1982b).

[5]Perry et al. (1981).

[6]Rossor et al. (1982d).

[7]Emson et al. (1980).

[8]Buck et al. (1981).

age of the patient. The results of some of these studies are summarized in Table 10-1.

In general these studies have not demonstrated major changes in concentrations of peptide immunoreactivities, although trends are towards a decline in the concentration. One drawback of many studies is that they have not been undertaken to assess specifically age-related changes and cover restricted age ranges and often involve only small numbers. Combined histological, immunohistochemical, and radioimmunoassay studies may be required to resolve many of the peptide correlates of central nervous system aging.

Cholecystokinin, vasoactive intestinal polypeptide and somatostatin are all found within cortical neurons (for review see Emson and Hunt, 1981) and there is additional evidence that neuropeptide Y may coexist with somatostatin in some cortical cells (Vincent et al., 1982). Cholecystokinin and vasoactive intestinal polypeptide are unchanged (Rossor et al., 1982b) although some alterations in cholecystokinin have been found in the more severe cases (Perry et al., 1983). In contrast, somatostatin has been found to be reduced in a number of studies (Davies et al., 1980; Rossor et al., 1980b; Perry et al., 1983); the greatest reduction is found in the temporal lobe, although widespread deficits were found by Davies et al. (1980).

The extent of the somatostatin deficit appears to be age related in that the abnormality is confined to the temporal lobe in the older at-death cases (Rossor et al., 1984). An age influence can also be discerned for the other neurotransmitter abnormalities. Thus in the older at-death patients the cholinergic abnormality spares the frontal cortex (Rossor et al., 1982c) and changes in GABA and noradrenaline are confined to the younger patient (Rossor et al., 1984); it is of interest that reductions in ChAT activity and somatostatin immunoreactivity are found in the temporal cortex irrespective of the age of death.

Peptides have also been examined in the dementias of Parkinson's disease and Huntington's disease. A proportion of patients with Parkinson's disease develop a dementia and in some, but by no means all, the histopathological features of Alzheimer's disease are found in the cerebral cortex. In those Parkinsonian patients with dementia Epelbaum et al. (1983) report losses of both somatostatin and ChAT activity from the frontal cortex.

Neuropeptides in Dementia

As with normal aging neuronal damage in Alzheimer's disease is relatively selective. The major neurotransmitter abnormality in this disease is found in the ascending cholinergic projection to the cerebral cortex. The loss of the cholinergic marker enzyme, choline acetyltransferase, from the cerebral cortex is now well established and can be related to damage to the ascending projection from the basal forebrain (for reviews see Rossor, 1982; Coyle et al., 1983). Loss of cells from the nucleus basalis of Meynert, the origin of the cholinergic projection, has been described (Whitehouse et al., 1982). Damage to the similar noradrenergic and serotonergic projections from the brain stem has also been demonstrated on neurochemical and histological grounds (Adolfsson et al., 1979; Bondareff et al., 1981; Cross et al., 1983; Mann and Yates, 1983).

Demonstration of abnormalities in these ascending systems has directed attention to subcortical structures in Alzheimer's disease, although analysis of peptides has not revealed any obvious abnormalities (Table 10-2). Vasopressin is of interest because of the reported effects in avoidance behavior paradigms in animals (De Wied, 1980). The peptide is found in a number of subcortical areas outside the neurohypophyseal system, including relatively high concentrations in the locus coeruleus (Sofroniew and Weindl, 1981), but no substantial changes are found in either Alzheimer's disease or Parkinson's disease (Rossor et al., 1980a, 1982a).

The observed abnormalities in the subcortical cholinergic and monoaminergic systems contrast with the localization of the main histological abnormalities to the cerebral cortex. Not only is there an abundance of senile plaques and neurofibrillary tangles but there is also good evidence for loss of cortical neurons (Terry et al., 1981; Mountjoy et al., 1983). An important question is whether the formation of tangles and loss of cells is specific to any particular group of cortical neurons. One approach is to

Table 10-2. Summary of changes in subcortical peptide immunoreactivities in Alzheimer's disease

Somatostatin	No change[1]
	↓ in hypothalamus[2]
Cholecystokinin	No change[3]
VIP	No change[3]
Neurotensin	↓ in amygdala (severe cases)[4,5]
TRH	No change[5,6]
LHRH	No change[6]
Substance P	No change[6]
met-ENK	No change[7]
Vasopressin	No change[8]

VIP = Vasoactive intestinal polypeptide; TRH = thyrotropin-releasing hormone; LHRH = luteinizing hormone-releasing hormone; met-ENK = met-enkephalin.

[1]Rossor et al. (1980b).

[2]Davies and Terry (1981).

[3]Rossor et al. (1982b).

[4]Perry et al. (1981).

[5]Biggins et al. (1983).

[6]Yates et al. (1983).

[7]Rossor et al. (1982d).

[8]Rossor et al. (1980a).

analyze neurotransmitters which are intrinsic to the cerebral cortex, and a number of peptides fulfill this role.

In Huntington's disease the major peptide changes occur in the striatonigral system where there are losses of met-enkephalin, cholecystokinin, and substance P (Emson et al., 1981) but, in contrast, dramatic increases in somatostatin (Aronin et al., 1983). Although shrinkage of the frontal lobes is often found in Huntington's disease, and is believed to relate to the dementia, there are no consistent changes in neurotransmitters, including cortical peptides, in this area.

Conclusion

Although reproducible changes can be observed in peptide immunoreactivities in aging and dementia the interpretation can be uncertain. First, there is the problem of the relationship of immunoreactivity to authentic peptide already referred to. A further problem is the interpretation of concentrations in the presence of shrinkage of tissue compartments, and finally, the relationship of loss of peptide to neuronal loss is unknown. In the presence of neuronal damage it is tempting to relate loss of peptide directly to loss of perikarya or processes, but altered levels within surviving neurons are an alternative explanation.

The most consistent peptide abnormality in dementia is that of somatostatin. It is of interest that a somatostatin deficit is found in Alzheimer's disease and Parkinson's disease with dementia, both of which have reductions in cortical ChAT activity, although there is no evidence of coexistence of somatostatin and ChAT in the same neurons (McKinney et al., 1982). In Alzheimer's disease the somatostatin deficit might relate to the observed loss of cortical neurons and thus reflect selectivity of the cell damage. However, although the concept of neurotransmitter-specific degenerative disease has been useful in Parkinson's disease, there is no particular reason why the neurotransmitter characteristics of a neuron should determine its vulnerability to damage and it remains to be seen how generally applicable the concept may be. Analysis of neuron-specific peptides is a useful means of addressing this question in aging and dementia.

References

Adolfsson, R., Gottfries, C.G., Roos, B.E., and Winblad, B.: Changes in brain catecholamines in patients with dementia of Alzheimer type. *Brit. J. Psychiat.* *135*, 216–223 (1979).

Aronin, N., Cooper, P.E., Lorenz, L.J., Bird, E.D., Sagar, S.M., Leeman, S.E., and Martin, J.B.: Somatostatin is increased in the basal ganglia in Huntington's disease. *Ann. Neurol.* *13*, 519–526 (1983).

Bartus, R.T., Dean, R.L., Beer, B., and Lippa, A.S.: The cholinergic hypothesis of geriatric memory dysfunction. *Science, 217*, 408–417 (1982).

Biggins, J.A., Perry, E.K., McDermott, J.R., Smith, A.I., Perry, R.H., and Edwardson, J.A.: Post-mortem levels of thyrotropic releasing hormone and neurotensin in the amygdala in Alzheimer's disease, schizophrenia and depression. *J. Neurol. Sci.* *58*, 117–122 (1983).

Bondareff, W., Mountjoy, C.Q., and Roth, M.: Loss of neurons of origin of the adrenergic projection to cerebral cortex (nucleus locus coeruleus) in senile dementia. *Neurology, 32*, 164–168 (1982).

Buck, S.H., Yamamura, H.I., Burks, T.F., and Rossor, M.: Substance P levels in the mammalian CNS in ageing. *Soc. Neurosci.* *7*, 605 (1981).

Cooper, P.E., Fernstrom, M.H., Rorstad, O.P., Leeman, S.E., and Martin, J.B.: The regional distribution of somatostatin, substance P and neurotensin in human brain. *Brain Research, 218*, 219–232 (1981).

Coyle, J.T., Price, D.L., and De Long, M.R.: Alzheimer's disease: a disorder of cortical cholinergic innervation. *Science, 219*, 1184–1190 (1983).

Cross, A.J., Crow, T.J., Johnson, J.A., Joseph, M.H., Perry, E.K., Perry, R.H., Blessed, G., and Tomlinson, B.E.: Monoamine metabolism in senile dementia of Alzheimer type. *J. Neurol. Sci.* *60*, 383–392 (1983).

De Wied, D.: Behavioural actions of neurohypophyseal peptides. *Proc. Roy. Soc. B.* *210*, 183–195 (1980).

Davies, P., Katzman, R., and Terry, R.D.: Reduced somatostatin-like immunoreactivity in cerebral cortex from cases of Alzheimer's disease and Alzheimer senile dementia. *Nature 288*, 279–280 (1980).

Davies, P., Terry, R.D.: Cortical somatostatin-like immunoreactivity in cases of Alzheimer's disease and senile dementia of the Alzheimer type. *Neurobiol. Ageing, 2*, 9–14 (1981).

Emson, P.C., Arregui, A., Clement-Jones, V., Sandberg, B.E.B., and Rossor, M.: Regional distribution of methionine-enkephalin and substance P-like immunoreactivity in normal human brain and in Huntington's disease. *Brain Research 199*, 147–160 (1980).

Emson, P.C., and Hunt, S.P.: Anatomical chemistry of the cerebral cortex. In Schmitt, F.O., Warden, F.C., Adelman, G., and Dennis, S.G. (Eds.), The Organization of the Cerebral Cortex, N.R.P. Colloquim, pp. 325–345. Cambridge: MIT Press, 1981.

Emson, P.C., Rossor, M.N., Hunt, S.P., Marley, P.D., Clement-Jones, V., Rehfeld, J., and Fahrenkrug, J.: Distribution and post-mortem stability of substance P, met-enkephalin, vasoactive intestinal polypeptide and cholecystokinin in normal human brain and Huntington's disease. In Rose, F.C. (Ed.), Metabolic Disorders of the Nervous System, pp. 312–321. Marshfield, MA, Pitman Publishing, Inc., 1981.

Epelbaum, J., Rubert, M., Moyse, E., Javoy-Agid, F., Dubois, B., and Agid, Y.: Somatostatin and dementia in Parkinson's disease. *Brain Research 278*, 376–379 (1983).

Hall, T.C., Miller, A.K.H., and Corsellis, J.A.N.: Variations in the human Purkinje cell population according to age and sex. *Neuropath. Appl. Neurobiol. 1*, 267–292 (1975).

Henderson, G., Tomlinson, B.E., and Gibson, P.H.: Cell counts in human cerebral cortex in normal adults throughout life using an image analysing computer. *J. Neurol. Sci. 46*, 113–136 (1980).

Iversen, L.L.: Neurotransmitters and CNS disease. *Lancet ii*, 914–918 (1982).

Krieger, D.T., and Martin, J.B.: Brain peptides. *New Eng. J. Med. 304*, 876–885, 944–951 (1981).

Mann, D.M.A., and Yates, P.O.: Serotonin nerve cells in Alzheimer's disease. *J. Neurol. Neurosurg. Psychiat. 46*, 96–98 (1983).

McGeer, P.L., McGeer, E.G., and Suzuki, J.S.: Ageing and extrapyramidal function. *Arch. Neurol. 34*, 33–35 (1977).

McKinney, M., Davies, P., and Coyle, J.T.: Somatostatin in not co-localized in cholinergic neurons innervating the cerebral cortex-hippocampal formation. *Brain Research 243*, 169 (1982).

Mountjoy, C.Q., Roth, M., Evans, N.J.R., and Evans, H.M.: Cortical neuronal counts in normal elderly controls and demented patients. *Neurobiol. Ageing 4*, 1–11 (1983).

Perry, E.K., Blessed, G., Tomlinson, B.E., Perry, R.H., Crow, T.J., Cross, A.J., Dockray, G.J., Dimaline, R., and Arregui, A.: Neurochemical activities in human temporal lobe related to ageing and Alzheimer-type changes. *Neurobiol. Ageing 2*, 251–256 (1981).

Perry, R.H., Candy, J.M., and Perry, E.K.: Some observations and speculations concerning the cholinergic system and neuropeptides in Alzheimer's disease. In Katzman, R. (Ed.), Biological Aspects of Alzheimer's Disease, pp. 351–361. Cold Spring Harbor, 1983.

Rossor, M.N.: Neurotransmitters and CNS disease: Dementia. *Lancet ii*, 1200–1204 (1982).

Rossor, M.N., Iversen, L.L., Roth, M., Hawthorn, J., Ang, V.T.Y., and Jenkins, J.S.: Arginine vasopressin and choline acetyltransferase in brains of patients with Alzheimer type senile dementia. *Lancet ii*, 1367–1368 (1980a).

Rossor, M.N., Emson, P.C., Mountjoy, C.Q., Roth, M., and Iversen, L.L.: Reduced amounts of immunoreactive somatostatin in the temporal cortex in senile dementia of Alzheimer type. *Neurosci. Lett. 20*, 373–377 (1980b).

Rossor, M.N., Hunt, S.P., Iversen, L.L., Bannister, R., Hawthorn, J., Ang, V.T.Y., and Jenkins, J.S.: Extrahypothalamic vasopressin is unchanged in Parkinson's disease and Huntington's disease. *Brain Research 253*, 341–343 (1982a).

Rossor, M.N., Emson, P.C., Iversen, L.L., Mountjoy, C.Q., Roth, M., Fahrenkrug, J., and Rehfeld, J.F.: Neuropeptides and neurotransmitters in cerebral cortex in Alzheimer's disease. In Corkin, S. et al. (Eds.), Alzheimer's disease: A report of progress, Ageing, Vol 19, pp. 15–24. New York: Raven, 1982b.

Rossor, M.N., Garrett, N.J., Johnson, A.L., Mountjoy, C.Q., Roth, M., and Iversen, L.L.: A post-mortem study of the cholinergic and GABA systems in senile dementia. *Brain 105*, 313–330 (1982c).

Rossor, M.N., Emson, P.C., Mountjoy, C.Q., Roth, M., and Iversen, L.L.: Neurotransmitters of the cerebral cortex in senile dementia of Alzheimer Type. In Hoyer, S. (Ed.), The Ageing Brain, Physiological and Pathophysiological Aspects, pp. 153–157. New York: Springer-Verlag, 1982d.

Rossor, M.N., Iversen, L.L., Reynolds, G.P., Mountjoy, C.Q., and Roth, M.: Early and late onset types of Alzheimer's disease are neurochemically distinct. *Brit. Med. J.* (in press).

Snyder, S.H.: Brain peptides as neurotransmitters. *Science 209*, 976–983 (1980).

Sofroniew, M.V., Weindl, A.: Central nervous system distribution of vasopressin, oxytocin and neurophysin. In Martinez, J.L. et al. (Eds.), Endogenous Peptides and Learning and Memory Processes. New York: Academic, 1981.

Terry, R.D., Peck, A., De Teresa, R., Schechter, R., and Horoupian, D.S.: Some morphometric aspects of the brain in senile dementia of the Alzheimer type. *Ann. Neurol. 10*, 184–192 (1981).

Vijayashanker, N., and Brody, H.: The neuronal population of the nuclei of the trochlear nerve and the locus coeruleus in the human. *Anat. Rec. 172*, 421–422 (1973).

Vincent, S.R., Johansson, O., Hölkefelt, T., Meyerson, B., Sachs, C., Elde, R.P., Terenius, L., and Kimmel, J.: Neuropeptide coexistence in human cortical neurons. *Nature 298*, 65–67 (1982).

Whitehouse, P.J., Price, D.L., Struble, R.G., Clark, A.W., Coyle, J.T., and De Long, M.R.: Alzheimer's disease and senile dementia: loss of neurons in the basal forebrain. *Science 215*, 1237–1239 (1982).

Yates, C.M., Harmer, A.J., Rosie, R., Sheward, J., Sanchez de Levy, G., Simpson, J., Maloney, A.F.J., Gordon, A., Fink, G.: Thyrotropin-releasing hormone, luteinizing hormone-releasing hormone and substance P immunoreactivity in post-mortem brain from cases of Alzheimer-type dementia and Down's syndrome. *Brain Research 258*, 45–52 (1983).

Chapter 11

Receptor-Mediated Alterations of Central Monoaminergic Transmission in Aged Wistar Rats

Wolfgang Kehr, Helmut Wachtel, and Karin Kurth

Summary

The in vivo release of brain catecholamines, the efficiency of feedback mechanisms controlling central catecholaminergic transmission, and the responsiveness of brain dopamine (DA) receptors to agonists and antagonists were studied in adult and senescent rats of the Wistar strain. After inhibition of monoamine oxidase the accumulation of 3-methoxy tyramine and normetanephrine was reduced in the forebrain of senescent animals despite elevated DA and NA levels indicating impaired catecholamine (CA) release. Consonantly, the locomotor stimulatory effect of the indirect CA agonist D-amphetamine was reduced in aged animals. However, the less pronounced hyperactivity induced by the direct DA agonists lisuride and propyl-transdihydrolisuride (propyl-TDHL) in senescent rats indicates decreased responsiveness of postsynaptic mesolimbic DA receptor as an additional causative factor. Apparently the responsiveness of postsynaptic nigrostriatal DA receptors is not altered by senescence as judged from the equal efficacy in adult and aged animals of haloperidol to cause catalepsy or of propyl-TDHL to induce stereotypies. Receptor-mediated feedback mechanisms controlling dopamine synthesis and metabolism appeared to be dampened in the senescent rats studied. The increase of dihydroxyphenylacetic acid induced by haloperidol as well as the stimulation of dopa synthesis induced by γ-butyrolactone was attenuated in senescent rats. In addition, the affinity of agonists to dopamine autoreceptors appeared to be reduced.

Introduction

There is an increasing body of evidence in humans that aging is associated with an impairment of dopaminergic, noradrenergic, serotonergic, and cholinergic transmission (Carlsson and Winblad, 1976; Gottfries and Winblad, 1980). Similar findings have been reported for rodents (Finch, 1973; McGeer et al., 1971; McGeer and McGeer, 1976; Meek et al., 1977; Samorajski, 1975). However, in our own studies on Wistar rats there was no indication for an age-related decrease of monoamine levels but rather an age-related increase of 5-hydroxytryptamine (5-HT) and noradrenaline levels was observed (Kehr, 1983). Also, noradrenaline and 5-HT synthesis were elevated in brain tissue of senescent Wistar rats, while dopamine synthesis was slightly reduced or unchanged, depending on the gender of the animals. These observation indicated that aging is not necessarily associated with degeneration of monoaminergic neurons or with a general impairment of monoamine synthesis or storage, and that with regard to aging in rats major strain differences appear to exist.

The present investigation aimed at elucidating the in vivo release of catecholamines, the responsiveness of postsynaptic neurons to dopamine receptor agonists and antagonists, as well as feedback mechanisms controlling catecholaminergic transmission in senescent rats of the Wistar strain. Furthermore, effects of a new and potent dopamine agonistic ergoline derivative with a long duration of action (Wachtel, 1983; Kehr et al., 1983) 6-*n*-propyl-transdihydrolisuride (propyl-TDHL) in adult and senescent rats will be described.

Material and Methods

Animals and Treatment Schedules

Male retired breeders or female Wistar rats bred at Schering AG, Berlin (originally derived from the Zentralinstitut für Versuchstierkunde, Hannover), or unexperienced young or adult rats of the same strain, were used in all experiments. Rats of the age of 26 months or older were considered aged or senescent, since the 50% survival point of the Wistar strain under investigation was found to be at 26 months of age (Kehr, 1983). The animals were kept under a constant light/dark cycle (light period from 6 A.M. to 6 P.M.) at an ambient temperature of 20–21 °C. They had free access to a standard diet (Altromin-R) and water. Drugs were administered intraperitoneally in a volume of 5 ml/kg body weight. Doses refer to the corresponding base. Control animals received the corresponding vehicle.

Drugs and Solutions

The following drugs were used: lisuride hydrogen maleate [lisuride; 3-(9,10-didehydro-6-methyl-8α-ergolinyl)-1,1-diethyl urea hydrogen maleate; Spofa, Prague, Czechoslovakia]; propyl-THDL tartrate [1,1-diethyl-3-(6-n-propyl-8α-ergolinyl) urea tartrate] prepared by Dr. G. Sauer, Department of Medicinal Chemistry, Schering AG, Berlin, Germany; γ-butyrolactone (Riedel-de Häen, Seelze, Germany); 3-hydroxybenzyl-hydrazine HCl (NSD 1015; Sandev Ltd., Harlow/Essex, England); apomorphine HCl (Sandoz AG, Basel, Switzerland); (+)-amphetamine sulfate (Merck AG, Darmstadt, Germany); haloperidol (Janssen AG, Düsseldorf, Germany); and pargyline HCl (Abbott, Chicago, U.S.A.). Haloperidol was suspended in isotonic saline solution with addition of 10% Cremofor EL (BASF, Ludwigshafen, Germany). All other drugs were dissolved in isotonic saline solution.

Behavioral Tests

Stereotyped behavior was determined according to Horowski and Wachtel (1976). Thirty min after i.p. administration of propyl-TDHL the animals were observed for 2 min for the presence of stereotyped behavior (continuous sniffing, licking, or gnawing movements for more than 30 sec within this time) by an experienced observer unaware of the previous treatment.

Locomotor activity was measured using infrared-light photocell motility meters (M/P 40 Fc; Motron Products, Stockholm, Sweden) as described by Modigh (1972). Every interruption of the photocell beam was recorded as one count. Individual rats were placed in a motility cage and the counts accumulating over 10 min intervals were recorded for up to 120 min.

Catalepsy was measured 120 min after i.p. administration of haloperidol by gently placing the animals' hind limbs on the upper plateau of a plastic step (height 6 cm, width 18 cm) and recording the time before the animals put both paws on the floor. Animals remaining in this imposed posture for $>$ 5 sec were considered cataleptic.

Motor coordination was assessed on a rotating rod essentially as described by Dunham and Miya (1957) and as modified by Jänicke (1982). Rats were trained to stay for $\geq$ 120 sec on a rod which was rotated at a speed of 20 rpm.

Biochemical Methods

Dopamine synthesis in rat striatum in vivo was assessed by measuring the accumulation of dopa following inhibiton of the aromatic amino acid decarboxylase with 3-hydroxybenzylhydrazine HCl (NSD 1015; 100 mg/kg i.p. 30 min before death) as described by Carlsson et al. (1972).

Catecholamine release was evaluated in rat brain in vivo by measuring the accumulation of 3-methoxytyramine and normetanephrine during 60 min after inhibiton of monoamine oxidase with pargyline, 75 or 150 mg/kg i.p. as described by Kehr (1981).

Dihydroxyphenylacetic acid (DOPAC) levels were measured in the dopamine-rich parts of the limbic system (n. accumbens, n. amygdaoideus centralis, olfactory tubercles, parts of the paleocortex) and the striatum by a radioenzymatic method described by Thiede and Kehr (1981).

Serum prolactin levels were determined using the radioimmunoassay kit for rat prolactin kindly provided by NIAMDD. Following decapitation blood from the trunk was collected in centrifuge tubes, allowed to clot at 4 °C, and centrifuged at 3000 g for 10 min. Serum was removed and stored at −20 °C until assay.

Lisuride levels in rat serum were determined by a radioimmunoassay as described by Hümpel et al. (1981).

Results

Catecholamine Release in Vivo as a Function of Age

3-Methoxytyramine and normetanephrine accumulating after inhibition of monoamine oxidase with pargyline served as indicators of dopamine and noradrenaline release in brains of 2-, 21-, and 30-month-old male rats. Parygline was injected i.p. at doses of 75 or 150 mg/kg 60 min before sacrifice. Both doses resulted in a comparable accumulation of the catecholamines among the various age groups (Table 11-1). However, despite high dopamine and noradrenaline levels, the accumulation of 3-methoxytyramine at 21 and 30 months of age was up to 40%, and the accumulation of normetanephrine up to 60%, lower than at 2 months of age (Table 11-1).

Effect of (+)-Amphetamine and Lisuride on Locomotor Activity

(+)-Amphetamine at a dose of 1.56 mg/kg s.c. stimulated locomotor activity markedly in young 2-month-old rats (Fig. 11-1). The stimulatory effect reached a maximum 50 min after drug administration. In 26-month-old rats the stimulatory effect was less pronounced. A maximum was reached at 40 min and the effect was shorter lasting as compared to the young animals. It has to be taken into consideration, however, that exploratory motility was very low in vehicle-treated 26-month-old control rats. The direct dopamine receptor agonist lisuride showed a biphasic effect on locomotor activity of 2-month-old rats (Fig. 11-2). At a dose of 0.1 mg/kg s.c. lisuride reduced exploratory motility during the first 20 min and stimulated locomotor activity between 40 and 120 min postappli-

Table 11-1. 3-Methoxytyramine (3-MT) and normetanephrine accumulation in forebrain of 2, 21, and 30-month-old male Wistar rats

	Dopamine (nmol/g)	3-MT (pmol/g)	Noradrenaline (nmol/g)	Normetanephrine (pmol/g)
2 months				
control	7.77 ± 0.13	n.d.	2.40 ± 0.09	n.d.
pargyline 75 mg/kg	9.54 ± 0.12[a]	380 ± 36	3.62 ± 0.14[b]	227 ± 39
pargyline 150 mg/kg	8.97 ± 0.10	387 ± 26	3.13 ± 0.10[a]	373 ± 25
21 months				
control	8.69 ± 0.44	n.d.	2.05 ± 0.09	n.d.
pargyline 75 mg/kg	10,04 ± 0.43	282 ± 24[d]	2.92 ± 0.11[b]	76 ± 46[c]
pargyline 150 mg/kg	9.74 ± 0.30	231 ± 30[d]	3.24 ± 0.07[b]	149 ± 27[d]
30 months				
control	8.23 ± 0.29	n.d.	3.23 ± 0.21[d]	n.d.
pargyline 75 mg/kg	10.27 ± 0.74[a]	301 ± 26[c]	4.54 ± 0.16[bd]	130 ± 12
pargyline 150 mg/kg	9.34 ± 0.46	242 ± 18[d]	4.47 ± 0.12[bd]	218 ± 44[c]

Pargyline was administered i.p. 60 min before death. Shown are the means ± S.E.M.; $n = 4$, each comprising forebrains of two rats. Statistics: analysis of variance, Tukey test: (a) $p < 0.05$, (b) $p < 0.01$ vs. respective age control, (c) $p < 0.05$, (d) $p < 0.01$ vs. respective treatment group of 2-month-old rats.

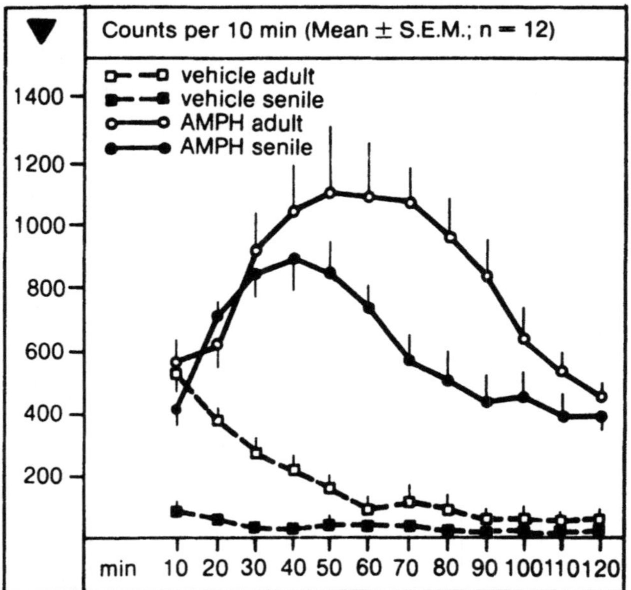

ANOVA/ Tukey test	10	20	30	40	50	60	70	80	90	100	110	120
□ vs ■	**	**										
○ vs □		**	**	**	**	**	**	**	**	**	**	**
○ vs ■	**	**	**	**	**	**	**	**	**	**	**	**
● vs □		**	**	**	**	**	**	**	**	**	**	**
● vs ■	**	**	**	**	**	**	**	**	**	**	**	**
○ vs ●	*					*	**	**	**			

* $p < 0.05$ ** $p < 0.01$

Figure 11-1. Effect of amphetamine (AMPH; 1.56 mg/kg s.c.) upon locomotor activity of adult (2-month-old) or senile (26-month-old) male rats.

cation. In 26-month-old rats the same dose of lisuride induced only a monophasic increase in locomotor activity. The increase was not as marked as in young rats. Lisuride-treated senescent animals showed about the same locomotor activity as young control rats.

Effect of Apomorphine and Lisuride on Striatal Dopamine Autoreceptors

Impulse generation in dopaminergic neurons was blocked by the administration of γ-butyrolactone, 750 mg/kg i.p., and dopamine synthesis was evaluated by measuring the accumulation of dopa following inhibition of the aromatic amino acid decarboxylase with NSD 1015, 100 mg/kg i.p. As shown in Figure 11-3 the stimulatory effect of γ-butyrolactone on striatal dopa accumulation of 35-month-old rats was less pronounced as compared to 2-month-old rats. However, the basal rate of dopa accumulation

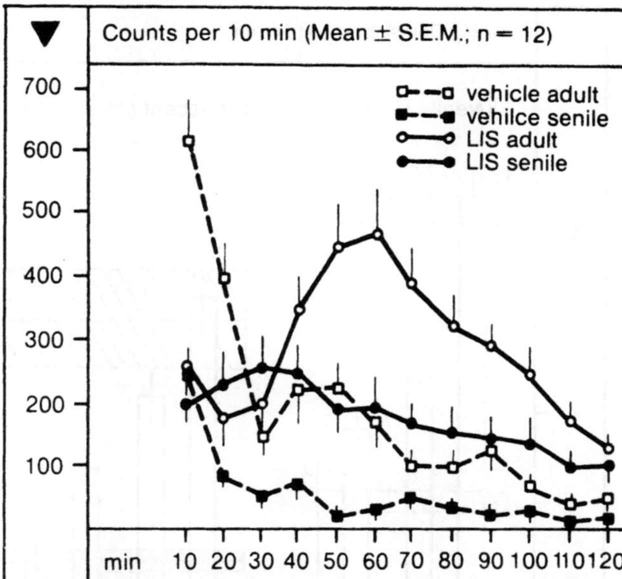

ANOVA/ Tukey test	10	20	30	40	50	60	70	80	90	100	110	120
□ vs ■	**	**	**	*	**							
○ vs □	**	**			**	**	**	**	**	**	**	
○ vs ■			**	**	**	**	**	**	**	**	**	*
● vs □	**	**										
● vs ■		*	**	*	*	*		*	*	*	*	
○ vs ●					**	**	**	**	**	*	*	

* $p < 0.05$ ** $p < 0.01$

Figure 11-2. Effect of lisuride (LIS; 0.1 mg/kg s.c.) upon locomotor activity of adult (2-month-old) or senile (26-month-old) male rats.

in striatum of senescent rats was 23% lower than in striatum of 2-month-old rats.

At the low dose of 0.05 mg/kg apomorphine had no effect on the γ-butyrolactone-induced increase of dopa. At the 0.5 mg/kg dose apomorphine reduced the effect of γ-butyrolactone on dopa in 2-month-old rats but not in 35-month-old rats. The inhibitory effect of lisuride 0.03 and 0.1 mg/kg on dopa accumulation of γ-butyrolactone-treated animals was similar in 2-month and 35-month-old rats. In this connection, however, attention has to be drawn to a separate experiment in which lisuride levels have been determined in serum of 2- and 33-month-old male rats 35 min after an injection of lisuride, 0.1 mg/kg i.p. and 30 min after NSD 1015, 100 mg/kg i.p. Serum levels in 2-month-old rats were 57 ± 4 nmol/l (mean ± S.E.M., $n = 12$; body weight 207 ± 2 g) and in 35-month-old rats 155 ± 18 nmol/l (mean ± S.E.M., $n = 12$; body weight 463 ± 9 g).

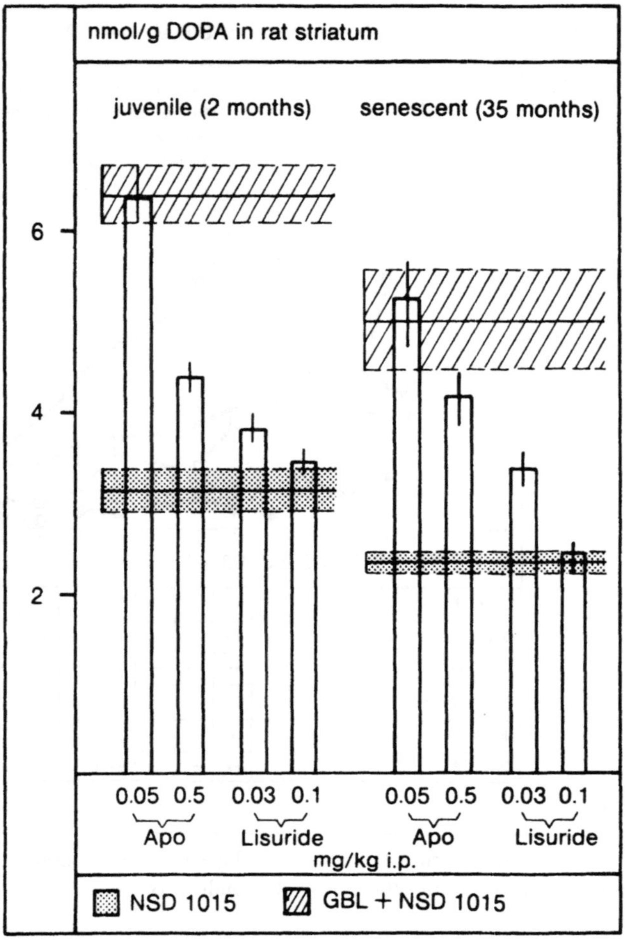

Figure 11-3. Autoreceptor-mediated inhibition of dopamine synthesis by dopamine agonists in striatum of juvenile and senescent rats following γ-butyrolactone administration. With the exception of NSD 1015-treated control animals all rats received an i.p. injection of γ-butyrolactone (GBL), 750 mg/kg 40 min and NSD 1015, 100 mg/kg i.p. 30 min before death. Apomorphine (APO) and lisuride were administered 5 min prior to NSD 1015. Shown are the means ± S.E.M., $n = 6$.

Effect of Haloperidol on Motor Functions and DOPAC Levels

Haloperidol was administered i.p. and locomotor activity was measured for 60 min starting at 30 min postapplicationem. As shown in Table 11-2 haloperidol reduced locomotor activity in adult animals in a dose-dependent manner. In senescent animals of 33–35 months of age the activity of vehicle-treated animals was more than 50% lower than in adult animals. In senescent rats, the response to haloperidol was reduced; i.e.,

Table 11-2. Effect of haloperidol on exploratory motility and mesolimbic DOPAC levels in adult (5-month-old) and senescent (33–35-month-old) female Wistar rats

	Locomotor Activity (counts per 60 min)		DOPAC, ng/g	
	adult	senescent	adult	senescent
Vehicle control	2640 ± 372	1244 ± 212	597 ± 27	503 ± 35
Haloperidol				
50 μg/kg i.p.	2523 ± 224	919 ± 114	662 ± 55	517 ± 35
200 μg/kg i.p.	713 ± 270[b]	818 ± 216	1098 ± 40[b]	789 ± 68[a]
1000 μg/kg i.p.	180 ± 49[b]	336 ± 112[b]	1075 ± 50[b]	769 ± 57[a]

Locomotor activity was measured between 30 and 90 min and DOPAC levels at 120 min after administration of haloperidol.

Shown are the means ± S.E.M.; $n = 10$. Statistics: analysis of variance, Dunnett test; significant differences vs. vehicle control: (a) $p < 0.05$, (b) $p < 0.01$.

only at the highest dose of 1 mg/kg was a reduction of locomotor activity observed.

Since parts of the limbic system (e.g., the n. accumbens) play an important role in the regulation of locomotor activity, the level of the main deaminated dopamine metabolite DOPAC was determined in the dopamine-rich part of the limbic system of the same animals 2 hr after drug or vehicle administration. Haloperidol, 200 and 1000 μg/kg in-

Table 11-3. Catalepsy induced by haloperidol and striatal DOPAC levels in adult (5-month-old) and senescent (33–35-month-old) female Wistar rats

	Incidence of Catalepsy		DOPAC, ng/g	
Treatment	adult	senescent	adult	senescent
Vehicle control	2/10	3/10	403 ± 64	302 ± 27
Haloperidol				
50 μg/kg i.p.	2/10	2/10	602 ± 106	453 ± 27
200 μg/kg i.p.	5/10	4/10	1252 ± 141[b]	562 ± 80[a]
1000 μg/kg i.p.	9/10	9/10	1120 ± 139[b]	879 ± 75[b]

Cycle state of adult rats: diestrus.

Shown are the number of cataleptic animals per group and mean DOPAC levels ± S.E.M., $n = 10$; Statistics: analysis of variance, Dunnett test; significant differences vs. respective vehicle control: (a) $p < 0.05$, (b) $p < 0.01$.

Catalepsy and DOPAC levels were measured 120 min after administration of haloperidol.

creased the DOPAC level in adult animals by 84% and 80%, and in senescent rats by only 57% and 53% respectively.

The incidence of catalepsy was determined at 2 hr after administration of haloperidol, 50–1000 μg/kg. As shown in Table 11-3 haloperidol was equipotent in inducing catalepsy in both age groups. Catalepsy induced by neuroleptics appears to be due to blockade of striatal dopamine receptors. Therefore DOPAC levels were measured in striatum of the same animals. In adult animals DOPAC levels were increased more than threefold (maximal effect) by haloperidol at a dose of 200 μg/kg which induced catalepsy in only 50% of the animals. In senescent rats the same dose of haloperidol increased DOPAC levels by only 86%, while in contrast to the limbic system a dose of 1 mg/kg further increased DOPAC levels to almost threefold of controls.

Effect of Propyl-TDHL on Motor Functions and Serum Prolactin Levels

The potent dopamine receptor agonist propyl-TDHL was administered to adult (4-month-old) and senescent (31-month-old) rats and the function of three different dopamine systems was evaluated—the mesolimbic system by means of locomotor activity, the striatal system by means of the occurrence of stereotyped movements, and the hypophyseal system by means of an effect on serum prolactin levels. Furthermore, the effect of subchronic pretreatment with propyl-TDHL (12.5 μg/kg s.c. once daily for 3 weeks) on rotarod performance was investigated in 30-month-old female rats in comparison with subchronically vehicle-pretreated age-matched controls.

As shown in Table 11-4 propyl-TDHL induced stereotyped behavior in a dose-dependent manner and to a similar extent in both age groups. Locomotor activity increased maximally after 50 μg/kg i.p., while a stimulation of locomotor activity in senescent animals was observed after the highest dose (200 μg/kg i.p.) only. Subchronic pretreatment with propyl-TDHL significantly improved motor coordination in senescent rats. Whereas only 46% (11 of 24 animals) of the subchronically vehicle-treated rats stayed on the rotarod at 20 rpm for ≥ 120 sec, there were 77% (17 of 22 animals) of the propyl-TDHL-treated rats ($p < 0.05$; Fisher's Exact Method, one-tailed), which reached the criterion.

Serum prolactin values were very high in senescent control animals, probably due to prolactin-secreting adenomas of the pituitary. Prolactin levels were reduced to normal values by propyl-TDHL at a low dose of 12.5 μg/kg i.p., indicating a high dopaminergic potency of the compound. There was also a tendency towards suppression of prolactin levels in young animals in which tonic dopaminergic inhibition of prolactin release is operating optimally thus leaving almost no additional margin for pharmacologic manipulation by dopamine agonists.

Table 11-4. Locomotor activity, stereotyped movements, and serum prolactin levels following administration of propyl-TDHL to adult (4-month-old) and senescent (31-month-old) female Wistar rats

	Incidence of Stereotyped Movements		Locomotor Activity (counts per 60 min)		Serum Prolactin Levels (μg/1)	
	adult	senescent	adult	senescent	adult	senescent
Vehicle control	0/10	0/10	1789 ± 165	1128 ± 112	32 ± 8.2	220 ± 36
Propyl-TDHL						
12.5 μg/kg i.p.	4/10	5/10	1258 ± 232	1310 ± 199	33 ± 16	25 ± 3[a]
50 μg/kg i.p.	7/10	7/10	3589 ± 969[a]	1518 ± 421	17 ± 0.6	55 ± 31[a]
200 μg/kg i.p.	9/10	10/10	3588 ± 681[a]	2768 ± 435[a]	19 ± 1.2	64 ± 28[a]

Sterotypies were measured 30 min, locomotor activity between 45 and 105 min, and prolactin levels 120 min after administration of propyl-TDHL. Shown are the number of stereotyped animals per group, mean activity counts and mean prolactin levels ± S.E.M., $n = 10$. Statistics: analysis of variance, Dunnett test; significant differences vs. respective vehicle control: (a) $p < 0.05$, (b) $p < 0.01$.

Discussion

Neurochemical evidence suggests that the function of monoaminergic neurons is modified during aging and particularly that dopaminergic transmission is impaired (c.f. Finch and Randall, 1981). Our own studies on male and female rats of the Han-Wistar strain revealed that in contrast to other strains catecholamine and 5-HT synthesis and storage was not impaired during aging (Kehr, 1983). The present study was aimed at studying the various steps of transmission which follow catecholamine synthesis and storage.

As far as the presynaptic part of transmission is concerned transmitter release appears to be one of the most relevant factors. Thus, we have tried to get an indication of catecholamine release in rat brain in vivo by measuring the accumulation of 3-methoxytyramine (3-MT) and normetanephrine, the *o*-methyl metabolites of dopamine and noradrenaline, which are formed exclusively outside catecholaminergic neurons.

Despite high dopamine and noradrenaline levels 3-MT and normetanephrine accumulated at a reduced rate in brains of 21- and 30-month-old rats, indicating reduced release of both catecholamines (Table 11-1). The reduced accumulation of 3-MT and normetanephrine may either be due to an impairment of the release process per se or to a reduction in firing rate of dopaminergic and noradrenergic neurons.

In accord with a decrease of catecholamine release the exploratory locomotor activity of senescent rats was markedly lower than in juvenile rats (Figs. 11-1 and 11-2). In addition, the stimulatory effect of the catecholamine-releasing agent (+)-amphetamine on locomotor activity was weak in senescent rats despite the fact that the absolute dose of (+)-amphetamine for senescent rats was higher due to about 2-times-greater body weight and despite the observation of Honecker and Coper (1975) and Hicks et al. (1980) that brain levels of (+)-amphetamine are higher in old than in young animals if the drug is administered per kg body weight.

Apart from reduced catecholamine release the weak effect of (+)-amphetamine can also be interpreted in terms of reduced responsiveness of the postsynaptic neurons. In fact, when the direct dopamine receptor agonist lisuride was administered the stimulatory effect on locomotor activity was much weaker in senescent rats than in young rats (Fig. 11-2), indicating that the responsiveness of the postsynaptic neurons to a dopamine agonist was indeed reduced. This interpretation got further support by the finding that lisuride levels in blood serum were about threefold higher in senescent as compared to juvenile rats.

Also, the inhibitory effect of the dopamine receptor antagonist haloperidol on locomotor activity appeared to be reduced in senescent rats (Table 11-2), which again would suggest that the postsynaptic dopamine receptors involved—most likely those of the mesolimbic system—were less sensitive to haloperidol. However, it has to be taken into consideration that the basal activity level of old rats was low as compared to adult rats.

However, the incidence of catalepsy induced by haloperidol appeared to be the same in adult and senescent rats. Since catalepsy has been associated with dopamine receptor blockade in the caudate nucleus the data suggest that the responsiveness of striatal postsynaptic dopamine receptors is less affected by the aging process than that of the postsynaptic mesolimbic receptors. This notion is supported by the fact that propyl-TDHL was equipotent in old and adult rats in inducing stereotyped movements, another symptom which is believed to be released by stimulation of striatal dopamine receptors (Table 11-4).

Stimulation of locomotor activity by propyl-TDHL, however, which is most likely due to stimulation of mesolimbic dopamine receptors, was weak in senescent rats as compared to adult rats.

How does the dopaminergic neuron react to dopamine receptor stimulation or blockade? The activity of dopaminergic neurons is under the control of a receptor-mediated feedback mechanism involving both postsynaptic receptors and autoreceptors.

The weak compensatory increase of striatal and mesolimbic DOPAC levels induced by haloperidol in senescent rat points to an age-related dampening of receptor-mediated activation of dopamine metabolism. The available data appear to indicate that the maximum increase of DOPAC is lower in senescent than in adult rats and that haloperidol is effective in the same dose range. However, haloperidol brain levels have to be determined before a definite conclusion can be drawn.

The local autoreceptor-mediated feedback system within the striatum has been studied following cessation of impulse generation in dopamine neurons by administration of γ-butyrolactone (Walters and Roth, 1976). Since under these conditions there is no release of dopamine, dopamine synthesis starts to increase in order to overcome the deficit of dopamine at receptor sites. In senescent animals the increase of striatal dopa synthesis was not as pronounced as in young animals (Fig. 11-3), suggesting that the autoreceptor-mediated feedback was not as active. As an alternative explanation the data could indicate that the capacity of the rate-limiting enzyme tyrosine hydroxylase was reduced.

The feedback inhibition induced by apomorphine was weaker in old rats and that of lisuride was similar in adult and senescent rats. Taking into consideration that lisuride plasma levels were threefold higher in old rats one must assume that the affinity of lisuride to dopamine autoreceptors was reduced in aged rats. In support of this contention lisuride failed to show an initial depression of locomotor activity in senescent rats, an effect which is generally elicited by direct dopamine agonist in adult rats (Fig. 11-2) and which is known to be mediated by dopamine autoreceptors (Strömbom, 1976).

Since dopaminergic and possibly also noradrenergic transmission is impaired in senescence, and since this may be the cause for motor dysfunctions and among others a cause for cognitive deficits, dopamine and noradrenaline receptor agonists should be of benefit for these pathological conditions.

Recently, we became interested in propyl-TDHL, an extremely potent dopamine agonist with a long duration of action (Wachtel, 1983; Kehr et al., 1983) which in addition has some adrenergic properties. The dopaminergic properties have been shown above and are further illustrated by the prolactin-lowering effect of very low doses in senescent rats (Table 11-4). Chronic treatment with propyl-TDHL improved the impairment of motor coordination in senescent rats, suggesting that this compound may also be of benefit in conditions of motor dysfunctions in humans.

References

Carlsson, A., Davis, J.N., Kehr, W., Lindqvist, M., and Atack, C.V.: Simultaneous measurement of tyrosine and tryptophan hydroxylase activities in brain in vivo using an inhibitor of the aromatic amino acid decarboxylase. *Naunyn Schmiedeberg's Arch. Pharmacol. 275*, 153–168 (1972).

Carlsson, A., and Winblad, B.: Influence of age and time interval between death and autopsy on dopamine and 3-methoxytyramine levels in human basal ganglia. *J. Neural Trans. 38*, 271–276 (1976).

Dunham, N.W., and Miya, T.S.: A note on a simple apparatus for detecting neurological deficit in rats and mice. *J. Amer. Pharmac. Assoc. 3*, 208–209 (1957).

Finch, C.E.: Catecholamine metabolism in the brains of aging male mice. *Brain Res. 52*, 261–276 (1973).

Finch, C.E., and Randall, P.K.: Aging and basal gangliar functions. *Ann. Rev. Gerontol. Geriatr. 2*, 49–87 (1981).

Gottfries, C.G., and Winblad, B.: Neurotransmitters and related enzymes in normal aging and in dementia of Alzheimer type (DAT). In Gurski, G.E. (Ed.), Determining the Effects of Aging on the Central Nervous System, pp. 7–18. Free University of Berlin, Schering AG, 1980.

Hicks, P., Strong, R., Schoolar, J.C., and Samorajski, T.: Aging alters amphetamine-induced stereotyped gnawing and neostriatal elimination of amphetamine in mice. *Life Sci. 27*, 715–722 (1980).

Honecker, H., and Coper, H.: Kinetics and metabolism of amphetamine in the brain of rats of different ages. *Naunyn-Schmiedeberg's Arch. Pharmacol. 291*, 111–121 (1975).

Horowski, R., and Wachtel, H.: Direct dopaminergic action of lisuride hydrogenmaleate, an ergot derivative, in mice. *Eur. J. Pharmacol. 36*, 373–383 (1976).

Hümpel, M., Nieuweboer, B., Hasan, S.H., and Wendt, H.: Radioimmunoassay of plasma lisuride in man following intravenous and oral administration of lisuride hydrogen maleate; effect on plasma prolactin level. *Eur. J. Clin. Pharmacol. 20*, 47–51 (1981).

Jänicke, B.: Die Motorik als Modell physiologischen Alterns bei der weiblichen Wistar-Ratte (Rattus Norvegicus). Dissertation, Free University Berlin, 1982.

Kehr, W.: 3-Methoxytyramine and normetanephrine as indicators of dopamine and noradrenaline release in mouse brain in vivo. *J. Neural Transm. 50*, 165–178 (1981).

Kehr, W.: Regulation of monoamine metabolism in young and old rats: effect of ergot derivatives. In Calne, D.B. et al. (Eds.), Lisuride and Other Dopamine Agonists. New York: Raven, 1983.

Kehr, W., Wachtel, H., and Schneider, H.H.: Dopaminergic and antidopaminergic properties of ergolines structurally related to lisuride. *Acta Pharmaceutica Suec. Suppl. 2*, 98–110 (1983).

McGeer, E.G., Fibiger, H.C., McGeer, P.L., and Wickson, V.: Aging and brain enzymes. *Exp. Gerontol. 6*, 391–396 (1971).

McGeer, E., and McGeer, P.L.: Neurotransmitter metabolism in the aging brain. In Terry, R.D., and Gershon, S. (Eds.), Neurobiology of Aging, pp. 389–403. New York: Raven, 1976.

Meek, J.L., Bertilsson, L., Cheney, D.L., Zsilla, G., and Costa, E.: Aging-induced changes in acetylcholine and serotonin content of discrete brain nuclei. *J. Gerontol. 32*, 129–131 (1977).

Modigh, K.: Central and peripheral effects of 5-hydroxytryptophan on motor activity in mice. *Psychopharmacologia 23*, 48–54 (1972).

Samorajski, T.: Age-related changes in brain biogenic amines. In Brody, H., Harman, D., and Ordy, J.M. (Eds.), Aging, Vol. 1, pp. 199–214. New York: Raven, 1975.

Strömbom, U.: Catecholamine receptor agonists: Effects on motor activity and rate of tyrosine hydroxylation in mouse brain. *Naunyn-Schmiedeberg's Arch. Pharmacol. 292*, 167–176 (1976).

Thiede, H.-M., and Kehr, W.: Conjoint radioenzymatic measurement of catecholamines, their catechol metabolites and DOPA in biological samples. *Naunyn-Schmiedeberg's Arch. Pharmacol. 318*, 19–28 (1981).

Wachtel, H.: Central dopaminergic and antidopaminergic effects of ergot derivatives structurally related to lisuride. In Calne, D.B. et al. (Eds.), Lisuride and Other Dopamine Agonists, pp. 109–125. New York: Raven, 1983.

Walters, R., and Roth, R.H.: Dopaminergic neurons: an in vivo system for measuring drug interactions with presynaptic receptors. *Naunyn-Schmiedeberg's Arch. Pharmacol. 296*, 5–14 (1976).

Chapter 12

Dopamine Receptors: Antiparkinsonian Activity and Molecular Mechanisms

Menek Goldstein, Jow Y. Lew, Abraham Lieberman, and Kjell Fuxe

Summary

Ergot derivatives such as bromocriptine, lergotrile, pergolide, and mesulergine relieve tremor and elicit abnormal involuntary movements in monkeys with ventromedial tegmental lesions. These ergots are of therapeutic value in patients with advanced Parkinson's disease, especially in those whose condition is complicated by diurnal oscillations in performance and/or who no longer respond to treatment with levodopa alone. Some nonergot dopamine agonists (e.g., LY 141865, EMD 23-448, AY 27-110) stimulate, at low doses, presynaptic, as well as supersensitive postsynaptic, dopamine receptors. Results obtained from studies in animal models suggest that these compounds might be effective antiparkinsonian agents.

In a separate study, we have investigated the properties of solubilized striatal D-2 dopamine receptors. Evidence has been obtained that the D-2 dopamine receptor is a glycoprotein, and that the ganglioside, GM-1, interacts with the lectin, WGA, at a similar site as the dopamine receptor.

Pharmacologic and biochemical studies have shown that ergot alkaloids exert central DA agonist activities (Fuxe et al., 1974; Goldstein, et al., 1978). Thus, in rats with unilateral lesions of the nigro-striatal dopamine (DA) neurons, ergot alkaloids induce turning behavior, and in monkeys with unilateral ventromedial tegmental (VMT) lesions, they relieve the surgically induced tremor and evoke abnormal involuntary movements (AIM) (Poirier and Sourkes, 1965; Goldstein et al., 1969). The antitremor activity and the occurrence of AIMs elicited by ergot derivatives are of longer duration than that produced by levodopa or by apomorphine (APO). The evaluation of antitremor activities of DA agonists in monkeys with VMT lesions were of predictive value in assessing their antiparkinsonian activity in man. We have utilized the pharmacologic data in monkeys with VMT lesions for selecting potent antiparkinsonian drugs. Since our recent studies indicate that selective presynaptic DA agonists stimulate supersensitive, but not normosensitive, DA receptors, we have evaluated their antiparkinsonian activity in monkeys with VMT lesions. In the first part of this chapter, we will summarize some of these studies.

In the second part we will focus on recent advances in the solubilization and purification of striatal DA receptors. The existence of multiple DA receptor subtypes in the CNS (Lew and Goldstein, 1979; Schwarcz et al., 1978) suggests that some DA agonists might selectively stimulate these receptors. To characterize various DA receptor subtypes, it is necessary to investigate their physicochemical properties. With this aim in mind, we have attempted to develop procedures for solubilization and purification of striatal DA receptors.

The Antiparkinsonian Activities of Ergot Derivatives

Bromocriptine (CB-154, 2 Br-α-ergocryptine)

The findings by Corrodi et al. (1973) that bromocriptine (CB-154) has pharmacologic properties similar to agents that stimulate DA receptors have suggested a therapeutic potential for ergot derivatives in Parkinson's disease and in other disorders associated with hypofunctions of central DA neuronal systems. We have investigated the antitremor activity of CB-154 in monkeys with unilateral VMT lesions (Miyamoto et al., 1974). A single administration of CB-154 results in a dose-dependent relief of tremor in monkeys with unilateral VMT lesions. Concomitant with the relief of tremor, the occurrence of AIMs was observed. Repeated administration of CB-154 enhanced the antitremor efficacy and the intensity of AIMs. We (Lieberman et al., 1976) and others (Calne et al., 1974) have evaluated the antiparkinsonian activity of CB-154 in man.

In an extensive clinical study we have treated 66 patients with advanced Parkinson's disease with CB-154. These patients were characterized by increasing disability despite optimal treatment with levodopa/carbidopa. Forty-five patients able to tolerate 25 mg/day or more of CB-154 (adequately treated group) experienced a significant decrease in rigidity, tremor, bradykinesia, and gait disturbance (Lieberman et al., 1976). The factors that limited the use of CB-154 were the development of mental changes and orthostatic hypotension. Despite the adverse effects, CB-

154, used in combination with levodopa, was found to be effective in Parkinson's disease.

Lergotrile (2-chloro-6 methylergoline-8β-acetonitrile mesylate)

The finding that lergotrile is a potent inhibitor of prolactin secretion (Lemberger et al., 1974) has prompted us to investigate its antitremor efficacy in monkeys with VMT lesions. The single administration of lergotrile resulted in a dose-dependent relief of the spontaneous tremor in monkeys with VMT lesions. Repeated administration of lergotrile reduced its antitremor effectiveness. Sedation and compulsive circling behavior towards the denervated side were observed in all monkeys after a single administration of the drug (Lieberman et al., 1975).

Subsequently, lergotrile was given to 53 patients with advanced Parkinson's disease. Thirty-nine patients experienced a significant decrease in rigidity, tremor bradykinesia, and total score without an increase in AIMs. Sixteen of these 39 patients improved by one or more stages. In some patients, the levodopa-elicited "on–off" effects were improved by cotreatment with lergotrile (Lieberman et al., 1975). Lergotrile had to be discontinued in 32 of the total of 53 patients because of adverse effects including hepatoxicity (10 patients), mental changes (12 patients), and orthostatic hypotension (8 patients).

Pergolide (8-β-8 [(methylthio)methyl]-propylergoline)

The hepatotoxicity elicited by lergotrile has prompted a search for other dopaminergic ergoline derivatives with less severe side effects. We have evaluated the antitremor efficacy of 25 ergoline derivatives in monkeys with unilateral VMT lesions. Some of the ergoline derivatives were more potent than bromocriptine or lergotrile in ameliorating tremor in monkeys (Goldstein et al., 1979). Among the tested ergoline derivatives, pergolide was found to be the most potent one (Goldstein et al., 1979). These findings have prompted us to initiate a clinical study on the antiparkinsonian activity of pergolide in man. Initially, pergolide was studied in 13 patients, and subsequently in 56 patients with advanced Parkinson's disease. The group included 45 patients with on–off phenomena. Pergolide, when combined with levodopa, resulted in a significant decrease in the overall disability (Lieberman et al., 1981; Lieberman et al., 1982). Treatment with pergolide also resulted in a significant increase in the number of hours in which the patients were in the "on" period (Lieberman et al., 1981). The major adverse effects necessitating discontinuation of pergolide were the occurrence of an organic confusional syndrome (6 patients), increased dyskinesias (4 patients), and cardiovascular abnormalities (3 patients) (Lieberman et al., 1982). Although treatment with pergolide had to be discontinued in some patients, nevertheless this drug is beneficial in many patients with advanced

Parkinson's disease, especially in those whose condition is complicated by diurnal oscillations in performance (on–off phenomena) and who are no longer responding to other treatment modalities.

Mesulergine (CU 32-085; 8-α-aminoergoline)

The finding that CU 32-085 exerts in vivo central DA agonist activity (Enz, 1981) prompted us to investigate its effects on tremor in monkeys with VMT lesions. The results of our study show that CU 32-085 relieves tremor more effectively when the drug is given orally instead of intraperitoneally (Goldstein et al., 1983a,b). Interestingly, CU 32-085 produces less severe AIMs than the previously tested ergot derivatives.

Recently we initiated a 6-month clinical trial with CU 32-085. Some patients with severe Parkinson's disease, and with a declining response to levodopa and diurnal oscillations in performance, have significantly benefited from the treatment with CU 32-085. In another group of patients with less severe Parkinson's disease, treatment with CU 32-085 made it possible to reduce the dose of levodopa by 54% and in a few patients, levodopa was completely replaced by CU 32-085. Adverse effects with CU 32-085 are (so far) minimal, and when they occur, are similar to those of levodopa.

The Antiparkinsonian Activity of Presynaptic DA Agonists

We have compared the activities of several DA agonists at presynaptic DA receptors in vivo with their potencies at postsynaptic DA receptors in vitro. Interestingly, the partial ergoline derivative LY 141865 has a low affinity for the postsynaptic DA receptors in vitro as measured by its potency to displace dopaminergic radioactive ligands from striatal membranes, but it effectively stimulates the presynaptic DA receptors in vivo (Rabey et al., 1981). We have recently tested the levorotatory isomer of LY 141865, namely LY 156258, for its potency to stimulate dopaminergic receptors. Preliminary studies indicate that the levorotatory isomer LY 156258 is at least twice as potent as the racemic mixture, LY 151865. Although both compounds have relatively low affinity for the normosensitive DA receptors, nevertheless both compounds at low doses effectively relieve tremor in monkeys with VMT lesions (LY 156258 is approximately twice as potent as LY 141865).

Two nonergot DA agonists, namely the indolyl-3-butylamine derivative EMD 223-448 (Seyfried et al., 1982; Yoshino, Matyjek and Goldstein, 1983), and the traponyl piperazine derivative AY 27-110 (Ahmed and Bagli, 1982), have a similar pharmacologic profile as the partial ergoline derivatives with respect to pre- and postsynaptic DA receptors. These compounds have low affinities for the postsynaptic DA receptors in vitro, but stimulate at low doses the presynaptic DA receptors in vivo (M. Goldstein, unpublished data). Furthermore, these two compounds effectively relieve tremor in monkeys with VMT lesions. Based on these results, we conclude that DA agonists with high affinity for presynaptic DA receptors exert stimulatory activities at postsynaptic supersensitive, but not normosensitive, DA receptors. One is therefore tempted to suggest that presynaptic DA agonists might be of therapeutic value in treatment of Parkinson's disease, and that they might produce fewer undesirable side effects than postsynaptic DA agonists.

Solubilization and Characterization of Striatal DA Receptors

The existence of at least two types of DA receptors in the striatum, one linked to adenylate cyclase (D-1) and another not linked (or negatively linked) (D-2), raises the question which of these mediates the antiparkinsonian activity. Although our data suggest that the antitremor activity in monkeys with VMT lesions is due to stimulation of D-2 DA receptors (Goldstein et al., 1983a,b), nevertheless the amelioration of some extrapyramidal dysfunctions might also be due to the stimulation of D-1 and/or of both D-1 and D-2 DA receptors. It seems, therefore, of importance to characterize the properties of the D-1 and D-2 DA receptors and to design drugs which selectively stimulate these receptors. We have developed a procedure for solubilization of striatal D-2 DA receptors, and we are now attempting to purify this receptor. The DA-receptor binding protein was solubilized with the detergent CHAPSO from bovine and rat striatal membranes (Lew, Fong, and Goldstein, 1981). Since some neurotransmitter receptors are glycoproteins, we have investigated their binding affinities to immobilized lectins. The DA receptor proteins were adsorbed on WGA-agarose column, and were selectively eluted with a solution containing N-acetylglucosamine (GlcNAc) (Lew et al., 1984). Thus, the DA receptor is a glycoprotein which contains either GlcNAc groups or sialic acid residues. The functional significance of the carbohydrate moieties of the DA receptor is not known.

Recently it was shown that treatment with the ganglioside GM-1 increases the survival of lesioned DA cell bodies and favors the recovery of synaptic functions. The lesion-induced supersensitivity of DA receptors is also decreased by chronic treatment with GM-1 (Agnati et al., 1983). GM-1 contains N-acetylgalactosamine and sialic acid residues, and therefore we have tested whether the prelabelled ^{3}H-Spi-receptor protein complex is eluted from the WGA-agarose column by this ganglioside. It is evident from Figure 12-1 that 0.25M solution of GM-1 elutes the receptor binding protein from the WGA-agarose column. These results indicate

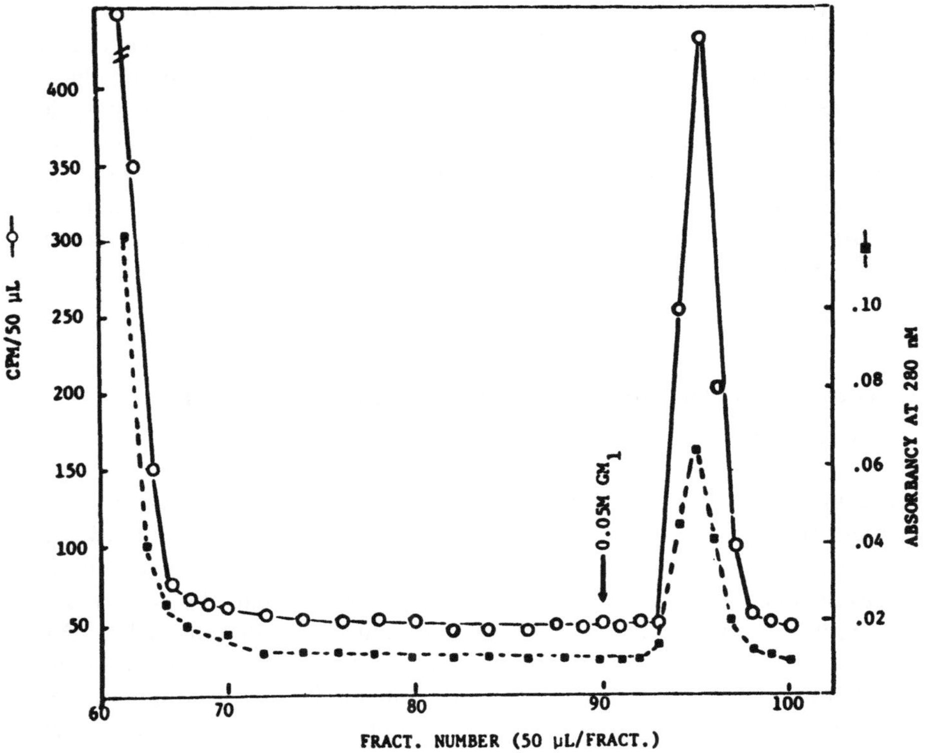

Figure 12-1. Chromatography of the CHAPSO-solubilized ^{3}H-Spi-receptor protein complex on WGA-agarose column. The ^{3}H-Spi-receptor protein complex was eluted with a buffer containing 0.25M GM-1. Circles indicate radioactivity; boxes indicate protein concentration.

that the ganglioside GM-1 and the DA receptor binding protein interact with the lectin WGA at the same or similar sites.

It is conceivable that gangliosides may affect the stability of DA receptors in vivo. It will be of interest to determine whether in aging brain gangliosides affect the sensitivity of DA agonists for the multiple DA receptors. The possible role of gangliosides in preventing the progression of Parkinson's disease merits investigation.

These studies were supported by grants NINCDS 06801 and NIMH 02717.

References

Agnati, L.F., Fuxe, K., Calza, L., Benfenati, F., Cavicchioli, L., Toffano, G., and Goldstein, M.: Gangliosides increase the survival of lesioned nigral dopamine neurons and favour the recovery of dopaminergic synaptic function in striatum of rats by collateral sprouting. *Acta Physiol. Scand.* (1983), 119:347–363, 1983.

Ahmed, F.R., and Bagli, J.: Troponoid. V. Crystallographic studies on AY-27110—a dopamine agonist of the troponylpiperazine series. *Can. J. Chem. 60*, 2687–2691 (1982).

Calne, D.B., Teychenne, P.F., Calveria, L.E., et al.: Bromocriptine in Parkinsonism. *Br. Med. J. 4*, 442–444 (1974).

Corrodi, H., Fuxe, K., Hokfelt, T., Lidbrink, P., and Ungerstedt, U.: Effect of ergot drugs on central catecholamine neurons: Evidence for a stimulation of central dopamine neurons. *J. Pharm. Pharmacol. 25*, 409–411 (1973).

Enz, A.: Biphasic influence of a 8α-amino ergoline, CU 32-085, on striatal dopamine synthesis and turnover *in vivo* in the rat. *Life Sci. 29*, 2227–2234 (1981).

Fuxe, K., Corrodi, H., Hokfelt, T., Lidbrink, P., and Ungerstedt, U.: Ergocornine and 2-Br-α-ergocryptine. Evidence for prolonged dopamine receptor stimulation. *Med. Bio. 52*, 121 (1974).

Goldstein, M., Battista, A.F., Nakatani, S., and Anagnoste, B.: The effects of centrally acting drugs on tremor in monkeys with mesencephalic lesions. *Proc. Natl. Acad. Sci. USA 63*, 1113 (1969).

Goldstein, M., Lew, J.Y., Nakamura, S., Battista, A.F., Lieberman, A., and Fuxe, K.: Dopaminephilic properties of ergot alkaloids. *Fed. Proc. 37*, 78–82 (1978).

Goldstein, M., Lew, J.Y., Engel, J., et al.: The dopaminephillic properties of ergoline derivatives. In Fuxe, K., and Calne, D.B. (Eds.), Dopaminergic Ergot Derivatives and Motor Function, pp. 253–260. Oxford: Pergamon, 1979.

Goldstein, M., Engel, J., Lieberman, A., Regev, I., Bystritsky, A., and Mino, S.: Therapeutic potentials of centrally acting dopamine and α_2-adrenoreceptor agonists. *J. Neural Transmission, Suppl. 18*, 257–263 (1983a).

Goldstein, M., Lew, J., Bystritsky, A., Lieberman, A., Engel, J., and Liljequist, S.: Multiple dopamine receptors: Interaction with α_2-adrenoreceptors. In Agnoli, A., Crepaldi, G., Spano, P.F. and Trabucchi, M., Aging Brain and Ergot Alkaloids, pp. 241–247. Aging, Vol. 23. New York: Raven, 1983.

Lemberger, L., Crabtree, R., Clemens, J., et al.: The inhibitory effect of an ergoline derivative (Lergotrile, Compound 83636) on prolactin secretion in man. *J. Clin. Endocrinol. Metab. 39*, 579–584 (1974).

Lew, J.Y., and Goldstein, M.: Dopamine receptor binding for agonists and antagonists in thermal exposed membranes. *Eur. J. Pharmacol. 55*, 429–430 (1979).

Lew, J.Y., Fong, J.C., and Goldstein, M.: Solubilization of the neuroleptic binding receptor from rat striatum. *Eur. J. Pharmacology 72*, 403–405 (1981).

Lew, J.Y., and Goldstein, M.: The solubilization and characterization of striatal dopamine receptors. *J. Neurochem. 42*:1298–1305 (1984).

Lieberman, A., Miyamoto, T., Battista, A.F., and Goldstein, N.: Studies on the antiparkinsonian efficacy of lergotrile. *Neurology 25*, 459–462 (1975).

Lieberman, A., Kupersmith, M., Estey, E., and Goldstein, M.: Treatment of Parkinson's disease with bromocriptine. *New Eng. J. Med. 295*, 1400–1404 (1976).

Lieberman, A., Goldstein, M., Leibowitz, M., Neophytides, A., Kupersmith, M., Pact, V., and Kleinberg, D.: Treatment of advanced Parkinson disease with pergolide. *Neurology 31*, 675–681 (1981).

Lieberman, A., Goldstein, M., Gopinthan, G., Leibowitz, M., Neophytides, A.,

Walker, R., Hiesiger, E., and Nelson, J.: Further studies with pergolide in Parkinson disease. *Neurology 32*, 1181–1184 (1982).

Miyamoto, T., Battista, A., Goldstein, M., and Fuxe, K.: Long-lasting antitremor activity induced by 2-Br-α-ergocryptine in monkeys. *J. Pharm. Pharmacol. 26*, 452 (1974).

Poirier, L.J., and Sourkes, T.L.: Influence of the substantia nigra on the catecholamine content of the striatum. *Brain 88*, 181 (1965).

Rabey, M.J., Passeltiner, P., Markey, K., Asano, T., and Goldstein, M.: Stimulation of pre- and postsynaptic dopamine receptors by an ergoline and by a partial ergoline. *Brain Res. 225*, 347–356 (1981).

Schwarcz, R., Creese, I., Coyle, J.T., and Snyder, S.H.: Dopamine receptors localized on cerebral cortical afferents to rat corpus striatum. *Nature (Lond.) 271*, 766–768 (1978).

Seyfried, C.A., Fuxe, K., Wolf, H.-P., and Agnati, L.F.: Demonstration of a new type of dopamine receptor agonist: an indolyl-3-butylamine. Actions at intact versus supersensitive dopamine receptors in the rat forebrain. *Acta Physiol. Scand. 116*, 465–468 (1982).

Yoshino, K., Matyjek, E.H., and Goldstein, M.: The effect of the indol-alkyl-piperdine derivative EMD 23-448 on pre- and postsynaptic central dopamine receptors. Abstract #538, *Fed.Proc. 42*, 384 (1983).

Chapter 13

Prolactin Studies in Senile Dementia of the Alzheimer Type

T. Samorajski

Summary

A comparison was made of serum prolactin levels in 54 healthy subjects and in 31 elderly nursing home patients who had dementia of mild to moderate severity. Both men and women showed a decline in serum prolactin levels with age. In the demented patients, prolactin levels were significantly higher than in age-matched controls. When dihydroergotoxine mesylate (Hydergine) or placebo was given to nursing home patients, significantly lower prolactin levels were found in Hydergine-treated patients compared to the control patients. A significant correlation was found between prolactin changes at 12 weeks and several categories of behavior measured by the Sandoz Clinical Assessment Geriatric Scale (SCAG). These results indicate that measures of circulating prolactin and possibly other hormones may prove useful in studies of neurotransmitter abnormalities in age-associated dementia and the response of elderly patients to various drug treatment strategies.

Introduction

There is good neurochemical evidence that the metabolism of neurotransmitter substances, primarily acetylcholine and dopamine, are modified during aging and as a consequence of Alzheimer's disease. Whether or not any of these changes in the brain are reflected as biochemical abnormalities in body fluids is unknown. A growing body of data indicates, however, that measurements of cholinergic and monoaminergic enzymes and associated metabolites in body fluids may be of some use in the diagnosis and treatment of age-associated psychiatric diseases such as depression and senile dementia of the Alzheimer type.

Hypothalamic biogenic amines have a major role in regulating pituitary function. Recent work on the localization of neurotransmitter substances in different regions of the brain has demonstrated that their concentration and turnover can change in response to different external and internal stimuli (Hökfelt et al., 1978). Endocrine stimuli alter anterior pituitary release by some kind of competition between the number of available molecules in the pituitary and turnover of one or more of the amines in the hypothalamus (Meites et al., 1977). Presumably, the three biogenic amines [dopamine (DA), norepinephrine (NE), 5-hydroxytryptophan (5-HT, serotonin)] and a variety of neuropeptides influence anterior pituitary hormone secretion by the release of peptidergic releasing or inhibiting factors (neurohormones) from nerve terminals in the hypothalamus into the portal circulation (Fig. 13-1).

In some elderly persons, the hypothalamus does not respond normally to electrical and chemical messages (Samorajski and Hartford, 1980). Consequently, many endocrine functions decline or fail during maturity and old age. Abnormalities in neurohormones and neurotransmitter constituents that may occur with aging and age-related mental diseases raise the possibility that measures of these substances in body fluids may help to establish the degree of organicity present in the brain and may be useful in assessing treatment outcome. Circulating neurohormones and neurotransmitter constituents currently under intensive study are shown in Table 13-1. The more common approach involves repetitive measures during a baseline period (1–4 weeks, drug free) often followed by a double-blind cross-over study with a trial drug.

The dexamethasone suppression test (DST) is perhaps the most common and reliable diagnostic test for primary or endogenous depression and as a prognostic test for clinical response to treatment with antidepressant medication (Brown, Haren, and Qualls, 1980; Carroll et al., 1981; Sternbach, Gwirtsman, and Gerner, 1981). In this test, cortisol levels are measured at intervals over 24 hours to establish the "escape" or "nonescape" of the cortisol response to dexamethasone. Dexamethasone (a synthetic form of cortisol) inhibits corticotropin releasing factor (CRF) in the hypothalamus and hense, ACTH release from the anterior pituitary. Raskind, Peskind, and Rivard (1981) reported that results of the dexamethasone suppression test may be abnormal in patients with Alzheimer-type dementia.

Probably more is known about the secretion of prolactin that any other hormone of the anterior pituitary. Agents in the hypothalamus that regulate prolactin release include a prolactin inhibitory factor (PIF) dopamine which can depress prolactin release, and acetylcholine which

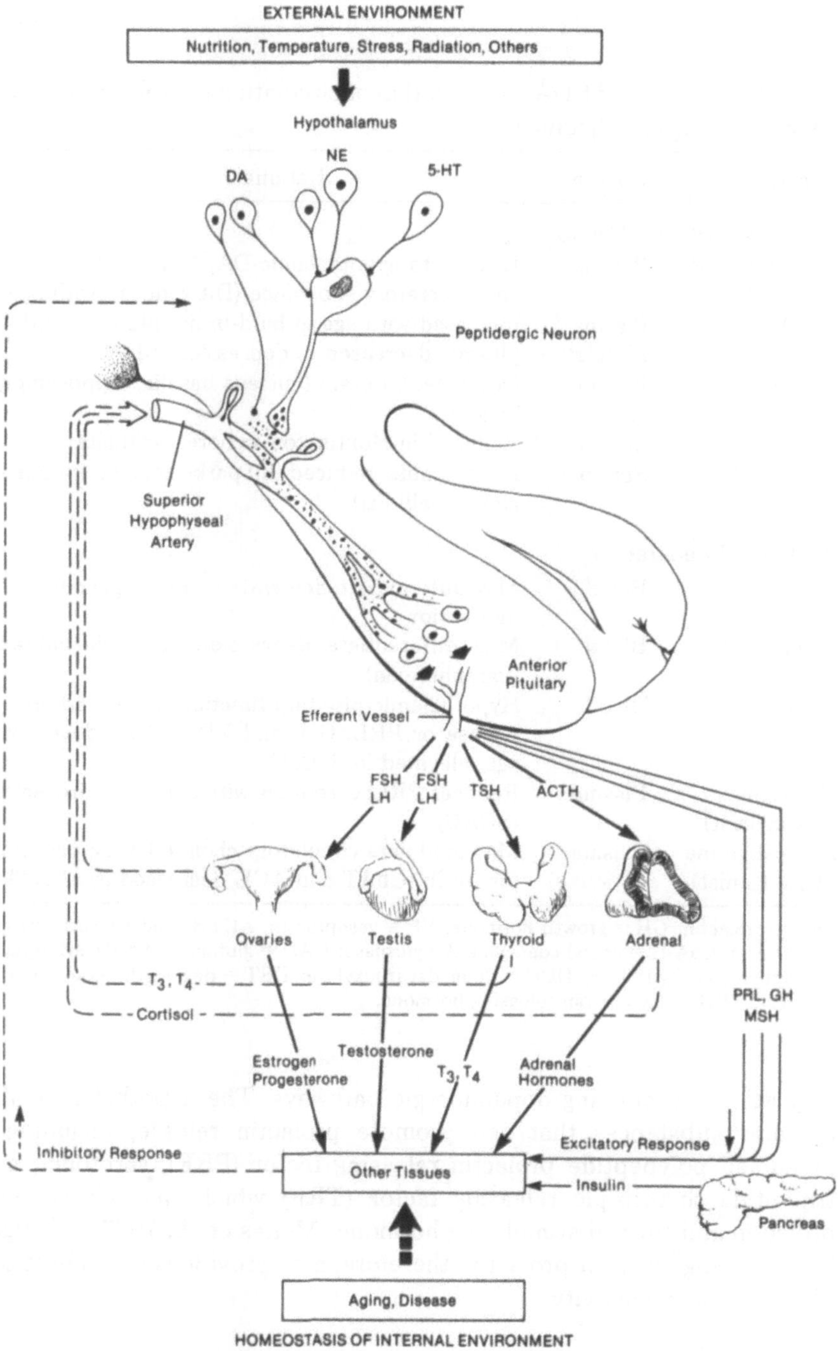

Figure 13-1. Diagrammatic illustration of external and internal environmental factors mediated by hypothalamic neurotransmitter and anterior pituitary and peripheral endocrine gland hormones. Various releasing or inhibitory factors and biogenic amines reach the anterior pituitary through the pituitary portal system derived from the superior hypophyseal artery. (Reprinted by permission from Fig. 3-1, page 51 in Busse, E.W., and Blazer, D.G. (Eds.), *Handbook of Geriatric Psychiatry*. Copyright 1980, Van Nostrand Reinhold Co., New York.)

Table 13-1. Age and SDAT modulation of circulating neurohormones and neurotransmitter substances

Constituent	Source	Rationale
A. Blood baseline strategy		
PRL, GH, VP, ACTH, LH	Plasma	Related to hypothalamic DA, 5-HT and neurosecretory substance (DA reduced with age)
MAO-B	Plasma Platelets	Increased with age in hind-brain, platelets and plasma; decreased in depression, SDAT
AcCoA-H	Plasma RBC	Decreased in brain (nucleus basalis, hippocampus) in SDAT
GAD	Serum	Reduced in Huntington's chorea (caudate)
TH, DDC	Serum	L-Dopamine reduced in parkinsonism (putamen, globus pallidus)
B. Acute dose strategy		
DST	Blood	May differentiate dementia and endogenous depression
TRH	Blood	May differentiate depression and schizophrenia (parapherenia)
L-dopa	Blood	Hypothalamic-pituitary function test based on release or PRL, GH, and VP (PRL reduced with age, elevated in SDAT)
Hydergine (DA agonist)	Plasma	Reduces PRL; correlates with clinical improvement (SCAG)
Physostigmine (ACh agonist)	Plasma	May modulate circulatory choline levels; precursor for AcCh (ChAT and ACE decreased in SDAT)

PRL = prolactin; GH = growth hormone; VP = vasopressin; ACTH = adrenocorticotropic hormone; AcCoA-H = acetyl-coenzyme A hydrolase; GAD = glutamic acid decarboxylase; TH = thyrosine hydrolase; DDC = dopa decarboxylase; DST = dexamethasone suppression test; TRH = thyrotropin-releasing hormone.

may act by stimulating dopaminergic pathways. The hypothalamus also contains substances that can promote prolactin release, including a presumed polypeptide prolactin releasing factor (PRF), serotonin, and tripeptide thyrotropic releasing factor (TRF) which can release both prolactin and thyroid-stimulating hormone (Meites et al., 1977). Changes in circulating levels of prolactin, therefore, may provide some indications of hypothalamic activity.

Results

We recently examined (Samorajski et al., 1983) the influence of age on prolactin levels in a group of healthy men and women (Fig. 13-2). Analysis of variance showed that younger women (21–50 years old) had a

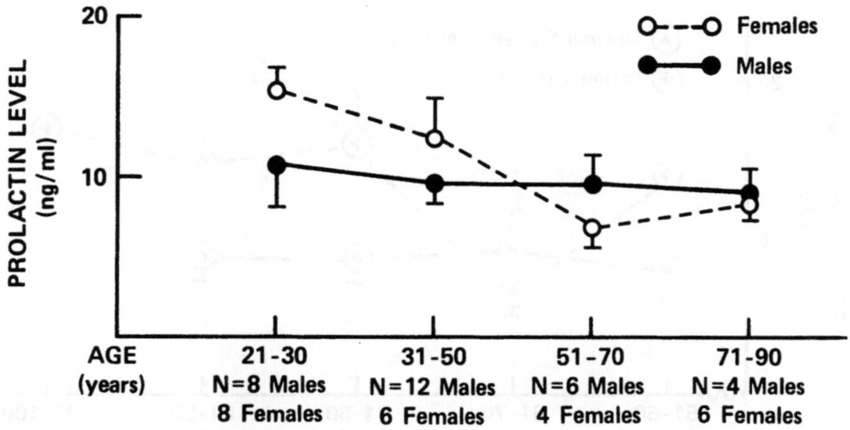

Figure 13-2. Serum PRL levels in normal men and women of various age groups. Data are expressed as mean ± S.E.M. The difference in younger (21–50) and older (51–90) women is significant at the $p < 0.025$ level (ANOVA). (Adapted from Samorajski, T., Ho, B., Kralik, P., and Hartford, J., 1982).

significantly higher prolactin level ($p < 0.025$) than the older women (51–89 years). A slight but insignificant serum prolactin decline with age was also found in men. Differences in serum prolactin levels of men and women were not significant and, consequently, the data for both were combined in subsequent comparisons.

We next determined serum prolactin levels of 31 mild-to-moderately demented patients and 21 age-matched controls (Fig. 13-3). In the 51–70-year-old group there were no apparent differences between the 3 patients and 10 controls. A comparison of the older controls and patients (ages 71–89 years; 26 patients and 11 controls) indicated that the patients had significantly higher prolactin levels ($p < 0.05$). The differences in serum prolactin levels among patients aged 71–80 years, 81–90 years, and 91–100 years were not significant.

In another study we examined the effects of the ergot alkaloid derivative dihydroergotoxine mesylate (Hydergine, Sandoz) on serum prolactin levels in Hydergine-treated and a placebo group at baseline (week 0) and at 6, 12, and 20 weeks of treatment (Fig. 13-4). In the Hydergine-treated patients, prolactin levels decreased significantly by weeks 6 and 12 ($p < 0.05$) and were lowest at 20 weeks. The placebo group did not show a significant change in prolactin levels during the 12-week period. We have previously shown that discontinuation of Hydergine treatment resulted in a return of PRL levels to pretreatment levels within 3–6 days (Samorajski et al., 1982).

Table 13-2 shows the relationship between changes in prolactin levels

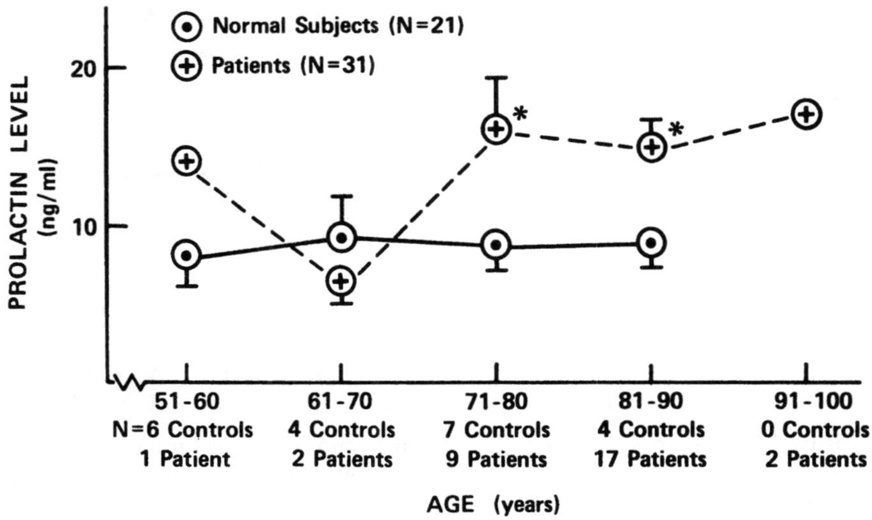

Figure 13-3. Serum PRL levels in SDAT patients and age-matched controls. Each value is the mean ± S.E.M.; $^*p < 0.05$ (ANOVA). (Adapted from Samorajski, T., Ho, B., Kralik, P., and Hartford, J., 1982).

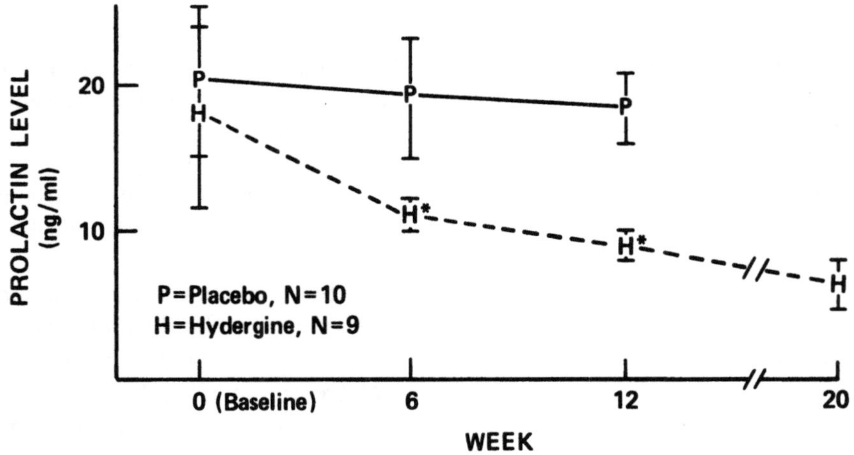

Figure 13-4. Serum PRL values at baseline (week 0) and after 6, 12, and 20 weeks of placebo (P) or Hydergine (H) treatment (2 mg three times per day). Each value is the mean ± S.E.M.; $^*p < 0.05$ (ANOVA). (Adapted from Samorajski, T., Ho, B., Kralik, P., and Hartford, J., 1982).

Table 13-2. Pearson product-moment correlation coefficients[a] for change in prolactin vs. change in SCAG factor composites

Item	Week 6 ($n = 9$)	Week 12 ($n = 5$)
1. Interpersonal relationships	0.11	0.14
2. Cognitive dysfunction	0.07	0.39
3. Affect	−0.64	−0.65
4. Apathy	0.00	0.51
5. Somatic functioning	−0.03	0.26
6. Self-care	−0.10	−0.33
7. Overall impression	−0.22	0.85
8. Average of 18 items	−0.15	0.54

[a]A positive correlation indicates that, as the prolactin level decreases, the SCAG variable improves. Reprinted by permission from Table 2, page 264 in Giacobini, E., Filogamo, G., Giocobini, G., and Vernadakis, A. (Eds.), *The Aging Brain: Cellular and Molecular Mechanism of Aging in the Nervous System.*

and composite scores on the Sandoz Clinical Assessment Geriatric Scale (SCAG), based on Pearson product-moment correlation coefficients. In this table a positive correlation indicates that, as the prolactin level decreased, clinical response improved. The correlation coefficients are based on values observed for all patients, that is, 9 patients completing 12 weeks of Hydergine treatment.

At week 6 the correlations were either negative or close to zero, indicating little relationship between changes in prolactin levels and changes recorded on the SCAG scale. At 12 weeks, the correlation of all factors except affect and self-care tended to be more positive. Values significantly different from zero include apathy, overall impression, and the total (average) of all items. Thus, at least at 12 weeks, improvement in SCAG ratings correlated positively with decreasing prolactin levels although the magnitude of the correlations were not large.

Individual SCAG scores of the 11 Hydergine-treated patients suggested that subjects could be categorized as either responders or nonresponders based on composite scores. Accordingly, 5 patients were identified as nonresponders and 6 as responding to Hydergine by the 12th week of treatment. Plasma Hydergine levels were determined at 6 and 12 weeks for both groups of patients and at 20, 28, and 34 weeks for the responders. There were no significant differences in Hydergine plasma levels between responders and nonresponders at any of the treatment intervals analyzed (Fig. 13-5).

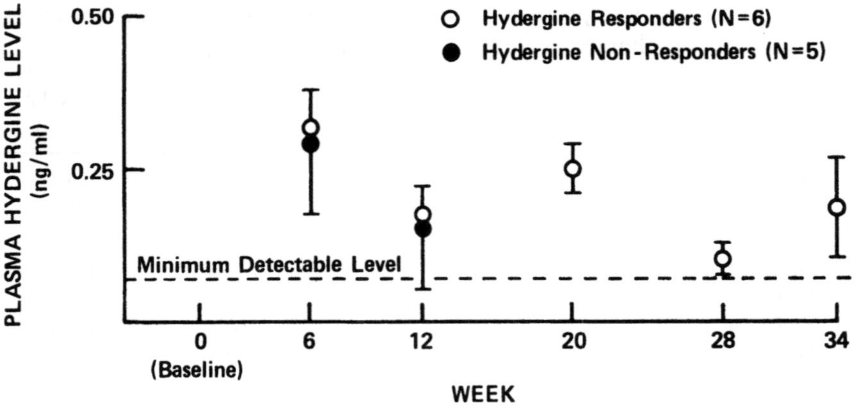

Figure 13-5. Serum Hydergine levels in SDAT patients identified as Hydergine responders and nonresponders at baseline (week 0) and 6, 12, 20, 28, and 34 weeks of treatment. Each value is the mean ± S.E.M. Differences between responders and nonresponders at 6 and 12 weeks were not significant.

Discussion

Serum prolactin levels in healthy men and women were found to decline with age (Fig. 13-2). An age-by-sex analysis failed to reveal significant differences between genders. One possible explanation for the decline in serum PRL with age may be that direct feedback to the pituitary gland from target organs may diminish as a consequence of structural and functional changes at the organ site. Perhaps the decrease in circulating prolactin levels with age in healthy men and women is the result of diminished signals from target organs to the lactotropes of the anterior pituitary. Another possibility is that there may be a significant change with age in the functional state of the dopaminergic tuberoinfindibular pathway. A decline with age in dopamine levels and activity in the hypothalamus of rodent brain has been reported (Samorajski and Rolsten, 1973; Finch, 1975). Yet another possibility is that there may be an age-related change in the function of the anterior pituitary cells. This problem remains to be resolved by future research.

Decreased function of the tuberinfindibular pathway may be particularly pertinent to the study of age-associated psychiatric diseases because of its influence on releasing excitatory or inhibitory factors associated with endocrine function. The secretion of prolactin (PRL) by the pituitary seems to be primarily controlled by dopaminergic (DA) inhibitory neurons (Gregerman and Bierman, 1981). A loss or imbalance of DA neurons in the hypothalamus associated with SDAT may result in a decrease of prolactin-inhibitory activity or an increase in prolactin-releasing activity, with a concomitant increase in the circulating PRL levels of SDAT patients as shown in Figure 13-3. Changes in the hypothalamic–pituitary axis may result, throughout the body, in further senescent changes associated with the mechanism of prolactin action in various biological systems (Horrobin, 1980).

Serum prolactin has been shown to be decreased by Hydergine at oral dosages of 1 mg three times per day (Gross et al., 1979). In our study, using 2 mg three times daily (Fig. 13-4) a progressive decline also occured in relation to treatment (6–20 weeks). Furthermore, results indicated some degree of correlation between changes in prolactin level and treatment outcome based on SCAG scores (Table 13-2).

Calculation of Pearson product-moment correlations at 6 and 12 weeks yielded some interesting differences. At 6 weeks, the correlations were either negative or close to zero. At 12 weeks, the correlations tended to be more positive, with correlation between apathy, overall impression, and lower prolactin levels approaching significance (Table 13-2). Gaitz and Hartford (1979) noted that the ergot alkaloids are relatively slow-acting at currently approved dosage levels. Some correlation between cognitive function and prolactin levels at 12 weeks was found in this study, but the interaction did not reach statistical significance. Our results suggest that Hydergine exerts its beneficial effects by improving the function of hypothalamic DA neurons, possibly in the same or a similar way that L-dopa compensates for the loss of nigrostriatal DA neurons in Parkinson patients.

An examination of the individual SCAG scores of the Hydergine-treated patients revealed that about one-half of these patients could be identified as responders and one-half as nonresponders. Individual SCAG scores and prolactin levels were not related. It seems then, that measurement of basal PRL serum levels at a single time point during treatment is not sufficient to differentiate responders from nonresponders before or during the course of Hydergine treatment. Studies of neuroendocrine abnormalities and clinical responses in neuropsychiatric patients may require that use of an acute-dose strategy that is, evaluation of neuroendocrine response at several (hourly) time points after an acute challenge dose of a test drug. The acute challenge strategy may be more useful for studying PRL response to Hydergine than chronic-basal-level assays because PRL levels are rapidly depressed or elevated by administration or withdrawal of Hydergine.

We also examined the possibility that circulating levels of Hydergine might be different among patients who responded to Hydergine and those who did not, but we found this not to be so at any treatment interval analyzed (Fig. 13-5). The data were too limited and variable to predict whether a "therapeutic window" exists for correlating Hydergine blood levels with treatment outcomes.

As aging seems to involve a progressive imbalance between neurotransmitters in the brain, the question of drug, precursor, and hormone treatment to delay the aging process and the onset of disease is an interesting one. If normal aging is a sequence of interlinked neuronal and endocrine transitions without intrinsic degenerative changes, it should be possible to control the processes involved through drugs, precursors, and/or hormones. Conversely, if a disease is caused by a deficiency of a critical neurotransmitter or an imbalance between related neurotransmitter systems, the condition might improve with the administration of a critical constituent. One example is parkinsonism, in which administration of L-dopa reverses some symptoms by restoring DA to the brain.

Impairments in sensory processes, intelligence, learning, and memory may constitute inevitable manifestations even of normal aging. Depression and mood disorders are equally or even more prominent symptoms of many elderly persons. The cognitive and emotional impairments increase in severity with clinical symptoms of senile dementia, Alzheimer's disease, and other organic brain syndromes. To counteract cognitive, emotional, and neurological disorders of aging, psychoactive drugs, neuropeptides, and dietary precursors for neurotransmitters appear as inevitable therapeutic agents (Samorajski, Hicks, and Ordy, 1980). Table 13-3 lists the most common drugs and precursors that have been or are being used to modulate cerebral function in the elderly.

Future Prospects

The current focus on neuropharmacologic research is almost exclusively on neurotransmitters and their enzymes. Nearly all possible drug and precursor effects on such brain functions as learning, memory, and affect have been associated with alterations at the neurotransmitter level. Unfortunately, synaptic processes are widely distributed throughout the body and a beneficial result at one site may be counteracted by an adverse side-reaction at another.

Neuropeptides may exist in the same nerve ending with the classical neurotransmitter and, like them, may have excitatory or inhibitory functions (Hökfelt et al., 1980). Although neuropeptides may also be widely distributed throughout the body, many are confined to specific neurons. Some neuronal neuropeptides are found only in the hypothalamic–pituitary axis and many act only as neurohormones on pituitary cells. The distribution of peptides in the brain suggests an influence on memory and other behavioral effects. If future research can more specifically identify impaired neurons, it may then be possible that a critical neuropeptide can be identified and processed for delivery to the region involved.

Table 13-3. Drug and precursor modulation of neurotransmitters in the elderly

Drug Precursor[a]	Behavior	Mechanisms	Condition[b]
		A. CNS stimulants, analeptics, anabolic agents	
Methylphenidate	Alertness	Metabolism: DA-Agonist	Senescence (all have adverse
Pipradol	Cognition	Metabolism	side effects)
Pyritinol	Affect	Metabolism	
Naftydrofuril	Cognition	Metabolism	
		B. Vasodilators, ergot alkaloids	
Papaverine	Alertness	Circulation	Senescence
Cyclandelate	Cognition	Circulation	SD
Hydergine	Affect	Circulation, metabolism	SD
		C. Modulators of cholinergic system ChAc-ACh-AChE	
Choline	Memory	Precursor	Senescence
Lecithin	Memory	Precursor	SD
Physostigmine	Memory	AChE-Inhibitor	SD
		D. Modulators of monoaminergic systems: DA, NE, 5-HT	
L-dopa	Tremors	DA-Precursor	Parkinsonism
Tyrosine	Affect	NE-Precursor	Senescence
Tryptophan	Sleep	5-HT Precursor	Insomnia
Pargyline	Depression	MAO-Inhibitor	SD
		E. Antipsychotic, anti-depressant, anti-anxiety agents	
Thioridazine	Antipsychotics	DA-NE receptors	Senescence
Amitriptyline	Antidepressants	NE-5-HT-uptake	Senescence
Diazepam	Anxiolytics	GABA-DA enzymes	Senescence
		F. Nootropic or "mind-acting"	
Piracetam	Cognition	Telencephalic GABA, RNA	Senescence
Centrophenoxine	Cognition	Cell loss, lipofuscin	Senescence
Neuropeptides	Memory	?	SD

SD = senile dementia; senescence = normal aging.

[a]Drug precursors listed constitute only a representative sample of major classes of compounds tested clinically in man.

[b]Efficacy may vary from significant improvement to no effect or impairment of performance.

Although there is as yet little direct evidence that neuropeptides figure importantly in aging, the hypothesis is an attractive one to explore. Another hope is that more specific and sensitive drugs, possibly combined with a neuropeptide antibody, may prove useful for arresting or even reversing currently untreatable conditions. Undoubtedly, many of the obstacles to adequate treatment of dementia will disappear when more precise definition of the chemistry involved in the processing of mood, memory, and emotion becomes available in the future. Finally, it is interesting to contemplate and, more importantly, to study how life-long habits might influence the aging process of the brain and the quality of old age among an increasing proportion of the world's total population.

Acknowledgments

The author thanks Ms. Susan Sansom for assistance in the preparation of this chapter. The support of Sandoz, Inc., East Hanover, N.J. in the conduct of this study is greatly appreciated. This paper is based substantially on a recent report to be published in *The British Journal of Clinical Practice* (symposium supplement).

References

Brown, W.A., Haren, R.J., and Qualls, C.B.: Dexamethasone suppression test identifies subtypes of depression which respond to different antidepressants. *Lancet II*, 928–929 (1980).

Carroll, B.J., Feinberg, M., Greeden, J.F., et al.: A specific laboratory test for the diagnosis of melancholia. *Arch. Gen. Psychiatry 38*, 15–22 (1981).

Finch, C.E.: Neuroendocrinology of aging: A view of an emerging area. *Bioscience 25*, 645–650 (1975).

Gaitz, C.M., and Hartford, J.T.: Ergot alkaloids in treatment of geriatric patients with dementia. In Nandy, K. (Ed.), Geriatric Psychopharmacology, pp. 213–224, New York: Elsevier/North Holland, 1979.

Gregerman, R.I., and Bierman, E.L.: Aging and hormones. In Williams, R.H. (Ed.), Endocrinology, p.p. 1192–1212. Philadelphia: W.B. Saunders, 1981.

Gross, R.J., Eisdorfer, C.E., Schiller, H.S., and Cox, C.: Effects of ergot alkaloids on serum prolactin in non-psychotic organic brain syndrome of the elderly. *Exp. Aging Res. 5*, 293–302 (1979).

Hökfelt, T., Elde, R., Fuxe, K., Johansson, O., Ljungdahl, A., Goldstein, M., Luft, R., Efeudic, S., Nilsson, G., Terenius, L., Ganten, D., Jeffcoate, L., Rehfeld, J., Said, S., Perez de la Mora, M., Possani, L., Tapia, R., Teran, L., and Palacios, R.: Aminergic and peptidergic pathways in the nervous system with special reference to the hypothalamus. In Baldessarini, R.J., and Martin, J.B. (Eds.), The Hypothalamus, pp. 69–136. New York: Raven, 1978.

Hökfelt, T., Johansson, O., Ljungdahl, A., Lundberg, J.M., and Schultzberg, M.: Peptidergic neurones. *Nature 284*, 515–521 (1980).

Horrobin, D.F.: Secretion, metabolic clearance, normal levels and environmental stimuli. In Prolactin, Vol. 8, pp. 13–23. St. Albans, Vermont: Eden, 1980.

Meites, J., Simpkins, J., Brani, J., and Advis, J.: Role of biogenic amines in control of anterior pituitary. *IRCS Med. Sci. 5*, 1–7 (1977).

Raskind, M., Peskind, E.R., and Rivard, F.: The dexamethasone suppression test in presenile and senile dementia of the Alzheimer's type. *Gerontologist 21*, 157 (1981).

Samorajski, T., and Hartford, J.: Brain physiology of aging. In Busse, E.W., and Blazer, D.G. (Eds.), Handbook of Geriatric Psychiatry, pp. 46–82. New York: Van Nostrand Reinhold, 1980.

Samorajski, T., Hartford, J., Kralik, P.M., Ho, B., and Smith, R.C.: Changes in serum prolactin, growth hormone, monoamine oxidase and acetyl-coenzyme A hydrolase with age and Hydergine. *British J. Clin. Practice* (Symposium Supplement 30) 9–16 (1983).

Samorajski, T., Hicks, P.B., and Ordy, J.M.: Metabolism of other neurotransmitters in degenerative syndromes associated with aging. In Tissot, R. (Ed.), États Déficitaires Cérébraux Liés à L'Âge, pp. 125–152, Georg: Librairie de L'Université, Genève, 1980.

Samorajski, T., Ho, B., Kralik, P.M., and Hartford, J.T.: Serum prolactin changes with age, senile dementia and dihydroergotoxin mesylate treatment. In Giacobini, E., Filogamo, G., Giacobini, G., and Vernadakis, A. (Eds.), The Aging Brain: Cellular and Molecular Mechanisms in the Nervous System, Vol. 20, pp. 259–269. New York: Raven, 1982.

Samorajski, T., and Rolsten, C.: Age and regional differences in the chemical composition of brain of mice, monkeys and humans. In Ford, D.H. (Ed.), Progress in Brain Research, Vol. 40, Neurobiological Aspects of Maturation and Aging, pp. 253–265. New York, Elsevier Scientific Publishing, 1973.

Sternbach, H., Gwirtsman, H., and Gerner, R.H.: The dexamethasone suppression test and response to methylphenidate in depression. *Am. J. Psychiatry 138*, 1629–1630 (1981).

Chapter 14

Prospects for Synergistic Drug Combinations for the Treatment of Senile Amnesias

Arthur Cherkin and James F. Flood

Summary

Memory impairment is the hallmark of senile dementias. Although no present treatment satisfactorily prevents, retards, or reverses memory failure, modest improvement has been achieved by pharmacologic means. Combination treatments tend to improve results; in our mouse model, cholinergic drugs show marked supra-additive effects on memory enhancement, with only additive effects on toxicity. The drugs include cholinomimetics (arecoline, deanol, oxotremorine) and anticholinesterases (edrophonium, tacrine). Supra-additivity occurs within and between these classes, using intracerebroventricular or subcutaneous injection. Maximal memory retention can be achieved with two-drug combinations at doses which are 95% reduced from single-drug doses; this suggests the potential for low-dose synergistic combination drugs for treating senile amnesias. Other insights include the observations that poweful supra-additivity occurs even in combinations of drugs with similar mechanisms of action; cholinergic drug dose–response curves are inverted U-shape; and the "therapeutic window" can be widened by appropriate drug combinations and dose ratios.

A typical concern of many elderly is failing memory. Moderate to severe memory failure, the hallmark of dementias, occurs in 5–15% of those over 65 years of age, associated with Alzheimer's disease, multiinfarct dementia, drug toxicosis, nutritional deficiencies, and many other conditions. The increasing prevalence of dementias, as the population ages, has attracted renewed attention to pharmacologic enhancement of memory. There is now abundant evidence of statistically significant improvement of psychometric memory scores by a variety of drugs, but the extent of functional clinical improvement has been disappointing (Bartus et al., 1982). As a result, there have been recent calls for new strategies for the treatment of senile dementias (Crook and Gershon, 1981; Reisberg et al., 1983; Roberts, 1983).

Our interest is in the memory dysfunctions associated with dementias. The strategy we chose in late 1980 includes a systematic search for strong supra-additivity in memory-enhancing drugs, with two motivations: basic science and preclinical. The basic science motivation is to add to our knowledge of memory mechanisms. Pharmacologic probes are widely used for the study of memory mechanisms (Kubanis and Zornetzer, 1981) but relatively little attention has been devoted to systematic exploration of drug combinations for this purpose. For example, seven reviews of the pharmacology of human memory (cited in Cherkin and Riege, 1983, p. 422) make no mention of drug combinations. The preclinical motivation is to provide insights which may lead to development of rational low-dosage combinations of drugs intended to rehabilitate failing memory to a clinically useful extent, and hopefully to disclose caveats for clinical trials of memory enhancers.

There are obvious disadvantages to the combination drug strategy. Polypharmacy is already the regrettable rule in the treatment of the elderly (Cooper, 1979; Salzman, 1981) and irrational drug combinations are properly criticized (Blaschke et al., 1981; Ouslander, 1981). Drug interactions are generally considered to be hazardous rather than beneficial (Blaschke et al., 1981). Drug combinations (e.g., Corkin et al., 1982; Drachman et al., 1982; Peters and Levin, 1979, 1982) have not yet led to a generally accepted treatment for senile amnesias. On the other hand, rational combinations can be extremely effective and widely used, as in the treatment of infections (Rudoy et al., 1974) and cancer (Carter and Slavik, 1974). The marked dose reductions (as much as 95%), which our results indicate may be feasible with appropriate combinations, can reasonably be expected to reduce side effects and toxic interactions with other drugs. Resort to combinations of memory enhancers has been suggested repeatedly in recent years (e.g., Bartus et al., 1982; Hollister, 1981; Roberts, 1982) and clinical trials with such combinations have reported improved results, as compared with the single drugs (e.g., Ferris et al., 1982; Peters and Levin, 1979, 1982; Reisberg et al., 1983).

In late 1980, we launched a research program to explore the interactive effects of drugs upon memory enhancement and upon toxicity. A systematic study in human subjects or in aged animals was manifestly not feasible, because of the very large number of subjects required for combination drug experiments. We therefore adopted a well-developed young adult mouse model (Flood et al., 1975, 1981, 1983). We decided also to start with cholinergic system drugs, for two reasons. First, the cholinergic hypothesis of geriatric memory dysfunction was under intensive laboratory and clinical study (Bartus et al., 1980; 1982). Second, we had extensive dose–response data for eight cholinergic drugs which enhance memory retention in the selected mouse model (Flood et al., 1981). The intracerebroventricular route of administration was explored first, in order to minimize the influence of any peripheral effects of the cholinergic drugs, followed by the subcutaneous route and currently the oral route.

The oral route differs profoundly from the two injection routes, from the point of view of memory mechanisms. The *injected* drugs were administered *after* training, to avoid any effects upon acquisition of the trained response. Then, the test for memory retention was delayed for 1 week after drug injection, to permit elimination of the drug and its metabolites, so that memory retrieval mechanisms would not be affected. In sum, the acute injection experiments were designed so that the drugs would operate upon memory consolidation and not upon information input or retrieval. In contrast, chronic oral administration is intended to resemble more closely the clinical situation, where a successful memory enhancer would preferably be administered by mouth, and would be present in the brain throughout information input, memory consolidation, storage, and retrieval. This is obviously a far more complex situation than is encountered with the acute injection techniques, the major effects of which are considered to be upon the consolidation process only.

At this time, we have completed our planned study of cholinergic drugs by the intraventricular and subcutaneous routes and have started the chronic oral studies. The major findings to date may be summarized as follows, for cholinergic drugs tested for enhancement of 1 week memory retention in young adult mice trained in an active-avoidance T-maze paradigm:

1. The dose–response curves are inverted-U shaped, for single drugs and for drug combinations.
2. Low doses enhance memory: high doses impair memory.
3. Memory enhancers interact at low doses to improve memory and at higher doses to impair memory, both in a supra-additive manner.
4. The ratio of drug doses in a combination is a critical variable in dose–response determinations.
5. Therapeutic windows are narrow for single drugs, requiring closely spaced doses to locate the memory enhancing range. The windows are wider for certain drug combinations.
6. The optimal dose for enhancing 1 week retention is higher than that for 3 hr retention.

Procedure

The experimental procedures were published in detail (Flood et al., 1975) and utilized in numerous experiments during the succeeding eight years (e.g., Flood et al., 1981, 1983). In brief, young adult mice are trained in 4 trials to run to the safe (no foot-shock) arm of a T-maze within 5 sec after a warning buzzer sounds; those who fail to enter the correct arm in 5 sec receive foot-shock until they do. Mice which learn too quickly or too slowly are discarded, in order to reduce within-group variance and thereby reduce the total number of mice required per experiment; this exclusion totals fewer than 20% of the mice. Immediately after training, the mice are injected with the drug solution or with saline, typically in groups of 20. One week later, the mice are tested for memory retention. The "recall score," which is the percentage of mice which meet the criterion of 1 correct response within 3 trials, is considered as the indicant of memory for the original training. The training conditions can be controlled so that the control mice (uninjected or saline-injected) are "undertrained" (20–30% recall score) or "overtrained" (70–80% recall score). This is accomplished by modifying the training parameters (e.g., number of training trials, buzzer strength, and foot-shock level). The undertrained mice remember the task for 3 hr but forget it in 1 week; they are therefore suitable for memory *enhancement* studies. Conversely, the overtrained mice remember well for 1 week and are suitable for memory *impairment* studies. All experiments are run with blind-coded injection solutions, to eliminate experimenter bias. Saline controls are included in a given run, if necessary for meaningful blind coding.

Results—Intracerebroventricular Route

The initial experiments with arecoline hydrobromide (ARE), edrophonium chloride (EDR; Tensilon®) and their combination (Flood et al., 1983) yielded a fortunate coincidence, namely, the entire dose–response curves for ARE and EDR proved to be identical (Fig. 14-1). Thus, a constant weight ratio of 1 ARE to 1 EDR could be utilized; 1 ng of ARE was equipotent with 1 ng of EDR at all doses tested. The ceiling response for memory retention (70–80% recall score) occurred at a dose of 100 ng of ARE or 100 ng of EDR. The same ceiling response for the two-drug combination occurred at a dose of 2.5 ng of ARE plus 2.5 ng of EDR, or a total of 5.0 ng (Fig. 14-2). This is a 95% reduction from the dose of either drug alone. This 20-fold potentiation, a total surprise, encouraged our subsequent detailed studies with other two-drug combinations of cholinergic agonists and anticholinesterases.

The dose–response curves of ARE and of EDR (Fig. 14-1) and of ARE + EDR (Fig. 14-2) proved to be typical of all the drugs subse-

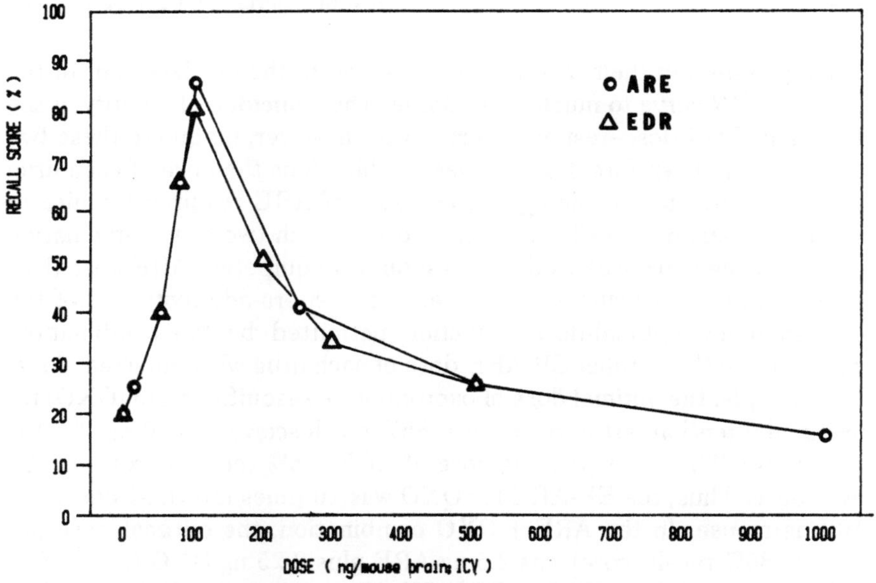

Figure 14-1. Dose–response curves of arecoline (ARE) and of edrophonium (EDR). The equipotency of ARE and EDR is coincidental. Administration was by intraventricular injection, within 1 min after training in a T-maze to avoid foot-shock applied 5 sec after sounding a warning buzzer. Retention of the trained avoidance was tested 1 week later, using a criterion of 1 avoidance response within 3 test trials. The ordinate represents the percentage of each group ($N = 20$) which met criterion.

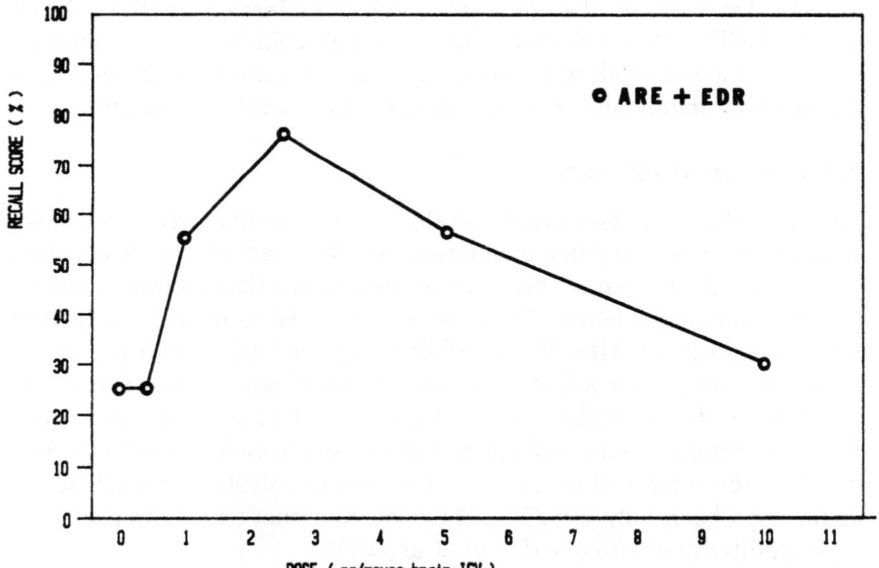

Figure 14-2. Dose–response curve of ARE + EDR, in combination. The abscissa indicates the dose of each drug: the total dose of the two equipotent drugs is double this value. Note that the optimal total dose (2.5 + 2.5 = 5.0 ng) is 1/20 of the optimal dose (100 ng) of either drug alone, shown in Fig. 14-1.

quently tested, in their inverted-U shape and in the displacement of the ARE + EDR curve to much lower doses. The coincidental identity of the ARE and EDR dose–response curves was, however, unique to these two components. Therefore, for all other combinations the dose of each drug was first converted to the equipotent dose of ARE required by mice to reach the maximal recall score. The dose of each two-drug combination could thus be expressed as the corresponding equipotent ARE dose (EP-ARE), to permit calculation of the extent of supra-additivity and of the corresponding optimal-dose reduction permitted by the combination, compared to the optimal EP-ARE dose of each drug when injected alone. For example, the optimal dose of oxotremorine sesquifumarate (OXO) for maximal retention test performance (85% recall score) was 10 ng of OXO per mouse. The corresponding dose of ARE (85% recall score) was 100 ng/mouse. Thus, the EP-ARE for OXO was 10 times the OXO dose, i.e., 100 ng/mouse. In the ARE + OXO combination, the optimal dose per mouse (85% recall score) was 2.5 ng ARE plus 0.25 ng OXO (2.5 ng EP-ARE), or a total dose of 5.0 ng EP-ARE. The potentiation factor was thus 100/5.0 = 20 and the dose reduction was 100 − 5 = 95 ng, a 95% reduction in the single drug EP-ARE dose. The same calculations were carried out for all drug combinations. The reductions in the optimal intraventricular dose for maximal retention test performance (recall scores of 75–85%) are summarized in Fig. 14-3. The potentiation factor of the three-drug combination (ARE + OXO + EDR) was 67, compared with 20 for each of the three two-drug combinations (ARE + EDR; OXO + EDR; ARE + OXO). The practical gain in dose reduction, however, was too small to encourage further exploration of three-drug or higher-order combinations in our present experimental paradigm.

Potentiation of Efficacy

The marked potentiation described above relates to the increased *potency* of two drugs when used in combination. Another view relates to increased *efficacy* of a given dose of each drug in the combination, as was shown for choline + piracetam in rats (Bartus et al., 1981). We selected noneffective individual doses of ARE (5 ng), EDR (5 ng) and OXO (0.5 ng), doses which have no greater effect than does saline. When we tested the three possible two-drug combinations, each using one-half of these noneffective doses, the retention test performance was raised to ceiling levels (75–85% recall). If the combined drugs had acted only additively, the recall scores would have been only 20–25%. Thus the combinations showed marked supra-additivity of efficacy (Flood et al., 1983).

Amnestic Effect of High Doses

High doses of ARE, EDR, and OXO appear to have no effect on memory retention, compared to saline controls, in "undertrained" mice, that is,

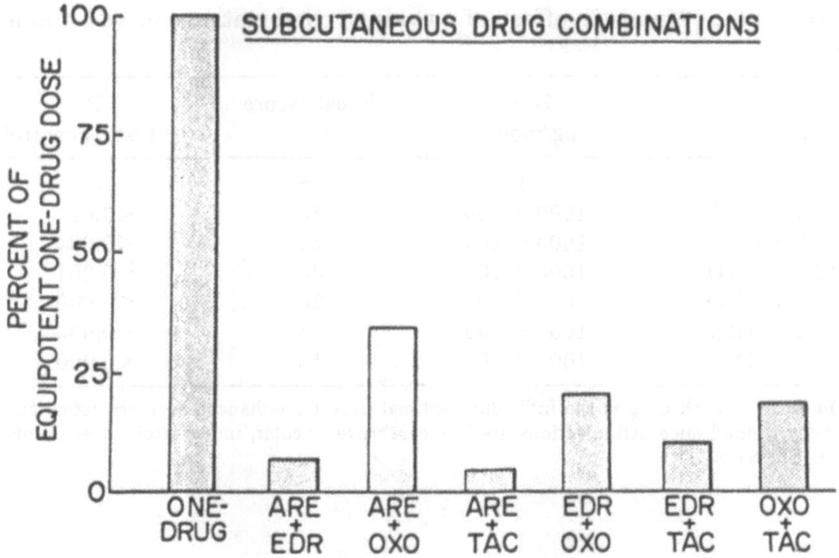

Figure 14-3. Reduced intraventricular doses of two-drug combinations required for peak response (75% or higher recall score). The doses in each optimal combination were converted to the equipotent dose of ARE (see text). The ordinate represents the percent of this one-drug dose, normalized to 100%. The first bar refers to ARE, EDR, or OXO, each administered by itself. (From Cherkin, A. and Flood, J.F.: Remarkable potentiation among memory-enhancing cholinergic drugs in mice. In Regelson, W. and Sinex, F.M. (Eds.), *Intervention in the Aging Process, Part A: Quantitation, Epidemiology, and Clinical Research*, pp. 225–245. New York: Alan R. Liss, 1983, with permission of the publisher.)

mice trained under the conditions which result in low recall test scores (20–25%) for controls 1 week later. When such high doses are tested in "overtrained" mice, which have control recall test scores of 75–85% 1 week later, they show a marked amnestic effect, with 10–40% recall scores (Cherkin and Riege, 1983; data of Flood et al.). Furthermore, the combinations of high-dose ARE + OXO, ARE + EDR, and OXO + EDR showed potentiation of the amnestic effect (Table 14-1).

Results—Subcutaneous Route

Subcutaneous administration of single drugs and two-drug combinations confirmed the findings by intracerebroventricular injection. As expected, the subcutaneous doses had to be increased (by factors of 440 for ARE alone to 3674 for ARE + OXO, on a molar basis) to achieve maximal retention test scores (Flood et al., 1984a). Also, the potentiation factors were somewhat lower and more variable for the subcutaneous injections,

Table 14-1. Amnestic effect of two-drug combinations in well-trained mice

Drugs	Dose (ng/mouse)	Recall Score (%)	P (χ^2 test vs control)
Control	0	85	—
DEA + ARE	1000 + 100	50	<0.02
DEA + EDR	1000 + 100	40	<0.004
DEA + OXO	1000 + 10	35	<0.001
EDR + OXO	100 + 10	20	<0.0001
EDR + ARE	100 + 100	15	<0.0001
ARE + OXO	100 + 10	10	<0.0001

The dose of each drug is the individual optimal dose for enhanced memory retention in weekly trained mice. All injections are intracerebroventricular, immediately after training. $N = 20$/group.

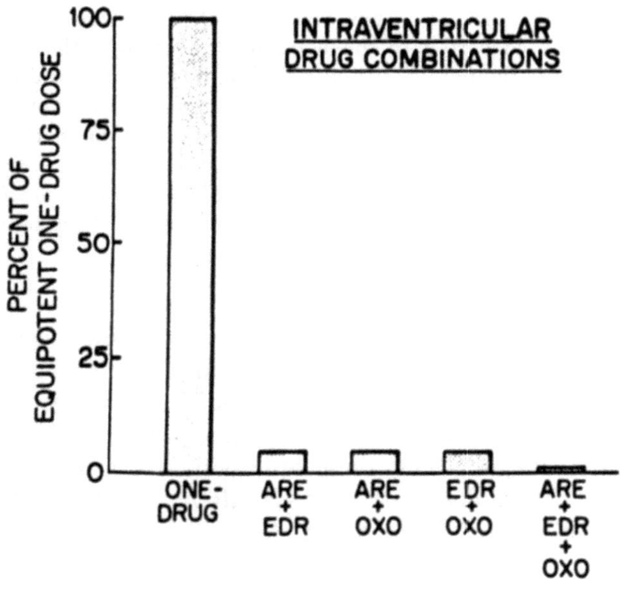

Figure 14-4. Reduced subcutaneous doses required for peak response (see legend, Fig. 14-3). The subcutaneous doses are much larger than the intraventricular doses (Fig. 14-3) but the potentiating effect of the drug combinations is similar. (From Cherkin, A. and Flood, J.F.: Remarkable potentiation among memory-enhancing cholinergic drugs in mice. In Regelson, W. and Sinex, F.M. (Eds.), *Intervention in the Aging Process, Part A: Quantitation, Epidemiology, and Clinical Research*, pp. 225–245. New York: Alan R. Liss, 1983, with permission of the publisher.)

as indicated by the dose-reduction values (Fig. 14-4). In addition, the subcutaneous dose–response curves for the single drugs ARE, EDR, OXO, and tacrine (TAC), shown in Figure 14-5, point up another problem, namely, the width of the "therapeutic window". For example, the ratio of the high and low doses of TAC which result in a 50% recall score is 96/30, or 3.2. The corresponding ratio for OXO is 146/11, or 13.3. The latter is clearly preferable from the preclinical point of view because it would presumably permit easier dose titration of individual subjects, to produce optimal memory retention. A wide therapeutic window is one of our desiderata in evaluating drug combinations for potential clinical trials.

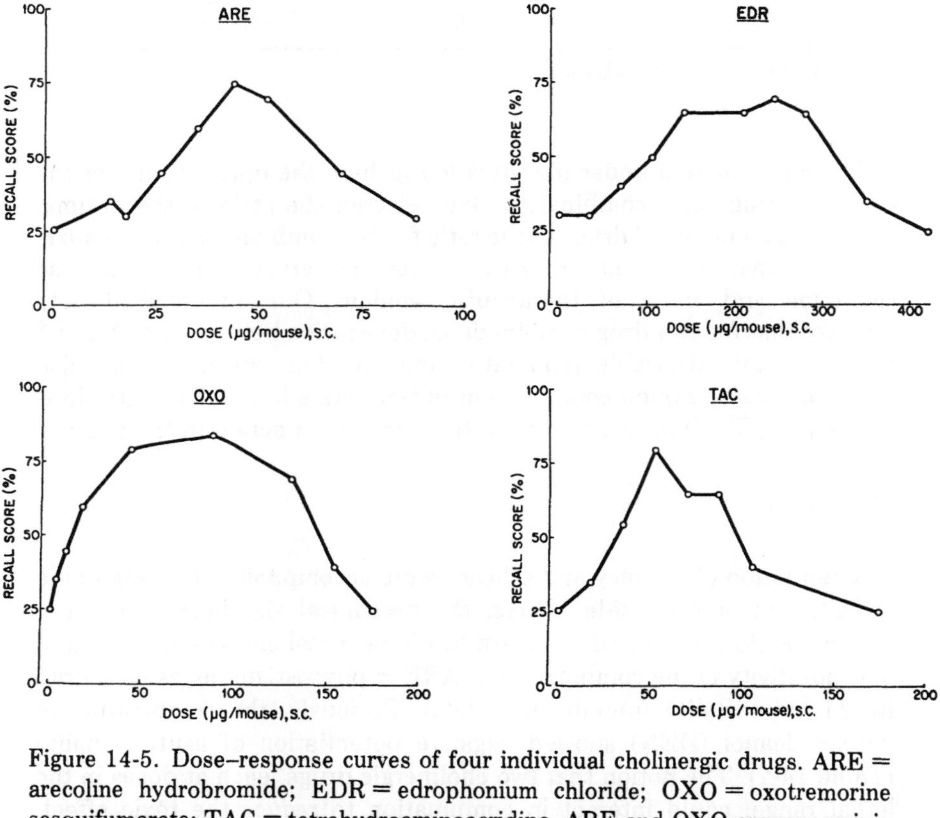

Figure 14-5. Dose–response curves of four individual cholinergic drugs. ARE = arecoline hydrobromide; EDR = edrophonium chloride; OXO = oxotremorine sesquifumarate; TAC = tetrahydroaminoacridine. ARE and OXO are muscarinic agonists; EDR and TAC are cholinesterase inhibitors. (From Cherkin, A. and Flood, J.F.: Remarkable potentiation among memory-enhancing cholinergic drugs in mice. In Regelson, W. and Sinex, F.M. (Eds.), *Intervention in the Aging Process, Part A: Quantitation, Epidemiology, and Clinical Research*, pp. 225–245. New York: Alan R. Liss, 1983, with permission of the publisher.)

Table 14-2. Infra-additivity of the lethality of subcutaneous arecoline + deanol in 2-day-old chicks ($N = 10$/gp). The deanol dose, 71 mg/chick in all cases, was approximately the LD_{10} when injected alone.

	ARE (mg/chick)	Observed Mortality (%) ARE	Observed Mortality (%) ARE + DEA	Predicted Additive Mortality (%)[a]
	79	50	10	67
	93	50	10	72
	110	60	60	76
	132	60	70	80
	157	60	40	84
Mean	114	56	38	76
χ^2		3.25	14.73	
P		0.11	<0.001	

[a]Calculated by log probit analysis.

Other parameters under investigation include the optimal ratio of the doses of drugs in a combination. We selected the ratio of the optimal doses of the individual drugs as the ratio for our combinations. We realize, however, that this is not necessarily best in terms of maximal dose reduction and width of therapeutic window. Our unpublished data indicate that for two-drug combinations, dose ratios between 1 to 1 and 1 to 8 are more desirable than ratios outside that range. We are also exploring how to exploit combinations of fast-acting (e.g., EDR) with slow-acting (e.g., TAC) drugs, to extend the duration of action in the brain.

Toxicity

If potentiation of potency and efficacy were accompanied by comparable potentiation of toxic side effects, the preclinical significance of these studies would be nullified. Pilot studies in neonatal chicks demonstrated only additivity in the combination of ARE + physostigmine, as measured by 24 hr mortality (unpublished data). Curiously, the combination of ARE + deanol (DEN) showed negative potentiation of acute lethality (Table 14-2). The notion that two cholinergic drugs, each at doses in the lethal range, could interact in combination to *reduce* the toxic effect, would not have occurred to us. This surprising finding, coupled with the surprisingly large extent of supra-additivity we had discovered, had an interactive effect upon our entire approach to designing combination drug experiments. That effect was to diminish our reliance upon the "facts" of today's pharmacology and toxicology and to increase our reliance upon running experiments which might be considered a priori to fly in the face of "reality."

The real interest with respect to toxicity is not in high-acute dose levels within the lethal range, which have limited relevance for our preclinical approach, but in the much lower chronic oral dose levels which are within the memory enhancing range. Here, behavioral toxicity studies are more appropriate and are now in progress. The test behaviors, applied to mice ingesting drugs and drug combinations in their drinking water for several months, include tests of sensory abilities (acoustic, visual, pain), motor abilities (stamina, coordination, activity), and general health (body weight, posture, gait, eye condition, and reflex and trophic reactions). These studies are in progress with young adult mice and will be extended to aged mice. Already we have found two unusual cases of negative interaction: the ARE + TAC and the OXO + TAC combinations impair rotorod performance less than do the individual drugs alone, each at the same dose as in its combinations.

Interpretation—Basic Science

The supra-additivity of memory enhancement in the case of a cholinomimetic (e.g., ARE or OXO) combined with an anticholinesterase (e.g., EDR or TAC) could be interpreted as reflecting the synergistic interaction between the exogenous agonist and the prolonged action of endogenous acetylcholine (ACh) resulting from its slower hydrolysis by the inhibited acetylcholinesterase. This of course presupposes that the ACh levels in the CNS of normal young adult mice is suboptimal for memory consolidation, which is suggested also by the improved memory in 13-month-old mice raised on a choline-enriched diet (Bartus et al., 1982).

The interpretation is more difficult for the supra-additivity observed in combinations of two cholinomimetics (ARE + OXO) or of two anticholinesterases (EDR + TAC). One possibility is that the supra-additivity has a pharmacokinetic basis: the effect of the combination is prolonged because one drug acts more slowly than the other. We have indirect evidence which is compatible with this interpretation (Flood et al., 1984b). When a noneffective dose of ARE by the intracerebroventricular route (50 ng) is injected three times after training (immediately, 90 min after, and 180 min after) the retention test score reaches ceiling (95% recall). Appropriate control groups showed no enhancing effect with 150 ng injected 180 min after training, or with two 50-ng injections, or with three saline injections. The results indicate that prolonging the duration of stimulating the cholinergic system can enhance memory processing during the 3 hr after training.

For the ARE + OXO combinations, supra-additivity could reflect the existence of subtypes of central ACh receptors. Briggs et al. (1982) have described two muscarinic agonist receptor subtypes in both young (6 mo) and old (24 mo) rat brain; this supports the subtype hypothesis. It may be added that Stanley and Drachman (1983) have recently reported two subpopulations of ACh receptors at the neuromuscular junction, one with a half-life of 0.78 days and a second with a half-life of 12.4 days.

The case for multiple forms of acetylcholinesterase, to explain supra-additivity of the anticholinesterases, is on firmer ground. At least four molecular forms of acetylcholinesterase have been identified (Massoulie and Bon, 1982) and it can be speculated that EDR and TAC have differential effects in inhibiting different forms of the enzyme.

Our data, while suggestive, do not permit identifying the mechanisms underlying the observed supra-additivity. We have started to explore this area in collaboration with neurochemical colleagues. It is of course entirely possible that two or more mechanisms are involved, including differential pharmacokinetics, multiple ACh receptor sites, multiple forms of acetylcholinesterase, and others.

Implications—Preclinical

Our point of view is that the year 2000 will see effective treatments for senile amnesias which may arise from the zinc-deficiency speculation of Burnet (1981), the transplantation of brain cells to replace deteriorated neurons (Bjorklund, 1983), or from developments unthought of today. But for those who agonize through their "36 hour days" in caring for demented family members, and for a society facing the enormous human, social, and financial burdens of caring for those who cannot be kept at home, there is a compulsion to do better than we have done with today's state of the art. Hence our interest in the strategy of a multimodel approach to treating geriatric memory dysfunction (Yesavage et al., 1981; Cherkin and Riege, 1983), including synergistic low-dose pharmacotherapy. If the insights emerging from our research with mice have any relevance to the clinical treatment of memory failure, they suggest the following caveats:

1. Dose–response curves may be inverted-U shaped, for single drugs and for drug combinations.
2. Low doses may enhance memory; high doses may impair.
3. Memory enhancers may interact to improve or to impair memory.
4. Memory enhancing drugs may interact with prescribed medications, with positive or negative effects upon memory.
5. Such interactions may convert memory enhancement to memory impairment.

6. Therapeutic windows may be narrow, requiring individual dose titration for each patient.
7. Treatments which are optimal for enhancing "short-term" memory may be suboptimal for enhancing "long-term" memory.

Keeping these caveats in mind, we venture to suggest to our practitioner colleagues a clinical treatment approach for the senile amnesias, as follows:

1. Identify and correct all "reversible dementias" by careful diagnosis.
2. For the future, assume that all cases are potentially treatable.
3. For today, accept a realistic limited treatment goal; namely, to enhance memory enough to preserve or restore independent functioning in a subgroup of responders.
4. Apply a multimodal approach, comprising synergistic drug combinations plus nonpharmacologic interventions, to provide optimal nutrition, socialization, sensory stimulation, exercise, and cognitive skills training.
5. Individualize drug dosage for each patient.
6. Identify a subgroup of reliable responders.
7. Follow up to maintain optimal individual drug dosage for the responders.
8. Modify treatments to identify additional responders.

References

Bartus, R.T., Dean, R.L., III, Beer, B., and Lippa, A.S.: The cholinergic hypothesis of geriatric memory dysfunction. *Science 217*, 408–417 (1982).

Bartus, R.T., Dean, R.L., III, Goas, J.A., and Lippa, A.S.: Age-related changes in passive avoidance retention: Modulation with dietary choline. *Science 209*, 301–303 (1980).

Bartus, R.T., Dean, R.L., III, Sherman, K.A., Friedman, E., and Beer, B.: Profound effects of combining choline and piracetam on memory enhancement and cholinergic function in aged rats. *Neurobiol. Aging 2*, 105–111 (1981).

Blaschke, T.F., Cohen, S.N., Tatro, D.S., and Ruben, P.C.: Drug–drug interactions and aging. In Jarvik, L.F., Greenblatt, D.J., and Harman, D. (Eds.), *Clinical Pharmacology and the Aged Patient*, pp. 11–26. New York: Raven, 1981.

Bjorklund, A., as reported by Kolata, G.: Brain grafting work shows promise. *Science 221*, 1277 (1983).

Briggs, R.S., Petersen, M.M, and Cook, P.J.: Muscarinic agonist receptor subtypes in aging rat brain. *Neurobiol. Aging 3*, 259–261 (1982).

Burnet, F.M.: A possible role of zinc in the pathology of dementia. *Lancet I*, 186–188 (1981).

Carter, S.K., and Slavik, M.: Chemotherapy of cancer. *Ann. Rev. Pharmacol. 14*, 157–183 (1974).

Cherkin, A., and Riege, W.H.: Multimodal approach to pharmacotherapy of senile amnesias. In: Cervos-Navarro, J., and Sarkander, H.I. (Eds.), *Brain Aging: Neuropathology and Neuropharmacology*, pp. 415–535. New York: Raven, 1983.

Cooper, S.J.: Behavioral studies of drug interactions. In Brown, K., and Cooper, S.J. (Eds.), Chemical Influences on Behaviour, pp. 533–597. London: Academic, 1979.

Corkin, S., Davis, K.L., Growdon, J.H., Usdin, E., and Wurtman, R.J.: Alzheimer's Disease: A Report of Progress in Research. New York: Raven, 1982.

Crook, T., and Gershon, T. (Eds.): Strategies for the Development of an Effective Treatment for Senile Dementia. New Canaan, Conn.: Mark Powley Associates, 1981

Drachman, D.A., Glosser, G., Fleming, P., and Longenecker, G.: Memory decline in the aged: Treatment with lecithin and physostigmine. *Neurology 32*, 944–950 (1982).

Ferris, S.H., Reisberg, B., Crook, T., et al.: Pharmacologic treatment of senile dementia: Choline, L-DOPA, piracetam, and choline plus piracetam. In Corkin, S. et al. (Eds.), *Alzheimer's Disease: A Report of Progress in Research*, pp. 475–481. New York: Raven, 1982.

Flood, J.F., Bennett, E.L., and Orme, A.E.: Relation of memory formation to controlled amounts of brain protein synthesis. *Physiol. Behav. 15*, 97–102 (1975).

Flood, J.F., Landry, D.W., and Jarvik, M.E.: Cholinergic receptor interactions and their effects on long-term memory processing. *Brain Res. 215*, 177–185 (1981).

Flood, J.F., Smith, G.E., and Cherkin, A.: Memory retention: Potentiation of cholinergic drug combinations in mice. *Neurobiol. Aging 4*, 37–43 (1983).

Flood, J.F., Smith, G.E., and Cherkin, A.: Memory enhancement: Supra-additive effect of subcutaneous cholinergic drug combinations in mice. *Psychopharmacology* (in press, 1984a).

Flood, J.F., Smith, G.E., and Cherkin, A.: Memory retention: Effect of prolonged cholinergic stimulation in mice. *Pharmacol. Biochem. Behav. 20*:161–163, 1984b.

Hollister, L.E.: An overview of strategies for the development of an effective treatment for senile dementia. In Crook, T., and Gershon, S. (Eds.), Strategies for the Development of an Effective Treatment for Senile Dementia. New Canaan, Conn.: Mark Powley Associates, 1981.

Kubanis, P., and Zornetzer, S.F.: Age-related behavioral and neurobiological changes: A review with an emphasis on memory. *Behav. Neural Biol. 31*, 115–172 (1981).

Massoulie, J., and Bon, S.: The molecular forms of cholinesterase and acetylcholinesterase in vertebrates. *Ann. Rev. Neurosci. 5*, 57–106 (1982).

Ouslander, J.G.: Drug therapy in the elderly. *Ann. Intern. Med. 95*, 711–722 (1981).

Peters, B.H., and Levin, H.S.: Effects of physostigmine and lecithin on memory in Alzheimer disease. *Ann. Neurol. 6*, 219–221 (1979).

Peters, B.H., and Levin, H.S.: Chronic oral physostigmine and lecithin administration in memory disorders of aging. In Corkin, S. et al. (Eds.), *Alzheimer's Disease: A Report of Progress*, pp. 421–426. New York: Raven, 1982.

Reisberg, B., London, E., Ferris, S.H., Anand, R., and de Leon, M.J.: Novel pharmacologic approaches to the treatment of senile dementia of the Alzheimer's type (SDAT). *Psychopharmacol. Bull. 19*, 220–225 (1983).

Roberts, E.: Potential therapies in aging and senile dementias. *Ann. NY Acad. Sci. 396*, 165–178 (1982).

Rudoy R.C., Nelson, J.D., and Haltalin, K.C.: In vitro susceptibility of Shigella strains to trimethoprim and sulfamethoxazole. *Antimicrob. Agents Chemother. 5*, 439–443 (1974).

Salzman, C.: Psychotropic drug use and polypharmacy in a general hospital. *Gen. Hosp. Psychiat. 3*, 1–9 (1981).

Stanley, E.F., and Drachman, D.B.: Rapid degradation of "new" acetylcholine receptors at neuromuscular junctions. *Science 222*, 67–69 (1983).

Yesavage, J.A., Westphal, J., and Rush, L.: Senile dementia: Combined pharmacologic and psychologic treatment. *J. Am. Geriatr. Soc. 29*, 164–171 (1981).

Chapter 15

Effects of Aging and Hypertension on Cerebral Blood Flow and Autoregulation in Normal Subjects and CVD Patients

Yukito Shinohara

Summary

The influence of age on cerebral blood flow (CBF) and cerebrovascular response was investigated using the atraumatic ^{133}Xe inhalation and intravenous injection methods in normal volunteers and the results were compared with those in patients with cerebral infarction. In normals, regional CBF decreased rather uniformly throughout the brain with advancing age. Cerebrovascular responses, particularly the autoregulatory mechanism, also seemed to deteriorate with advancing age, particularly in CVD patients. Multivariate analysis indicated that age was the most important among 15 parameters and laboratory test data for determining CBF in normals. In patients with cerebrovascular disease (even in the chronic stage), age was relatively unimportant.

A possible explanation of the CBF reduction in healthy aged people is the reduction of oxygen and glucose metabolism, together with pathologic changes of the cerebral vessels. The decline of cerebrovascular response may also be attributable to pathologic changes of cerebral vessels, as well as of the autonomic nervous system.

Introduction

Cerebral blood flow in humans has been studied extensively in a variety of pathologic and physiologic conditions during the last 20 years. However, the effects of aging on cerebral blood flow (CBF) and cerebrovascular response are still a matter of debate. Little and conflicting information is available on the effect of aging on the blood flow and its regulation in the brain. Some studies (Scheinberg et al., 1953; Fazekas et al., 1955; Kety, 1956; Dekorninck et al., 1977) have shown a decline of CBF in normal subjects. For example, Kety (1956) suggested that progressive CBF reduction occurs through adolescence, adulthood, and senescence. In contrast, other investigators (Shenkin et al., 1953; Lassen et al., 1960; Gottstein et al., 1979; Olesen, 1974) did not find significant differences in CBF between young and old normal subjects. The inconsistency between these results is probably related in part to the traumatic and invasive nature of the techniques used in early studies of CBF measurement in humans, as pointed out by Melamed et al. (1980). The development of a noninvasive technique for CBF measurement now permits a safe approach to this problem. The purpose of this presentation is to describe the influence of age on CBF measured using an atraumatic method in normal volunteers.

Subjects and Methods

The subjects studied were 46 normal volunteers, aged 18–92 years, who were healthy and free of any neurological signs and symptoms including headache and so on. Physical examinations, including blood pressure, auscultation of heart sounds, blood cell count, liver function tests, electrolytes, and so on, also showed no abnormalities. In almost all normal volunteers, CT examinations were also performed and the results were considered to be normal in relation to the age of the subjects. In other words, the subjects studied were considered to be completely normal in a strict sense.

CBF was measured by the atraumatic ^{133}Xe inhalation method and/or intravenous injection method. The mean values of gray matter flow or initial slope index for 32 areas of both hemispheres were considered as representative of the CBF in the normals.

Results and Comments

Figure 15-1 shows the relationship between age and blood flow in the brain in normals. The vertical axis shows mean gray matter blood flow in the brain, which was measured using the ^{133}Xe inhalation method. It is clear that increases of age and reduction of mean gray matter blood flow

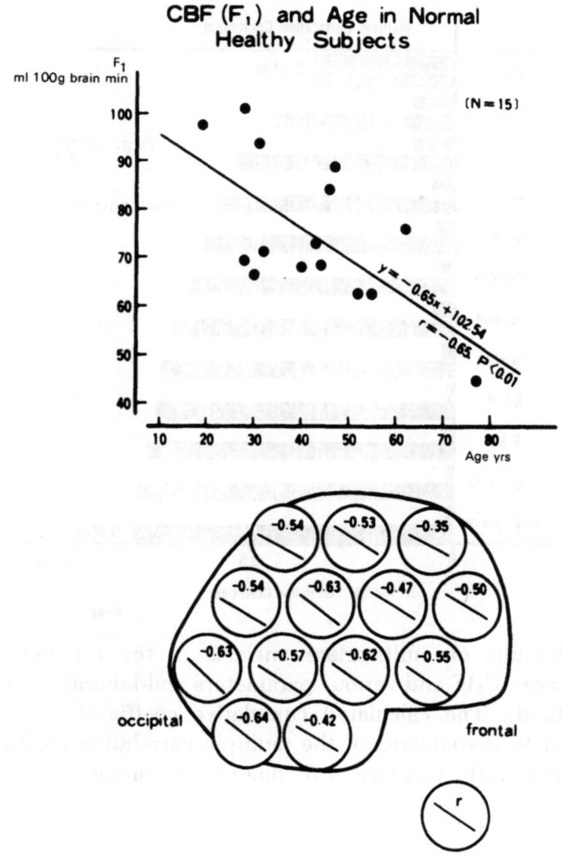

Figure 15-1. Relationship between gray matter blood flow (F_1) in the brain and age of normal volunteers (^{133}Xe inhalation method). The upper part shows the correlation obtained for 15 subjects, and the lower part shows the mean values of flow reduction in various regions of the brain.

are well correlated. This result is in good agreement with that of Melamed et al. (1980), who reported a decline of CBF with normal aging using the same ^{133}Xe inhalation method. As shown in the lower part of Figure 15-1, the reduction of blood flow with age was observed in all parts of the brain through the frontal to occipital areas, and the degree of reduction was similar in all parts (Shinohara et al., 1983). This result indicates that there is a significant correlation between age and CBF, but it was not determined whether age is the most important of the various factors affecting CBF. To investigate this point, the influence on CBF of 15 parameters and laboratory test data were evaluated by means of multivariate analysis. The parameters and laboratory test data chosen for this study were age, blood pressure, fasting, blood sugar, blood urea nitrogen, and so on.

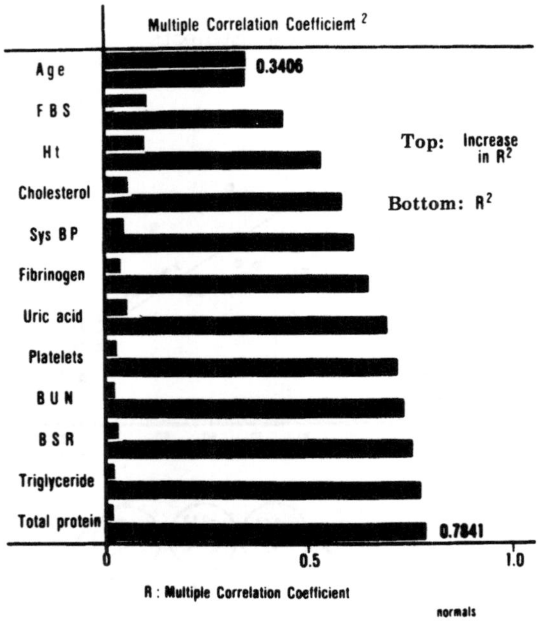

Figure 15-2. Results of multivariate analysis of the relationship in normal volunteers between CBF and various parameters and laboratory test data (^{133}Xe inhalation method). The calculated cumulative coefficients of determination, which are equal to the squares of the multiple correlation coefficients (R^2) are shown, together with the increase of R^2 due to each factor.

Figure 15-2 shows the calculated cumulative coefficients of determination which are equal to the squares of the multiple correlation coefficients. The largest coefficient of determination, 0.34, was that for age, followed by FBS and Ht. Thus, age appeared to be the most important among these parameters for determining CBF in normals.

It is known that pulmonary function can be influenced by aging. Thus, the relation between the ^{133}Xe concentrations in expired air and arterial blood was investigated. As shown in Figure 15-3, in a patient with impaired pulmonary function, the ^{133}Xe concentration in arterial blood did not coincide with that in expired air. When ^{133}Xe was injected intravenously, as shown in the lower part of Figure 15-3, the ^{133}Xe concentration in the arterial blood and that in expired air showed a good coincidence. To avoid the effect of aging on pulmonary function and values of CBF as measured by the ^{133}Xe inhalation method, some investigations were performed using the ^{133}Xe intravenous injection method. As shown in Figure 15-4, the correlation between mean gray matter blood flow and age of the subject was again statistically significant. The result of multivariate analysis showed that the largest coefficient of

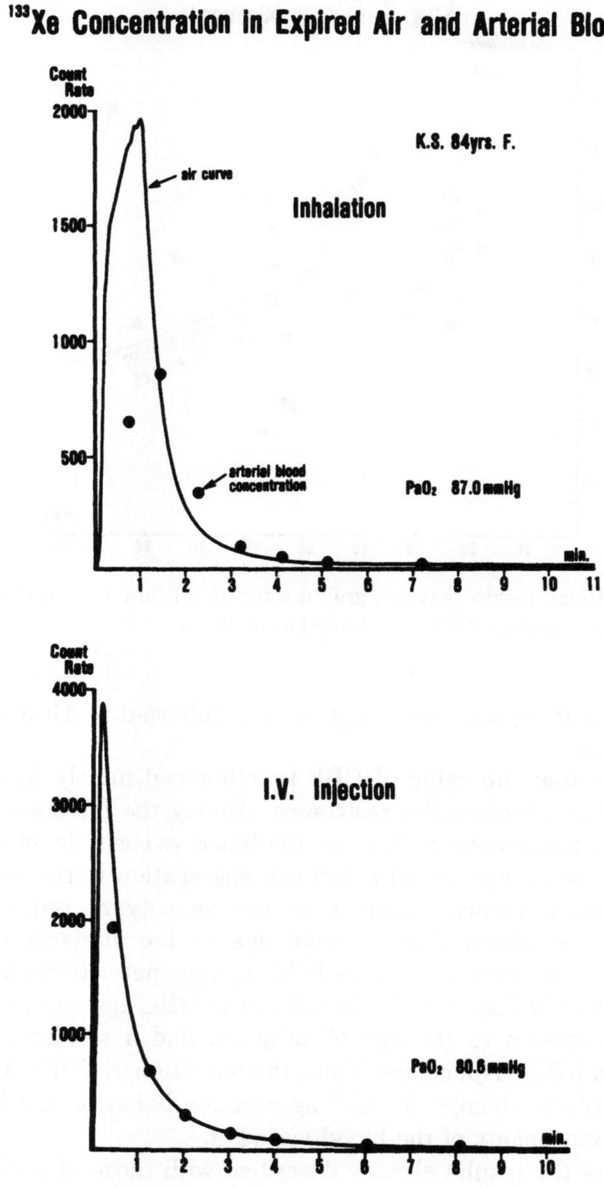

Figure 15-3. Concentrations of ^{133}Xe in expired air and arterial blood of a patient with impaired pulmonary function after ^{133}Xe inhalation (upper) and ^{133}Xe IV injection (lower).—, ^{133}XE in expired air; ●, ^{133}XE in arterial blood.

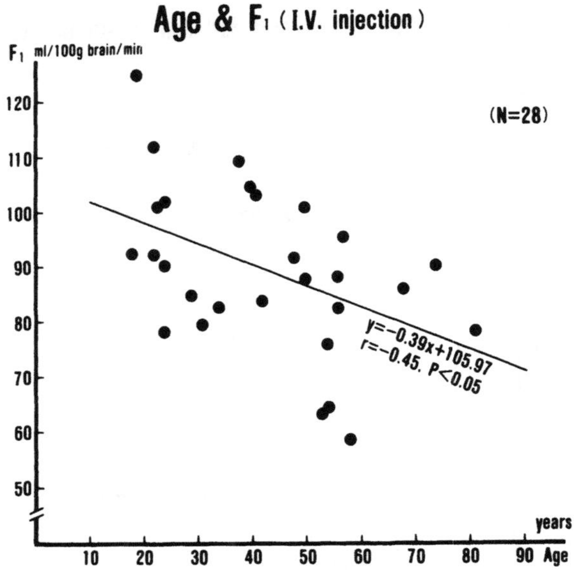

Figure 15-4. Relationship between gray matter blood flow (F_1) in the brain and age of normal volunteers (^{133}Xe IV injection method).

determination (0.36) was again that for age, followed by Ht and systolic blood pressure.

It is known that the value of CBF is influenced mainly by perfusion pressure and cerebrovascular resistance. Among the factors which may affect the cerebrovascular resistance, the blood viscosity is influenced to some degree by change of red blood cell aggregation in the vessels. To investigate the influence of aging on the velocity of red blood cell aggregation, the relationship between age of the subjects and RBC aggregation was examined using an RBC aggregometer (Kobatake et al., 1979). As shown in Figure 15-5, the velocity of RBC aggregation in whole blood is not related to the age of subjects, and a similar result was obtained with RBC suspensions. Thus, the reduction in CBF with aging is not attributable to changes in RBC aggregation behavior and Ht, which are major determinants of the blood viscosity.

To compare the results already described with those of patients with cerebrovascular disease, similar investigations were performed in 59 CVD patients. For this study the volume of low density area (LDA) on CT film was added as a new parameter, and in fact it showed the largest coefficient of determination (0.22), followed by Ht and so on in the acute stage of CVD (which is less than 28 days after onset). Age was, naturally, not the most important factor for determining CBF in these patients. For CBF in the diseased hemisphere in the chronic stage of CVD, LDA remains the most important parameter for determining CBF, followed by MABP, and

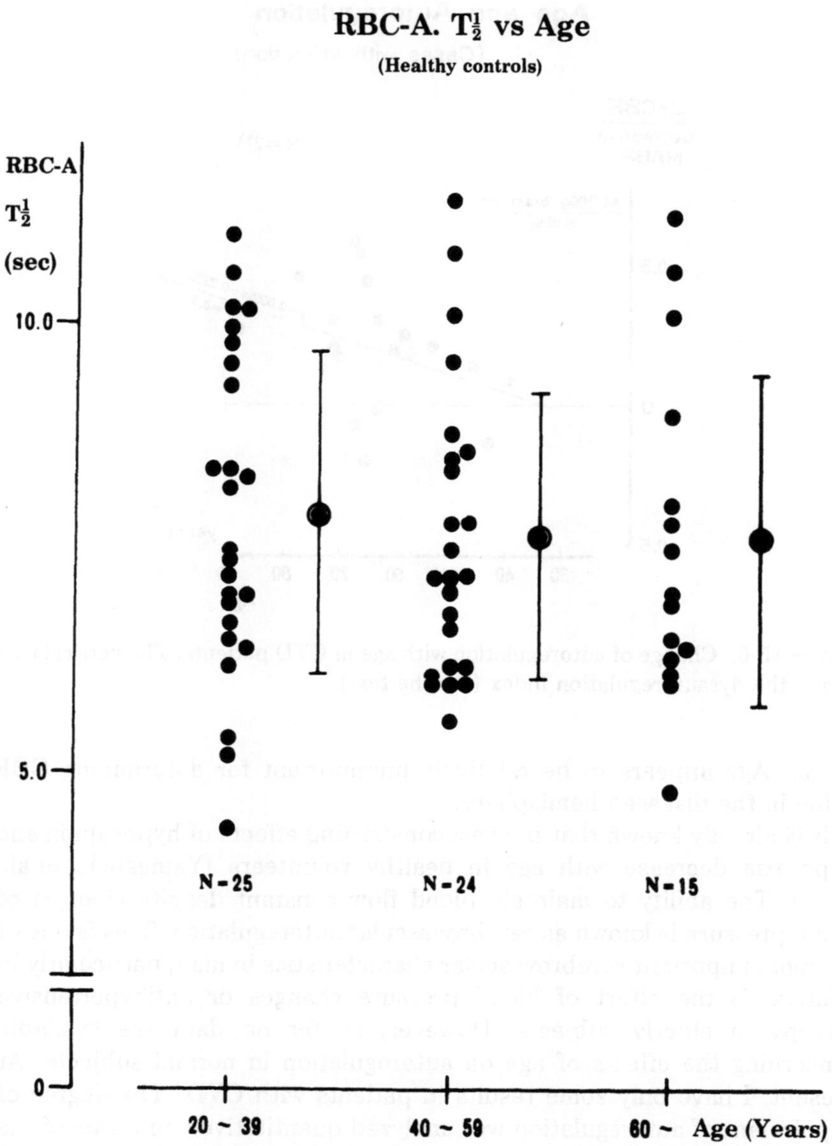

Figure 15-5. Dependence of the velocity of red blood cell aggregation ($T_{½}$) in whole blood on age in normal subjects. The subjects ($N = 64$) were grouped into three age ranges.

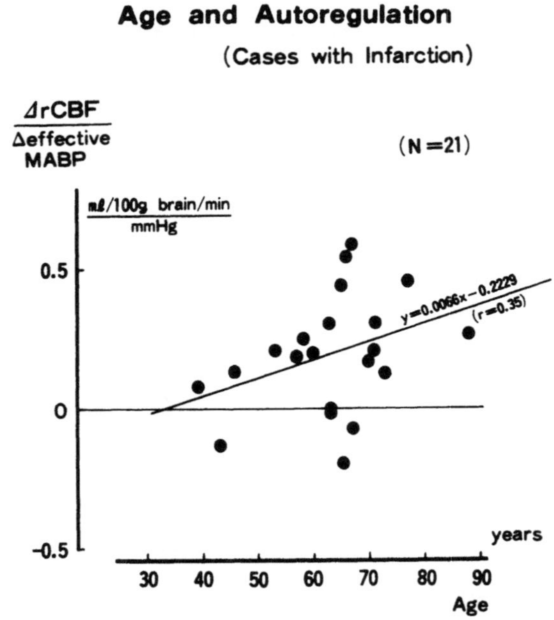

Figure 15-6. Change of autoregulation with age in CVD patients. The vertical axis shows the dysautoregulation index (see the text).

so on. Age appears to be relatively unimportant for determining CBF value in the diseased hemisphere.

It is already known that the vasoconstricting effects of hypocapnia and hyperoxia decrease with age in healthy volunteers (Yamaguchi et al., 1979). The ability to maintain blood flow constant despite changes of blood pressure is known as cerebrovascular autoregulation. This is one of the most important cerebrovascular characteristics in man, particularly in relation to the effect of blood pressure changes or antihypertensive therapy in elderly subjects. However, so far no data are available concerning the effects of age on autoregulation in normal subjects. At present, I have only some results in patients with CVD. The degree of impairment of autoregulation was analyzed quantitatively in terms of the dysautoregulation index, which is equal to CBF decrease per 1 mmHg fall in effective perfusion pressure on head-up tilting. The effective perfusion pressure was measured from a catheter inserted into the internal carotid artery. As shown in Figure 15-6, the results indicated that impairment of autoregulation becomes greater with increasing age, although a statistically significant correlation was not obtained.

Figure 15-7 shows the effect of hypertension on autoregulation in CVD patients in two age groups. Statistical analysis was not carried out since the numbers of subjects were too small, but there is some indication that

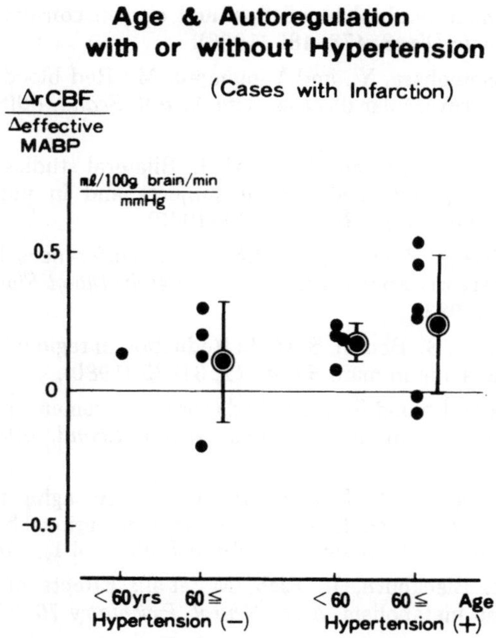

Figure 15-7. The effects of hypertension and age on autoregulation in CVD patients. The vertical axis shows the dysautoregulation index (see the text).

hypertensive patients over 60 years of age have more severe impairment of autoregulation.

The reason why there is CBF reduction in healthy aged people is still obscure. Although there is still much controversy, the reduction of oxygen and glucose metabolism with advancing age which has been observed by some investigators (Metter et al., 1983; Rapoport et al., 1983) using positron emission tomography may be one of the factors, together with pathologic change of the cerebral vessels. The decline of cerebrovascular response is also attributable to the pathologic changes of the cerebral vessels and possibly also the autonomic nervous system.

References

Dekorninck, W.J., Calay, R., and Hongne, J.C.: CBF in elderly with chronic cerebral involvement. In Ingvar, D.H., Lassen, N.A. (Eds.), Cerebral function, metabolism and circulation. *Acta Neurol. Scand. 56*(Suppl 64), 412–413 (1977).

Fazekas, J.F., Kleh, J., and Finnerty, F.A.: Influence of age and vascular disease on cerebral hemodynamics and metabolism. *Am. J. Med. 18*, 477–485 (1955).

Gottstein, U., and Held, K.: Effects of aging on cerebral circulation and metabolism in man. *Acta Neurol. Scand. 60*(Suppl 72), 54–55 (1979).

Kety, S.S.: Human cerebral blood flow and oxygen consumption as related to aging. *J. Chronic Dis. 3*, 478–486 (1956).

Kobatake, K., Shinohara, Y., and Yamamoto, M.: Red blood cell aggregation in occlusive cerebrovascular disease. *Acta Neurol. Scand. 60*(Suppl 72), 612–613 (1979).

Lassen, N.A., Feinberg, I., and Lane, M.H.: Bilateral studies of cerebral oxygen uptake in young and aged normal subjects and in patients with organic dementia. *J. Clin. Invest. 39*, 491–500 (1960).

Metter, E.J., Riege, W.H., Kuhl, D.E. et al.: Differences in regional glucose metabolic intercorrelations with aging. *J. Cereb. Blood Flow Metabol. 3*(Suppl 1), s482–484 (1983).

Melamed, E., Lavy, S., Bentin, S. et al.: Reduction in regional cerebral blood flow during normal aging in man. *Stroke 11*, 31–35 (1980).

Olesen, J.: Cerebral blood flow. Methods for measurement, regulation, effects of drugs and changes in disease. *Acta Neurol. Scand. 50*(Suppl. 57), 1–134 (1974).

Rapoport, S.I., Duara, R., Horwitz, B. et al.: Brain aging in 40 healthy men: rCMRglc and correlated functional activity in various brain regions in the resting state. *J. Cereb. Blood Flow Metabol. 3*(Suppl 1), s484–485 (1983).

Scheinberg, P., Blackburn, I., Rich, M. et al.: Effects of aging on cerebral circulation and metabolism. *Arch. Neurol. Psychiatry 70*, 77–85 (1953).

Shenkin, H.A., Novak, P., Goluboff, B. et al.: The effects of aging, arteriosclerosis and hypertension upon the cerebral circulation. *J. Clin. Invest. 32*, 459–465 (1953).

Shinohara, Y., Takagi, S., and Kobatake, K.: Effect of aging on CBF and autoregulation in normal subjects and CVD patients. *Eur. Neurol. 22*(Suppl 2), 36–37 (1983).

Yamaguchi, F., Meyer, J.S., Sakai, F. et al.: Effects of normal human aging on cerebral vasoconstrictive responses to hypocapnia with demonstration of ischemic threshold. *Acta Neurol. Scand. 60*(Suppl. 72), 88–89 (1979).

Part IV

Imaging Techniques

Chapter 16

Imaging Techniques of the Aging Brain

R. Nick Bryan

Some practical thoughts concerning imaging techniques for patients who have Alzheimer's disease are presented, followed by a somewhat negative, biased overview of the value of current imaging procedures for these diseases. Finally, a new technique that will inevitably be applied to these patients, nuclear magnetic resonance (NMR) imaging, is discussed.

Nuclear magnetic resonance has not been tested significantly in this patient population. To be frank, the practical value of the use of imaging techniques, that is, static imaging techniques, for elderly patients who are or are not demented remains to be proved. Imaging techniques have been used mainly for diagnosing problems other than such basic disease processes as Alzheimer's disease. We look for meningiomas, butterfly glioblastomas, subdural hematomas, and for hydrocephalus which is often the communicating type, either idiopathic or the result of subarachnoid hemorrhage. Unfortunately, that is basically the only practical value of today's imaging techniques for the demented patient. Although they are valuable, they are simply not very helpful for diagnosing the intrinsic process of Alzheimer's disease.

Multi-infarct dementia is another common clinical situation for which the computed tomography (CT) scan or a comparable type of imaging examination may be helpful. CT is one way to differentiate multi-infarct dementia from Alzheimer's disease. In conjunction with history and physical examination, a CT scan is about 90% accurate in diagnosing

---

This is an edited version of Dr. Bryan's presentation at the *Aging 2000* symposium.

multi-infarct dementia. The problem is, of course, that many of these patients may have a combination of brain atrophy of aging and perhaps actual Alzheimer's disease added to previous vascular insults and strokes. CT yields an overview but it does not tell us anything about the patient's functional capacity, and that is an unfortunate aspect of this imaging technique. CT is a static image of the gross anatomy, and that is about all.

In general, in patients who may have Alzheimer's disease, we look for gross atrophy of the brain. We apply that term loosely in clinical neuroradiologic practice to a process that results in volume loss of the brain and a secondary increase in the volume of cerebrospinal fluid in the subarachnoid spaces and the ventricles. A typical CT scan of a patient who indeed has Alzheimer's disease will show prominent cerebral sulci and large lateral ventricles. Patients with dementia, regardless of etiology, have difficulty complying with the requirements for doing a satisfactory CT scan. The problem is more serious when NMR studies, that take even longer, are undertaken.

The problem is that all changes observed on the CT scan are not specific to Alzheimer's disease. Normal CT scans of different patients show quite a variety in ventricular size, all within normal limits depending on the patient's age. It is a statistical fact that ventricles and cerebral sulci normally grow larger as people age. In fact, the first thing we teach students and residents about CT scans is that if a CT scan of a patient older than 45 does not show some evidence of volume loss or atrophy, one should suspect that it is, in fact, an abnormal CT scan for a patient of that age. Such patients may have cerebral swelling or a subtle subdural hematoma. Volume loss is a normal phenomenon. Wide variations occur, and they are all within the limits of normal. Scans may show very large sulci, but the patient may have no neuropsychological evidence of dementia of any kind. But it is also found that patients who are finally given a clinical diagnosis of Alzheimer's disease may have a normal-looking scan for their age. Other patients may have a little more atrophy, but that is basically what we expect to see in most 65–75-year-old patients. In the individual patient, one simply cannot distinguish the normal aging process from atrophy of a pathologic nature, like Alzheimer's disease, on the basis of that patient's CT scan.

Some patients show changes in the deep white matter when the central part of the scan around the lateral ventricles appears black rather than gray. That is normal, and can loosely be termed leukoencephalopathy. This pattern is quite common in older patients, and is probably more common in patients with a variety of central nervous system (CNS) dysfunctions. These have never been categorized well, either in terms of the etiology of the CT appearance or its functional correlates. The NMR scan shows us much more because the technique is more sensitive to the appearance of white matter. I suspect that in older age groups, including those with Alzheimer's disease, we will see changes that suggest white matter disease. The significance of these changes in regard to anatomic and functional correlates is still poorly understood.

Several years ago we attempted to quantify the volumetric spaces of the central nervous system. Using a three-dimensional computerized program, one can calculate the intracranial bony volume from a series of scans. After many esoteric, computer-demanding steps, one can calculate ventricular volume, subarachnoid space volume, and total CSF volume (from which intracranial volume has been subtracted), all of which gives total brain volume and a calculation of the average brain CT number. Several research groups in this country have done this, the general result being two Gaussian distributions with a very high overlap. A slight difference in the mean between the population of normal aged versus demented Alzheimer's disease-impaired patients has been noted, but the overlap is so broad that, in an individual patient's case, it is of little practical use. Furthermore, as one becomes familiar with the way these volumetric analyses are done, one finds a minimum of 10–15% of procedural error in these numbers, no matter how they are obtained. The basic technique yields a 10–15% statistical slope, which is far greater, in fact, than the separation of the Gaussian curve. No matter how hard one works on it, one simply cannot get information helpful for individual patients in terms of volumetric analysis of the central nervous system, mainly because it is not a functional approach. The normal brain atrophies. The CT scan gives no clue to function because it shows only electron density of the brain, which has no functional correlate. I believe we will need something like an imaging and a functional assessment such as positron emission tomography (PET) scanning.

Now I shall discuss the next kind of test in vogue, nuclear magnetic resonance, which will be used to evaluate essentially all diseases, but particularly those of the central nervous system. NMR began as the result of a brief report of his research by Felix Bloch, a physicist at Stanford University (1946). His three formulas were extraordinarily elegant and persuasive, and they remain the foundation of essentially all NMR phenomena we work with today. From those three differential equations one can understand essentially everything that has been done since 1946. The article that really directed biomedical, and particularly clinical, emphasis on NMR was a cover article in *Science* by Raymond Damadian (1976), who was at that time at the State University of New York–Downstate Medical Center. The cover was an NMR picture of a hepatoma in the liver of a live rat. Like me, you may not have been overly impressed with that image. Intellectually, it is an important picture because of what the NMR scanning technique offers us in an anatomic sense. It is extraordinary. It is better than working with a cadaver because it reveals more anatomic information than can be gained at the dissecting table.

Why do these images work, and why do they look so good? Comparing CT scans and NMR images, we get much better anatomic resolution with the NMR. There is a greater difference in the NMR parameters between different tissues than in X-ray parameters. X rays measure electron density, but there is little difference between different tissues. NMR provides better contrast between tissues. There is a wide difference, for example, between gray matter and white matter in the brain. The electron-density difference between gray and white matter, which is what the CT scan measures, is about 0.05%, while there is a 100% difference in NMR T_1. There is a tremendous amount of contrast in the system. An NMR scan will clearly show the brain stem, fourth ventricle, pons, and medullla. There is more contrast between the spinal fluid and the brain than with CT. This obviously is the way NMR studies will be applied to elderly patients. Volumetric measures made with CT will be repeated with NMR to define brain versus spinal fluid. Although NMR measures will be better, the answers will still be incomplete. There will be a broad overlap among elderly patients with dementia and those without dementia, but it is a technological advance.

The real future of NMR lies not in the images that reveal strokes, multiple sclerosis, tumors, and blood flow, but in other problems we want to address. We want to do in vivo spectroscopy. We do not want to settle for pictures. We want to look at the functional component of the brain, and we can do this with NMR. First using phosphorus-31, we can look in vivo at adenosine-5′-triphosphate (ATP) and its primary metabolites such as creatine phosphate and inorganic phosphate. This is about one thousand times harder to do than to make an image from protons, but it will be possible in the future. It has already been done with patients who have a muscular disease. When such a patient places an arm into the magnet, one sees five peaks: Peaks 1, 2, and 3 indicate the three phosphates in ATP; peak 4 is the phosphate in creatine phosphate, the high energy reservoir; and peak 5 is inorganic phosphate that shows the pH of tissue. The procedure is totally noninvasive. This study was performed on a patient with McArdle's syndrome who has an enzymatic defect that prevents the transfer of phosphate from creatine phosphate to ATP appropriately. The NMR study showed the creatine phosphate peak functioning abnormally, using up too much of the compound. With NMR, we are able to look at metabolism in vivo, and that is what we want to do in evaluating these patients. We have some preliminary scans that strongly suggest that the real future potential of NMR lies in evaluation of diseases that are of much interest to geriatricians who will use NMR imaging with its functional chemical spectroscopy.

References

Bloch, F.: Nuclear induction. *Physiol. Rev. 70*, 460 (1946).

Damadian, R., Minkoff, L. Goldsmith, M., et al.: Field focusing nuclear magnetic resonance (FONAR): Visualization of a tumor in a live animal. *Science 194*(4272), 1430–1432 (1976).

Chapter 17

Computerized Tomography (CT) and Positron Emission Tomography (PET) in Normal and Pathologic Aging

Mony J. de Leon, Steven H. Ferris, and Ajax E. George

Summary

Cognitive deterioration in the elderly caused by Alzheimer's disease (AD) represents a great sociological, medical, and economic burden. Although the etiology of the disease remains obscure, there is increasing understanding of the pre- and postmortem brain changes. In vivo computed tomography (CT) studies have shown structural changes in the AD brain that are consistent with the reported gross postmortem findings. These CT changes which are associated with the magnitude of the cognitive dysfunction include increasing ventricular size, increasing sulcal prominence, and decreased discrimination between gray and white matter. However, many of these changes occur with normal aging, thus limiting their diagnostic value. Positron emission tomography (PET) studies have found that regional glucose utilization is significantly reduced in AD. This metabolic diminution is strongly related to the magnitude of the cognitive deficit. Importantly, PET studies have not demonstrated a clear normal aging effect and therefore highlight the potential of PET as a diagnostic tool. With the development of short-lived isotopes, PET studies will increasingly use test–retest paradigms to study the capacity of the aging and diseased brain to respond to chemical and behavioral perturbations. Such studies may further enhance the diagnostic utility of PET in AD.

Cognitive deterioration in the elderly represents an immense medical and sociological burden. It has been estimated that at least 10% of the aged, a total of more than three million persons, will eventually suffer severe mental deterioration (U.S. Bureau of Census, 1971; Kay, 1972; Redick et al., 1973). A much larger number will experience sufficient cognitive decline to impede their activities and compound the normal problems of aging. More than half of the residents in nursing homes have been classified as senile (U.S. Department of Health, Education, and Welfare, 1979). The true cost to society, in terms of loss of skilled labor, nursing and medical care, institutional requirements, etc., is difficult to estimate. The cost to individuals and their families is incalculable and often tragic.

Neuropathology

A general lack of understanding of the underlying etiology of cognitive decline in the elderly has hindered attempts to find effective treatments. However, our knowledge of the clinical symptomatology, natural history, neurochemistry, and neuropathology which accompany the evolution of senile dementia, has increased over the past several years. The autopsy studies of Tomlinson et al. (1970) and others contributed prominently towards a change in our conception of senile dementia. Senile dementia is now generally classified into dementia due to Alzheimer's disease (AD), multi-infarct dementia (MID), or mixed causes, including both AD and MID. AD is now thought to account for more than 50% of all cases of senile dementia (Hachinski et al., 1974).

Histopathological studies have revealed that senile plaques, neurofibrillary tangles, and granulovacuolar degeneration are more likely to be found in the brains of patients with senile dementia of the Alzheimer type than in the brains of age-matched cognitively normal controls (Blessed et al., 1968; Tomlinson and Kitchner, 1972). Recent studies have also provided preliminary evidence for selective regional neuronal losses in AD. Both Terry et al. (1981) and Mountjoy et al. (1983) found reductions of the larger-size neurons, most notably in both frontal and temporal cortex. Whitehouse et al. (1982) reported significant neuronal loss in the nucleus basalis of Meynert. Other recent experimental evidence has indicated that lesions in this group of basal forebrain cells will produce substantial and widespread reductions in cortical levels of choline acetyltransferase, suggesting that this subcortical lesion may account for some of the cholinergic and intellectual dysfunctions characteristic of AD (Johnston et al., 1981).

Gross pathological evaluations of AD patients have revealed frontal and temporal shrinkage of the cerebral convolutions with widening of the cortical sulci and ventricular dilitation (Tomlinson et al., 1970). However, such atrophic changes demonstrated in these brains are not specifically diagnostic of AD.

Computed Tomography in AD

Several of these pathological features have been observed during life using computed tomography (CT). Our early studies demonstrated using a rank-ordering procedure for CT scans that both ventricular and sulcal enlargements are associated with increasing cognitive impairment (de Leon et al., 1979). This finding has since been replicated by others (Jacoby and Levy, 1980; Gado et al., 1982). A recent review of CT studies of AD (de Leon and George, 1983) concluded that ventricular changes are more prominent than sulcal changes. In addition, there has been some CT evidence for regionally specific, possibly subcortical, changes in AD. We found that the width of the third ventricle is the best linear ventricular correlate of measures of cognitive impairment, and also the best correlate of total ventricular volume (de Leon et al., 1980; George et al., 1981b; George et al., 1983). We also found for 28 sampled brain regions in 35 AD patients that decreasing thalamic attenuation values were the most consistent correlates of cognitive decline (de Leon and George, 1983). Bondareff et al. (1981) found comparable changes in the caudate nucleus.

Improved gray matter–white matter discrimination is possible with current-generation CT equipment. This advance has led to the study of additional CT variables. A study by Naeser (1980) has shown that attenuation changes in white matter are associated with cognitive impairments in presenile Alzheimer's disease. Our results suggest a similar but much weaker trend in AD (George et al., 1981a; de Leon et al., 1982). We were the first to report and have since replicated on over 120 patients and controls that as AD patients were more cognitively impaired, the subjective discriminaton between gray matter and white matter decreased (George et al., 1981a). The best ventricular predictor of this parenchymal change was the width of the third ventricle. Our findings also suggest that gray-white discriminability is not strongly correlated with ventricular size or cortical sulcal prominance and therefore represents an additional CT parameter in the assessment of AD-related changes.

Despite correlational data, CT studies of AD have not established diagnostic criteria for AD. Accounting for this situation is the lack of CT-pathologic correlation studies to define the pathology of the CT changes. Furthermore, CT studies have generally been conducted with small samples, inconsistent patient inclusion and exclusion criteria, and few longitudinal studies have been reported.

Brain Metabolism

In vivo attempts to study the alterations in brain functions associated with cognitive decline in aging have included the study of cerebral blood flow (CBF) and brain metabolism. The study of human CBF and metabolism began with the Kety-Schmidt technique (1948). With the development of diffusable isotopes and extracerebral scintillation detectors, studies of CBF and metabolism in normal aging and in senile dementia (organic brain syndrome) have produced contradictory results. Several investigations indicated that CBF and cerebral metabolism decreased with age

(Kety, 1956; Lassen et al., 1960; Naritomi et al., 1979). However, others have found that when subjects are carefully screened, there are no changes with advancing age (Butler et al., 1965; Fujishima and Omae, 1980). With respect to the study of the degenerative dementias, nearly all investigations have reported decreases in CBF and/or cerebral metabolism relative to age-matched control subjects (Freyhan et al., 1951; Hagberg and Ingvar, 1976; Ingvar and Gustafson, 1970; Lassen et al., 1960; Obrist et al., 1970; Simard et al., 1971; Yamaguchi et al., 1980).

The development of positron emission tomography (PET) and the tracer ^{18}F-2-deoxy-2-fluoro-D-glucose (FDG) and $^{15}O_2$ (oxygen) permits for the first time the tomographic and regional study of cerebral metabolism. A recent PET study of normal aging reported diminishing metabolic rates of oxygen only up until the fifth decade (Lammertsma, 1981; Fieschi and Lenzi, 1983). PET studies of glucose metabolism in normal aging have resulted in contradictory findings. The UCLA group (Kuhl et al., 1982) reported "definite," but highly variable, diminutions with aging. This aging change was most apparent in the ratio of frontal to parietal regional metabolic rates (hypofrontality). Our data (de Leon et al., 1983a), those of Rapoport et al. (1983), and the UCLA group in a later study (Hawkins et al., 1983) suggest the absence of specific glucose metabolism changes in normal aging. Our PET-FDG studies of AD revealed highly significant diminutions in metabolism relative to aged controls (Ferris et al., 1980; de Leon et al., 1983a). We also found that these metabolic diminutions were associated with the degree of intellectual deficit. More recently a study using PET and the $^{15}O_2$ technique demonstrated diminished oxygen utilization and CBF in AD relative to controls and a correlation between this diminution and intellectual deficit (Frackowiak et al., 1981). Others using PET-FDG have reported that regional diminutions are associated with specific symptoms in AD (Chase et al., 1983).

Brain Structure–Brain Metabolism Correlations

Interestingly, in the absence of age-associated changes of regional glucose utilization, we find evidence for structural brain changes on computed tomography. Numerous studies have reported age-related structural brain changes (see de Leon and George, 1983, for review). Using a rank-ordering procedure de Leon et al. (1984) studied a combined group of CT scans from young and elderly normal volunteers with respect to ventricular dilitation and also cortical sulcal prominence. For ventricular dilitation, 69% of the elderly had ranks greater than the median rank, and 71% of the young had scores below the median rank. For the measure of cortical change, 91% of the elderly were above the median, and 92% of the young were below the median. These percentage distributions are significantly different ($p < 0.05$). In addition to rank ordering, we also estimated ventricular size using linear and volumetric measurements. The measurements indicated consistently significant increases in ventricular size with age. Interestingly, examination PET scans from these subjects indicated no age-related changes in glucose metabolism, nor any significant sulcal size or ventricular size by glucose metabolism (CT-PET) correlations. These data, therefore, suggest structural but not metabolic brain changes in normal aging.

In contrast with the results for normal aging, we have identified structure–function correlations in AD. In particular, we have obtained CT attenuation values for the same regions studied with PET (de Leon et al., 1983c). The results indicate that only the temporal lobes and the thalami, as measured by CT, show correlation with the regional metabolic rates from widespread areas of the brain. Such patterns of correlation may be of diagnostic importance. In addition, these results appear to be consistent with the known temporal lobe pathology of AD, and with the demonstrated role of the thalamus as a relay center and possible role of the thalamus in memory dysfunctions.

We have also learned that the ventricular enlargements and enlarged cortical sulci in AD are associated with marked metabolic diminutions. In particular, using linear measures relative to controls, there is an 11% increase in ventricular size in AD (a comparable increase was found between our young and old normals) that is accompanied by a 20% decrease in metabolic rate. Overall, in our studies of normal aging and dementia we infer that in AD the metabolic deficit proportionately exceeds the structural changes, but in normal aging the structural changes appear to occur without any metabolic changes. These results suggest that PET is potentially more useful than CT in the in vivo diagnosis of AD (de Leon et al., 1983b).

Our PET dementia studies have recently taken a major step forward. With the improved spatial resolution and sensitivity of the PET VI system compared with the earlier PET III, more brain regions are amenable to accurate study. In addition, PET VI has four rings of detectors enabling the scanning of seven brain slices simultaneously. Of tremendous importance is the availability of ^{11}C-deoxy-glucose (^{11}CDG). Since this glucose metabolism tracer has a half-life of 20 min (as compared to the 110 min of FDG), it enables one patient to receive two PET studies in a single day. Therefore, with PET VI and ^{11}CDG, we are currently expanding the applications of PET by studying brain function during active cognitive processing (functional mapping) and during perturbation by various pharmacologic probes (e.g., amphetamine, physostigmine). Where previous PET studies of aging and dementia have examined the brain in a passive resting state, it is possible that both age and disease-related changes may be enhanced during perturbation. Such changes would facilitate the development of in vivo diagnostic criteria for AD.

References

Bondareff, W., Baldry, R., and Levy, R.: Quantitative computer tomography in senile dementia. *Arch. Gen. Psychiat. 38*, 1365–1368 (1981).

Blessed, G., Tomlinson, B.E., and Roth, M.: The association between quantitative measures of dementia and of senile change in the cerebral grey matter of elderly subjects. *Br. J. Psychiatry 114*, 797–811 (1968).

Butler, R.N., Dastur, D.K., and Perlin, S.: Relationships of senile manifestations and chronic brain syndromes to cerebral circulation and metabolism. *J. Psych. Research 3*, 229–238 (1965).

Chase, T.N., Foster, N.L., Fedio, P., DiChiro, G., Brooks, R., and Patronas, N.J.: Alzheimer's disease: Local cerebral metabolism studies using the ^{18}F-fluorodeoxyglucose-positron emission tomography technique. In Samuel, D., Algeri, S., Gershon, S., Grimm, V.E., and Toffano, G. (Eds.), Aging of the Brain, pp. 143–154. New York: Raven, 1983.

de Leon, M.J., Ferris, S.H., Blau, I., George, A.E., Reisberg, B., Kricheff, I.I., and Gershon, S.: Correlations between CT changes and behavioral deficits in senile dementia. *Lancet 8147*, 859–860 (1979).

de Leon, M.J., Ferris, S.H., George, A.E., Christman, D.R., Fowler, J.S., Gentes, C., Reisberg, B., Gee, B., Emmerich, M., Yonekura, Y., Brodie, J., Kricheff, I.I., and Wolf, A.P.: Positron emission tomographic studies of aging and Alzheimer's disease. *Am. J. Neuroradiology 4*, 568–571 (1983a).

de Leon, M.J., Ferris, S.H., George, A.E., Reisberg, B., Christman, D., Kricheff, I.I., and Wolf, A.: Computed tomography and positron transaxial tomography evaluations of normal aging and Alzheimer's disease. *J. Cereb. Blood Flow Metab. 3*, 391–394 (1983b).

de Leon, M.J., Ferris, S.H., George, A.E., Reisberg, B., Kricheff, I.I., and Gershon, S.: Computed tomography evaluations of brain–behavior relationships in senile dementia of the Alzheimer's type. *Neurobiol. Aging 1*, 69–79 (1980).

de Leon, M.J., Ferris, S.H., George, A.E., Rosenbloom, S., Christman, D.R., Gentes, C.I., Reisberg, B., Kricheff, I.I., and Wolf, A.P.: Regional correlation of PET and CT in senile dementia of the Alzheimer's type. *Am. J. Neuroradiology 4*, 553–556 (1983c).

de Leon, M.J., and George, A.E.: Computed tomography in aging and senile dementia of the Alzheimer's type. In Mayeux, R., and Rosen, W. (Eds.), Recent Advances in Neurology: The Dementias, Vol. 38, pp. 103–122. New York: Raven, 1983d.

de Leon, M.J., George, A.E., Ferris, S.H., Christman, D.R., Fowler, J.S., Gentes, C., Brodie, J., Reisberg, B., and Wolfe, A.P.: Positron emission tomography and computed tomography assessments of the aging human brain. *J. Comput. Assist. Tomogr. 8*, 88–94 (1984).

de Leon, M.J., George, A.E., Ferris, S.H., Rosenbloom, S., Gentes, C.I., and Reisberg, B.: Grey matter and white matter CT correlates in senile dementia of the Alzheimer's type. Presented at the Aharon Katzir-Katchalsky Conference on the Aging of the Brain, Mantua, Italy, March 1982 (unpublished).

Ferris, S.H., de Leon, M.J., Wolf, A.P., Farkas, T., Christman, D.R., Reisberg, B., Fowler, J.S., MacGregor, R., Goldman, A., George, A.E., and Rampal, S.: Positron emission tomography in the study of aging and senile dementia. *Neurobiol. Aging 1*, 127–131 (1980).

Ferris, S.H., de Leon, M.J., Wolf, A.P., George, A.E., Reisberg, B. Christman, D.R., Yonekura, Y., and Fowler, J.S.: Positron emission tomography. In Mayeux, R., and Rosen, W. (Eds.), Advances in Neurology: The Dementias, Vol. 38, pp. 123–129. New York: Raven, 1983.

Fieschi, C., and Lenzi, G.L.: The aging brain and its metabolic balance: Positron emission tomography results and prospects. In Samuel, S., Algeri, D.,

Gershon, S., Grimm, V.E., and Toffano, G. (Eds.), Aging of the Brain, Vol. 22, pp. 123–131. New York: Raven, 1983.

Frackowiak, R.S.J., Pozzilli, C., Legg, N.J., du Boulay, G.H., Marshall, J., Lenzi, G.L., and Jones, T.: Regional cerebral oxygen supply and utilization in dementia—A clinical and physiological study with oxygen-15 and positron tomograpy. *Brain 104*, 753–778 (1981).

Freyhan, F.A., Woodford, R.B., and Kety, S.S.: Cerebral blood flow and metabolism in psychoses of senility. *J. Nerv. Ment. Dis. 113*, 449–456 (1951).

Fujishima, M., and Omae, T.: Brain blood flow and mean transit time as related to aging. *Gerontology 26*, 104–107 (1980).

Gado, M., Hughes, C.P., Danziger, W., Chi, D., Jost, G., and Berg, L.: Volumetric measurements of the cerebrospinal fluid spaces in demented subjects and controls. *Radiology 144*, 535–538 (1982).

George, A.E., de Leon, M.J., Ferris, S.H., and Kricheff, I.I.: Parenchymal CT correlates of senile dementia (Alzheimer's disease): Loss of gray–white matter discriminability. *Am. J. Neuroradiology 2*, 205–211 (1981a).

George, A.E., de Leon, M.J., Rosenbloom, S., Ferris, S.H., Gentes, C.I., Emmerich, M., and Kricheff, I.I.: CT ventricular volume and its relationship to cognitive impairment in dementia. Presented at the annual meeting of the American Aging Association, New York, September 1981 (1981b; unpublished).

George, A.E., de Leon, M.J., Rosenbloom, S., Ferris, S.H., Gentes, C., Emmerich, M., and Kricheff, I.I.: The relationship of CT ventricular volume in cognitive deficit. *Radiology 149*, 493–498 (1983).

Hachinski, V.C., Lassen, N.A., and Marshall, J.: Multi-infarct dementia: A cause of mental deterioration in the elderly. *Lancet 2*, 207–210, 1974.

Hagberg, B., Ingvar, D.M.: Cognitive reduction in presenile dementia related to regional abnormalities of the cerebral blood flow. *Br. J. Psychiatry 128*, 209–222 (1976).

Hawkins, R.A., Mazziotta, J.C., Phelps, M.E., Huang, S.E., Kuhl, D.E., Carson, R.E., Metter, R.J., and Riege, W.H.: Cerebral glucose metabolism as a function of age in man: Influence of the rate constants in the fluorodeoxyglucose method. *J. Cereb. Blood Flow Metabol. 3*, 250–253 (1983).

Ingvar, D.H., and Gustafson, L.: Regional cerebral blood flow in organic dementia with early onset. *Acta Neurol. Scand. 46*(43), 42–73 (1970).

Jacoby, R.J., and Levy, R.: Computed tomography in the elderly. 2. Senile dementia: Diagnosis and functional impairment. *Br. J. Psychiatry 136*, 256–269 (1980).

Johnston, M.V., Young, A.C., and Coyle, J.T.: Laminar distribution of cholinergic markers in neocortex: Effects of lesions. *J. Neurosci. Res. 6*, 597–607 (1981).

Kay, D.W.K.: Epidemiological aspects of organic brain disease in the aged. In Gaitz, C.M. (Ed.), Aging and the Brain, pp. 15–26. New York: Plenum, 1972.

Kety, S.S.: Human cerebral blood flow and oxygen consumption as related to aging. *J. Chron. Dis. 3*, 478–436 (1956).

Kety, S.S., and Schmidt, C.F.: The nitrous oxide method for the quantitative determination of cerebral blood flow in man—Theory, procedure, and normal values. *J. Clin. Invest. 27*, 476–483 (1948).

Kuhl, D.E., Metter, E.J., Riege, W.H., and Phelps, M.E.: Effects of human aging on patterns of local cerebral glucose utilization determined by the [^{18}F] fluorodeoxyglucose method. *J. Cereb. Blood Metabol. 2*, 163–171 (1982).

Lammertsma, A.A., Frackowiak, R.S.J., Lenzi, G.L., Heather, J.D., Pozzilli, S., and Jones, T.: Accuracy of the oxygen-15 steady state technique for measuring CBF and $CMRO_2$: Tracer modelling statistics and spatial sampling. *J. Cereb. Blood Flow Metabol. 1*(Suppl 1), S3–S4 (1981).

Lassen, N.A., Feinberg, I., and Lane, M.H.: Bilateral studies of cerebral oxygen uptake in young and aged normal subjects and in patients with organic dementia. *J. Clin. Invest. 39*, 491–500 (1960).

Mountjoy, C.Q., Roth, M., Evans, N.J.R., and Evans, H.M.: Cortical neuronal counts in normal elderly controls and demented patients. *Neurobiol. Aging 4*, 1–11 (1983).

Naeser, M.A., Gebhardt, C.T., and Levine, H.L.: Decreased computerized tomography numbers in patients with presenile dementia. *Arch. Neurol. 37*, 401–409 (1980).

Naritomi, H., Meyer, J.S., Sakai, F., Yamaguchi, F., and Shaw, T.: Effects of advancing age on regional cerebral blood flow—Studies in normal subjects and subjects with risk factors for atherothrombotic stroke. *Arch. Neurol. 36*, 410–416 (1979).

Obrist, W.D., Chivian, E., Cronquist, S., and Ingvar, D.H.: Regional cerebral blood flow in senile and presenile dementia. *Neurology 20*, 315–322 (1970).

Rapoport, S.I., Duara, R., London, E.D., Margolin, R.A., Schwartz, M., Cutler, N.R., Partanen, M., and Shinowara, N.L.: Glucose metabolism of the aging nervous system. In: Samuel, D., Algeri, S., Gershon, S., Grimm, V.E., and Toffano, G. (Eds.), Aging of the Brain, Vol. 22, pp. 111–121. New York: Raven, 1983.

Redick, R.W., Kramer, M., and Taube, C.A.: Epidemiology of mental illness and utilization of psychiatric facilities among older persons. In Busse, E.W., and Pfeifer, E. (Eds.), Mental Illness in Later Life, pp. 199–231. Washington, D.C.: American Psychiatric Association, 1973.

Simard, D., Olesen, O.B., Paulson, O.B., Lassen, N.A., and Shinhoj, E.: Regional cerebral blood flow and its regulation in dementia. *Brain 94*, 273–288 (1971).

Terry, R.D., Peck, A., DeTeresa, R., Schecter, R., and Horoupina, D.S.: Some morphometric aspects of the brain in senile dementia of the Alzheimer type. *Ann. Neurol. 10*, 184–192 (1981).

Tomlinson, B.E., Blessed, G., and Roth, M.: Observations on the brains of demented old people. *J. Neurol. Sci. 11*, 205–242 (1970).

Tomlinson, B.E., and Kitchner, D.: Granulovacuolar degeneration of hippocampal pyramidal cells. *J. Pathol. 106*, 165–185 (1972).

U.S. Bureau of the Census: Statistical Abstract of the U.S. 1971 Census, 92nd Edition. Washington, D.C.: U.S. Government Printing Office, 1971.

U.S. Department of Health, Education, and Welfare, Public Health Service: Chronic conditions and impairments of nursing home residents. In Vital Health Statistics. Washington, D.C.: U.S. Government Printing Office, 1969.

Whitehouse, P.J., Price, D.L., Struble, R.G., Clark, A.W., Coyle, J.T., and DeLong, M.R.: Alzheimer's disease and senile dementia: Loss of neurons in the basal forebrain. *Science 215*, 1237–1239 (1982).

Yamaguchi, F., Meyer, J.S., Yamamoto, M., Sakai, F., and Shaw, T.: Noninvasive regional cerebral blood flow measurements in dementia. *Arch. Neurol. 37*, 410–418 (1980).

Part V

Experimental Neuropathology

Chapter 18

Cholinergic Deficiencies in Senile Dementia of the Alzheimer Type

Joseph T. Coyle

I shall focus on the cholinergic system that may be affected in Alzheimer's dementia and senile dementia of the Alzheimer type. One of the interesting questions that arises with regard to subcortical neuronal systems and their role in these disorders concerns the surprising evidence of recent neuropathological studies that suggest a rather modest loss of neurons in the cerebral cortex. It is clear that the cortex, hippocampus, and related limbic structures are the sites heavily affected by such pathological stigmata as plaques, tangles, and granular vacuolar degeneration. In studies in which objective cell-counting techniques have been used, Terry and his colleagues* found that thinning of the cerebral cortex is minimal and loss of cells is difficult to document. The largest cells are, however, selectively affected, and recent findings by the Cambridge group from substantial numbers of age-matched controls and pathologically diagnosed demented patients again support documentable, but not overwhelmingly large, cell loss in various areas of the cortex.

Let me explain briefly some of the markers and characteristics of the cholinergic nervous system. Cholinergic synapses have a high affinity for choline uptake that concentrates choline in the nerve terminal. They possess the enzyme choline acetyltransferase, which reacts with choline and acetyl coenzyme A to generate acetylcholine, but, of course, they store substantial amounts of acetylcholine for release. The presence of

*This is an edited version of Dr. Coyle's presentation at the *Aging 2000 Symposium*. References were unavailable for this chapter at press time.

acetylcholine and the enzyme choline acetyltransferase is a sine qua non of cholinergic neurons. In addition, they have acetylcholinesterase activity which is also found in postsynaptic neurons. Although cholinergic neurons are rich in acetylcholinesterase, the enzyme is not specifically associated with them. In the postsynaptic receptors, the cerebral cortex, and the hippocampus, the muscarinic receptor appears to be the dominant form.

Interest in the role of cholinergic neurons in the pathophysiology of Alzheimer's dementia originated in the success of investigators who revealed selective transmitter deficits in Parkinson's disease, and subsequently in Huntington's disease. Other research groups then began to look for cholinergic markers in the brains of patients who had died of Alzheimer's dementia. At the same time, taking a psychopharmacologic approach, Drachman noted what had long been known in the literature, that drugs that block central muscarinic receptors may produce memory impairments, especially in recent and working memory. Drachman compared the effects of low doses of scopolamine, a selective antagonist of central muscarinic receptors, on the performance of young healthy individuals and that of aged persons. He found a striking parallel between the effects of scopolamine on cognition of young adults and the normal cognitive impairments seen in the aged. The drug had striking effects on working memory, preserving verbal IQ as opposed to the performance IQ.

More direct evidence came from studies done initially by several groups in England, namely, Davies, Roth et al., and the Perrys, among others. They assayed the actvity of choline acetyltransferase in various areas of the cerebral cortex and the hippocampus in patients with pathologically diagnosed Alzheimer's dementia and compared the enzyme's activity to that of age-matched controls. They found striking reductions in the activity of choline acetyltransferase, on the order of 80–90%, depending on brain region, the hippocampus consistently being the most severely affected. To put it in perspective, this is equivalent to the reductions in dopamine and tyrosine hydroxylase activity that have been noted in the striatum of Parkinsons's disease patients.

One of the problems with the findings was that the source of cholinergic innervation in the cortex was unclear. Profound reduction in cholinergic markers would, of course, be consistent with a localization in the cerebral cortex if one believed that the primary lesion was in cortical neurons. The controversy arose from the fact that, more than 20 years ago, Hebb and co-workers showed that if one undercut the cerebral cortex, which would presumably cause degeneration of axons going into the cortex, this resulted in a striking loss of choline acetyltransferase activity in the overlying cortex. This could, however, be a retrograde degeneration caused by the cross-sectioning of axons from the cholinergic neurons of the cortex. Lewis, using acetylcholinesterase histochemical techniques, then suggested that the basal forebrain's large neurons, which stained intensely for this enzyme, were the source of innervation. In an elegant study, Butcher and colleagues showed that other neurons that used dopamine and norepinephrine as their neuronal transmitter clearly did not use acetylcholine, but stained similarly intensely for acetylcholinesterase activity. More recent studies with cortical transections suggested that these did not reduce choline acetyltransferase activity in the cortex, while polyclonal antibody immunohistochemical studies suggested that there were actually cholinergic neurons in the cerebral cortex. It was unclear, therefore, whether cholinergic neurons were located inside or outside the cortex.

We became interested in these questions several years ago for completely different reasons—not because of our interest in aging, but because we wanted to study the development of aminergic innervation in the cerebral cortex. We conducted some research with specific cytotoxins injected into various areas of the brain. These substances caused a selective pattern of degeneration that kills neurons whose cell bodies are at the injection site but spares fibers passing through or terminating in the region. The study avoided some of the interpretation problems associated with gross destructive lesions. If one makes a lesion in an area and then measures the activity, for example, of choline acetyltransferase in the cortex, the reduced activity then presumably reflects the degeneration of neuronal cell bodies in the injection area that projected to the cortex.

Although we examined many areas with the lesioning technique, we found that injections of the cytoxin in the ventral medial aspects of the globus pallidus caused a striking decrease in choline acetyltransferase activity in the ipsilateral cerebral cortex of the rat one week after injection. In examination of marker for the GABAergic neurons known to be intrinsic to the cortex, glutamate decarboxylase indicated that it was not affected, which suggested that the choline acetyltransferase decrease was not caused by direct damage to the cerebral cortex. More intensive studies of these lesions in the ventral medial globus pallidus showed commensurate reductions in all presynaptic markers for the cholinergic neurons (activity of choline acetyltransferase, levels of endogenous acetylcholine, uptake process for choline, and acetylcholinesterase activity). This suggested that acetylcholinesterase is highly associated with cholinergic projection to the cerebral cortex.

Declines in acetylcholinesterase activity were first reported 20 years ago by Pope in the cortex of Alzheimer's dementia patients. There was no reduction in GABAergic markers in the cerebral cortex and no reduction in the markers for noradrenergic, histaminergic, or serotonergic axons which passed close by or through the lesioned area, indicating that the lesion was highly specific to neurons whose cell bodies were located there.

These neurons are part of the basal forebrain magnocellular complex.

They are among the largest neurons in the brain and stain intensely for acetylcholinesterase. The critical issue is how these projections to the cerebral cortex are organized and how much they contribute to the total cholinergic innervation of the cortex.

There are two ways to look at these questions. One is by a quantitative lesion technique, in which one can determine the relative contribution of these neurons to the cholinergic markers in the cerebral cortex. The other, more qualitative and topographic, involves retrograde transport studies. In the quantitative studies one simply lesions various areas of the basal forebrain complex. The more rostral group would, in the rat, be equivalent to the nucleus basalis. When one looks at the various areas of the cerebral cortex and hippocampal formation in the rat, one sees that lesions that affect the basal complex produce striking reductions in choline acetyltransferase in the frontal and parietal cortex, somewhat smaller reductions in the occipital cortex, and none in the hippocampus. Conversely, lesions in the diagonal-band medial septum do not affect the frontal cortex, have mild effects in the parietal cortex, greater effects in occipital cortex, and striking ones in the hippocampal cortex. If one adds up the losses in choline acetyltransferase produced with just these two large lesions, one can account for between 60 and 80% of cholinergic innervation of the cerebral cortex by these neurons.

The retrograde tracing technique allows one to look more precisely at the brain's topography, as opposed to dropping little bombs on it. The technique involves injections of very small quantities of a tracer, either a fluorescent dye or horseradish peroxidase. If a neuron sends an axon to innervate the injected area, neuronal terminals will take up the marker and transport it back to the cell body after a period of time. If an adjacent neuronal cell body projects an axon to some completely different area, this would, of course, not be labeled by the tracer and, in this way, one can see the topography of these projections precisely. Illuminated under fluorescence, cells stained by tracer provide information about their projections to the various areas of the cortex, hippocampal formation, and limbic system.

These studies have been conducted in rats and in great detail in primates, especially by Mesulum. Mesulum recently coupled these studies with immunocytochemical techniques to visual choline acetyltransferase in cholinergic cell bodies. He divided this complex into basically four groups. CH-1, the medial septum, projects a hippocampal formation almost exclusively. CH-2, the vertical limb of the diagonal band, goes to the hippocampus and hypothalamus. CH-3, the horizontal limb of the diagonal band, goes to the olfactory bulb, and CH-4, which is the nucleus basalis of Meynert in the substantia innominata, projects to the entire cerebral cortex and to the amygdala. These projections are located in the basal forebrain, overlying the hypothalamus, below the basal ganglia extending up to the septum, and they account for between 70 and 90% of the cholinergic innervation of the cerebral cortex.

Information about the source of cholinergic innervation of the cerebral cortex made it possible to examine this cell group in postmortem brains of senile dementia patients. Choline acetyltransferase deficiency in the cerebral cortex does not necessarily mean that the neurons projecting into the cerebral cortex have degenerated; the degeneration might be the result of defective transport of this enzyme. Whitehouse and Price at Johns Hopkins Medical Institution studied the nucleus basalis of middle-aged and old patients who had had Alzheimer-type dementia. Their index case, compared to an age-matched control, is that of a man who died after a 15-year history of Alzheimer-type symptomatology, whose family had a history of dementia, and who, on neuropathologic examination, exhibited the pathologic stigmata of Alzheimer's dementia. They showed that the nucleus basalis complex, compared to that of the age-matched control, contained a strikingly reduced number of cell bodies. The loss of cells was examined in the nucleus basalis tissue from several other patients and, with a subjective but blind rating, or assessment of cell density, or counts of cells and comparable sections, striking reductions in the number of cell bodies in the nucleus basalis of Meynert were evident.

Rossor looked at choline acetyltransferase activity in the substantia innominata and several other brain regions in patients who had died with neuropathologically diagnosed Alzheimer's dementia. He found that in the nucleus basalis of controls, mean choline acetyltransferase activity was approximately 82 nmol/mg/min, whereas in the Alzheimer's dementia patients it was 26 nmol/mg/min, about a 70% decrease. One does not find comparable reductions in the putamen or hypothalamus, so that, looking at cell loss quantitatively by neurochemical analysis, there seems to be a striking decrement in cholinergic neuron markers in the basal forebrain complex of the nucleus basalis in patients who had Alzheimer-type dementia.

A problem one confronts is trying to connect the neuropathology of this disorder with its neurochemical pathology, and there may be some relationships, especially with regard to plaques. We know that plaque density correlates with cognitive impairments in patients tested in vivo, and, according to Perry's postmortem assessments, with choline acetyltransferase reductions in the cerebral cortex. Struble and Price found rich acetylcholinesterase reactivity in young plaques in the cortex, somewhat less activity in slightly more mature plaques, and not much activity in what they described as mature plaques with heavy amyloid deposits. It would be simplistic to say that the cholinergic neurons are the only neuronal systems that may be affected by plaques, but some association between these neuropathologic stigmata and neurochemical abnormalities is likely.

Considerable evidence exists of reduced glucose utilization and oxygen consumption in the cerebral cortex of Alzheimer patients. The significant reduction in glucose utilization and oxygen consumption in the cortex of demented individuals would be consistent with a global and nonspecific impairment in cell function of the cerebral cortex. If one looks at the ability of cortical tissue to consume glucose in vitro, however, there is no evidence of reduction.

Bowen was able to accumulate biopsy samples from neuropathologically diagnosed living patients with Alzheimer's dementia. Bowen studied CO_2 production from radioactive glucose in brain biopsy samples from age-matched controls and Alzheimer patients. He found an increased CO_2 production in the patients. One wonders, therefore, whether cholinergic input in the cerebral cortex might play a role in impairing or reducing cerebral neuronal activity as manifested by decreased glucose turnover. We conducted a study with Lund at the Aging Institute in which we lesioned the nucleus basalis of rats and subjected the animals to Sokoloff's 2-deoxyglucose autoradiographic technique. We noted a reduction in glucose turnover in the cortex, ipsilateral to the lesion as compared to contralateral. If one compares lesion to sham lesion, one sees a decrease in glucose turnover that is reversed by administration of oxytremarine, a direct-acting muscarinic receptor agonist. Much interest and hope have been raised by the possibility that one might be able to treat cholinergic deficits in the cortex and hippocampus by administering drugs that enhance cholinergic neurotransmission. Recent studies have pointed to mildly positive results as, for example, one by Davies of the effects of physostigmine. But none of these studies found dramatic effects, in no way of the magnitude seen with L-dopa in treatment of dopamine deficiency in Parkinson's disease.

Conclusion

On the basis of neuroanatomic and neurophysiologic studies, it is clear that one should not equate the cholinergic system too readily with the nigrostriatal dopaminergic system, which seems to be highly collateralized. That is like saying that the cholinergic system is like oak trees in a forest, with overlapping axon terminals and individual neurons innervating literally millions and millions of cells, whereas retrograde tracing studies suggest that these cholinergic inputs are much more topographic in organization, more like plane trees in a forest. If one administers a drug that works presynaptically in the dopaminergic system, there may be sufficient remaining fiber input to the striatal cells so that the remaining fibers may serve as a substrate for the indirectly acting drugs, whereas a loss of cholinergic neurons may leave spaces so that there is no presynaptic substrate. In addition, the dopaminergic neurons are tonically active, their firing rate fairly constant over time. Neurophysiologic studies suggest, on the other hand, that the cholinergic neurons are phasically active, firing irregularly in bursts, and with periods of quiet that are related to specific behaviors. I question whether or not drugs that act broadly at muscarinic receptors, or presynaptically at cholinergic neurons, will be able to replace effectively the spatially and temporally discrete information conveyed by the neurons in the nucleus basalis.

Chapter 19

Noncortical Transmitter-Specific Neurons in Senile Dementia of the Alzheimer Type

William Bondareff

Summary

The benchmark of senile dementia of the Alzheimer type (SDAT) is an abundance of neuritic plaques and neurofibrillary tangles in the cerebral cortex. Noncortical neurons, some of which are associated with specific neurotransmitters, are also involved. The latter, including neurons of the nucleus locus ceruleus (noradrenergic), nucleus basalis complex (cholinergic), and nuclei of the brainstem raphe (serotonergic), innervate target regions in the cerebral cortex and selective noncortical regions of the brain known to be involved in "higher" cortical functions. Neuronal pathology in the noncortical noradrenergic and cholinergic nuclei appears to affect the cortical distributions of norepinephrine and acetylcholine and may also influence the distribution of plaques and tangles in target regions. These interrelationships between noncortical, transmitter-specific neurons and the target neurons they innervate are age related. Their clinical expression may contribute to the severity of symptoms in the early onset subtype of Alzheimer's disease.

Comparisons of clinical, biological, and sociological literature are complicated by the multiple meanings given to disorders of cognition. In the following, *senile dementia of the Alzheimer type* (SDAT) refers to a specific disease characterized by dementia sometime during the course of the disease in a person who succumbs at an age of at least 60–65 years and in whose cerebral cortex abundant neurofibrillary tangles and neuritic plaques can be demonstrated. Abundant is defined according to criteria outlined by Tomlinson (1982). No distinction is made between SDAT, dementia of the Alzheimer type (DAT), and Alzheimer's disease (AD) as the definition, which is the same in each, rests on a bottom line of abundant plaques and tangles in the cerebral cortex.

SDAT is a specific neuronal disorder in which neurons are involved not only as a result of the disease, but also as a result of aging. Involved neurons are found in the cerebral cortex and in several noncortical regions of the brain as well. They may show a variety of abnormalities—structural, chemical, and functional—including death, and disease-related neuronal death has been demonstrated in certain parts of the cerebral cortex, locus ceruleus, amygdala, hippocampus, and substantia innominata. Age-related loss of neurons, although found in different regions or nuclei than in SDAT, can also be demonstrated in the cerebral cortex, amygdala, and hippocampus. Age-related neuronal loss has not been demonstrated in nucleus basalis (Meynert) or related nuclei of the substantia innominata in humans (Chui, Bondareff, and Zarow, in press) but has been found in nucleus locus ceruleus (Vijayashankar and Brody, 1979).

In SDAT neuronal loss is probably demonstrated most reliably in nucleus locus ceruleus. The neurons of this prominent nucleus, which are large and contain neuromelanin, are readily visualized and can be counted with automated methods of image analysis throughout the entire rostral–caudal extent of the nucleus. With such methods, two populations of surviving neurons were shown in SDAT patients (Bondareff, Mountjoy, and Roth, 1982). In one there was a loss of only 20% of neurons as compared with nondemented persons of comparable age; in the other, a severe loss of 80–85% of total neurons was found. Patients in whom neuron loss was extensive were found to be relatively younger at the time of death, severely demented, and often women.

Neuronal loss has also been demonstrated in the nucleus basalis complex in patients dying with SDAT. "Nucleus basalis complex" refers to a group of neurons, largely in the substantia innominata, which includes the nucleus of the diagonal band (Broca), medial septal nucleus, and nucleus basalis (Meynert). Large, fusiform neurons are found largely, but not exclusively, in the latter. Because the distribution of these large neurons and morphologically discrete nuclei may vary in specimens isolated for biochemical analyses, the relationship between biochemical and anatomical data may be uncertain. As Henke and Lang (1983) demonstrate, results from different laboratories may be difficult to compare. The large, fusiform neurons in the substantia innominata lie ventral to globus pallidus. The loss of these neurons in SDAT, described by Whitehouse et al. (1982) appears to be minimal and perhaps even absent in older patients, but is severe (70–90% of normal counts) in younger patients.

Patients dying with SDAT have well-documented decrements of both cholinergic and noradrenergic transmitters or in the activities of transmitter-associated regions of the brain and in several noncortical nuclei. Choline acetyltransferase (ChAT) activity has been shown to be diminished in the hippocampus, mammillary body, amygdala, and caudate nucleus in SDAT patients (see Table 19-1) and decrements of norepinephrine (NE) have been shown in the hippocampus and hypothalamus (Table 19-1). In addition, decreased amounts of serotonin (5HT), dopamine (DA), and somatostatin have been found (Table 19-1). These regions of the brain, as well as areas of cerebral cortex which also show diminished levels of ChAT, NE, 5HT, and DA in SDAT patients, are all associated with functions collectively described as "higher cortical," namely language, memory, cognition, emotional expression, and social interaction. They are innervated, primarily, by ascending neuronal pathways, which take their respective origins from nuclei which, like nucleus locus ceruleus and nucleus basalis, actively synthesize a neurotransmitter.

ChAT is synthesized by neurons of the nucleus basalis, diagonal band (of Broca), and septal nuclei. In SDAT, ChAT activity declines in the cholinergic neurons which innervate cortical and other regions associated with "higher" functions. A noradrenergic ascending projection originates similarly in the nucleus locus ceruleus which is the major, if not exclusive, source of NE in "higher" centers. Dopamine-β-hydroxylase activity, essential in the synthesis of NE, has been shown histochemically to decline in SDAT (Iversen et al., 1983). The presence of numerous neuritic plaques and neurofibrillary tangles in neurons of the nucleus basalis and nucleus locus ceruleus, and in the neurons of the raphe (from which originate ascending serotonergic axons) and substantia nigra (from which originate ascending dopaminergic axons) in SDAT (Ishii, 1966) further indicates involvement of these nuclei.

It is, therefore, apparent that at least four noncortical, transmitter-specific nuclei, together with their ascending axons and terminals, are involved in SDAT. Neurons of these four nuclei—the nucleus basalis complex, nucleus locus ceruleus, nuclei of the brainstem raphe, and the substantia nigra—have ascending projections with divergent terminals, diffusely distributed to cerebral cortex and other "higher" target centers. The distributions of terminals of these four ascending projection systems, although not known with certainty in humans, are summarized in Figure 19-1, largely as deduced from experimental animal studies. Having established the dimensions of lesions involving these four neuronal projection systems in SDAT, their cellular pathology can be discussed generally.

Each system, in essence, consists of three parts: perikaryon, ascending axon, and axon terminals, represented diagrammatically in Figure 19-2.

Table 19-1. Selective bibliography of transmitter substances which decline in SDAT

	Transmitters				
Brain Region	ChAT	NE	DA	5-HT	Somatostatin
Cerebral cortex	Davies (1979) Rossor et al. (1982a)	Adolfsson et al. (1979) Iversen et al. (in press)	Mann et al. (1980) Iversen et al. (in press)	Carlsson (1981)	Rossor et al. (1980)
Hippocampus	Davies (1979) Rossor et al. (1982a)	Mann et al. (1980) Carlsson (1981)		Carlsson (1981)	Rossor et al. (1980)
Amygdala	Davies (1979) Rossor et al. (1982a,b)				
Hypothalamus	Davies (1979) Yates et al. (1982)	Yates et al. (1981) Mann et al. (1980)	Carlsson et al. (1980)	Carlsson et al. (1980)	
Mammillary body	Davies (1979)				
Caudate	Davies (1979) Rossor et al. (1982a)	Carlsson (1981)	Adolfsson et al. (1979) Mann et al. (1980)	Carlsson (1981)	
Nucleus basalis	Rossor et al. (1982b)				
Locus ceruleus	Rossor et al. (1982a)				
Substantia nigra	Rossor et al. (1982a)				

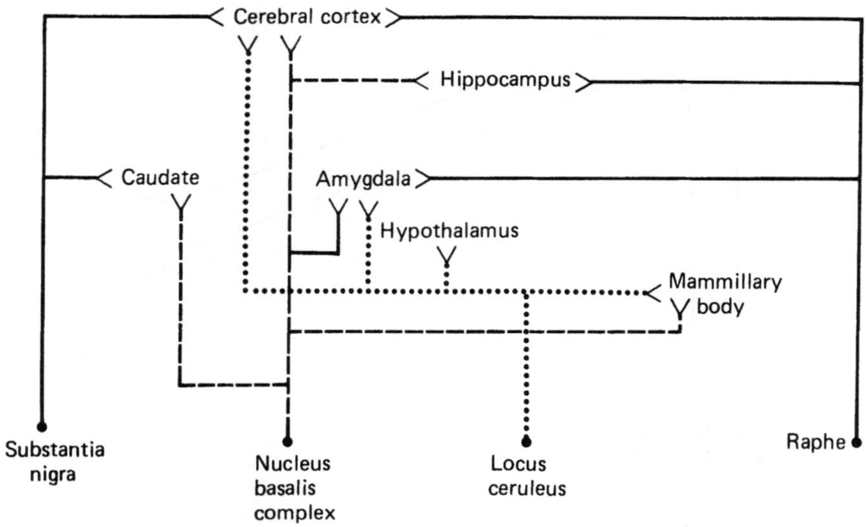

Figure 19-1. Diagram of ascending transmitter-associated projection systems. Neurons of origin in substantia nigra (dopaminergic), nucleus basalis of Meynert and associated nuclei of the substantia innominata (cholinergic), nucleus locus ceruleus (noradrenergic), and raphe (seratonergic) innervate widely distributed target areas associated with "higher" cerebral cortical functions.

Damage to any one part would compromise the whole and result in the depletion of a specific neurotransmitter in the target region of the brain. Damage to the perikaryon, for example, has been proposed by Mann et al. (1980), who report finding the volume of nuclei and the amount of cytoplasmic RNA decreased in surviving neurons of locus ceruleus in SDAT patients. It is possible, as the work of these authors suggests, that the observed depletion of cytoplasmic RNA is associated with the accumulation in these neurons of neuromelanin. These provocative findings suggest impairment of neurotransmitter metabolism by locus ceruleus neurons in SDAT.

The possibility that ascending axons (Fig. 19-2) might be selectively involved in lesions of ascending neuronal systems in SDAT is suggested by Rossor (1981) who describes neurons of these four systems as components of an "isodendritic core." Although anatomical peculiarities of isodendritic core axons have been noted, it is unclear how they might impair transmitter metabolism or transport in SDAT. Impaired axoplasmic transport, however, is also suggested by the accumulation of neurofibrillary tangles in the perikarya of these neurons (Tomlinson, 1982), as the relationship betwen neurofibrils and axoplasmic transport is well established. However, a relationship between neurofibrillary tangles

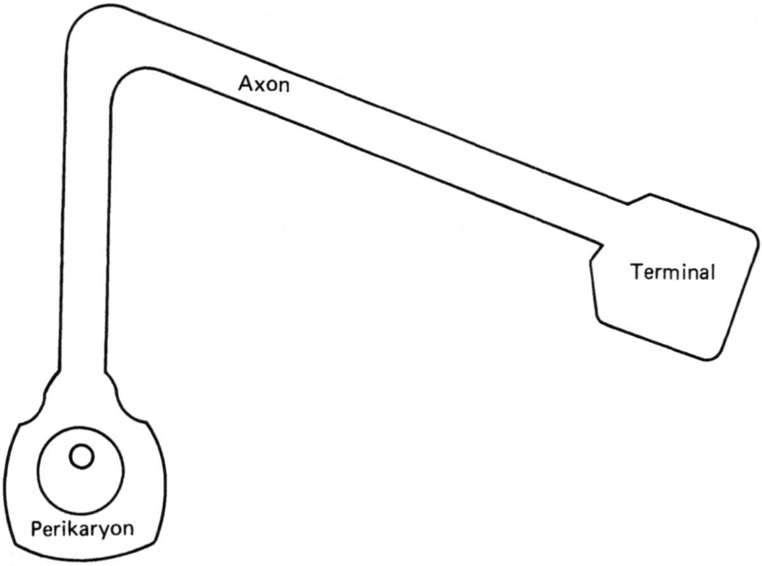

Figure 19-2. Diagram of an ascending transmitter-associated neuron. The neuron, whose perikaryon (soma) is located in a noncortical nucleus, has an axon which ends in a presynaptic terminal in a "higher" target area.

and axoplasmic transport has not been established. The possibility that presynaptic axon terminals might be sites of selective impairment is suggested by findings of Benton et al. (1982) that uptake of NE and 5-HT by terminals isolated from cerebral cortex is reduced in SDAT patients. The latter is supported by the recently reported observation of Candy et al. (1983) that nucleus basalis perikarya remain strongly cholinesterase (AChE) positive in SDAT, while their target sites in cortex are virtually depleted of AChE.

Neuronal pathology in SDAT appears to summate with changes that appear to be more related to age than to SDAT per se and involve neurons in transmitter-specific, noncortical nuclei and in the target areas which these nuclei innervate. Most noticeably, they include the accumulation with age of lipofuscin and nueromelanin. Although presumed to be cytotoxic, especially in monoamine-synthesizing neurons, neither lipofuscin nor neuromelanin has been shown convincingly to disrupt cellular function, but it is reasonable to speculate that quinones and molecular oxygen produced in the synthesis of neuromelanin from catecholamine may indeed be cytotoxic. Other age-related changes demonstrated in various parts of the brain which might involve transmitter-specific ascending projection systems and the regions of the brain they innervate are summarized in Table 19-2. These changes, especially the age-related loss of neurons, in part add to and in part modify neuronal changes related to SDAT.

Effects of age on the expression of neuronal pathology in SDAT have been discussed (Bondareff, 1983). Rossor et al. (1981) found depletion of ChAT activity in the frontal lobe cortex of SDAT patients dying at a younger age to be significantly greater than in those who died older. Bird et al. (1983) found this excessive depletion of frontal lobe ChAT activity

Table 19-2. Documented age-related changes in the human central nervous system

	Structure	Age Range	Change
Gross Anatomy			
Weight	Whole brain	18–20 mo to 95–96 yr	Decrease
Dimensions	Cerebellum	20–30 yr to 80–90 yr	Decrease
	Cerebrum		
length and width	Pons	21–30 yr to 60–90 yr	No change
height	Cerebrum	21–30 yr to 60–100 yr	Decrease
Volume	Brain	20–29 yr to 80–89 yr	Decrease
	Vent, cochlear nucl.	50 yr to 90 yr	Decrease
	Dentate nucl.	24 yr to 99 yr	Decrease
Dimensions	Lateral ventricles	9 mo to 90 yr	Increase
Width	Brain gyri	Adult to 75 yr	Increase
Intimal thickness	Brain arteries	1 yr to 90 yr	Increase
Histology and Cytology			
Neurons, numbers of	Cerebellum	60 yr to 100 yr	Decrease
	Inferior olivary nucleus	Birth to 89 yr	No change
	Locus ceruleus	Birth to 86 yr	Decrease
	Cranial nerve nuclei	Birth to 89 yr	No change
Synapses, numbers of	Cerebral cortex	15–54 yr to 65–89 yr	No change
Lipofuscin	Inferior olivary nucleus	11 d to 91 yr	Increase
Melanin	Substantia nigra	Birth to 60 yr	Increase
Cytoplasmic RNA	Inferior olivary nucleus	11 d to 90 yr	Decrease
Neurofibrillary tangles and senile plaques	Cerebral cortex	70–80 yr to 90–100 yr	Increase
Dendrites	Cerebral cortex	58 yr to 96 yr	Decrease
	Parahippo. Gyr.	44 yr to 81 yr	Increase

in younger SDAT patients to correlate with the incidence of myoclonus. Although a preferentially greater deficit in the amount cortical NE and the number of locus ceruleus neurons was not found in younger SDAT patients by Iversen et al. (1983), a greater loss of locus ceruleus neurons was found by Bondareff et al. (1982). Perry et al. (1981) were unable to correlate loss of locus ceruleus neurons with cortical ChAT activity and questioned whether impairment in the ascending noradrenergic projection system necessarily accompanies impairment in the ascending cholinergic system. This apparent controversy brings into focus the hypothesized existence of multiple subtypes of SDAT (clinical, histological, and/or biochemical subtypes meeting the same histopathological criteria) and the role of age in their expression.

Other effects of age on neuronal pathology in SDAT include greater numbers of neuritic plaques and neurofibrillary tangles and substantially greater neuronal loss in the noncortical transmitter-specific nuclei of younger SDAT victims. These effects of age, summarized in Table 19-3, suggest that SDAT may exist in one of two clinically distinct subtypes: AD-1, a more prevalent subtype of late onset, and AD-2, a relatively uncommon, more pernicious subtype of early onset.

The obvious similarity between the presumed subtypes of SDAT and those of diabetes mellitus (adult and juvenile onset) prompts the speculation that early-onset SDAT (AD-2) is initiated by a severe loss of neurons in noncortical nuclei. Because the disease process must quickly overrun the capacity of surviving neurons to innervate target neurons, behavior is soon impaired and the disease runs a rapidly deteriorating course. Late-onset SDAT (AD-1) appears to summate more insidiously

Table 19-3. Clinical and neurobiological characteristics of two subtypes of Alzheimer's disease (SDAT) (see Bondareff, 1983)

	AD-1	AD-2
Age of onset	Old age	Middle age
Clinical course	Insidious	Rampant
Parietal lobe impairment	++	+++
Motor signs	+	++
Ventricular enlargement	+	++
Neurofibrillary tangles	+++	++++
Loss of neurons		
nucleus locus ceruleus	+	+++
nucleus basalis	?	+++
Decreased ChAT		
cerebral cortex	+	+++
substantia innominate	+	+++

Severe (+++), moderate (++) and slight (+).

with age-related changes and becomes significantly symptomatic later as compensatory mechanisms fail and subcortical neurons are unable to maintain normal functioning of target structures.

The involvement of transmitter-specific ascending systems indicates that SDAT is not simply accelerated aging. It appears to be a disorder in which the involvement of selective noncortical nuclei and the structures they innervate, modified by age, results in an incapacitating impairment of higher cortical functions.

References

Adolfsson, R., Gottfries, C.G., Roos, B.E., and Winblad, B.: Changes in brain catecholoamines in patients with dementia at Alzheimer's type. *Br. J. Psychiatry 135*, 216–223 (1979).

Benton, J.S., Bowen, D.M., Allen, S.J., Hoan, E.A., Davison, A.N., Neary, D., Murphy, R.P., and Snowden, J.S.: Alzheimer's disease as a disorder of isodendritic core. *Lancet I*, 456 (1982).

Bird, T.D., Stranaban, S., Sumi, S.M., and Raskind, M.: Alzheimer's disease: choline acetyltransferase activity in brain tissue from clinical and pathological subgroups. *Ann. Neurol. 14*, 284–293 (1983).

Bondareff, W., Mountjoy, C.Q., and Roth, M.: Loss of neurons of origin of the adrenergic projection to cerebral cortex (nucleus locus ceruleus) in senile dementia. *Neurol. 32*, 164–168 (1982).

Bondareff, W.: Age and Alzheimer's disease. *Lancet I*, 1447 (1983).

Candy, J.M., Perry, R.H., Perry, E.K., Irving, D., Blessed, G., Fairbairn, A.F., and Tomlinson, B.E.: Pathological changes in the nucleus of Meynert in Alzheimer's and Parkinson's diseases. *J. Neurol. SA 54*, 277–289 (1983).

Carlsson, A.: Aging and brain neurotransmitters. In Crook, T., and Gershen, S. (Eds.), Strategies for the Development of an Effective Treatment for Senile Dementia. pp. 93–104. New Canaan, Conn.: Mark Powley Assoc., 1981.

Carlsson, A., Adolfsson, R., Aquilonius, S.-M., Gottfries, C.-H., Oreland, L., Svennerholm, L., and Winblad, B.: Biogenic amines in human brain in normal aging, senile dementia, and chronic alcoholism. In Goldstein, M. et al. (Eds.), Ergot Compounds and Brain Function: Neuroendocrine and Neuropsychiatric Aspects. New York, Raven Press, 1980.

Chui, H., Bondareff, W., and Zarow, C.: Neurobiology of Aging (in press).

Davies, P.: Neurotransmitter-related enzymes in senile dementia of the Alzheimer type. *Br. Res. 171*, 319–327 (1979).

Henke, H., and Lang, H.: Cholinergic enzymes in neocortex, hippocampus and basal forebrain of non-neurological and senile dementia of Alzheimer-type patients. *Br. Res. 267*, 281–291 (1983).

Iversen, L.L., Rossoe, M.N., Reynolds, G.P., Hills, R., Roth, M., Mountjoy, C.Q., Foote, S.L., Morrison, J.H., and Bloom, F.E.: Loss of pigmented dopamine-B-hydroxylase positive cells from locus ceruleus in senile dementia of Alzheimer's. *Neurosci. Lett.* 39:95–100 (1983).

Ishii, T.: Distribution of Alzheimer's neurofibrillary changes in the brain stem and hypothalamus of senile dementia. *Acta Neuropath. 6*, 181–187 (1966).

Mann, D.M.A., Lincoln, J., Yates, P.O., Stamp, J.E., and Toper, S.: Changes in the monamine containing neurones of the human CNS in senile dementia. *Brit. J. Psychiat. 136*, 533–541 (1980).

Perry, E.R., Tomlinson, B.E., Blessed, G., Perry, R.H., Cross, A.J., and Crow, T.J.: Neuropathological and biochemical observations on the noradrenergic system in Alzheimer's disease. *J. Neurol. Sci. 51*, 279–287 (1981).

Rossor, M.N.: Parkinson's disease and Alzheimer's disease as disorders of the isodendritic core. *Br. Med. J. 283*, 1588–1590 (1981).

Rossor, M.N., Emson, P.C., Mountjoy, C.Q., Roth, Sr. M., and Iversen, L.L.: Reduced amounts of immunoreactive somatostatin in the temporal cortex in senile dementia of Alzheimer type. *Neurosci. Lett. 20*, 372–377 (1980).

Rossor, M.N., Garret, N.J., Johnson, A.L., Mountjoy, C.Q., Roth, M., and Iversen, L.L.: A post-mortem study of the cholinergic and GABA systems in senile dementia. *Brain 105*, 313–330 (1982a).

Rossor, M.N., Iversen, L.L., Johnson, A.J., Mountjoy, C.Q., and Roth, M.: Cholinergic deficit in frontal cerebral cortex in Alzheimer's disease is age dependent. *Lancet II*, 1422 (1981).

Rossor, M.N., Svendsen, C., Hynt, S.P., Mountjoy, C.Q., Roth, M., and Iversen, L.L.: The substantia innominata in Alzheimer's disease: and histochemical and biochemical study of cholinergic marker systems. *Neurosci. Lett. 82*, 217–222 (1982b).

Tomlinson, B.E.: Plaques, tangles and Alzheimer's disease. *Psych. Med. 12*, 449–459 (1982).

Vijayashankar, N., and Brody, H.: A quantitative study of the pigmented neurons in the nuclei coeruleus and subcoeruleus in man as related to aging *J. Neuropath. Exp. Neurol. 38*, 490–497 (1979).

Whitehouse, P.J., Price, D.L., Struble, R.G., Clark, A.W., Coyle, J.T., and DeLong, M.R.: Alzheimer's disease and senile dementia—loss of neurons in the basal forebrain. *Science 215*, 1237–1239 (1982).

Yates, C.M., Ritchie, I.M., Simpson, J., Maloney, A.F.J., and Gordon, A. Noradrenaline Alzheimer-type dementia and Down's syndrome. *Lancet II*, 39–40 (1981).

Chapter 20

Neuropathology of the Aging Brain and Dementia of the Alzheimer Type

Henryk M. Wisniewski and George S. Merz

Summary

The two most prominent histopathological changes found in high numbers in the Alzheimer's disease (AD) brain are the neurofibrillary tangle and the neuritic and amyloid plaque. Each of these lesions is characterized by an accumulation of proteinaceous fibrous profiles (the paired helical filaments) and amyloid fibers, respectively. These structures are not only distinguishable from each other but from all of the normal cellular filaments as well. Both lesions are also found, in low numbers, in the brains of aged, but otherwise clinically normal, individuals. This quantitative difference between age-associated pathology and the AD brain implies that the cause(s) responsible for the lesions may be fundamentally the same and differ only in degree.

The association of plaques with scrapie and other slow, unconventional virus infections supports the hypothesis of an infectious etiology for Alzheimer's disease.

The list of pathological changes in the aged brain is long and involves all elements of the central nervous system, the nerve cells and their processes, glia, meninges, and vessels (Wisniewski and Terry, 1973a). Until 1966, there were no good quantitative studies to show which of these lesions were associated with loss of cognitive function and dementia. Studies carried out by Ball and Nuttall (1977), Roth et al. (1966), and Tomlinson et al. (1970), revealed that with an increased number of neurofibrillary changes, neuritic plaques, and granulo-vacuolar degeneration, the chance of showing clinical signs and symptoms of dementia increases. Because Alzheimer (1907) was first to report a case of profound dementia associated with a brain characterized by large numbers of neurons with neurofibrillary changes and neuritic plaques, this condition was called Alzheimer's disease. Because his patient was a 51-year-old woman, the disease was also characterized as a presenile dementia.

Only subsequently was it found that the same type of morphological changes were also present in large numbers in cases of senile dementia. Because slow progressive intellectual deterioration and memory loss are the most characteristic clinical features of both of these conditions, the question of a distinction between Alzheimer's disease and senile dementia arose. Some authors believe that all patients with this characteristic clinical behavior (intellectual deterioration and memory loss, restlessness, wandering, verbal output decrease, aphasia, apraxia, agnosia, echolalia, logoclonia) and the typical histologic alterations should be classified under the eponym Alzheimer's disease (AD). Others, while recognizng the morphological similarities between the two conditions, prefer, on clinical grounds, to refer to the disease occurring at age 40–65 with predominant parietal lobe deficits (aphasia, agnosia, apraxia) as Alzheimer's disease or presenile dementia. Those over age 65 with more global deterioration of the cortical functions are said to have senile dementia of the Alzheimer type (SDAT).

The plaques and tangles found in AD/SDAT are also found in much lower numbers in normal old individuals. Until recently neuropathologists had not determined how many plaques and/or neurons with tangles should be considered as a "normal" age-associated process and at which point the diagnosis of SDAT should be made.

During the recent National Institutes of Health/American Association of Retired Persons (NIH/AARP) sponsored "Workshop on the Diagnosis of Alzheimer Disease," it was agreed that in any microscopic field encompassing 1 mm^2 of tissue, the following are the neuropathological criteria for the diagnosis of Alzheimer disease:

1. In any patient *less than 50 years of age*, the number of neuritic plaques and neurofibrillary tangles seen anywhere in the neocortex should be greater than 2–5 per field. This enables the anatomical pathologist to establish a very firm diagnosis, even in medicolegal cases and in the absence of any helpful clinical history.
2. In any patient *between age 50 and 65 years*, there will be some number of tangles, but the number of plaques must be 8 or greater per field. This will again permit a diagnosis with a very high degree of confidence (± 95%).
3. For any patient *between 66 and 75 years of age*, some tangles will still be present, but the number of neuritic plaques must be greater than 10 per field.

4. In any patient *older than 75 years*, tangles may sometimes not be found in the neocortex, but the number of plaques should exceed 15 per microscopic field.

Implicit in the neuropathological criteria listed above is the view that the presence of neurons with neurofibrillary changes and plaques in small numbers is accepted as "normal" in older people.

This raises several questions: Are the morphological changes found in the CNS of clinically normal individuals pathological? If the changes are pathological, is normal aging a disease? How different is the aging process from pathological findings seen in various diseases? Finally, how does the presence of these morphological changes in normal aging affect our thinking about the pathogenesis and etiology of SDAT?

In our opinion, a biochemical, morphological, and functional approach to senescence requires recognition of the fact that all measurable and visible variations from the state where structure is normal and function is maximal are, by definition, pathologic. If by reason of their number and location, these pathologic changes elicit a clinical expression, then there is disease. Although gerontologists seem to avoid discussion of disease, one might argue that "normal aging" is simply that stage of pathology without clinical expression.

None of the many changes found in the aged brain can be considered specific for aging, since they all may be present in pathologic situations in some young and middle-aged brains. The situation is somewhat analogous to that in oncology, where even though the majority of cancers occur in people over 50, their development cannot be considered solely as a consequence of cellular senescence. However, genetically programmed, time-dependent changes in the cell, plus exposure to environmental insults, may open the way to an increased incidence of pathologic alterations. Therefore, one might say that the aged cell is an environment in which certain pathologic changes can more readily develop.

Neurofibrillary Changes

Neurofibrillary changes refer to an excessive accumulation of fibrous profiles in the perikarya of neurons. Neurons with neurofibrillary changes are found, in varying numbers, in many and unrelated human diseases (Wisniewski et al., 1979). In the light microscope the affected nerve cells are best visualized by silver-staining techniques. Ultrastructural studies of the neurons with neurofibrillary tangles reveal that, in the majority of human diseases, the tangles are composed of abnormal structures called paired helical filaments (PHFs) (Wisniewski et al., 1976). Each filament in the pair is 10–12 nm in diameter and is helically wound around its partner, thereby giving an overall PHF profile that is 20–24 nm in diameter. The helical feature of the PHF results in the repeating "nodes" at regular 80 nm intervals. Recent negative-staining studies of PHF and supra-ultrathin sections of the PHF revealed that each of the 10 nm filaments making the PHF is made of four protofilaments. However, the ultrastructure of the PHF protofilaments and those of the 10 nm normal neurofilaments is different (Wisniewski and Wen, in prep.). The PHFs are uniquely pathologic and as indicated above their morphology is quite unlike the normal neurofilaments, neurotubules, and microfilaments that are typical of the normal neuron.

One of the remarkable features of PHFs is their resistance to various fixatives and to postmortem autolysis. Although the basis for this is not known it is probably related to another characteristic of the PHF. When the neurofibrillary tangles are stained with congo red they exhibit a characteristic green–red birefringence when viewed with polarized light. This is also a property of amyloid, another pathologic fiber. In the case of the systemic amyloid it is known that this property is a consequence of a β-pleated configuration of the constituent proteins (Glenner, 1980). Although a β-pleated configuration has not yet been established for the PHF, it seems likely to be the case. Another feature probably contributing to the stability of the tangle is seen in recent studies which show that in some neurons the PHFs are tightly packed into what are described as paracrystalline arrays in which the individual PHFs are connected by "crossbridges" (Metuzals et al., 1982).

Administration of various chemicals such as aluminum salts in some animal species and spindle inhibitors in all animal species leads to the formation of neurofibrillary changes that, in the light microscope, resemble those seen in SDAT. However, electron microscopy revealed that these induced tangles are composed of 10 nm unpaired, straight filaments that are indistinguishable from normal neurofilaments (Wisniewski et al., 1968; Wisniewski et al., 1970; Wisniewski et al., 1981a).

Biochemical studies of purified PHFs confirms the morphological observation that such profiles are very resistant to various degradation conditions (Selkoe, 1982). They can, however, be degraded by a combination of sonication and repeated cycles of heating to 100°C in sodium dodecyl sulfate and β-mercaptoethanol (Iqbal et al., 1984). Polyacrylamide gel electrophoresis of this material revealed a high-molecular-weight polypeptide band and several bands in the 45,000–62,000 dalton range. These bands are also found in normal control preparations but in much lower amounts. The origin of these polypeptides is not known but it appears that they are not new or novel (Iqbal et al., 1982). Rather, it is likely that they are the product of an impaired degradation process in which a normal cellular component accumulates perhaps as a result of incomplete degradation of cell protein(s). This could well be the result of a quantitative or qualitative abnormality in protein-degrading enzymes, which leads to the polymerization of proteins and their storage in a manner analogous to the formation of lipofuscin granules from lipids and amyloid fibers in the systemic amyloidosis.

Immunohistochemical studies have shown that antisera prepared against microtubule preparations cross-reacts with antigens present in neurofibrillary tangles (Grundke-Iqbal et al., 1979; Yen et al., 1981). Other work has shown that some antisera prepared against neurofilament components also immunostain AD/SDAT neurofibrillary tangles (Gambetti et al., 1980; Dahl et al., 1982). These immunohistochemical studies must be interpreted with caution because of what appears to be the trapping of nonconstituent proteins within the tangle. Evidence for this comes from recent work showing that (1) the blood/brain barrier is compromised in SDAT such that the tangles (and plaques) contain both albumin and gamma globulins, and (2) both tangles and plaques are stained with antibodies to prealbumin (Wisniewski and Kozlowski, 1982; Shirahama et al., 1982). Thus light-microscopic immunocytochemistry alone is unlikely to provide an unequivocal candidate for the PHF precursor protein.

Neuritic (Senile) Plaques

Neuritic (senile) plaques are complex structures made of both neuronal and nonneuronal elements. They were first observed by Blocq and Marinesco in 1892, and named senile plaques by Simchowicz (1911). Since Bielschowsky's (1911) and Divry's (1934) reports, it has been known that amyloid is present in these plaques. The metallic impregnation methods show also that the glial elements, particularly the microglia and astrocytes, are part of the plaque structure. However, because of the limitations of light-microscope techniques in identifying the various elements of the neuropil the origin and nature of the silver-positive rods and granules seen in the plaques was not known. Subsequent ultrastructural studies showed that the granular structures were the dystrophic, regenerating, and degenerating unmyelinated neuronal processes (neurites). At this point it should be recalled that early investigators like Fisher (1907) were of the opinion that nerve cell processes are involved in plaque formation. Bouman (1934), influenced by the silver-staining methodology, postulated that the buds and knots represented regenerating neurites. As already mentioned these observations were confirmed by electron-microscopic studies as well as recent examination of the plaques using the Golgi method (Probst et al., 1983). Many varieties of plaques have been described, but in general the following types are recognized: (1) typical, classical, or mature plaques with a central core of amyloid surrounded by microglia, phagocytes, and astrocytes, and silver-positive rods and granules which represent dystrophic regenerating and degenerating neurites; (2) primitive, atypical, or immature plaques in which the amyloid is dispersed between the reactive cells and regenerating and dystrophic neurites; and (3) compact, burned-out or amyloid plaques that are made almost entirely by the deposits of amyloid.

One of the unanswered questions of plaque pathogenesis concerns the relationship between the amyloid deposition and the neuritic pathology. According to one hypothesis the first change which leads to plaque formation is the deposition of a "thread-like substance" (i.e., amyloid fibers) in the brain tissue. The second phase of the process is characterized by a reaction on the part of the nerve fibers (Marinesco and Minea, 1912; Divry, 1934; Schwartz, 1970). A second hypothesis states that pathologic changes in other CNS components (e.g., blood vessels, glia, and neurons with neurofibrillary change) were responsible for the initiation of plaque formation. According to this view the amyloid originated either from the disintegration of the nerve cells or the necrobiosis of neurologia (Simchowicz, 1911; Ferraro, 1931; Bouman, 1934). The observation that, in the cortex, dystrophic neurites (in clusters no larger than 2 or 3) were found without amyloid lent to the belief that amyloid is not the initiator of plaque formation (Terry and Wisniewski, 1970; Wisniewski and Terry, 1973b). On the strength of this observation we proposed that the primary dystrophic and degenerative changes in neurites attracted microglia which, activated by the local pathology of the neuropil, started to produce amyloid. Subsequent studies of the pattern of degeneration of cortical terminals undergoing Wallerian degeneration due to undercutting or spindle-inhibitor-induced terminal pathology revealed that none of these changes led to amyloid deposition and plaque formation (Wisniewski and Terry, 1970; Ghetti and Wisniewski, 1972). Also, in studies of infantile neuroaxonal dystrophy in humans in which there are many dystrophic neurites in the cortex, amyloid deposition has not been observed as a component of the pathology (Seitelberger, 1971; Jellinger, 1973). Thus, neuritic dystrophy and degeneration per se is not sufficient to initiate plaque formation.

Another approach to plaque pathogenesis was suggested by the finding that infection of genetically susceptible strains of mice with selected scrapie agents leads to the formation of neuritic and amyloid plaques in the central nervous system (CNS) (Wisniewski et al., 1975; Bruce et al., 1976). Because of a suggestion of an immune response to scrapie infection (Collis et al., 1979) it was proposed that the formation of a neurotoxic immune complex might be responsible for the dystrophic and degenerative changes in neuropil and the formation of amyloid fibers (Wisniewski et al., 1975). Furthermore, observation of alterations in the blood/brain barrier (BBB) of scrapie-infected mice (Wisniewski et al., 1981b) provided the means by which such complexes might gain access to the CNS. Subsequent studies, however, showed that the BBB is also changed in scrapie-infected mice that do not form plaques. Therefore chronic change in the BBB was not sufficient to explain plaque formation. Regardless of the role of BBB changes and/or presumed immune complexes ultrastructural studies revealed that the first changes appear to be related to the hypersecretory activity of microglia which release proteinacious material into the extracellular space (Wisniewski et al., 1982; Moretz et al., 1983). It is in this milieu that assembly of amyloid fibers takes place. This concept envisions that the primary etiologic and pathogenetic events are associated with the CNS amyloidogenesis and that the neuritic abnormalities are a secondary phenomenon. At this point the factor(s) leading to the formation of the amyloidogenic protein are not known. One possibility is that etiologic factors such as an infectious agent might alter the biology of microglia/pericytes such that they become "producer cells" in which amyloidogenic proteins arise as a new protein not normally expressed or as an overproduction of a native protein normally present in the cell. A second option is that the amyloidogenic protein is derived from either the bloodstream or elsewhere in the brain. In this case the microglia behave as "processor" cells and alter the protein(s) in such a way that it now polymerizes into fibers that are deposited locally.

Studies have shown that in SDAT there is a cortical cholinergic deficiency (Davies and Maloney, 1976) which is a consequence of the destruction of the cholinergic neurons of the diagonal band of Broca (dbB) and the nucleus basalis of Meynert (nbM) that project into the cortex (Whitehouse et al., 1981, 1982).

The studies of the nuclei of the basal forebrain led to the belief that the neuronal loss in these nuclei may play a role in the pathogenesis of neuritic plaques (Struble et al., 1982). It was postulated that "due to an unidentified pathogenetic process (for example, a toxin, transmissible agent, genetic factor, or age-related event) a dbB or nbM neuron first begins to show abnormalities in distal intracortical axons; these acetylcholine esterase (AChE)-rich neurites form immature plaques. With time some of these neurites degenerate; these polypeptides, liberated into the microenvironment of the neuropil, may contribute to the amyloid core. Thus, the mature plaque shows argentophilic AChE-positive neurites and amyloid. Eventually, the AChE-containing neurites disappear, leaving an amyloid plaque as the only evidence of this process" (Price et al., 1982). However, if this is really the case one would expect to find that, in the end stage of the disease, most if not all of the plaques would be of the burned-out or amyloid type. In fact, this type of plaque is not very common in the cortex of SDAT victims. What one sees is the predominance of the primitive (or immature), and classical (or mature) plaques. In other words, at the time of death there are many abnormal neurites in spite of all the extensive loss of cholinergic terminals.

Other evidence pointing to the fact that dbB or nbM neurites are not necessary for initiation of the plaque formation is the presence of neuritic plaques in the cerebellar cortex where these nuclei do not project (Pro et al., 1980). Our recent study shows that Alzheimer plaques occur more frequently than expected, not only within defined subcortical nuclei (including nucleus basalis of Meynert) but also within the subcortical fiber system (Rudelli et al., 1984). This study showed also that the peripheral "halo" portion of the plaque where the abnormal neurites are found is determined by the neuropil response to the amyloid deposits, irrespective of the presence or absence of the cholinergic terminals. There are also cases with predominant perivascular distribution of plaques and there is no evidence of selective perivascular projection from nbM or dbB. Finally, data from the scrapie experiments show that the formation of plaques is closely associated not with the distribution of the cholinergic terminals but with the distribution of the infective agent. This conclusion is derived from several studies showing that in experimental scrapie in mice the distribution of plaques in brain with different inoculation routes is similar to the distribution of infectivity. For example, there are considerably more plaques in the inoculated hemisphere than in the contralateral hemisphere (Bruce and Fraser, 1981). A relation between amyloid formation and infectivity is also implied by the finding that large masses of amyloid are found in the needle track formed by the intracerebral inoculation of scrapie into mice (Wisniewski et al., 1981c). These data have led us to propose the following sequence of events in the pathogenesis of neuritic and amyloid plaque formation.

1. Microglia and pericytes make amyloidogenic protein(s) which are subsequently assembled into amyloid fibers.
2. In areas rich in terminals Wallerian-like and dystrophic changes in the neurites occur due to the neurotoxic effect of certain enzymes associated with the amyloidogenic proteins and/or compressive neuropil degeneration.
3. Regenerative changes in the neuropil lead to the formation of many sprouting, strongly silver-positive neurites.
4. A healing process leads to the removal of the dystrophic neurites and the disappearance of reactive cells, leaving behind the amyloid deposits which constitute "burned out" or amyloid plaques.

According to this hypothesis the presence of amyloid deposits (plaques) without the abnormal neuritic component in areas rich in terminals can either be the result of the finished healing process (burned-out plaques) or the result of rapidly formed amyloid deposits. In the latter situation, the host neuropil has had no chance to respond or for reasons not clear did not respond to the toxic and/or compressive amyloid deposits with the formation of the dystrophic and regenerating neurites.

As indicated above in SDAT there is a cortical cholinergic deficiency. This is believed to be a consequence of the destruction of the cholinergic neurons of the dbB and the nbM that project into the cortex (Whitehouse et al., 1981; Price et al., 1982). In the authors' opinion "the clear association between loss of cholinergic innervation and most, if not all, of the symptoms of Alzheimer's disease has significant implications for diagnosis, treatment, and, one may hope, ultimately prevention of the disease" (Coyle et al., 1982). The authors further point out that this view suggests that in SDAT there is a defect paralleling that seen in Parkinson's disease. In our view such a primary "monotransmitter" pathology is not likely to be the case in SDAT. The topography of the SDAT lesions is much broader than in Parkinson's disease where, by and large, only pigmented nuclei are affected. In contrast, SDAT involves the neocortex, hippocampal formation, amygdala, and basal forebrain nuclei. This broader distribution of lesions obviously affects more than one transmitter system. Recent studies show that somatostatin-mediated and noradrenegic systems are also affected in SDAT (Davies et al., 1980; Wood et al., 1982; Adolfsson et al., 1979; Mann et al., 1980). Therefore, if one were to find a way to overcome the cholinergic deficiency in SDAT one might see some improvement in cognitive function but not full recovery of their mental functions. Thus, one should not expect a repetition of the success of L-dopa therapy seen in Parkinson's disease. Besides, it is now evident that the L-dopa therapy did not stop the progress of Parkinson's disease. Concentration on how to treat the symptoms of Parkinson's disease appeared to detract the scientist and the funding agencies from the studies into causes of Parkinson's disease. This mistake should not be repeated with Alzheimer's disease.

Based on the data discussed above and recent observations that point to a compromised blood/brain barrier in Alzheimer's disease, we proposed the following two pathogenetic scenarios of Alzheimer's disease:

AD/SDAT Pathogenesis Scenario I

1. Primary protein pathology in neuronal and nonneuronal elements.
2. Expressed as overproduction and/or impaired degradation of specific protein leading to formation of B-pleated protein(s).
3. Resulting in PHF formation in neurons and amyloid deposition by microglia.
4. Causing other protein derangements such as disturbance of trophic factors and neuron loss, neurotransmitter deficiency, and alteration in enzymes regulating transendothelial transport which is manifested as a compromised BBB.

AD/SDAT Pathogenesis Scenario II

1. Primary pathology of blood/brain barrier leading to changes in permeability.
2. Expressed as chronic leakage of serum proteins into the CNS including enzymes which affect protein degradation.

3. Resulting in PHF formation, amyloid deposition, neurotransmitter deficiency, and neuronal loss.

According to our hypothesis both the primary protein pathology and the change in BBB results when genetically susceptible individuals are infected with one of the unconventional, scrapie-like infectious agents.

References

Adolfsson, R., Gottfries, C.G., Roos, B.E., and Winblad, B.: Changes in the brain catecholamines in patients with dementia of the Alzheimer type. *Br. J. Psychiat. 135*, 216–223 (1979).

Alzheimer, A.: Uber eine eigenartige Erkrankung der Hernrinde. *Zentralbl. Nervenheilkunde Psychiatrie 18*, 177–179 (1907).

Ball, M.J., and Nuttall, K.: Neurofibrillary tangles, granulovascuolar degeneration in the hippocampus with ageing and dementia. *Acta Neuropathol.* (Berlin) *37*, 111–118 (1977).

Bielschowski, M.: Zur Kenntnis de Alzheimerischen Krankheit (prasenilen Demenz mit Herdsymptomen). *J. Psychol. Neurol. 18*, 273–292 (1911).

Blocq, P., and Marinesco, G.: Sur les lesions et la pathogenie de l'epilepsie dite essentielle. *Sem. Med. 12*, 445–446 (1892).

Bouman, L.: Senile plaques. *Brain 57*, 128–142 (1934).

Bruce, M.E., Dickinson, A.G., and Fraser, H.: Cerebral amyloidosis in scrapie in the mouse: Effect of agent strain and mouse genotype. *Neuropathol. Appl. Neurobiol. 2*, 471–478 (1976).

Bruce, M.E., and Fraser, H.: Effect of route of inoculation on the frequency and distribution of cerebral amyloid plaques in scrapie mice. *Neuropathol. Appl. Neurobiol. 7*, 289–298 (1981).

Collis, S.C., Kimberlin, R.H., and Millson, G.C.: Immunoglobulin G concentration in the sera of Hardwick sheep with natural scrapie. *J. Comp. Pathol. 89*, 389–396 (1979).

Coyle, J.T., Price, D.L., and DeLong, M.R.: Brain mechanisms in Alzheimer's disease. *Hospital Practice 17*, 55–63, 1982.

Dahl, D., Selkoe, D.J., Pero, R.T., and Bignami, A.: Immunostaining of neurofibrillary tangles in Alzheimer's senile dementia with a neurofilament antiserum. *J. Neurosci. 2*, 113–119 (1982).

Davies, P., Katzman, R., and Terry, R.D.: Reduced somatostatin-like immunoreactivity in cerebral cortex from cases of Alzheimer's disease and Alzheimer senile dementia. *Nature 288*, 279–280 (1980).

Davies, P., and Maloney, A.J.F.: Selective loss of central cholinergic neurons in Alzheimer's disease. *Lancet 2*, 1403 (1976).

Divry, P.: De la nature de l'alteration fibrillaire d'Alzheimer. *J. Belge Neurol. Psychiatr. 34*, 197–201 (1934).

Ferraro, A.: The origin and formation of senile plaques. *Arch. Neurol. Psych. 25*, 1042 (1931).

Fisher, O.: Miliare Nekrosen mit drusigen Wuckerunger der Neurofibrillen, eine regelmassige Veranderung der Hirnrinde bei senile Demenz. *Monatsschr. Psychiat. Neurol. 22*, 361–372 (1907).

Gambetti, P., Velasco, M.E., Dahl, D., Bignami, A., Roessmann, U., and Sindley, S.D.: Alzheimer neurofibrillary tangles: An immunohistochemical study. In Amaducci, L., Davison, A.N., and Antuono, P. (Eds.), Aging of the Brain and Dementia, pp. 55–63. New York: Raven, 1980.

Ghetti, B., and Wisniewski, H.M.: On degeneration of terminals in the cat striatal cortex. *Brain Res. 44*, 630–635 (1972).

Glenner, G.: Amyloid deposits and amyloidosis. *New Eng. J. Med. 302*, 1283–1292, 1333–1343 (1980).

Grundke-Iqbal, I., Johnson, A.B., Wisniewski, H.M., Terry, R.D., and Iqbal, K.: Evidence that Alzheimer neurofibrillary tangles originate from neurotubules. *Lancet 1*, 578–580 (1979).

Iqbal, K., Grundke-Iqbal, I., Merz, P.A., and Wisniewski, H.M.: Alzheimer neurofibrillary tangle: Morphology and biochemistry. *Exp. Brain Res.* (Suppl.) *5*, 10–14 (1982).

Iqbal, K., Zaidi, T., Thompson, C.H., Merz, P.A., and Wisniewski, H.M.: Alzheimer paired helical filaments: Bulk isolation solubility and protein composition. *Acta Neuropathol.* (Berlin) *62*, 167–177(1984).

Jellinger, K.: Neuroaxonal dystrophy: Its natural history and related disorders. In Zimmerman, H.M. (Eds.), Progress in Neuropathology, Vol. II, pp. 129–180. New York: Grune & Stratton, 1973.

Mann, D.M.A., Lincoln, J., Yates, P.U., Stamp, J.E., and Toper, S.: Changes in the monoamine containing neurons of the human CNS in senile dementia. *Br. J. Psychiat. 136*, 533–542 (1980).

Marinesco, G., and Minea, J.: Untersuchungen uber die senilen plaques. *Monatsschi f. Psych. u. Neuc. 31*, Eng. H. 79 (1912).

Metuzals, J., Montpetit, V., Clapin, D.F., and Nelson, R.F.: Arrays of paired helical filaments in Alzheimer's disease. In Proc. of the Electron Microscopy Society of America, Washington, D.C., 1982, pp. 348–349. Baton Rouge: Claitor's Publ. Div., 1982.

Moretz, R.C., Wisniewski, H.M., and Lossinsky, A.S.: Pathogenesis of neuritic and amyloid plaques in scrapie—ultrastructural study of early changes in the cortical neuropil. In Samuel, D., Algeri, S., Gershon, S., Grimm, V.E., and Toffano, G. (Eds.), Aging of the Brain, pp. 61–79. New York: Raven, 1983.

Price, D.L., Whitehouse, P.J., Struble, R.G., Clark, A.W., Coyle, J.T., DeLong, M.R., and Hedreen, J.C.: Basal forebrain cholinergic systems in Alzheimer's disease and related dementias. *Neurosci. Commentaries 1*, 84–92 (1982).

Pro, J.D., Smith, Maj. C.H., and Sumi, S.M.: Presenile Alzheimer's disease: Amyloid plaques in the cerebellum. *Neurology 30*, 820–825 (1980).

Probst, A., Basler, V., Bron, B., and Ulrich, J.: Neuritic plaques in senile dementia of the Alzheimer type: A Golgi analysis in the hippocampal region. *Brain Res. 268*, 249–254 (1983).

Roth, M., Tomlinson, B.E., and Blessed, G.: Correlation between scores for dementia and counts of senile plaques in cerebral gray matter of elderly subjects. *Nature 206*, 109–110 (1966).

Rudelli, R.D., Ambler, M.W., and Wisniewski, H.M.: Morphology and distribution of Alzheimer neuritic (senile) and amyloid plaques in striatum and diencephalon. *Acta Neuropathol.* (submitted for publ.).

Schwartz, P.: Amyloidosis: Cause and Manifestations of Senile Deteriorations. Springfield, Illinois: Charles C. Thomas, 1970.

Seitelberger, F.: Neuropathological conditions related to neuroaxonal dystrophy. *Acta Neuropathol.* (Berlin) (Suppl V), 17–29 (1971).

Selkoe, D.J.: Molecular pathology of the aging human brain. *Trends in Neuroscience 5*, 332–336 (1982).

Shirahama, T., Skinner, M., Westermark, P., Rubinow, A., Cohen, A.S., Brun, A., and Kemper, T.L.: Senile cerebral amyloid: Prealbumin as a common constituent in the neuritic plaque, in the neurofibrillary tangle, and in microangiopathic lesion. *Am. J. Pathol. 107*, 41–50 (1982).

Simchowicz, T.: Histologische studien uber die senile demenz. *Nissl-Alzheimer's Arbeiten 4*, 267–444 (1911).

Struble, R.G., Cork, L.C., Whitehouse, P.J., and Price, D.L.: Cholinergic innervation in neuritic plaques. *Science 216*, 413–415 (1982).

Terry, R.D., and Wisniewski, H.M.: The ultrastructure of the neurofibrillary tangle and the senile plaque. In Wolstenholme, G.E., and O'Connor, M. (Eds.), Alzheimer's Diseases and Related Conditions, Ciba Foundation Symposium, London, pp. 145–168. London: Churchill, 1970.

Tomlinson, B.E., Blessed, G., and Roth, M.: Observations on the brains of demented old people. *J. Neurol. Sci. 11*, 205–242 (1970).

Whitehouse, P.J., Price, D.L., Clark, A.W., Coyle, J.T., and DeLong, M.R.: Alzheimer disease: Evidence for selective loss of cholinergic neurons in the nucleus basalis. *Ann. Neurol. 10*, 122–126 (1981).

Whitehouse, P.J., Price, D.L., Struble, R.G., Clark, A.W., Coyle, J.T., and DeLong, M.R.: Alzheimer's disease and senile dementia: Loss of neurons in the basal forebrain. *Science 215*, 1237–1239 (1982).

Wisniewski, H.M., Bruce, M.E., and Fraser, H.: Infectious etiology of neuritic (senile) plaques in mice. *Science 190*, 1108–1110 (1975).

Wisniewski, H.M., and Kozlowski, P.B.: Evidence for blood–brain barrier changes in senile dementia of the Alzheimer type (SDAT). *Ann. New York Acad. Sci. 396*, 119–129 (1982).

Wisniewski, H.M., Lossinsky, A.S., Moretz, R.C., and Vorbrodt, A.W.: Neuritic plaque formation and blood–brain barrier (BBB) changes in scrapie. *J. Neuropathol. Exp. Neurol. 40*, 1342 (1981b).

Wisniewski, H.M., Moretz, R.C., and Lossinsky, A.S.: Evidence for induction of localized amyloid deposits and neuritic plaques by an infectious agent. *Ann. Neurol. 10*, 517–522 (1981c).

Wisniewski, H.M., Narang, H.K., and Terry, R.D.: Neurofibrillary tangles of paired helical filaments. *J. Neurol. Sci. 27*, 173–181 (1976).

Wisniewski, H.M., Shelanski, M.L., and Terry, R.D.: Effects of miotic spindle inhibitors on neurotubules and neurofilaments in anterior horn cells. *J. Cell Biol. 38*, 224–229 (1968).

Wisniewski, H.M., Sinatra, R.S., Iqbal, K., and Grundke-Iqbal, I.: Neurofibrillary and synaptic pathology in the aged brain. In Johnson, J.E. Jr. (Ed.), Aging and Cell Structure, Vol. 1, pp. 104–142. New York: Plenum, 1981a.

Wisniewski, H.M., and Terry, R.D.: An experimental approach to the morphogenesis of neurofibrillary degeneration and the argyrophilic plaque. In Wolstenholme, G.E., and O'Connor, M. (Eds.), Alzheimer's Diseases and Related Conditions, Ciba Foundation Symposium, London, pp. 223–243. London: Churchill, 1970.

Wisniewski, H.M., and Terry, R.D.: Morphology of the aging brain, human and animal. *Progress in Brain Research 40*, 167–186 (1973a).

Wisniewski, H.M., and Terry, R.D.: Reexamination of the pathogenesis of the senile plaque. In Zimmerman, H.M. (Ed.), Progress in Neuropathology, Vol. II, pp. 1–26. New York: Grune & Stratton, 1973b.

Wisniewski, H.M., Terry, R.D., and Hirano, A.: Neurofibrillary pathology. *J. Neuropathol. Exp. Neurol. 29*, 163–176 (1970).

Wisniewski, H.M., Vorbrodt, A.W., Moretz, R.C., Lossinsky, A.S., and Grundke-Iqbal, I.: Pathogenesis of neuritic (senile) and amyloid plaque formation. In Hoyer, S. (Ed.), The Aging Brain—Physiological and Pathological Aspects, Experimental Brain Research, Supplementum 5, pp. 3–9. New York: Springer-Verlag, 1982.

Wisniewski, H.M., and Wen, G.Y.: Substructures of Alzheimer type of paired helical filaments (in preparation).

Wisniewski, K., Jervis, G.A., Moretz, R.C., and Wisniewski, H.M.: Alzheimer neurofibrillary tangles in diseases other than senile and presenile dementia. *Ann. Neurol. 5*, 288–294 (1979).

Wood, P.L., Etienne, P., Lal, S., Gauthier, S., Cajal, S., and Nair, N.P.V.: Reduced lumbar CSF somatostatin levels in Alzheimer's disease. *Life Sci. 31*, 2073–2079 (1982).

Yen, S.C., Gaskin, F., and Terry, R.D.: Immunocytochemical studies of neurofibrillary tangles. *Am. J. Pathol. 104*, 77–89 (1981).

Part VI

Prevention and Treatment of Physical Disorders

Chapter 21

Interaction of Aging and Disease

John W. Rowe

Summary

The normal aging process has a varied and important clinical impact. The physiology of the elderly differs from that of young individuals in specific predictable ways which result in age differences in the presentation and response to treatment of a broad array of disorders. This chapter reviews specific interactions between aging and disease states that may serve as models for an approach to the elderly patient.

A thorough knowledge of age-related physiologic changes that occur in man, in the absence of disease, is critical to a proper understanding of disease in old age since these physiologic changes form the substrate for the influence of age on the presentation of disease, its response to treatment, and the complications that ensue (Rowe and Besdine, 1982).

Before discussing the interaction of normal aging with disease states, it is appropriate to emphasize two major factors which play dominant roles in the expression of disease in the elderly. One principle relevant to both geriatric medicine and gerontological physiology is the marked variability that accompanies advanced age (Freis and Crapo, 1981). Decades of study of normal and abnormal aging have shown, perhaps more clearly than anything else, that the older people become, the less like each other they become. The marked variability in the clinical manifestations of a given illness in the elderly is due in part to (1) variability in the underlying physiologic changes, (2) the other diseases that the individual has accumulated over time, (3) the pattern of response to illness and interaction with health care professionals that is characteristic of the individual, and (4) the varying degrees of severity of pathophysiologic processes. A second major principle has to do with the critical importance of nonbiomedical factors in the determination of the clinical manifestations of disease late in life. More than any other segment of our society, the elderly manifest differing degrees of disability and loss of function depending on behavioral and sociological factors (Besdine, 1980).

The Continuum of Interaction Between Physiology and Pathology in the Elderly

A robust understanding of the varying interaction of the normal aging process with a variety of stresses and pathologic mechanisms is required to provide the proper framework for evaluation of the elderly patient. The interaction of age and disease varies from a lack of interaction on one end of the spectrum to the extreme example where the changes that occur with age actually represent disease inasmuch as they have direct, predictable, and adverse clinical sequelae. Several specific clinically relevant points along the continuum can be identified.

Variables that Do Not Change with Age

Perhaps the most important type of change that occurs with age, from a clinical standpoint, is no change at all. Too frequently clinicians are apt to ascribe a disability or abnormal physical or laboratory finding to "old age," when the actual cause is a specific disease process. Several examples of this category can be identified. In the first subset there is no effect of age on the variable under study. An example of this lack of change may be seen in hematocrit or packed-red-cell volume. This measurement is routinely obtained in many clinical settings, since a significant lowering of hematocrit defines the presence of anemia, a common and important medical illness of varying cause. Very frequently elderly individuals will be found to have low hematocrit levels and the clinician will categorize the patient as having "anemia of old age." The physician may fail to pursue the underlying basis of the anemia in his belief that the normal aging process has induced the anemia and that no investigation or treatment is warranted. However, data from several sources, including the Framingham Study, indicate that in healthy community-dwelling elders there is no change with age in hematocrit (Gordon and Shurtleff, 1973, Figure 7). Thus a lower hematocrit in an elderly individual cannot be ascribed to "anemia of old age," but deserves a proper investigation and treatment. Three common, often treatable, causes of anemia in the elderly include (1) nutritional deficits, particularly iron deficiency; (2) pernicious anemia or vitamin B-12 deficiency, which develops as levels of intrinsic factor fall in advanced age as a consequence of atrophy of the gastric mucosa; and (3) iron deficiency anemia secondary to blood loss, often from intestinal malignancies. Anemia and gastrointestinal blood loss are frequently the initial clinical evidences of an otherwise asymptomatic colonic carcinoma, which, if detected early, can be very effectively treated surgically.

A second circumstance in which there is no change in a clinical variable with age relates to factors in which a balanced physiologic change results in a lack of measurable change. An example of such a circumstance might be seen in the circulatory levels of many hormones, including testosterone. While the circulating level in blood of testosterone appears not to decline in healthy community-dwelling elderly men (Sparrow, Bosse, and Rowe, 1980; Harman and Tsitouras, 1980), studies indicate that this is the result of a balanced 25–30% decline in both testosterone production and catabolism rates (Vermuelen, Rubens, and Verdonk, 1972). Similar changes have been identified with regard to cortisol (West, Brown, Simons, Carter, Kumagai, and Englebert, 1961), thyroxine (Gregerman, Gaffney, and Shock, 1962) (Oddie, Myhill, Pirnique, and Fisher, 1968), aldosterone (Flood et al., 1967), and probably also exist for insulin (Minaker, Rowe, Pallotta, and Sparrow, 1982; Reaven, Greenfield, Mondon, Rosenthal, Wright, and Reaven, 1982). The clinically relevant fact remains that the variable most frequently measured does not change with age, and deviation from the normal range for all adults should be viewed as clearly abnormal, independent of age.

Physiologic Changes by Which Specific Diseases Become Less Likely or Severe with Age

While aging is characteristically considered to be associated with a greater prevalence or severity of disease, it is quite possible that the physiologic changes associated with normal aging result in many diseases being less likely or less severe in advanced age. Clearly, some disorders that appear to be based in altered immune system response, such as systemic lupus erythematosis, myasthenia gravis, and multiple sclerosis, are seen much more commonly in younger individuals than in older individuals. It is feasible that the changes that occur in the immune system with age, with marked decrease of function of T-lymphocytes and other aspects of immune competence might result in a less robust immunologic response to the inciting agent or event in these disorders (Gillis, Kozak, Durante, and Weksler, 1981).

Similarly, some diseases which occur in old age as well as younger adults clearly run a less virulent natural history in the elderly. One example may be carcinoma of the breast. Many cancer specialists feel that carcinoma of the breast runs a more virulent and more aggressive course in premenopausal than postmenopausal women. In addition, the likelihood of breast carcinoma responding well to hormonal therapy increases with the number of years after menopause. Thus elderly individuals with this disease might be expected, on the average, to enjoy a more favorable clinical course than their younger counterparts.

Physiologic Changes that Alter the Presentation of a Disease

This poorly understood area has long been recognized as of major importance to the practice of geriatric medicine. Many diseases that occur in both young and old adults have manifestly different clinical presentations and natural histories in the two age groups. Unlike the example of breast cancer, which was discussed above, these disorders should not necessarily be looked upon as being less severe or more severe in the elderly, but just different. One example of such a disorder is hyperthyroidism. Younger individuals with hyperthyroidism often present as agitated, anxious, and hyperkinetic with a palpable goiter (enlarged thyroid gland), elevated heart rate and blood pressure, hyperactive deep tendon reflexes, and almost ubiquitous complaints of weight loss and irritability. Conversely, it is well recognized that many elderly individuals with hyperthyroidism, manifested by elevations of circulating thyroid hormone to levels equivalent to those seen in younger individuals, will have a strikingly different clinical presentation. In these individuals irritability and hyperkinesis are infrequent and goiter is very rare (Davis and Davis, 1974). Deep tendon reflexes may be normal or even hypoactive, and the patient generally presents a deactivated or "apathetic" as opposed to activated clinical picture. The treatment of hyperthyroidism with generally the same modalities available to younger individuals results in the same general excellent prognosis in both young and old individuals. The major clinical importance of this difference relates to the education of physicians in the recognition of hyperthyroidism in the elderly. Many physicians not familiar with the special presentation of thyroid hormone excess in the elderly will not detect the disease and thus will allow its adverse physiologic and pathologic sequelae to continue untreated, thus permitting continued morbidity and, perhaps, mortality.

A second example of a common disorder which presents much differently in the elderly than in young adults is uncontrolled diabetes mellitus. In children and in young adults uncontrolled diabetes is generally manifested by a syndrome termed diabetic ketoacidosis. This is characterized by elevations of blood glucose, commonly to levels between 300 and 500 mg/dl and the presence of a severe metabolic acidosis associated with markedly elevated levels of circulating ketones. Conversely, elderly individuals with uncontrolled diabetes will frequently present with a syndrome termed hyperosmolar nonketotic coma, which is characterized by striking elevations of blood glucose, often to levels over

1000 mg/dl, and a relative or absolute lack of circulating ketones or acidosis. The elderly present with obtundation and coma secondary to the marked hyperosmolality induced by the elevated glucose levels, while younger individuals are more likely to present with manifestations of severe metabolic acidosis.

Other disorders in which the presentation is strongly influenced by age without necessarily making the disorder more or less severe include depression, acute glomerulonephritis, and rheumatoid arthritis.

Physiologic Changes that Increase the Likelihood or Severity of a Disease

This large and important category encompasses those abnormalities which are most commonly recognized as resulting from an interaction of age and disease and which account for the increasing morbidity and mortality of disease in old age. Age-related reductions in the function of numerous organs place elderly individuals at special risk for enhanced morbidity from diseases in those organs.

Finch has recently proposed a mechanism whereby normal age-related changes in brain neurotransmitters may influence the onset or severity of a variety of degenerative central nervous system diseases (Finch, 1980; Finch and Morgan, in press). In the case of Parkinson's disease he points out that normal human aging has been associated with progressive reductions in basal ganglia levels of dopamine as well as dopamine receptors and key enzymes required for dopamine synthesis (Finch and Morgan, in press; Severson et al., in press; McGeer, McGeer, and Suzuki, 1977; McGeer and McGeer, 1978). These decreases may interact with pathophysiologic changes to account for the increasing prevalence of Parkinson's disease in late life, whether secondary to viral encephalitis or associated with a genetic predisposition. While several models may be postulated for the interaction of aging and Parkinson's disease, Schwab notes that the onset of the disease many years after acute encephalitis (Schwab et al., 1956) and the enhanced susceptibility of old individuals to extrapyramidal side effects of neuroleptic agents (Ayd, 1961) are consistent with the development of age-related subclinical dopaminergic deficits.

Normal aging is associated with a marked reduction in pulmonary function, as reflected in the forced vital capacity and other measures of lung function. Healthy individuals in the ninth decade of life frequently will have lung function equal to only one-half of that of their 30-year-old counterparts. Thus an acute pulmonary disease, such as bacterial pneumonia, will be much more likely to induce a serious clinical manifestation in the elderly because of the markedly lessened pulmonary functional reserve. Over the past decade very significant advances have been made in our understanding of the marked reduction in immune competence that occurs with age. Immunosenescence is likely responsible, in some ways, for the increased severity of infections in the elderly. Thus, an elderly individual with pneumonia may be less likely to contain and control that infection in his respiratory tract than a young individual. Failure of immune function may result in dissemination of that infection to many organs and a much more serious if not life-threatening clinical illness may develop.

A similar argument holds for function in many other organs, including the kidneys. Normal renal function in the elderly is approximately 40% less than in young healthy adults (Rowe et al., 1976). Thus the loss of one kidney due to obstruction, vascular occlusion, or trauma in the elderly would be much more likely to result in a clinically significant reduction in glomerular filtration rates and overall renal function than the loss of function in one kidney in a healthy young individual.

In elderly individuals, multiple pathology or the simultaneous presence of diseases in several organs or organ systems is often the rule rather than the exception. In many cases physiologic changes that occur with age interact with multiple pathology to induce specifically geriatric syndromes. The high prevalence in the elderly of falls may be viewed as such a case. Several studies have demonstrated a marked increase in postural sway or decrease in the capacity to maintain upright posture with advancing age, particularly in women (Sheldon, 1963; Hasselkus and Shambes, 1975; Exton-Smith, 1976). Recent evidence suggests that this may be related to age-associated changes in the mechanoreceptors in the cervical spine (Wyke, 1979). Regardless of the mechanisms of this age-related effect, elderly individuals by virtue of their decreased capacity to maintain upright posture are at particular risk for the development of falling under a variety of circumstances which would not result in falls in younger individuals. Thus ice on the front step, a poorly lit stairway at home, or a moist bathtub without a rubber mat may all result in a near fall in a young individual and a serious fall in the elderly. The risk of the elderly to develop a serious consequence of this fall is enhanced by another age-related change which is also particularly common in elderly women, loss of bone mass or osteopenia. Thus hip fracture is essentially a disease of elderly women, and in most instances is induced by a fall under circumstances which would not have induced a fall or fracture in younger individuals.

A final example of a mechanism whereby age-related alterations in function increase the prevalence of a disease relates to the development of accidental hypothermia in frail elderly. This disorder has a high mortality rate and can be seen not only in individuals exposed to unheated rooms in the winter, but in individuals in heated rooms who appear to spontaneously develop marked lowering of body temperature. This disorder is essentially absent in healthy young individuals and occurs with increasing frequency with advancing old age. While the mechanisms of accidental hypothermia are poorly understood, alterations in sympathetic nervous system responsiveness seem likely to be a major contributor.

Physiologic Changes Which Mimic Specific Diseases

Some changes that occur with aging may be seen to mimic specific clinical entities, thus causing confusion regarding the diagnosis of specific diseases in the elderly. Perhaps the best and most widely recognized instance of this is the decrease in carbohydrate economy that occurs with advancing age in the absence of diabetes mellitus (Davidson, 1979). Normal aging appears to be associated with a decrease in the sensitivity of peripheral tissues to the effects of insulin (Defronzo, 1979; Rowe, Minaker, Pallotta, and Flier, 1983). This change is reflected by decreased performance on oral or intravenous glucose tolerance tests.

The oral glucose tolerance test finds frequent clinical application as a means of diagnosing the presence of chemical diabetes mellitus. In this test fasting individuals are given a standard oral dose of glucose and the plasma glucose level is checked at regular intervals over the next 2 hr. The level of blood sugar 2 hr after ingestion of a glucose challenge can be used to determine whether an individual is normal or has impaired glucose tolerance with very high levels being diagnostic of diabetes mellitus. Many medical textbooks include criteria for the diagnosis of diabetes mellitus on the oral glucose tolerance test which are based solely on studies of healthy young control populations.The changes in glucose tolerance with age, independent of diabetes or other confounding diseases, are so dramatic that over 50% of individuals over 60 years of age would be diagnosed as diabetic if age-adjusted criteria were not employed (Davidson, 1979). Unfortunately, too frequently physicians and other health professionals are unaware of the need for age adjustment in this as well as other types of clinical tests, thus resulting in a tendency for the overdiagnosis of diabetes in the elderly.

Physiologic Changes Which Have a Direct Clinical Impact

For many decades gerontologists and geriatricians have drawn a very clear line between the changes that occur with age and those that are associated with specific disease states. We have staunchly defended the view that age is not a disease, but a normal process that must be clearly understood in order to adequately diagnose and treat the increasing burden of illness that will befall a rapidly enlarging population. Substantial data in several different areas suggest that this approach is no longer tenable. There is no question that some physiologic changes that are aspects of normal aging itself have clearly adverse clinical sequelae. While a change may represent "normal aging" inasmuch as it is present in the entire population and cannot be avoided, one should not assume that this "normal" change is necessarily harmless.

While one can argue about the specific criteria for the definition of a "disease," one generally acceptable definition would include any process that results in clear adverse clinical sequelae measured as either morbidity or mortality. Under this definition there are clear changes that occur with advancing age which appear to be normal characteristics of the aging process and which would also qualify as diseases. Of the potentially very long list of such processes, three will be briefly reviewed.

More than any other biological changes, menopause seems clearly to be accepted as age related. While menopause is thus clearly "normal" it has become abundantly clear that this normal change is associated with increased risk for certain diseases such as osteoporosis and atherosclerosis, as well as symptomatic clinical manifestations such as hot flashes which are associated with sleep disturbances and are so frequent and severe as to be disabling in many individuals (Hannan, 1927; McKinlay and McKinlay, 1973).

A second change that occurs with normal aging which has direct adverse clinical consequences is cataract formation. Post-translational modifications of central lens proteins with advancing age result in increasing opacity as well as decreasing flexibility of the lens, which is manifested in decreasing capacity to accomodate to near vision (Weale, 1963). While the reasons for the development of cataracts in some individuals and not others are not clearly understood, they probably lie in the marked physiologic variability that was previously commented on as being characteristic of most if not all changes that occur with advancing age. Lens opacification or cataract is a common cause of blindness in older Americans. Thus this normal age-related change, in its most extreme form, would seem to clearly represent a disease.

A third characteristic type of change with advancing age that would appear to have direct clinical consequences is arteriosclerosis. This thickening of the walls of major arteries must be distinguished from atherosclerosis, which represents the development of placques on the vessel intima which encroach on the lumen. Arteriosclerosis appears to be a normal consequence of age-related changes in the extracellular material in arterial walls and is reflected in decreased compliance and increased stiffening of vessels with advancing age (O'Rourke, 1970). This is manifested in increased systolic blood pressure. Epidemiologic studies, including the Framingham study, have identified increases in systolic blood pressure as a major risk factor for several types of vascular disorders, most notably cerebrovascular disease or stroke (Kannel et al., 1970; Kannel et al., 1981). Thus, increases in systolic pressure, which appear to be consequences of normal age-related changes in vessel walls, carry with them an increased risk for serious morbidity or mortality.

References

Ayd, F.J.: A survey of drug-induced extra-pyramidal reactions. *J. Am. Med. Assoc. 175*, 1054–1060 (1961).

Besdine, R.: Geriatric medicine. In Eisdorfer, C. (Ed.), Annual Review of Gerontology and Geriatrics, Vol. 1, pp. 135–153. New York: Springer-Verlag, 1980.

Davidson, M.B.: The effect of aging on carbohydrate metabolism: a review of the English literature and a practical approach to the diagnosis of diabetes mellitus in the elderly. *Metabolism 28*, 688–705 (1979).

Davis, P.J., and Davis, F.G.: Hyperthyroidism in patients over the age of 60 years. Clinical features in 85 patients. *Medicine 53*, 161 (1974).

Defronzo, R.A.: Glucose intolerance and aging: evidence for tissue insensitivity to insulin. *Diabetes 28*, 1095–1101 (1979).

Exton-Smith, A.N.: Lecture to Conference on Geriatric Medicine. University of Western Ontario, Canada (unpublished).

Finch, C.E.: Relationships of aging changes in the basal ganglia to manifestations of Huntington's chorea. Ann. Neurology 7, 406–411 (1980).

Finch, C.E., and Moran, D.: Aging and schizophrenia: a hypothesis relating asynchrony in neural aging processes to the manifestations of schizophrenia and other neurologic diseases with age. In NIMH Symposium on Aging and Schizophrenia (in press). Rockville, Md.

Flood, C. et al.: The metabolism and secretion of aldosterone in the elderly subjects. *J. Clin. Invest. 46*, 960 (1967).

Fries, J.F., and Crapo, L.M.: The emergence of chronic, universal disease. In Vitality and Aging, pp. 79–96. San Francisco: W.H. Freeman, (1981).

Gillis, S., Kozak, R., Durante, M., and Weksler, M.E.: Immunological studies of aging. Decreased production of and response to T cell growth factor by lymphocytes from aged humans. J. Clin. Invest. *67*(4), 937–42 (1981).

Gordon, T., and Shurtleff, D.: Means at each examination and inter-examination variation of specific characteristics: Framingham Study-Exams 1–10. In Kannel, W.B. (ed.), The Framingham Study: An Epidemiological Investigation of Cardiovascular Disease, DHEW Publication No-NIH74-478. Washington, D.C.: U.S. Government Printing Office, 1973.

Gregerman, R.I., Gaffney, G.W., and Shock, N.W.: Thyroxine turnover in euthyroid man with special reference to changes with age. J. Clin. Invest. *41*, 2065–2074 (1962).

Hannan, J.H.: The Flushings of the Menopause. London: Bailiere, Tindall & Cox, 1927.

Harman, S.M., and Tsitouras, P.D.: Reproductive hormones in aging men. Measurement of sex steroids, basal leutineizing hormone and Leydig cell response to human chorionic gonadotropin. J. Clin. Endocrinol. Metab. *51*, 35–40 (1980).

Hasselkus, B.R., and Shambes, G.M.: Aging and postural sway in women. J. Gerontol. *30*, 661–667 (1975).

Kannel, W.B. et al.: Epidemiologic assessment of the role of blood pressure in stroke—the Framingham study. JAMA *214*, 301 (1970).

Kannel, W.B. et al.: Systolic blood pressure, arterial rigidity, and the risk of stroke. JAMA *245*, 1229 (1981).

McGeer, P.L., McGeer, E.G., and Suzuki, G.S.: Aging and extrapyramidal function. Arch. Neurol. (Chicago) *34*, 33–35 (1977).

McGeer, P.L., and McGeer, E.G.: Aging and neurotransmitter systems. In Finch, C.E., Poster, D.E., and Kenny, A.D. (Eds.), Parkinson's Disease: II. Aging and Neuroendocrine Relationships, pp. 41–58. New York: Plenum, 1978.

McKinlay, S.M., and McKinlay, J.B.: Selected studies of the menopause. *J. Biosocial Science* 5, 533–555 (1973).

Minaker, K.L., Rowe, J.W., Pallotta, J., and Sparrow, D.: Clearance of insulin: influence of steady state insulin level and age. Diabetes *31*, 132–135 (1982).

Oddie, T.H., Myhill, J., Pirnique, F.G., and Fisher, D.A.: Effects of age and sex on the radioiodine uptake in euthyroid subjects. J. Clin. Endocrinol. *28*, 776–782 (1968).

O'Rourke, M.F.: Arterial hemodynamics in hypertension. Circ. Res. *6* (Suppl. 2), 1234 (1970).

Reaven, G.M., Greenfield, M.S., Mondon, C.M., Rosenthal, M., Wright, D., and Reaven, E.: Does insulin removal rate from plasma decline with age? *Diabetes 31*, 670–674 (1982).

Rowe, J.W., Tobin, J.D., Andres, R.A., Norris, A., and Shock, N.W.: The effect of age on creatinine clearance in man. J. Gerontol. *31*, 155–163 (1976).

Rowe, J.W., and Besdine, R.W.: Preface. In Rowe, J.W., and Besdine, R.W. (Eds.), Health and Disease in Old age. Boston: Little, Brown & Co., 1982.

Rowe, J.W., Minaker, K.L., Pallotta, J., and Flier, J.S.: Characterization of the insulin resistance of aging. J. Clin. Invest. *71*, 1581–1588 (1983).

Schwab, R.S., Doshay, L.J., Garland, H., Bradshaw, P., Garvey, E., and Crawford, B.: Shift to older age distribution in Parkinsonism. *Neurology 6*, 783–790 (1956).

Severson, J.A., Marcussen, J., Windblod, B., and Finch, C.E.: Age-related loss of dopaminergic binding sites in human basal ganglia. J. Neurochem. (in press).

Sheldon, J.H.: The effect of age on the control of sway. Gerontol. Clin. *5*, 129–138 (1963).

Sparrow, D., Bosse, R., and Rowe, J.W.: The influence of age, alcohol consumption, and body build on gonadal function in men. J. Clin. Endocrinol. Metab. *51*, 508–512 (1980).

Vermeulen, A., Rubens, R., and Verdonk, L.: Testosterone secretion and metabolism in male senescence. J. Clin. Endocrinol. Metab. *34*, 730–735 (1972).

Weale, R.A.: The Aging Eye. New York: Harper and Row, 1963.

West, C.D., Brown, H., Simons, E.L., Carter, D.B., Kumagai, L.F., and Engelbert, F.L.: Adrenocorticol function and cortisol metabolism in old age. J. Clin. Endocrinol. Metab. *21*, 1197–1207 (1961).

Wyke, B.: Cervical articular contributions to posture and gait: Their relation to senile disequilibrium. Age and Aging *8*, 251–258 (1979).

Chapter 22

Rational and Successful Health Care of Tomorrow's Elderly: An Academic Perspective

Richard W. Besdine

Summary

Inadequate reporting of illness by the elderly, coupled with the passivity of our medical apparatus, make it highly probable that disease will be far advanced before the aged patient gets into the health care system. During the delay between onset and detection, it is possible for multiple pathologies to interact, harming the patient and producing irrevocable disability in spite of eventual excellent care. For some elderly patients, delay is lengthened because of neglect of a number of nonspecific but serious problems, including immobility, incontinence, and cognitive loss, any or all of which may herald major functional decline. These risks, which delay treatment and allow irretrievable losses for elderly sick people, might be avoided by adding an active case-finding surveillance mechanism for the elderly to our current passive health care system.

Illness, Behavior, and Disease in Old Age

As we discuss, plan, and implement health care services for the inexorably aging current and future cohorts of Americans, it is crucial to draw upon any useful existing data identifying unique characteristics of elderly individuals which might suggest alterations of the structure of health care delivery and of the education of health care providers for the elderly.

Demography

The first important area is the demographic imperative, indicating that there has been and will continue to be a sharp increase of older Americans whose health care demands special attention. Like Europe before us, and developing nations in the future, the United States' elderly population is increasing. Many factors have collaborated over the past century to "age" our society. Understanding the graying of America provides the clinician with an important perspective. The longest-living humans live no longer today than they did centuries ago. Maximum human life span (approximately 100 years) has not changed, but average life expectancy has increased dramatically. Previously unimagined numbers of people are surviving into extreme old age, many with the burdens of disease, social disadvantage, emotional vulnerability, and the poverty such burdens create. Average life expectancy in America has increased by more than 25 years during the 20th century, from 47 years in 1900 to 73 years in 1980. For each four months elapsed since 1900, the average American has gained more than 1 month of life. In 1900 fewer than 3 million people were 65 years of age or older, only 4% of the population. Now, in less than a century, the more than 25 million elderly individuals comprise nearly 12% of our population.

Because all individuals who will become 65 years of age and older in the next 50 years have already been born, demographic projections about aging are relatively secure. During this period the elderly population will double, reaching more than 50 million individuals. If during this period the total U.S.A. population grows at the projected 40%, more than 1 in 5 citizens will be over 65 years of age. The "old-old" (over the age of 75) subset of elderly will increase even faster, from 35% of the over-65 population to 45%; and those 85 years of age and older will triple from 2 million to 6 million individuals.

The increase in average life expectancy can be attributed to three distinct phenomena. Usually occurring first chronologically, and most important in developing countries, is improvement in infant survival, which had its major impact in the U.S.A. during the first one-third of this century. Better nutrition and medical care of pregnant women and improved delivery techniques have enhanced the chance for survival of live births. Better sanitation, an improved standard of living, better nutrition, prevention and treatment of infectious diseases, and progress in medical care have all sharply increased the survival rate for children born in the United States. Once these children reach adulthood, they are very likely to survive to old age. If the average life expectancy in a society is 50 years, for each infant who dies in the first year of life, someone lives to be 100 years old. As large numbers of these previously dying infants survive, average life expectancy jumps sharply.

Table 22-1. United States age-specific mortality

	1958–1968	1969–1978
65–74	−10%	−12%
75–84	−8%	−10%
>85	−3%	−25%

The second contribution to longevity in America came with a better environment and improved medical care, especially through the development of antibiotic treatment for infections. For example, death rates from tuberculosis and bacterial pneumonia, major killers of the young, fell dramatically between 1930 and 1950. Thus, cohorts of young adults, enlarged by increased survival of infants, were kept large by the decrease in death rates among young adults themselves.

The most recent contribution to longevity in the United States comes from the aged themselves. In the generation from 1958 to 1978, declines in absolute and relative deaths within the cohorts 65 years of age and older occurred for the first time (Rice, 1981). Deaths per 100,000 population declined dramatically (Table 22-1). These improved survival rates for Americans already old show no suggestion of slowing or stopping, implying that limits have not yet been reached. The cause(s) for this new longevity have not been identified with certainty, but major gains in life expectancy among the old come from reduction of incidence and mortality of heart diseases and stroke, the two major killers of elderly persons. Declines in age-specific coronary and stroke mortality during the period of improved survival appear in Table 22-2 (Walker, 1983).

During the same period, major life style and dietary changes occurred for Americans (Table 22-3), and mass detection and treatment programs for hypertension were implemented.

It is likely that the decline in death rates has some relationship to lifestyle, diet, and treatment of hypertension among Americans, but strict causality cannot be invoked since the individuals who survived had already attained substantial longevity prior to the changes. In addition,

Table 22-2. United States age-specific mortality, 1963–1981

	Coronary Mortality	Stroke Mortality
65–74	−37%	−53%
75–84	−30%	−50%
>85	−26%	−44%

Table 22-3. Per capita United States consumption, 1963–1980

Cigarettes	−27%
Eggs, milk, cream, butter	−23%
Animal fat and oil	−39%
Vegetable fat and oil	+58%
Fish	+23%

Medicare and Medicaid legislation were implemented in 1965–1966, and also appear to have contributed to health improvements for the old.

Whatever the ultimate explanations, greater longevity for Americans resulting from increased survival in all three stages of life is a present reality with major implications for our society and its health care system.

Use of Health Services

Disability, doctor visits, and disease are more prevalent in the elderly and generate increased use of health care services. The prevalence of disease and disability rises sharply with age and is highest in the very segment of the elderly population increasing the most rapidly of all, the old-old. This rapidly growing group of increasingly old and infirm citizens is making demands on the traditional health care delivery system that are qualitatively different from any experienced before. These demands will continue to escalate, and the strain on the health care system will increase disproportionately since the elderly, having more illness, use more services. Although only 11% of the population, Americans over age 65 account for 40% of all acute hospital bed days, use 25% of all prescription drugs purchased, and spend 30% of our $287 billion health budget and more than 50% of the $80 billion federal health expenditure. This disproportionate use of health resources by elderly Americans, though notable, should not be regarded as unfair or unjustified. The escalating disease burden coincident with aging produces the accelerated need for and use of health care. In view of the major use of services by the elderly, any special characteristics exhibited by elder persons, healthy or ill, represent crucial features to be considered in the planning and implementation of present and future services for aged Americans.

Characteristics of Illness and Disease in Old Age

Nonreporting. The first unusual feature exhibited by ill old people is a striking phenomenon partly responsible for the late detection and thus discouraging prognosis and outcome of many diseases in the elderly. Old persons have been repeatedly shown not to report illness to their health care providers. Legitimate symptoms heralding serious but often treatable disease are concealed, or at least not reported by elderly patients. The first suggestion that older persons did not seek medical attention when suffering health-related functional decline came from Scotland. In the 1950s and 1960s, several pioneer geriatricians screened elderly individuals, seeking information about illness behavior, suspecting that verifiable differences might underlie the clinical impressions that old people did not seek medical care promptly when ill (Anderson, 1966; Williamson et al., 1964). The findings in these and subsequent corroborating studies were surprising, even to the investigators. An iceberg of concealed disease was discovered among Scottish elderly enrolled in the British National Health Service, which appeared to have the necessary features to provide adequate service to the elderly: doctors responsible for each older person's outpatient care; free care; and numerous, accessible doctors' offices. Yet startling numbers of problems hitherto unknown to and untreated by the patient's responsible physician were discovered. Nor were the problems esoteric, requiring sophisticated diagnostic methodology. Frequently encountered disorders included congestive heart failure, correctable hearing and vision deficits, tuberculosis, urinary dysfunction, anemia, chronic bronchitis, claudication, cancers, nutritional deficiencies, uncontrolled diabetes, foot disease hampering mobility, dental disease impeding nutrition, dementia, and depression.

Further questioning of subjects and review of primary data led to some clear explanations for this apparently self-destructive illness behavior of elderly Scots. Older people perceive pain, malaise, and disability adequately, but choose to conceal their distress or at least not seek treatment. The most common explanation for symptom tolerance and nonreporting was the pervasive belief that old age is inextricably associated with illness, functional decline, and feeling sick. Old and young, lay and professional, men and women, all believe that to be old is to be ill. Obviously this "ageist" view of health and disease guarantees that older individuals, even when afflicted with the same symptoms that impel the middle-aged sick into the mainstream of the health care system, will not seek care, will suffer in silence the progression of many diseases, and endure the functional losses engendered by untreated illness. That old age in the absence of disease is a time of good health and persisting function has been documented by numerous studies of normal aging (Finch and Hayflick, 1977), but while our society labors in ignorance of gerontologic information, elders will continue expecting decline and dysfunction. A useful geriatric maxim is that sick old people are sick because they are sick, not because they are old. Although decline in numerous physiologic functions characterizes normal human aging, these declines are gradual, and their functional impact is ameliorated by the decades over which they occur and by the remaining, if diminishing, reserve capacities of the individual. Thus, major functional decline, especially if abrupt in an individual already old, is usually attributable to disease, not age.

A second explanation for old people not reporting illness was that the high prevalence of depression, coupled with the many losses common in late life, interfered with the desire to regain vigor. A third block to reporting illness was found to be intellectual loss. Though never normal, the increasing prevalence of cognitive loss with age is doubly dangerous to the detection of disease. Cognitively impaired individuals have a diminished ability to complain and are also evaluated less enthusiastically for associated medical disease or even reversible disease producing the intellectual loss itself (NIA Task Force, 1980). A fourth explanation for symptom concealment by elderly patients was fear that something would be found and generate diagnostic or therapeutic interventions that in themselves would produce functional loss and jeopardize independent living. Finally, today's octogenarians, having grown up when health care systems produced less salubrious interventions, may be reluctant to seek care even in the present. A recent American study confirms and further illuminates the phenomenon of incomplete reporting of disease symptoms by the elderly (Brody and Kleban, 1981). Community-dwelling independent old people were found to conceal one-half of their symptoms, and when they did complain, more than one-half the complaints were voiced to family members or friends rather than health care providers. Sadly, these informants tend to agree with elderly patients that symptoms, once occurring in old age, are inevitable and untreatable.

The abundant documentation that disease is not being reported by the elderly appears to contradict a clinical rule of thumb that identifies hypochondriasis as common among aged patients. Many clinicians caring for elderly patients cite an individual or two who tries their patience and goodwill with endless complaints rooted in trivial or nonexistent illness. Yet when studied, the hypochondriacal, doctor-shopping, old person appears to be one more unverifiable mythical figure in people's ideas about aging (Costa and McCrae, 1980). Not only is hypochondriasis less common among older people, but when elders do complain, important disease is found underlying their complaints substantially more often than in younger, nonhypochondriacal individuals (Stenback, Kumpulainen, and Vauhkonen, 1978).

Multiple pathology. A second characteristic of illness in old age, important in planning geriatric health care and predisposing elderly individuals to functional decline based on late detection of potentially treatable diseases, is the common occurrence of illness clustering in aged patients. Usually called multiple pathology, the existence of several concurrent diseases in an old person who either is not obviously ill or is under treatment for a different problem has a profound negative influence on health and functional independence in old age. A random sample of community-dwelling subjects over 65 years of age found nearly 3.5 important disabilities per person (Williamson et al., 1964). An earlier study of elderly patients being admitted to hospitals documented six pathological conditions per person (Wilson, Lawson, and Brass, 1964). A recent American clinical experience tabulated common problems often coexisting in elderly individuals (Besdine, 1980); these were congestive heart failure, depression, dementia, chronic renal failure, angina pectoris, osteoarthritis/osteoporosis, gait disorders, urinary incontinence, constipation, arterial and venous insufficiency in the legs, diabetes mellitus, chronic pain, sleep disturbance, multiple drug regimens, and anemia.

The number of pathologic conditions in an individual is strongly related to age, often rising to more than a dozen in the very old. If the entire spectrum of multiple pathologic conditions is not identified and carefully considered, virtually any diagnostic or therapeutic initiative is as likely to produce harm as benefit. In the absence of obvious flare-up of one problem, major danger still exists for the patient with multiple pathology. Korenchevsky (1961) first pointed out the destructive, insidious virulence of unattended multiple pathologies in the uncomplaining elderly patient. Undetected, untreated diseases create ricochetting stress in several organ systems or tissues, producing deterioration of a previously diseased but compensated physiologic function. As each overburdened organ fails, there is created "what rapidly becomes an irreversible concatenation of deteriorations, passing multiple points of no return, leading to infirmity, dependence, and, if uninterrupted, death" (Besdine, 1980).

Thus, multiple pathologic conditions exert detrimental influence on elderly individuals in at least two important ways. In the first instance, the diagnostic evaluation or treatment of one identified illness interacts adversely with one or several occult conditions, producing iatrogenic harm. For example, an old man with ankle edema and pulmonary congestion of mild heart failure is given a potent diuretic which rapidly clears a liter of excess fluid from his circulation and improves the identified problem of heart failure. The rippling secondary effects are not beneficial. The abrupt diuresis overwhelms the emptying capacity of his bladder, previously compromised by prostatic enlargement, and produces acute urinary retention. The secondary kidney damage and pain of retention produces acute confusion, worsened by early memory loss of Alzheimer's disease. The diuretic raises already high but previously asymptomatic levels of blood sugar and uric acid due to occult diabetes and gout, respectively. Each of these now becomes symptomatic with impaired consciousness and dehydration of hypersmolar diabetes, and the exquisitely painful foot of gout. The second adverse impact of occult disease interaction can be summarized as disease–disease relationships. An example is the old woman with unreported urinary tract infection producing frequent urgent urination which exceeds the mobility limit of her degenerative osteoarthritis and makes her incontinent. Uncorrected poor vision and urine on the floor cause a fall with a fracture of her osteoporotic hip, and secondary decompensation of heart failure. The retrospective identification of previously unidentified disorders that have led to fixed functional losses in a once-independent elder is a truly depressing but improvable aspect of geriatric medical care.

Disease in old age. The third category of important differences between young and old individuals relevant to planning health care for the elderly is in the behavior of clinical illness itself (Besdine, 1982). Disease in old age has two special features that must be considered in the organization of health services as well as in provision of individual care for the elderly. First, there is a group of disorders, some rare and some common, which usually occur only in aged individuals. These conditions are easily enumerable (Table 22-4), and comprise a straightforward component of geriatric medicine.

The second group of diseases, in addition to being much larger than the first, introduces a complexity with major implications for geriatric care.

Table 22-4. Diseases and disorders usually found only in the elderly

1.	Diabetic hypersmolar nonketotic coma
2.	Stroke
3.	Polymyalgia rheumatica and giant cell arteritis
4.	Metabolic bone disease
5.	Degenerative joint disease
6.	Hip fracture
7.	Dementia syndrome
8.	Falls
9.	Paget's disease
10.	Gammopathies
11.	Chronic lymphatic leukemia
12.	Tuberculosis
13.	Herpes zoster
14.	Basal cell carcinoma
15.	Parkinsonism
16.	Angioimmunoblastic lymphadenopathy with dysproteinemia
17.	Normal pressure hydrocephalus
18.	Pressure sores
19.	Accidental hypothermia
20.	Urinary incontinence
21.	Arteriosclerotic heart disease and its complications
22.	Amyloidosis
23.	Solid tumor, especially prostate, colon, breast, and lung
24.	Carpal tunnel syndrome
25.	Hearing and vision impairment
26.	Colonic angiodysplasia

Table 22-5. Nonspecific or altered presentation of disease in old age

1.	Refusal to eat or drink
2.	Falling
3.	New incontinence
4.	Dizziness
5.	Acute confusion
6.	New onset or abrupt worsening of dementia
7.	Weight loss
8.	Failure to thrive

These are diseases which, though occurring in patients of all ages, behave differently in the elderly. A fundamental principle of geriatric medicine is that virtually any disease with a classic complex of signs or symptoms frequently presents in old age with few or none of the characteristic findings. The classic presentation is often replaced by one or more nonspecific problems, which may be misidentified as due to aging rather than disease (Table 22-5). The appearance of any of these findings in an elderly person heralds the onset or worsening of disease and should never be attributed to old age alone. In addition to altered disease presentation, altered clinical course, unpredicted responses and reaction to treatment, and unexpected outcomes, including recovery, characterize disease in elderly persons. Certain disorders are particularly likely to be obscured in the elderly (Table 22-6) and should be considered in perplexing clinical situations.

The underlying cause for these altered characteristics of common diseases in old age has not been definitely identified, but certain observations are relevant. The interaction of disease with the bio-behavioral alterations produced by normal aging is one factor exerting powerful influence upon the appearance of disease in elderly persons. Additionally, aging appears to reduce physiologic reserve asymmetrically,

Table 22-6. Disorders likely to present nonspecifically in old age

1.	Depression
2.	Drug intoxication
3.	Myxedema
4.	Alcoholism
5.	Myocardial infarction
6.	Pulmonary embolism
7.	Pneumonia
8.	Cancer
9.	Surgical abdomen
10.	Thyrotoxicosis, masked or apathetic

making certain organ systems and tissues most vulnerable to the altered homeostasis produced by disease, regardless of the locus of the disorder. Thus, the phenomenon of "weak-link" systems emerges, and locomotion, cognition, and continence frequently are disrupted in old persons with new or exacerbated disease occurring in any organ system.

Interaction of Illness Behavior with Health Care

As disease progresses undetected and untreated in the elderly, prolonged disability, long and expensive therapeutic interventions, and permanent functional losses become increasingly likely. Delays in diagnosis and treatment are especially pernicious for the elderly patient. Yet continuing delay in initiation of health care is exactly what is to be expected from the interaction of elderly individuals with our health care system. Our health care system is passive, especially for elderly people, and lacks prevention-oriented or early detection efforts. American medical care of the critically ill, elderly hospitalized patient is the best in the world. Science and technology are most expertly blended to help the sick. But American hospital beds, HMOs, physicians' offices, emergency rooms, and neighborhood health centers all wait passively for the symptomatic patient to activate the system. For the most part, this passive system of health care provision is adequate for children, who have parental advocates, and for young and middle-aged adults who have the need to work and earn, impelling them to seek medical relief of function-impairing symptoms. But aged persons, without advocates and usually without jobs, burdened by society's and their own ageist views of functional loss in the elderly, cannot be relied upon to initiate appropriate health care for themselves, especially early in the course of an illness when intervention is most likely to have a favorable outcome. Our health care system relies on the patient to enter the system and initiate care; and that is precisely the one illness behavior most often missing in aged individuals.

References

Anderson, W.F.: The prevention of illness in the elderly: the Rutherglen experiment in medicine in old age. Proceedings of a conference held at the Royal College of Physicians of London. London: Pitman, 1966.

Besdine, R.W.: Geriatric medicine: an overview. *Ann. Rev. Gerontol. Geriatr. 1*, 135 (1980).

Besdine, R.W.: Data base of geriatric medicine. In Rowe, J.W., and Besdine, R.W. (Eds.), *Health and Disease in Old Age*, pp. 1–14. Boston: Little, Brown and Co., 1982.

Brody, E.M., and Kleban, M.H.: Physical and mental health symptoms of older people: who do they tell? *J. Am. Geriat. Soc. 29*, 442–449 (1981).

Costa, P.T., Jr., and McCrae, R.R.: Somatic complaints in males as a function of age and neuroticism: a longitudinal analysis. *J. Behav. Med. 3*, 245 (1980).

Finch, C.E., and Hayflick, L.: *Handbook of the Biology of Aging*. New York: Van Nostrand Reinhold, 1977.

Korenchevsky, V.: *Physiological and Pathological Aging*. New York: Basel/Karger, 1961.

National Institute on Aging Task Force. Senility reconsidered: treatment possibilities for mental impairment in the elderly. *JAMA 244*, 259 (1980).

Rice, D.: Living Longer: Demographic Changes and Health Care. Washington, D.C.: National Center for Health Statistics, Division of Vital Statistics, 1981.

Stenback, A., Kumpulainen, M., and Vauhkonen, M.L.: Illness and health behavior in septaugenarians. *Gerontologist 33*, 57 (1978).

Walker, W.J.: Changing U.S. Lifestyle and declining vascular mortality—a retrospective. *N. Engl. J. Med. 308*, 649–651 (1983).

Williamson, J. et al.: Old people at home: their unreported needs. *Lancet 1*, 1117 (1964).

Wilson, L.A., Lawson, I.R., and Brass, W.: Multiple disorders in the elderly. *Lancet 2*, 841 (1962).

Part VII

Interface of Psychiatry and Medicine

Chapter 23

Psychiatry versus Medicine: Am I My Brother's Keeper?

Harvey L. Ruben

Summary

Who should treat the demented patient? How should psychiatry, medicine, and neurology relate to each other concerning these multiproblemed people? Many psychiatrists believe that only internists or neurologists should manage the brain-diseased individual. But internists and neurologists rarely have the time, the training, or the inclination to get involved with the behavioral, familial, and social problems of these poor sufferers. About one-third of patients in medical and surgical units in general hospitals are over the age of 65, and the prevalence of brain disease in these patients is estimated at from 30 to 50%. Yet many of them are not adequately treated for this problem. Practical and political issues related to who should treat the demented persons determine how to develop a meaningful professional collaboration around the management of these patients.

All of us involved with the elderly know the statistics: The aged in America comprise 11% of our population. They account for 40% of our acute hospital days. Thirty percent of the $160+ billion spent on medical care, and more than 50% of the $40 billion federal health budget accrue to the elderly. They buy 25% of all prescription drugs. Nursing home care cost $10 billion in 1976, $21.6 billion in 1980, and is expected to reach $75 billion in 1990. The 1.4 million nursing home beds in this country exceed the 850,000 acute beds by more than 50%. Of those nursing home beds, 1.1 million are occupied by the elderly. Although only 5% of the elderly are in nursing homes at any one time, 25% will spend some time in a nursing home, and those over the age of 80 are more likely to die in a nursing home than in their own homes. Of those 5% in a nursing home, 60–70% are suffering from some form of dementing illness (Besdine, 1980).

Of those patients seen on consultation liaison services in general hospitals, 30% are over the age of 60. These are medical and surgical patients in whom the prevalence of mental disorders is estimated as between 40 and 50%. In 1980 over 26% (nearly 10 million) of the patients discharged from nonfederal short-term hospitals were elderly, and they accounted for 38% of the total hospital beds used and had an average hospital stay of about 30% longer than those under the age of 65. Delirium is found to occur in 30–50% of all the elderly patients at some point during their acute hospitalizations. Dementia with or without delirium is found in at least 10% of these patients. Affective and anxiety disorders have been found in as many as 30% of these patients (Lipowski, 1983).

So here we have it: A population of elderly people who have a high prevalence of both physical and emotional disorders, who are utilizing health care services and dollars at a much higher rate than any other segment of the population. Next will be discussed what in the crudest terms we behavioral scientists refer to as turf—"Who is going to take control?" This presentation is, in part, a report of the work of the Task Force on the Interface of Psychiatry and Medicine in Geriatrics of the Council on Aging of the American Psychiatric Association. More importantly, however, it is a discussion of the answer to that critical question, "Who's going to take charge?"

The Task Force had its inception in the Spring of 1982. The Board of Trustees of the APA gave the Council on Aging, under the Chairmanship of Dr. Charles M. Gaitz, the go-ahead on setting up this task force. APA President Dr. Keith Brodie appointed Dr. Marshall Folstein, our Chairman, and Dr. Jonathan Lief of Boston, and myself, as committee members to study this area. Our purpose was "to further identify and clarify the knowledge base about clinical relationships and research questions at the interface of psychiatry and medicine in geriatrics." This was obviously a very large task, and as we met over the next year to discuss how to deal with this issue it became clear to us that we had to more narrowly define the scope of our work if we were to produce anything that was meaningful. We commenced by interviewing as many people as we could, psychiatrists, internists, neurologists, and nonphysicians dealing with the elderly in a variety of settings, in order to develop some sense of how various people were viewing this issue. Dr. Folstein had an opportunity to discuss the issue at a World Health Organization meeting with psychiatrists from France, Germany, East Germany, the Soviet Union, Bulgaria, and England. He learned that although psychiatrists in those countries had much greater training in both neurology and medicine than we in America, they, too, had failed to agree about who should take responsibility for the demented patient and how such patients should be cared for. It became clear to us as we narrowed our topic that this was a very pertinent issue. Who should care for the demented patient? How would medicine, neurology, and psychiatry interface in managing these individuals? We realized that we could not treat the cognitive impairment of the demented individual, but we could deal with the functional deficits, with the disturbed behavioral symptoms, and with the families of these patients. And we knew that this was a very important role for psychiatrists. Thus, we decided to use dementia (and particular Alzheimer's disease) as a departure point in the discussion of all the issues related to the interface of medicine and psychiatry in geriatrics.

It is interesting to note that in terms of dealing with dementia, we decided that Alzheimer's disease would be a main area of interest in our study with the hope that we would be able to offer some reasonable recommendations for training psychiatrists, physicians, and other health professionals in dealing with these multiproblemed patients. Some 6 months later we were quite pleased to learn that the new Secretary of Health and Human Services, Margaret Heckler, had declared a federal offensive on Alzheimer's disease because this increased the public relevancy of the work we as a task force were doing.

In order to gather additional information so that we could better focus our endeavors, we continued to survey various groups of health professionals, including psychiatrists, neurologists, internists, psychologists, nurses, and administrators. It became alarmingly clear to us on the task force that the general consensus was that psychiatrists at best had a limited role in the management of demented patients. Since demented patients usually had multiple medical problems, at the very least it was believed that they needed to be managed by internists. Since they often might have some more esoteric neurologic illness such as a supranuclear palsy or a brain tumor, a neurologist was needed, especially to interpret the CAT scan, the EEG, and other neurologic procedures. Neuropsychologists were necessary to help evaluate the patient in order to determine their functional strengths and weaknesses. Many internists believed that their colleagues who were dealing with the elderly should have requisite knowledge of psychopharmacology and "counseling" to be able to manage agitation, depression, and the other emotional problems of the demented patients.

In the case of the patients who had no current need for active medical intervention but who remained disoriented, demented, and possibly with other psychiatric symptoms, the typical internist saw these patients as being "nonmedical" and relegated them to the care of psychiatrists (if they were available) or social workers and nurses. Even most general psychiatrists surveyed seem to believe that there is no role for the psychiatrist in the management of the demented patient, but rather that these were medical and neurological issues. This obviously was a very sensitive area which evoked a great deal of emotion. When asked why there was no role for the psychiatrist in these areas, these individuals seemed to believe that there was no issue of psychotherapy for these patients and that, in addition, they had not been trained to deal with the management of these patients or their families.

Thus it became very clear to us that if our task force was going to have any impact whatsoever, we would have to educate both our own colleagues and members of our allied health professions about the potential role of the psychiatrist in the management of the demented individual. In an attempt to do this we developed a questionnaire for both psychiatrists and internists (see Appendix) which served both to assess their attitudes, but also to sensitize them to the fact that a psychiatrist might be involved in dealing with demented patients. This questionnaire was recently included in the registration packet of all attendees at the 1983 APA Fall Committee Meetings in Washington, and we are currently collating the results. We chose to focus our attention on dementia, because it has become one of the most pressing psychiatric problems in the current decade and its promises to become even more pressing with the continued aging of our population as we move into the next century. Thus once we have worked out the interface issues in this area, it should become much more simple to collaborate in other areas.

We continue to grapple with the issue of what kind of psychiatrist could best deal with the demented individual. Our deliberations have ranged from thinking that it might be appropriate to develop a subspecialty within geriatric psychiatry to deal with the demented patient (what Dr. Marshal Folstein referred to as the geriatric dementia doctors or the GERDEMDOCS). Perhaps it would be more appropriate to train all general psychiatrists in the management of demented patients, so that they would be comfortable dealing with patients in a hospital, a nursing home, or a home care setting. Currently, our task force agrees that there should be two levels of training for psychiatrists to prepare them for dealing with these patients. On the one hand, there should be intensive training during geriatric psychiatric fellowships in order to enable the geriatric psychiatrist to have special expertise in this area. In addition, all general psychiatric residencies should include a reasonable amount of exposure to these patients so that the average psychiatrist can feel comfortable in handling such individuals in his or her practice should the need arise.

The geriatric psychiatrist should have perhaps a PGY-4 and PGY-5 year which is specifically aimed at giving him or her an intensive experience in dealing with the psychiatric, psychopharmacologic, neurological, and medical issues of managing these patients. Such a physician could be the primary physician for the demented patient either in the home, the nursing home, or the hospital. These psychiatrists would also be able to manage the family and relate to the support system of the patient in order to develop a total treatment plan. They would have to be well versed in community resources such as day care programs, Meals-on-Wheels, visiting nurses, and so forth. An important and timely consideration is the fact that such a psychiatrist would have little difficulty making a reasonable living anywhere in this country in these increasingly difficult economic times.

Considering the training of general psychiatrists, we believe that the general psychiatric resident should spend some time dealing with demented patients and their families in a skilled nursing facility, on the consultation liaison service of a general hospital, and in the outpatient department. This would make the average psychiatrist conversant with these issues and more comfortable in managing these patients in both an inpatient and outpatient facility.

Another set of recommendations of the task force deals with an approach that we believe should be taken by the American Psychiatric Association. The President should make a statement to the effect that dementia is a serious psychiatric problem and requires the attention of all psychiatrists. Questions about the management of the demented patient should be included in the examinations of the American Board of Psychiatry and Neurology. All APA journals should publish articles dealing with research and clinical issues relating to dementia. Our annual meeting should have a reasonable number of sessions dealing with geropsychiatry scheduled so that interested psychiatrists could attend all of them if they wished. The APA should establish relationships with other professional societies, organizations, and agencies dealing with aging and the aged in an attempt to help resolve some of the turf issues that have arisen. The APA and the American Medical Association should establish a joint task force to develop guidelines for managing demented patients with special emphasis on the use of medications and restraints in inpatient and skilled nursing facilities. The constitution and bylaws of the APA should be revised to include the management of the demented patient in the list of the kinds of patients and problems that are treated by psychiatrists. Finally, the APA should make recommendations to the directors of residency training programs about including the material we have been discussing in the general residency curriculum as a way to further these ends.

So far we have been discussing an approach to defining and enhancing the interface of psychiatry and medicine in geriatrics which has been pursued by our task force. This may sound like a rather academic discussion to you, and, of course, it must be. However, there are other very real issues relating to this interface that we should consider before I conclude. At the beginning of my discussion I mentioned the issue of turf—"Who's in charge?" A very real factor which motivates turf discussions happens to be our own economic self-interests. To the extent that we are motivated by financial gain (which we all are to varying degrees) this further confounds the interface and is, of course, at the core of the turf issue. As a friend of mine who is an excellent internist said to me a few weeks ago at a staff meeting in a skilled nursing facility, "Why should I bring in a psychiatric consultant to see my patient (who is agitated and who is on psychotropic medications) when the state will only pay me to see the patient once a month and when Medicare will pay you to see the patient once a week?" Of course, my friend was incorrect. Medicare will pay you and me a maximum of \$312.50 a year for all the visits we make to patients in skilled nursing facilities. So although we can go once, twice, or three times a week (as often as we wish and as often as is medically indicated), the patient who has this level of need will use up his or her Medicare psychiatric benefit in a very short period of time so that most of our visits will be pro bono. What I could not say to my friend, for had I, I would surely have done irreparable harm to our "personal interface" was that I, of course, am better prepared to manage the agitation and psychotropics that he is. Rather, I suggested to him that whenever the patient's behavior became a problem for the nurses or other patients, I would be happy to see the patient and take over the psychotropic drug management.

The obvious critical issue in terms of interface is the monetary issue. The answer to the question, "Who is going to manage the demented patient?," is, in one sense, simply the one who is going to make the money. Unfortunately, there is currently not much money available to manage these patients, and an important part of our interface with the medical, neurological, and other involved health professionals is forming an effective alliance so that we can adequately present to the federal and state governments the need for more money being directed for the care of these individuals. Secretary Heckler's assault on Alzheimer's disease is a very excellent beginning, but is aimed mainly at research and demonstration projects. A much more appropriate and immediate step in the United States is to influence the federal government (the Social Security Administration) to liberalize Medicare benefits for the management of all the emotional problems of the elderly, in addition to the management of demented individuals who, as we have seen, constitute the largest segment of the emotionally disturbed elderly. Once we are successful in doing this, I think we will be surprised to find out how much easier it will be to motivate residency training directors and chairpersons of the departments of psychiatry to get involved in this area. As a cynic, I must say that where the dollars are is where the attention flows, and the more money we can bring into this area the more likely we are going to get the attention of our colleagues.

The need for psychiatrists to be involved in the management of demented patients is obvious. In my own professional life, for 6 years I have been involved with the elderly as a psychiatric consultant in nursing homes, as the treating psychiatrist on inpatient units, and as the consulting psychiatrist on the consultation liaison service. It is astonishing to me how often our medical brethren mismanage problems of the demented patients. Agitated elderly come from teaching wards of major hospitals loaded up with Valium; depressed, dying elderly patients are refused antidepressant therapy by their internists who say that, of course, they should be depressed; patients being treated with a potpourri of psychotropics on inpatient services which cause them to become acutely delirious. I firmly believe that when more money is available to treat these patients, they will become more interesting—to internists, to neurologists, to psychiatrists, to any physician who has to make a living while practicing medicine.

Thus the work of our task force and of the Council on Aging of the American Psychiatric Association, and all of us in the health professions, is to help sensitize our legislators, our patients, their families, and the public at large to the importance of adequate insurance coverage and adequate expenditure of federal research, programmatic, and training funds to ensure that well-trained, knowledgable health care professionals of every discipline are appropriately involved in managing the demented elderly. Psychiatry vs. medicine: Am I my brother's keeper? I hope not. I hope rather that I am only one of his first colleagues to recognize the importance of our collaboration in these important areas so that we can further the physical and emotional health of all our patients and their families.

Appendix: APA Questionnaire for Psychiatrists and Internists

Purpose: To survey attitude and practice of internists and psychiatrists concerning demented patients.

1.	In the past month did you evaluate or manage a demented patient?	NO	YES
2.	Is your training adequate to care for a demented patient?	NO	YES
3.	Do you want more knowledge regarding the care of demented patients?	NO	YES
4.	Do you care for any patients in nursing homes?	NO	YES
5.	Are psychiatrists needed in nursing homes?	NO	YES
6.	Is there anything a psychiatrist can do for a demented patient?	NO	YES
7.	Is the care of demented patients an appropriate task for a psychiatrist?	NO	YES
8.	Would you consult with a specialist in geriatric medicine concerning a demented patient?	NO	YES

9. Estimate the percentage of your time spent in any of the following:

   Private Office ______
   Hospital ______
   University ______
   Nursing Home ______
   Other (Specify) ______

10. Please tell us about yourself:

    Age: ______
    Sex: ______
    Speciality: __________
    Board Certified: __________

11. Comments: ____

____

____

References

Besdine, R.: Geriatric medicine: An overview. *Ann. Rev. Gerontol. Geriatr. 1*, 135–153 (1980).

Lipowski, Z.J.: The need to integrate liaison psychiatry and geropsychiatry. *Am. J. Psychiatry 140*, 1003–1005 (1983).

Chapter 24

Toward an Interface of Mental and Physical Health Phenomena in Geriatrics: Clinical Findings and Questions

Gene Cohen

Summary

The admonition to attend to the "whole" person is part of the preamble of many discussions on geriatrics. This attention, it is pointed out, requires an understanding of the interaction of biological with psychosocial factors as they affect health, illness, and overall functioning in the older patient. The discussion that follows examines such interactions from a particular vantage point by looking at examples within various systems of the body, including the cardiovascular, pulmonary, gastrointestinal, endocrine, immune, and central nervous systems. Within this framework several paradigms will be considered: psychiatric factors that precipitate physical health problems; physical health problems with psychiatric consequences; and the effect of concurrent mental and physical health problems on one another. In the process, clinical relationships and research questions will be identified.

While the admonition to attend the "whole" person in geriatrics has been widely disseminated, translations of this counsel into clinical practice and clinical research have been less well delineated. In the discussion that follows, this area will be looked at from a particular vantage point.

Specifically, an attempt will be made to examine areas where clinical relationships and issues can be identified at the interface of mental and physical health phemonena in the care and study of aging patients. This vantage point can be expanded by looking at a range of related paradigms, illustrated as follows:

1. Psychiatric factors that precipitate physical health problems, e.g., depression → poor nutrition and/or dehydration
2. Physical health problems with psychiatric sequelae, e.g., hearing loss → delusions
3. Psychosocial factors influencing the course of a medical disorder, e.g., living alone → nursing home placement for stroke patient
4. Concurrent mental and physical health problems influencing the course of one another, e.g., paranoid state + congestive heart failure (CHF) → paranoia about medicines, being poisoned, interring with proper management of CHF
5. Mental or physical health problems as a consequence of pharmacologic treatment, e.g., (a) reserpine in treatment of hypertension → depression; (b) amitriptyline in treatment of depression → glaucoma

The above paradigms are not meant to be comprehensive, but representative of various major "interface" considerations that emerge. Moreover, the information that follows should not be seen as reflecting a complete picture of the growing body of knowledge in the field of geriatrics, where the terrains of psychiatry and internal medicine come closer together. Instead, this information is presented as a more extensive illustration of the large number of clinical relationships and research questions that can be recognized or can come to mind when one focuses in more closely on any of the systems of the body. In this context, the following material will ideally spark new curiosity in clinicians and researchers alike to look for interacting mental and physical health factors in treatments or investigation relevant to older individuals.

The material is grouped in two ways. First, two systems of the body—the pulmonary and cardiovascular systems—are examined from several perspectives in identifying specific relationships that reflect the interface of physical and psychosocial factors affecting health in the elderly. Given the number of medical problems of a cardiopulmonary nature that older people experience, these particular systems were seen as a useful starting point.

Second, a more general discussion then follows where one can appreciate how this same type of search for interfacing physical and psychosocial phenomena can be carried out in any and all of the remaining systems of the body, whether endocrinologic, gastrointestinal, musculoskeletal, etc.

The Pulmonary/Respiratory System

Opportunities for prevention in medicine are increasingly being sought, particularly for primary prevention, where the onset of a given disease can be prevented. Understanding the potential effect of certain psychiatric risk factors on normal physiologic mechanisms of defense along the aging respiratory tract can likely help the clinician lower the incidence of serious pulmonary disease in the older population. The elderly are, for example, at greater and more serious risk for developing lower respiratory tract infections like pneumonia (Freeman, 1978). Hence, it is desirable to identify factors that could make older persons more susceptible to such infections in any effort to reduce susceptibility in general. The psychiatric arena, however, is less often considered in the search for risk factors, though it may represent one of the greater sources. Consider the following potential and not unusual scenario that can occur with a specific group of older patients.

A number of older people who become depressed (depression is more frequent with the elderly than with any other age group; Gurland, 1976) may turn to alcohol (Simon, 1980). Excess alcohol use in the elderly may then interfere with the normal respiratory tract mechanisms of defense against infection in at least four ways, apart from the central effect on the respiratory center in the brain stem.

1. The cough reflex, already somewhat altered in old age, may then be further impaired by alcohol, thereby reducing the elimination of infected material along the nasopharynx (Berkowitz et al., 1973).
2. Dehydration associated with alcohol excess could lead to reduced amounts of mucus along the respiratory tract which would otherwise play a greater role in capturing inhaled particles for removal via coughing or swallowing.
3. With aging it appears that alcohol has a greater effect on retarding cilia movement along the respiratory tree where these cilia facilitate the upward and outward expulsion of infected or irritating particles.
4. Along the respiratory tract can be found macrophages which kill bacteria. How these macrophages are affected with aging is not entirely clear, but it is known that alcohol abuse has a toxic effect on macrophages causing loss of bactericidal capacity—no doubt worse in the older person, who has greater sensitivity to alcohol (Freeman, 1978).

Thus, by intefering with the cough reflex, mucus level, ciliary movement, and macrophage activity, alcohol excess can place the older person at greater risk for pulmonary infection. This creates a further responsibility on the part of the clinician to be more concerned about depression and/or alcohol abuse in the elderly, especially in those older persons who already have a chronic pulmonary disease or a history of frequent or recurrent respiratory tract infections.

Chronic Obstructive Pulmonary Disease

An interesting example of the incorporation of psychodynamic considerations into medical treatment can be seen in the range of interventions for chronic obstructive pulmonary disease (COPD) associated with severe emphysema and/or bronchitis. Elderly patients in particular with severe COPD may develop anxiety and depression secondary to both their disability and a sense that they no longer have control over their bodies. This latter feeling of loss of control can be quite discouraging, with a risk of the patient "giving up." The treatment plan should, therefore, provide an opportunity for the patient to feel that he or she can still take some control over what will happen. Exercise is an approach that simultaneously offers a sense of control as well as a specific medical intervention.

When people become breathless with exertion, they tend to avoid exercise. However, this results in a further loss of fitness which may itself contribute to subsequent exertional dyspnea. Some improvement in breathing might actually result with careful and graduated exercise. The impact of exercise is probably on the muscles of the chest and abdomen that facilitate smoother breathing, rather than on the lungs. When this is explained to the patient, he has an incentive to gradually initiate exercises (Woolf and Svero, 1969). At the same time exercise provides a concrete opportunity for the patient to take action, to participate actively in the treatment program. It can provide an activity, a diversion, a hope, and, ideally, a sense of satisfaction and improvement.

Psychiatric Symptoms as Signals of Underlying Pulmonary Problems in Older Patients

To see changes in memory function or concentration as a corollary of aging results in missing many early signals of treatable disorders in the elderly. Difficulty concentrating, like abdominal pain, can be associated with numerous underlying causes. One such cause of this cognitive dysfunction in the elderly is a subclinical pneumonia. Older people are more at risk for developing pneumonia following a respiratory tract infection, and the manifestations of the disease may be more varied with them (Reichel, 1978). For example, some elderly individuals may not develop a fever as soon a younger adults with the disease. Laboratory studies may also be misleading, with the white blood cell count potentially not elevated to suspicious levels. Moreover, the pneumonia may begin to set in after an upper respiratory tract infection seems to have resolved; in other cases, there is no suggestion at all of a respiratory tract disturbance. With a subclinical pneumonia, an older patient may experience a subtle interference of adequate oxygenation of blood due to impaired lung function. Inadequately oxygenated blood supply to the brain can then lead to trouble in intellectual functioning. The patient with congestive heart failure with an incipient pneumonia is even more at risk for this to occur since there is also difficulty in efficient pumping of the blood. The point again is that given the frequency of lower respiratory tract infections in the elderly, the list of differential diagnoses for altered cognitive functioning should include pulmonary, and particularly cardiopulmonary, disorders.

Moving from pneumonia to a far less common problem, the role of psychiatric symptomatology signaling an underlying pulmonary problem, is again dramatically illustrated in the case of the "sleep apnea syndrome" (Manson, 1978; Guilleminault et al., 1977). Symptoms include deterioration of intellectual facility, daytime somnolence, personality changes, morning headache, and impotence. An important nighttime clue is the acute onset of loud snoring. Rather than an organic brain syndrome of unknown etiology, which would often be considered in the older patient, the cause is attributed to upper airway obstruction, due to largyngeal dysfunction, leading to apneic periods and hypoxia. What causes the laryngeal problem is not understood, and no structural abnormality is apparent. Several severe cases have been treated surgically by creating a permanent tracheostomy resulting in complete disappearance of symptoms. More recently, a growing number of reports in the literature have implicated hypnotics as another precipitating factor in sleep apnea (Kripke et al., 1982).

Psychiatric Symptoms Associated with Drug Treatment of Pulmonary Infections and Tuberculosis

Toxic psychosis related to parenteral use of penicillin was first described in the literature in 1948 (Johnson, 1979; Kline & Highsmith, 1948). The psychosis can be associated with an allergic reaction, though it need not be. It has been pointed out that if a psychotic reaction should occur, drug treatment generally is not necessary, since most patients have a rapid recovery. In some cases, however, brief phenothiazine administration may be indicated.

Isoniazid, a first-line antituberculosis drug, has been associated with insidious impairment of memory and concentration as well as with acute delirium—all of which may be related to pyridoxine deficiency that can accompany isoniazid use. This risk should especially be kept in mind with the elderly, and attention paid to appropriate prophylaxis and treatment (e.g., pyridoxine supplements).

A number of the less frequently used drugs in the treatment of tuberculosis can have side effects related to mental status. Cycloserine, for example, can have toxic manifestations ranging from nervousness, irritability, and somnolence, to psychosis. As in the case of isoniazid, the problems may be due to an accompanying pyridoxine deficiency.

Ethionamide, another infrequently used antituberculous drug, can induce depression, while use of the agent rifampin can be followed by fatigue and ataxia. An important drug–drug interaction had also been reported with Rifampin treatment of TB in methadone addicts, with the antituberculous medication being found to aggravate methadone withdrawal symptoms (Manson, 1978).

The Cardiovascular System

Cardiac Disease and Neurotic Disorders in Old Age

The relationship of a person's overall physical health to his or her mental health is always an intriguing issue, even more so in later life. With the high degree of morbidity and mortality associated with diseases of the heart and blood vessels in the elderly, clinical relationships and research questions relevant to the cardiovascular system are especially important. For example, a highly significant association of cardiac disorder with late-onset neurotic reactions was shown in a random community sample (Bergmann, 1971, 1978). Also, it has been suggested in this regard that autonomic overactivity, in conjunction with basic atherosclerotic pathology, may have a deleterious effect on the long-term prognosis of cerebrovascular and ischemic heart disease (Bull, 1969). Moreover, the role of stress in accelerating the atherosclerotic process has long been suspected and continues to be an area of research interest (Moylan and Flye, 1978). There is also some evidence suggesting that regardless of diagnostic category, acutely ill older people with reactive affective disorders require more time to recover from physical health problems than patients not suffering from reactive mental disorders (Bergmann and Eastham, 1974); the investigators in that study suggest that it might be fruitful to examine the possibility of recognition and treatment of neurotic and emotional upset in the acutely ill elderly, and to test the hypothesis that psychiatric treatment speeds up recovery and reduces mortality in nondemented older persons.

Psychiatric Symptoms Associated with Drug Treatment of Cardiovascular Problems in the Elderly

Antihypertensive agents. Given the high prevalence of hypertension in the elderly and the higher vulnerability to adverse drug reactions in general with older people, antihypertensive agents demand particular attention.

With the development of psychiatric symptoms by those taking these drugs, the matter of differential diagnosis arises. The clinician must decide whether or not the symptoms are caused by the drugs, or if they are coincidental, representing the concurrent emergence of independent mental disorder. Treatment ramifications are apparent.

Diuretics remain the most frequently used medication for older patients with high blood pressure. It is reported that as many as 40% of patients taking diuretics will complain of fatigue (Hammond and Kirkendall, 1979; Bullpitt and Dollery, 1973). Fatigue is, of course, a major symptom of depression which, like hypertension, is very common in the elderly. Hence, despite the frequency of fatigue as a side effect of diuretic use in the elderly, its presence should also push the clinician to rule out depression.

Diuretics can induce hyponatremia, which has been reported to produce clinical depression, the likelihood being greater when reserpine is administered along with the diuretic (Lewis, 1971). The effect of diuretics on sodium levels demands even more careful attention with the patient being considered for lithium treatment for major mood disorders, since lithium also is associated with lowering the sodium level. Thus, administering lithium in combination with a diuretic that lowers sodium can lead to a drug–drug interaction causing renal dysfunction from marked hyponatremia, or such a combination could adversely affect lithium treatment of depression in the elderly (Lutz, 1975).

Thiazide diuretics can have hypercalcemia as a side effect (Duarte et al., 1971). An increase of serum calcium may be associated with a diversity of symptoms, including anorexia, constipation, and lethargy, which may raise the suspicion of depression. Moreover, elevated calcium levels may be associated with depression itself.

Apironolactone, triamterene, and other diuretics lead to potassium retention. If potassium levels rise too high, various medical problems can occur, including insidious confusion which could be misinterpreted as senility (Goodman and Gillman, 1975).

When prescribing diuretics, another interaction is the potential for orthostatic hypotension, resulting in falls and possibly fractures when phenothiazines or tricyclic antidepressants are being used to treat psychiatric disorders in older persons. This is due to the fact that the volume depletion induced by diuretics, in combination with orthostatic hypotension associated with various psychotropic medications, can lead to a more pronounced lowering of blood pressure, especially upon rising from a sitting or reclining position.

Apart from diuretics, there is a range of other drugs used for treating hypertension that can produce psychiatric side effects, affect psychiatric treatment, or lead to adverse drug–drug interactions when used in conjunction with certain psychotropic medications in the elderly.

Reserpine is used less frequently than before to treat hypertension.

Nonetheless, there is a significant association of depression with its use (6% to 20%, depending on the study) with insidious onset even at relatively low dosages (0.25 mg/day) (Goodwin et al., 1972; Cole and Davis, 1975). Furthermore, the onset of depression may be delayed for more than a year; in such cases, the clinician may be hesitant to implicate the drug as the cause of the mood disorder. Other symptoms that might signal the development of depression with reserpine are nightmares and trouble concentrating. If reserpine is stopped, the depression goes away, but may return if the drug is resumed. The increased risk of depression with this drug when sodium-depleting diuretics are used was alluded to above.

Methyldopa is one of the more commonly used antihypertensive agents with depression reported in as many as 10% of patients (Hammond and Kirkendall, 1979). Drowsiness, sedation, impotence, and difficulty with ejaculation are other problems that may be reported that might raise questions of an emotional or psychosomatic nature (Hammond and Kirkendall, 1979). Concentration or memory problems may appear insidiously in some patients, with studies showing prolonged reaction time to stimuli among subjects taking methyldopa.

Some important drug–drug interactions reported with methyldopa include the following: Serum lithium levels have been reported raised when methyldopa was also being taken, thus having ramifications for the treatment of manic depressive disorders in older patients who are also being treated for high blood pressure (Byrd, 1975). There are cases where it appears that the effectiveness of methyldopa is reduced with the concurrent use of tricyclic antidepressants (Tester-Dalderup, 1977). Meanwhile, the use of monoamine oxidase (MAO) inhibitors for depression concurrently with methyldopa may cause a rise in blood pressure (Van Rossum and Hurkmans, 1963). In another report, the combination of methyldopa with haloperidol was described as causing acute dementia in two patients (Bergmann and Eastham, 1974).

It also has been said that the antihypertensive effect of guanethidine is blocked by phenothiazines and tricyclic antidepressants. Such combinations could precipitate a hypertensive crisis in those being treated for high blood pressure with guanethidine.

Drugs used in the treatment of cardiac dysfunction in the elderly. Propranolol is one of the drugs frequently prescribed in the treatment of certain cardiac arrhythmias. Patients on high doses of propranolol for long periods of time may be at risk for depression (Waal, 1967). Other CNS effects are infrequent, but should still be mentioned. These include nightmares, trouble sleeping, dizziness, confusion, illusions, visual hallucinations, and paranoid symptoms (Fleminger, 1978; Fraser and Carr, 1976; Holland and Kaplan, 1976).

The digitalis glycosides used in the treatment of congestive heart failure and cardiac arrhythmia are among the most frequently prescribed drugs for the elderly. "Of all the drugs in the pharmacopoeia the digitalis glycosides have amongst the narrowist therapeutic ratios (ratio of optimal to toxic dose) of any drug (Doherty et al., 1979). Neuropsychiatric symptoms include headache, visual disturbances, delirium, paranoid symptoms, aphasia, confusion, and hallucinations (Doherty et al., 1979).

Cardiac disease, drug treatment and concurrent depression in the elderly. While it is generally appreciated how prevalent depression is in the elderly, it is less well recognized how frequent atypical manifestations of depression are presented in later life (Cohen, 1977). In such cases, the clinician may overlook clues that point to an incipient mood disorder as the underlying problem. For example, the older patient with congestive heart failure who appears to be deteriorating may not in fact be having an exacerbation of the cardiac disease. Rather, the decline may reflect a covert feeling of having given up, acted out by taking less medicine or even stopping it. Instead of a compliance issue, one could be looking at indirect suicidal maneuvering with a masked depression. Hence, a change in physical status or level of functioning demands a differential diagnostic approach that takes into consideration psychodynamic issues as well.

General Discussion

The Gastrointestinal System

An important clinical question with the older person presenting with gastrointestinal (GI) complaints is whether the distress is physical or functional (due to psychological factors). Biases vary greatly in this area, with some clinicians viewing the elderly as experiencing a very high degree of hypochondriacal GI symptoms, whereas others feel that the frequency of organic causes of GI problems is quite significant. In an attempt to add clarity to this question an interesting study was conducted where 300 patients over age 65 who presented with GI complaints at the outpatient department of a medical center were studied comprehensively for at least a year following their initial visit (Sklar, 1978). Findings are listed below:

10% had gastrointestinal malignancy.

8% had gall bladder disease.

6% had duodenal ulcer.

3% had gastric ulcer.

3% had diverticulosis of the colon.

14% had a wide variety of problems with an organic basis.

56% had functional gastrointestinal distress, with no anatomical changes to account for them. This category included problems like irritable colon, spastic colitis, gastritis, heart burn, nausea, diarrhea, constipation, and other psychophysiologic problems.

The findings, in short, are significant in both directions, functional as well as organic, with around 50% in each group. The obvious conclusion is that the burden on the practitioner—internist or psychiatrist—in evaluating a patient with GI problems is to conduct a comprehensive differential diagnostic workup, since both groups have a high prevalence rate in the elderly. Moreover, there is always the possibility that functional and organic GI problems can coexist.

The Endocrine System

Hypoglycemia and diabetes. Several points can be made about hypoglycemia that reflect interfacing medical and psychiatric concerns. Hypoglycemia can, for example, produce symptoms that resemble those of anxiety or depression (Martis and Rose, 1965). It is also possible to have hypoglycemia only at night, and in such cases the patient might complain of nightmares or headache on awakening, symptoms which again might suggest psychic distress rather than a metabolic problem or too much insulin in the case of the diabetic who becomes hypoglycemic while sleeping.

Looking further at diabetes in the elderly, very different explanations can be drawn upon for similar clinical manifestations. The patient who looks melancholic might indeed have a depression in reaction to his or her diabetes. On the other hand, chronic mild hypoglycemia (such as from overmedication with insulin as alluded to above) may make the patient look lethargic or dispirited and, therefore, give the impression of being depressed. If the hypoglycemia is not recognized and the patient is instead misdiagnosed as having a depression, he might be treated with tricyclic antidepressants which can actually aggravate the underlying hypoglycemic state.

The thyroid. While it is increasingly understood that hypothyroidism in the elderly can present with a clinical picture that mimics depression, it is far less recognized that a state called paradoxical or apathetic hyperthyroidism can occur in older patients and also mimic depression (Davis, 1978). Meanwhile, the patient being treated for depression with lithium could develop hypothyroidism as a side effect of the drug; this hypothyroid condition could then resemble depression which might lead the clinician to increase the lithium level, thinking that the depression is being undertreated, and in the process make the patient more hypothyroid.

Gonadotropins. An interesting research question is raised by the following relationship that could be perceived as either an important correlation, or as simply a coincidence. The relationship pertains to the frequency of depression among women in later life and the levels of FSH (follicular stimulating hormone) and LH (lutenizing hormone) released by the pituitary after menopause. Epidemiologic studies suggest that the frequency of depression among women rises in later life until about the age of 70, when it appears that a slight drop begins to be noticed (Gurland, 1976). At the same time, FSH and LH levels rise after menopause until around age 70, when they begin to fall somewhat (Brown, 1978). Is this correlation potentially significant in suggesting a relationship between gonadotropin levels and depression among women in later life, or is it basically happenstance that both changes described above occur around age 70 in older females? If there were a relationship between the two, it might also explain why some women who are depressed at the time of menopause respond to estrogen treatment, while others do not. The explanation along these lines might point out that differential responses could be related to the timing of estrogen administration, since earlier use would suppress the elevation of FSH and LH, whereas a delay would substantially increase the amount of estrogen required for feedback suppression (McPherson et al., 1975). Again, the significance of this relationship remains a research question.

Metabolism and nutrition. Questions commonly arise about the role of adequate nutrition in relation to a sound mind and mental health in later life. While much research remains to be done in this area, the more apparent areas for intervention involve preventing deficiency states. Classic examples here include the situation of the elderly alcoholic who has been neglecting a proper diet and becomes at greater risk of developing a thiamine deficiency, and therefore Korsakoff's psychosis characterized by short-term memory deficits and confabulation. Vitamin B_{12} deficiency can occur, though much less frequently than popular opinion assumes; mental changes found include apathy, irritability, moodiness, depression, and, less commonly, paranoid features, delusions, hallucinations, confusion, and dementia. Pyridoxine (vitamin B_6) deficiency with associated neuropsychiatric symptoms was discussed earlier as a possible side effect of isoniazid treatment of tuberculosis. The uncommon neurological disorder called Marchiafava-Bignami disease associated with chronic alcoholism and possibly nutritional factors (this remains a research question) manifests signs of dementia, aphasia, and apraxia which can resemble those of Alzheimer's disease, once more pointing out the need for rigorous differential diagnosis (Dale, 1980).

From a different perspective, some interesting points and questions can be raised about vitamin D needs and metabolism in later life. Ordinarily, vitamin D deficiency is quite unusual, especially in the United States where supplements of the vitamin are in so many foods. However, vitamin D is metabolized in the liver by enzymes whose rate of action can be increased by a variety of drugs commonly taken individually or in combinations by the elderly. Such drugs used for psychotropic purposes include barbiturates, chlordiazepoxide, meprobamate, imipramine, chlorpromazine, haloperidol, chloral hydrate, and glutethimide, among others (Thompson, 1979). Hence, if a drug speeds up the metabolism of vitamin D, then the minimal need for the vitamin increases. With chronic barbiturate use, for example, the daily requirement of vitamin D may increase tenfold. Moreover, vitamin D is the "sunshine vitamin," where exposure to sunlight is necessary for proper metabolism—a factor that becomes more critical with older persons who may have less exposure to sunshine. The risk for vitamin D deficiency increases further with depressed older persons who by becoming withdrawn may not obtain adequate nutritional intake (taking in less of the vitamin), stay more indoors (away from sunlight), and perhaps by consuming excess alcohol (another liver enzyme inducer).

All of these concerns about vitamin D in the elderly take on larger importance because of the considerably greater risks of musculoskeletal aches and pains and fractures in general with older people—risks that are increased with vitamin D deficiency due to this vitamin's critical role in bone and skeletal integrity (Barzel, 1978). Clearly, much more research in this area would be beneficial both in further clarifying the risk factors and in quantifying them.

Nutritional questions also arise around Alzheimer's disease. Though no etiologic relationship has been found in terms of poor nutrition leading to Alzheimer's disease, the use of the food substance lecithin has been tried, for treatment purposes, alone and in combination with physostigmine. Its therapeutic benefit, however, has not been clearly demonstrated (Funkenstein et al., 1981; Thal et al., 1983).

Immune System. One of the potentially most dramatic new research frontiers in geriatrics deals with the impact of psychiatric disorder and stress on the immune system's role in maintaining physical health. Given the generally more delicate balance between systems of the body along with lesser organ reserve in the aging organism, the matter of immunologic activity and autoimmunity in later life are eliciting growing interest and concern.

Although no mechanism of action has been clearly delineated, it is nontheless known that emotional stress can influence the function of the immune system. A parallelism, for example, has been shown between the intensity and duration of behavioral disturbances and a fall in circulating antibody titers (Stein et al., 1976). Examples of stress and psychiatric disturbance altering the course of, and vulnerability to, a wide variety of diseases are abundant (Stein et al., 1980). In this regard, emotional factors have been implicated in severe peridontal disease (gingivitis) (Moulton et al., 1952), which becomes of greater concern in later life; studies have described psychological variables influencing the rate of recovery from influenza (Imboden et al., 1961); in cancer research it has been reported that both cell-mediated and humoral immune responses may play a part in the cause and course of certain neoplasms (Stutman, 1975); investigations are going on where the roles of the immune system and autoimmune phenomena are being looked at in relation to Alzheimer's disease (Eisdorfer, 1978).

The central nervous system. In looking at the central nervous system we can find numerous examples of brain disease affecting the mind and behavior. One need only to peruse the section on organic mental disorders in *DSM-III* of the American Psychiatric Association; the elderly in particular are more at risk for such disorders. The focus here, though, will be on only one of these organic mental disorders or organic brain syndromes—Alzheimer's disease. Alzheimer's disease is a disorder of unknown cause, a progressive dementia with a characteristic neuropathological picture, while its clinical diagnosis is one of exclusion where all other causes of dementia must first be ruled out.

Alzheimer's disease offers several illustrations of interfacing mental and physical phenomena. To begin with, its diagnosis is difficult to make, with various psychological disorders, such as depression or paranoia, masquerading as Alzheimer's physical brain disease. Then, there are the major symptoms of the disorder, most of which represent mental and behavioral disturbances—from memory trouble to agitation to wandering. All of these symptoms elicit the consideration of behavioral interventions. Moreover, there are psychiatric problems which cause excess disability in the Alzheimer patient. Just as severe depression and paranoia in the elderly can be confused with Alzheimer's disease, so too they can accompany the disorder, bringing about disability in excess of that caused by the intellectual dysfunction done. These concomitant psychiatric symptoms can respond to treatment, resulting in overall improvement of the patient at that stage in his or her illness. Thus, interfacing psychological aspects of this physical brain disease can complicate diagnosis, aggravate the clinical course, and play a major part in intervention strategies.

Alzheimer's disease as a central nervous system disorder illustrates the risks of inaccurate diagnosis and excess disability in overlooking the impact of psychological phenomena on brain disease as well as the opportunities for improved clinical management by utilizing available psychiatric interventions (Miller and Cohen, 1981; Wells, 1982; Cohen, 1983).

Conclusion

The preceding material obviously only scratches the surface of the enormous territory of clinical relationships and research questions at the interface of mental and physical health phenomena in geriatrics. But ideally it has made the idea of exploring that territory more relevant to clinician and researcher alike.

References

American Psychiatric Association. DSM III: Diagnostic and Statistical Manual of Mental Disorders, 3rd ed. Washington, D.C.: APA, 1980.

Barzel, U.S.: Common metabolic disorders of the skeleton in aging. In Reichel, W. (Ed.), Clinical Aspects of Aging, pp. 277–287. Baltimore: Williams and Wilkins, 1978.

Bergmann, K.: The neuroses of old age. In Kay, D.W.K., Walk, A., (Eds.), Recent Developments in Psychogeriatrics. A Symposium. *Br. J. Psychiatry 6* (Spec. Publ.), 39–50 (1971).

Bergmann, K.: Neurosis and personality disorder in old age. In Post, A.I.D., (Ed.), Studies in Geriatric Psychiatry, pp. 41–75. New York: John Wiley & Sons, 1978.

Bergmann, K., and Eastham, E.J.: Psychogeriatric ascertainment and assessment for treatment in an acute medical ward setting. *Age Ageing 3*, 174–188 (1974).

Berkowitz, H., Reichel, J., and Shim, C.: The effect of ethanol on the cough reflex. *Clin. Sci. Mol. Med. 45*, 527–531 (1973).

Brown, A.D.G.: Gynaelogical disorders in the elderly. In Brocklehurst, J.C. (Ed.), Textbook of Geriatric Medicine and Gerontology, pp. 326–337. New York: Churchill Livingstone, 1978.

Bull, G.M.: A comparative study of myocardial infarction and cerebral vascular accidents. *Gerontology* (Basel) *11*, 193–205 (1969).

Bulpitt, C.J., and Dollery, C.T.: Side effects of hypotensive drugs evaluated by a self-administered questionnaire. *Br. Med. J. 3*, 485–487 (1973).

Byrd, G.J.: Methyldopa and lithium carbonate. Suspected interaction (Letter). *JAMA 233*, 20 (1975).

Cohen, G.D.: Approach to the geriatric patient. *Med. Clin. N. Am. 61*, 855–866 (1977).

Cohen, G.D.: Alzheimer's disease—The human concept. In Katzman, R. (Ed.), Biological Aspects of Alzheimer's Disease, Banbury Report 15, pp. 3–6. New York: Cold Spring Harbor Laboratory, 1983.

Cole, J.D., and Davis, J.M.: Reserpine-induced depression. In Freedman, A., Kaplan, H.I., and Sadock, B.J. (Eds.), Comprehensive Textbook of Psychiatry II, Vol. 2, p. 1952. Baltimore: Williams and Wilkins, 1975.

Dale, A.J.D.: Organic mental disorders associated with disturbances in metabolism, growth, and nutrition. In Kaplan, H.I., Freedman, A., Sadock, B.J. (Eds.), Comprehensive Textbook of Psychiatry III, Vol. 2, pp. 1405–1413. Baltimore: Williams and Wilkins, 1980.

Davis, P.J.: Endocrines and aging. In Reichel, W. (Ed.), The Geriatric Patient, pp. 82–90. New York: H.P. Publishing Co., 1978.

Doherty, J.D., deSoyza, N., Kane, J.J., Murphy, M.L., Scovil, J., and Watson, J.: Cardiac glycosides. In Levenson, A.J. (Ed.), Neuropsychiatric Side Effects of Drugs in the Elderly—Aging, Vol. 9, pp. 39–48. New York: Raven, 1979.

Duarte, C.G., Winnacker, J.L., Becker, K.L. et al.: Thiazide-induced hypercalcomia. *New Engl. J. Med. 284*, 828–830 (1971).

Eisdorfer, C., Cohen, D., and Buckley, C.C. III: Serum immunoglobulins and cognition in the impaired elderly. In Katzman, R. et al. (Eds.), Alzheimers Disease: Senile dementia and Related Disorders—Aging, Vol. 7, pp. 401–407. New York: Raven, 1978.

Fleminger, R.: Visual hallucinations and illusions with propranolol. *Br. Med. J. 1*(6121), 1182 (1978).

Fraser, H.S., and Carr, A.C.: Propranolol psychosis. *Br. Med. J. 129*, 508–509 (1976).

Freeman, E.: The respiratory system. In Brocklehurst, J.C. (Ed.), Textbook of Geriatric Medicine and Gerontology. New York: Churchill Livingstone, 1978.

Funkenstein, H.H., Hicks, R., Dysken, M.W., and Davis, J.M.: Drug treatment of cognitive impairment in Alzheimer's disease in the late-life dementias. In Miller, N.E., and Cohen, G.D. (Eds.), Clinical Aspects of Alzheimer's Disease and Senile Dementia—Aging, Vol. 15, pp. 139–160. New York: Raven, 1981.

Goodwin, F.K., Ebert, M.H., and Bunney, W.E., Jr.: Mental effects of reserpine in man: A review. In Shader, R.I. (Ed.), Psychiatric Complications of Medical Drugs, pp. 73–102. New York: Raven, 1972.

Goodman, L.S., and Gillman, A.: The Pharmacological Basis of Therapeutics. New York: Macmillan, 1975.

Guilleminault, C., Eldridge, F.L., Tilkian, A. et al.: Sleep apnea due to upper airway obstruction: A review of 25 cases. *Arch. Int. Med. 137*, 296–300 (1977).

Gurland, B.J.: The comparative frequency of depression in various adult age groups. *J. Gerontol. 31*, 283–292 (1976).

Hammond, J.J., and Kirkendall, W.M.: Antihypertensive agents in neuropsychiatric side effects of drugs in the elderly. In Levenson, A.J. (Ed.), Neuropsychiatric Side Effects of Drugs in the Elderly—Aging, Vol. 9, pp. 44–68. New York: Raven, 1979.

Holland, O.B., and Kaplan, W.M.: Propranolol in the treatment of hypertension. *New Engl. J. Med. 294*, 930–936 (1976).

Imboden, J.B., Carter, A., and Leighton, E.C.: Convalescence from influenza: A study of the psychological and clinical determinants. *Arch. Intern. Med. 108*, 115 (1961).

Johnson, A.H.: Antibiotics. In Levenson, A.J. (Ed.), Neuropsychiatric Side Effects of Drugs in the Elderly—Aging, Vol. 9, pp. 27–38. New York: Raven, 1979.

Kline, C.L., and Highsmith, L.S.: Toxic psychosis resulting from penicillin. *Ann. Intern. Med. 28*, 1057–1058 (1948).

Kripke, D.F., Ancoli-Israel, S., and Okudaira, N.: Sleep apnea and nocturnal myoclonus in the elderly. *Neurobiology of Aging 3*, 329–336 (1982).

Lewis, W.H.: Iatrogenic psychotic depressive reaction in hypertensive patients. *Am. J. Psychiatry 127*, 1416–1417 (1971).

Lutz, E.G.: Lithium toxicity precipitated by diuretics. *J. Med. Soc. N.J. 72*(5), 439–440 (1975).

Manson, R.M.: Respiratory tract and mediastinium. In Krupp, M.A., and Chatton, M.J. (Eds.), Current Medical Diagnosis and Treatment, pp. 112–159. Los Altos, Calif.: Lange Med. Pub., 1978.

Martis, V., and Rose, F.C.: Hypoglycaemia. Philadelphia: F.A. Davis, 1965.

Miller, N.E., and Cohen, G.D. (eds.): Clinical Aspects of Alzheimer's Disease and Senile Dementia—Aging, Vol. 15. New York: Raven, 1981.

Moulton, R., Ewen, S., and Thieman, W.: Emotional factors in peridonal disease. *Oral Surg. 5*, 833 (1952).

Moylan, J.A., and Flye, M.W.: Peripheral vascular disease in the geriatric patient. In W. Reichel (Ed.), Clinical Aspects of Aging, pp. 91–104. Baltimore: Williams and Wilkins, 1978.

McPherson, J.C. III. Costoff, A., and Mahesh, V.B.: Influence of estrogen–progesterone combinations on gonadotropin secretion in castrate female rats. *Endocrinology 97*, 771–779 (1975).

Reichel, J.: Pulmonary problems in the elderly. In Clinical Aspects of Aging, pp. 85–90. Baltimore: Williams and Wilkins, 1978.

Simon, A.: Alcoholism. In Birren, J.E., and Sloane, R.B. (Eds.), Handbook of Mental Health and Aging, pp. 661–664. Englewood Cliffs, N.J.: Prentice-Hall, 1980.

Sklar, M.: Gastrointestinal diseases in the aged. In Reichel, W. (Ed.), Clinical Aspects of Aging, pp. 173–181. Baltimore: Williams and Wilkins, 1978.

Stein, J., Schiavi, R., and Camerino, J.: Influence of brain and behavior on the immune system. *Science 191*, 435–440 (1976).

Stein, M., Schleifer, S., and Keller, S.: Immune disorders. In Kaplan, H.I., Freedman, A., and Sadock, B.J. (Eds.), Comprehensive Textbook of Psychiatry III, Vol. 2, pp. 1961–1972. Baltimore: Williams and Wilkins, 1980.

Stutman, O.: Immunodepression and malignancy. *Adv. Cancer Res. 22*, 261–422 (1975).

Tester-Dalerup, C.B.M.: Hypotensive drugs. In Dukes, M.N.G. (Ed.), Side Effects of Drugs, pp. 164–179. Amsterdam: Excerpta Medica, 1977.

Thal, L.J., Masur, D.M., and Fuld, P.A.: Memory improvement with oral physostigmine and lecithin in Alzheimer's disease. In Katzman, R. (Ed.), Biological Aspects of Alzheimer's Disease, Banbury Report 15, pp. 461–469. New York: Cold Spring Harbor Laboratory, 1983.

Thompson, J.H.: Sites and mechanisms of drug interactions. In Levenson, A.J. (Ed.), Neuropsychiatric Side Effects of Drugs in the Elderly—Aging, Vol. 9, pp. 5–25. New York: Raven, 1979.

Van Rossum, J.M., and Hurkmans, J.A.T.M.: Reversal of the effect of beta-methyldopa by monoamine oxidase inhibitors. *J. Pharm. Pharmacol. 15*, 493–499 (1963).

Waal, H.J.: Propranolol-induced depression. *Br. Med. J. 2*, 50 (1967).

Wells, C.: Chronic brain disease: An update on alcoholism, Parkinson's disease, and dementia. *Hosp. Community Psychiatry 33*, 11–126 (1982).

Woolf, C.R., and Svero, J.T.: Alteration in lung mechanics and gas exchange following training in chronic obstructive lung disease. *Diseases of the Chest 55*, 37–44 (1969).

Part VIII

Pharmacotherapy of Mental Illness in the Elderly

Chapter 25

Pharmacotherapy of Mental Disorders of Old Age

Leo E. Hollister

Summary

The three major mental disorders of old age are the three "D's": depression, dementia, and delirium. While present-day treatment of depression leaves much to be desired, one does not feel powerless to treat the depressed elderly patient unless they are overwhelmed by serious illnesses or social disasters. Delirium, if recognized, can also be managed successfully. Often it is self-limited, even without specific treatment. It is dementia which remains the crucial challenge.

The treatment of dementia has been disappointing. Except for the possible modest benefits of antipsychotics, antidepressants, and anti-anxiety drugs for symptomatic control, little evidence supports the idea that some drugs specifically ameliorate the course.

Thus, as we approach the year 2000, we have no assurance that we possess the means either to prevent or to treat this most devastating mental illness of old age. Fortunately, this ignorance has been recognized. An energetic campaign is underway to remedy this situation.

Present predictions are that early in the 21st century approximately 20% of persons in the United States will be over 65 years of age. One should expect to see during the next two or three decades a substantial increase in the prevalence of mental disorders of old age. Let us now consider each of these as well as what pharmacologic interventions may be helpful.

Depression

Depression is probably the most common mental disorder of the aged. Several reasons account for its prevalence in this age group. First, it is the most common mental disorder of adult life; as more adults survive longer it remains relatively frequent. Second, the elderly have many psychosocial reasons to become depressed. Loss of health, of companionship, of vigor, of social position, and of income not only become more frequent as one gets older but accumulate with the previous losses of a lifetime. Third, a somewhat speculative reason, is that the biological substrate for depression, a diminution in availability of aminergic neurotransmitters, is more likely in the elderly due to increased activity of monoamine oxidase (MAO) in aging brains (Eckert et al., 1980).

Diagnosis

Whatever the reason for the depression, its management is not much different from that in earlier years of life. If the depression is not severe and is clearly related to some identifiable loss, it may heal spontaneously with time. No more than supportive therapy may be needed. On the other hand, a severe depression, especially if it occurs in a person with episodes of depression earlier in their life, may require urgent treatment, possibly with electroconvulsive therapy. Thus, the distinction between "reactive" and "endogenous" depressions is as important in the elderly as it is in younger persons.

Depression in the senium may produce many of the characteristic symptoms of depression of earlier onset (anxiety, bodily complaints, guilt, feelings of worthlessness, and disturbances of such vital bodily functions as sleep, appetite, sexual drive, and motor activity). Atypical manifestations in the elderly may include marked social withdrawal, confusion, severe hypochondriasis, delusions of persecution, and hostile behavior. These features may mislead the unwary to think that the patient has an organic brain syndrome rather than true depression (Wells, 1979). Some of the distinguishing features of depressive pseudodementia and true dementia are shown in Table 25-1.

Although suicide is not one of the ten leading causes of death in persons over 55 years of age because many other causes of death are frequent, the total number of suicides in the elderly is still much higher than in other age groups. Any elderly depressed patient should be evaluated for the risk of suicide and appropriate preventive steps taken if that risk appears to be high. The sense of hopelessness in depressed elderly is greater than at other ages not only because they realize that time is running out but also because they are often simultaneously afflicted with incurable physical disorders.

Table 25-1. Some characteristics distinguishing depressive psuedodementia from true dementia

Pseudodementia	Dementia
Onset defined, duration brief, rapid progression	Onset poorly defined, long duration, slow progression
Previous psychiatric disorder	Less likely to have previous psychiatric disorders
Awareness of cognitive loss, does not try	Unaware, struggle to perform tasks
Distressed, affective changes predominate	Unconcerned, affect labile and shallow
Uncommon nocturnal worsening	Nocturnal accentuation of dysfunction common
Attention, concentration may be preserved	Faulty attention and concentration
"Don't know" answers typical	Near-miss answers frequent
Global memory loss	Recent memory more impaired than remote memory
Does both poorly and well on performance tasks	Does badly on all tasks of similar difficulty
Anxiety, guilt, social withdrawal common	Less anxiety and guilt, tries to maintain social contact

Treatment for physical disorders may expose the elderly patient to drugs that may secondarily cause depression. Antihypertensives are most prone to produce depression, but a variety of other drugs to which the elderly may be exposed also have such potential (Whitlock and Evans, 1978). One may do the elderly depressed patient a great favor by eliminating all such drugs and discovering a readily reversible depression.

Treatment

Any antidepressant drug may be suitable. One might think that MAO inhibitors should be first-choice drugs for elderly patients based on the known increase of the activity of this enzyme in the aging brain. The efficacy of MAO inhibitors for treating depressions in the aged has not been specifically tested. The risks of such treatment are greater than in younger persons. Fragile arteries in the elderly may be less able to stand the stress of acutely elevated blood pressure, should an interaction with foods or other drugs occur. On the other hand, the orthostatic hypotension which regularly follows use of MAO inhibitors may lead to more serious consequences when falls occur in patients with fragile bones. Consequently, these drugs are seldom considered as first choices.

Tricyclic antidepressants are usually employed first, but they must be used with great caution. The generally slower ability of older persons to eliminate drugs may lead to higher plasma concentrations of these drugs when the same dose is given as would be appropriate for a younger person (Thompson, Moran, and Nies, 1983).

Pharmacodynamic effects may also be increased, due to increased sensitivity of receptors or decreased ability to exploit compensatory mechanisms. Thus, serious side effects of these drugs tend to be more common in the elderly. Sedation and mental confusion are mental side effects that may confound the diagnosis and suggest that patients are really demented when in fact they are not. Urinary retention and constipation can lead to serious consequences in the elderly. Some tricyclics tend to produce much orthostatic hypotension, with adverse consequences already mentioned. The concomitant presence of cardiovascular disease has been a source of concern, but the only two absolute contraindications for the use of tricyclics are an acute myocardial infarction and intraventricular block (Hollister, 1978). Most elderly patients can be treated with tricyclics safely if the drugs are used judiciously.

Judicious use of these drugs follows the familiar adage about drug use in general among elderly: "Start low, go slow." Initial doses of a tricyclic antidepressant that might be 75 mg/day in robust middle-aged persons should be reduced to 10–30 mg/day in the elderly. Frequently 50 mg/day is adequate, and in the absence of any major side effects, full doses of 150 mg/day may be used. Routine monitoring of plasma concentrations of tricyclics is not yet justified but a strong case can be made for checking plasma concentrations in the elderly to make sure that the levels are on the conservative side.

If the clinical response is good, maintenance treatment is reasonable in the elderly. The dose to use for effective maintenance is still not decided. Some clinicians prefer to use whatever dose was required to produce the remission, while others prefer to reduce the dose to one-half or one-third the therapeutic dose. The latter procedure has much to commend it, if it works.

A poor clinical response to tricyclics would be an indication for a trial of an MAO inhibitor. It is probably better to go immediately to the other class of drug than to try a second or third tricyclic. If one of the latter group does not work, it is not too likely that another will. Doses of the MAO inhibitor should also be conservative, beginning with 15 mg/day of phenelzine or 10 mg/day of tranylcypromine. Augmentation of doses should be gradual, with similar increments.

Lithium may be highly effective for maintenance treatment, especially if side effects of tricyclics are bothersome or if maintenance with tricyclics of MAO inhibitors is not effective. Doses should be small, as lithium elimination in the elderly is much slower due to the "physiologic" decrease in renal function that is universal with aging. Frequent monitoring of serum lithium concentrations is desirable. Carbamazepine may also be useful for maintenance but little systematic experience has been developed for this drug in elderly patients.

The "second generation" antidepressants should be tried only when both older classes of drugs fail. Their increase in safety as compared with older drugs has become less evident as more experience with them develops. Amoxapine may be suitable for treating delusional depressions, where its combination of antidepressant and antipsychotic actions may be desirable. The utility of maprotiline and trazodone in elderly patients has not been fully evaluated.

Elderly patients should not be denied the potential benefit from electroconvulsive therapy simply because of their age. With full anesthesia, the risks of this procedure are slight. Benefits might be large, as many patients refractory to other approaches have responded to this modality. One might combine antidepressants with ECT to try to reduce the course of treatment and to sustain remission better.

Course

Recent experience has suggested a pessimistic view of the outcome of depression in elderly patients (Murphy, 1983). Only one-third of 124 elderly patients diagnosed as depressed had shown a good response after one year's follow-up. However, a substantial amount of the poor outcome was related to concomitant physical illnesses, which lead to death in over one-seventh of the group. Only 3% wound up with a diagnosis of dementia. Thus, the outcome for patients who are more salvageable, using the various treatments mentioned, might be considerably greater.

Dementia

About 10% of people over 65 years of age suffer from dementia, with the prevalence increasing to about 22% for those over 80 years of age. As the percentage of the total population over age 65 is steadily increasing in the developed countries of the world, with those aged 75 years or over increasing more than twice as fast as the general population, one can anticipate an imminent quiet epidemic of dementia (Editorial, 1978).

One of life's greatest disasters, to the afflicted person as well as to his family, is the onset of severe mental impairment in the elderly person. The course is often a long-term decline toward death without dignity.

Physicians are the ones usually first called upon to see whether they can do something to mitigate the condition.

Diagnosis

The earliest changes are usually cognitive. Recent memory is impaired, although the patients' preserved remote memory allows them to enjoy their anecdotage. The general level of alertness wanes: activities that formerly gave pleasure are no longer pursued. Impaired judgment may become evident as an additional manifestation of decreased intellectual function. With advancing pathologic change, signs become more severe. Frank disorientation and confusion replace the initial slight memory loss. The patient becomes truly demented.

Changes in personality and behavioral disturbances occur along with the failing cognitive functions. Patients may become irritable, hostile, or emotionally labile to those close to them, causing perplexity and distress to those who feel ill-used. Motivation and initiative may become completely lost, leading to a vegetative existence. Patients become obstreperous, cooperate poorly, and shun social contact. They care little about their common daily hygiene.

The insidious onset of such symptoms in a patient over 65 years of age is most likely senile dementia (Alzheimer's disease). Nonetheless, depression and dementia share many common clinical manifestations, so chances for misdiagnosis exist. Depression (pseudodementia) is potentially treatable, while true dementia is difficult if not impossible to reverse. Thus, proper diagnosis is of great importance to the patient (Schmidt, 1974).

Another common mental disorder in the elderly is delirium. As it most often occurs in the context of medical or surgical illnesses, and as it is usually quickly reversible, it is seldom listed as a diagnosis. Delirium also shares many common aspects with dementia but the differential diagnosis is not likely to be as difficult as it is between depression and dementia. The natural curse of delirium usually settles any argument.

The yield of reversible cases of dementia has been variously estimated to be from 10 to 25% (Wells, 1978). Intensive investigation of 200 patients with a provisional diagnosis of dementia revealed that 33 patients had a potentially treatable disorder, while 20 patients had depression, an eminently treatable disorder (Smith and Kiloh, 1981). This rather high yield of potentially reversible dementia was doubtless due to the fact that only 55 patients in this series were over age 65 years. If one focuses on these patients, one finds that the diagnosis of dementia was confirmed in 53, only two having potentially reversible illness (normal-pressure hydrocephalus and hypothyroidism). Two other patients had dementia of known and fairly obvious cause (Huntington's disease and trauma), while the remaining 49 had dementia of unknown cause, presumably

Table 25-2. Questions of mini-mental-status questionnaire

1. What is the date today? (month, day, year)
2. What day of the week is it?
3. What is the name of this place?
4. What is your telephone number? or
   What is your street address? (if no telephone)
5. How old are you?
6. When were you born?
7. Who is now President?
8. Who was President just before?
9. What was your mother's maiden name?
10. Subtract 3 from 20 and keep on subtracting.

Eight or more errors—severe mental impairment
Three to seven errors—mild to moderate impairment
Up to two errors—normal functioning

Alzheimer's disease or multi-infarct dementia. Thus, the number of salvageable patients over age 65 with a diagnosis of dementia may be somewhat smaller than previous estimates.

A mini-mental-status examination has been proposed as a way to judge the degree of mental impairment (Pfeiffer, 1975) (Table 25-2). Other variations have included questions such as "What is my name?," but it is important to ask questions that the patient has a reasonable chance to answer correctly. Other tests have been devised specifically to detect cognitive incapacity in medically ill patients (Jacobs et al., 1977). It is not certain that such tests would discriminate between a demented and a delirious patient.

Treatment

The treatment of Alzheimer's disease may be directed at the management of certain symptoms (that is, symptomatic) or at the presumed cause of the basic disorder (that is, specific) (Hollister, 1975).

Symptomatic treatment. Symptomatic treatment includes the use of antipsychotic, antidepressant, and antianxiety drugs. Antipsychotic drugs are probably the most useful. Their main benefits are seen in three areas: restoration of a normal sleep–wake cycle, curbing irritable or agitated behavior, and improving self-care. The gains are modest but often clinically valuable. Although low-potency drugs such as thioridazine were favored in the past, recently the trend has been to use high-potency drugs, such as haloperidol or thiothixene.

The benzodiazepines are extraordinarily safe drugs and may be used in the elderly to curb anxiety, which by itself does not require the other psychotherapeutic drugs. Diazepam (Valium) is probably the best choice, despite a theoretical advantage for oxazepam (Serax), which requires less metabolism. These drugs are best used in single daily doses taken either as needed or in the evening. In the latter case the drug may suffice for any accompanying sleep disturbance. Small doses, probably no more than the equivalent of 2–5 mg of diazepam daily, and interrupted treatment periods—a few days on, a few days off—are desirable.

Specific treatment. Specific treatment aimed at correcting some postulated cause of senile brain disease includes the use of stimulant or analeptic drugs, cerebral vasodilators, drugs averred to improve brain metabolism, drugs with a variety of special actions, and the experimental use of precursors of various neurotransmitters (Table 25-3).

1. *Stimultants.* Although stimulants may increase the acquisition of new information in the normal elderly, no beneficial effects have been proven during chronic treatment of patients. Pentylenetetrazole (Metrazol) was widely used in the past but is now considered to be a somewhat obsolete treatment.

Table 25-3. Presumed specific drug treatment of psychoses associated with old age

Stimulants, analeptics
Pentylenetetrazole—alone or combined
Methylphenidate, pipradrol—amphetamine surrogates
Magnesium pemoline—a weak, long-acting stimulant
Cerebral vasodilators
Papaverine—usually orally
Cyclandelate
Anticoagulants—to prevent thrombosis
Stimulants of cerebral metabolism
Co-dergocrine mesylates—widely used
Nafronyl—experimental
Drugs with special actions
Gerovital H-3—procaine hydrochloride
Precursors or augmentors of neurotransmitters
5-hydroxytryptophan—for serotonin
Levodopa—possibly with carbidopa, for catecholamines
dimethylaminoethanol, choline, lecithin—for acetylcholine
Tetrahydroaminacrin, physostigmine
Nootropics
Piracetam

2. *Cerebral vasodilators*. According to current belief, dilatation of cerebral vessels, even if it could be achieved, would probably not be helpful for most elderly persons with senile brain disease. Since vasodilation is not likely to be selective but general, one could argue that these drugs might actually divert blood away from the brain. In any case they do not seem to be of much value. Papaverine, cyclandelate (Cyclospasmol), and cinnarizine (not available in the United States at this writing) are some of the most widely used drugs of this type, but proof of efficacy from well-controlled clinical studies is scanty (Yesavage et al., 1975). Anticoagulants have been tried in an attempt to prevent vascular thrombosis, but such use is not of proven efficacy.
3. *Drugs increasing brain metabolism*. A number of drugs that formerly were believed to act as cerebral vasodilators are now averred to act by increasing brain metabolism. Increased cerebral blood flow may follow as a consequence of increased carbon dioxide production in the brain. The oldest such drug is ergoloid mesylates (Hydergine), a combination of three ergot alkaloids. This drug has been studied more extensively than any of the others. Controlled studies have produced more favorable than negative conclusions regarding the efficacy of the drug as compared with papaverine and placebo (Yesavage et al., 1979). The favorable results reported from treatment are not consistent from one study to another. Furthermore, they are more likely to be statistically than clinically significant. Most studies have evaluated the drug over 12 week treatment periods, a time that may still be inadequate for all of the benefits of drug therapy to become evident. The usual daily dosage of ergoloid mesylates was 1 mg given sublingually three times daily. An orally administered 1 mg tablet has also been marketed. Even the daily dose of this drug has not been established. Over the years, doses have been progressively increased, with recent evidence suggesting that a 6 mg dose is better than the smaller dose (Yoshikawa et al., 1983). Doses as high as 12 mg/day have been used with few side effects.

   Nafronyl is a new compound which is also said to act by increasing brain metabolism; the increased carbon dioxide production leads to local vasodilation. It is marketed in Europe, and most controlled clinical trials comparing the drug to placebo have been favorable (Yesavage et al., 1979). Studies in the U.S.A. to date have been inconclusive.
4. *Drugs with special actions*. Although almost every vitamin and hormone has been used in the past for treatment of the elderly demented, the absence of any proof of efficacy indicates the futility of such treatment. A nostrum called Gerovital H-3 has caught the current fancy. It is procaine in a presumed special pharmaceutical preparation making it suitable for intramuscular administration. Because local hydrolysis of procaine given in this fashion is probably complete within

minutes, it is difficult to see how much of the drug could get access to the systemic circulation and to the brain. Procaine has been found to inhibit monoamine oxidase weakly, but if that is its only mechanism of action, other drugs are readily available that are more potent, longer lasting, and more effective orally. One cannot help believing that Gerovital H-3 works only as an expensive placebo (Olsen, Hank, and Jarvik, 1978).

5. *Precursors of neurotransmitters*. If monoamine oxidase activity increases in the aging brain, one might expect that a deficiency of biogenic amine neurotransmitters might occur. Furthermore, some patients with Parkinson's disease in which dopamine deficiency is present also have clinical evidence of dementia and pathological evidence of Alzheimer's disease. Thus, it is tempting to speculate that repletion of dopamine may help patients with senile brain disease. Initial clinical trials with the dopamine precursor, levodopa, have not been very encouraging. The same has been true for more limited trials with the serotonin precursor, 5-hydroxytryptophan (Meyer et al., 1977).

Involvement of acetylcholine in senile brain disease is somewhat more compelling. Neurochemical evidence suggests that both acetylcholine and choline acetylase are depleted in aging brains. Scopolamine, an anticholinergic drug, is well known to produce delirium, and some of the confusional states resemble those seen in patients with senile brain disease. The scopolamine-induced delirium is reversible with physostigmine, a centrally active cholinesterase inhibitor. This model may be oversimplistic, as the scopolamine-induced changes in thinking are nonspecific, and it is not at all certain that their reversibility in persons with normal brains by replenishing acetylcholine can be duplicated in demented patients. An initial clinical trial with the presumed acetylcholine precursor dimethylaminoethanol (Deanol, Deaner) produced only slightly encouraging results (Ferris et al., 1977).

Subsequent controlled clinical trials with Deanol have shown no significant benefit (Fisman, Merskey, and Helmes, 1981). Trials with other precursors, such as choline and lecithin, have also been negative (Etienne et al., 1981). Attempts have been made to use acetylcholinesterase inhibitors, such as tetrahydroaminocrin and physostigmine, with mixed results (Blass and Weksler, 1983). Intravenous physostigmine has been shown to improve memory processes in patients with Alzheimer's when given acutely (Davis and Mohs, 1982). It remains to be seen whether orally administered drug will do as well, as that would be the only feasible way to use physostigmine as a therapeutic agent. Approaches to treatment with precursors are based on the assumption that the synthetic enzyme is still adequate. This assumption is somewhat shaky in view of the fact that diminished choline acetyltransferase has been a routine finding in brains from Alzheimer's patients. The use of acetylcholinesterase inhibitors assumes that acetylcholine is only relatively deficient and that cholinergic receptors are preserved, again shaky assumptions. At present, approaches using various methods for increasing acetylcholine have not been encouraging.

6. *Nootropics*. This term denoted a class of drugs assumed to stimulate cognitive function. Piracetam is the model drug in this group. It resembles a cyclized form of gamma-aminobutyric acid (GABA), a major neurotransmitter. Animal results with the drug were impressive and a variety of human trials have shown benefit in patients. Most of these clinical trials have originated overseas, but some have been done in North America by reputable investigators (Lehmann, 1983). The drug continues to excite much interest and a variety of chemical homologs have been synthesized by various drug companies.

Delirium

Delirium is characterized by fluctuating levels of awareness, in contrast to dementia. Tremors, restlessness, confusion, stupor, decrease in the amount of sleep with day–night sleep reversal, and visual hallucinations are also common manifestations. Rapid pulse, flushed skin, dilated pupils, and intense emotional states are also seen. The onset is usually abrupt, and the usual course is relatively brief, leading either to recovery or death. Delirium may appear in an already demented person during the course of an incidental illness (Task Force, 1980).

Treatment

It is much easier to treat a patient with delirium or depression than one with dementia. The importance of not overlooking a remediable cause cannot be emphasized too much. Management of a delirious old person is based primarily on treating the underlying causes, which may be multiple (Dunn and Ari, 1973). Reassurance, maintaining familiar surroundings, having family members present, and keeping some lights on at night are some environmental aspects that may lessen confusion. Although sedative drugs should be kept to a minimum, restlessness or irritability from lack of sleep may require some kind of sedation. A small dose of an antipsychotic drug repeated during the day along with a conventional sedative-hypnotic at night may afford relief. One might use haloperidol 2 mg orally three times daily followed by diazepam 5 mg at night. More aggressive or disturbed behavior may require larger doses of the antipsychotic.

References

Blass, J.P., and Weksler, M.E.: Toward an effective treatment of Alzheimer's disease. *Ann. Int. Med. 98*, 251–253 (1983).

Davis, K.L., and Mohs, R.C.: Enhancement of memory processes in Alzheimer's disease with multiple-dose intravenous physostigmine. *Am. J. Psychiatry 139*, 1421–1424 (1982).

Dunn, T., and Arie, T.: Mental disturbance in the old person. *Br. Med. J. 4*, 413–416 (1973).

Eckert, B., Gottfries, C-G., Von Knorring, L., Oreland, C., Wiberg, A., and Winblad, B.: Brain and platelet monoamine oxidase in mental disorders. I. Schizophrenics and cycloid psychotics. *Prog. Neuropsychopharmacol. 4*, 57–68 (1980).

Editorial. Dementia—the quiet epidemic. *Br. Med. J. 1*, 1–2 (1978).

Etienne, P., Dastor, D., Gauthier, S., Ludwick, R., and Collier, B.: Alzheimer disease: Lack of effect of lecithin treatment for three months. *Neurology 31*, 1552–1554 (1981).

Ferris, S.H., Sathanathan, G., Gershon, S., and Clark, M.A.: Senile dementia: treatment with deanol. *J. Am. Geriatric Soc. 25*, 241–244 (1977).

Fisman, M., Merskey, H., and Helmes, E.: Double-blind trial of 2-dimethylaminoethanol in Alzheimer's disease. *Am. J. Psychiatry 138*, 970–972 (1981).

Hollister, L.E.: Drugs for mental disorders of old age. *J. Am. Med. Assoc. 234*, 195–198 (1975).

Hollister, L.E.: Tricyclic antidepressants. *New Engl. J. Med. 299*, 1106–1109, 1168–1172 (1978).

Jacobs, J.W., Bernhard, M.R., Delgado, A., and Strain, J.J.: Screening for organic mental syndromes in the medically ill. *Ann. Int. Med. 86*, 40–46 (1977).

Lehmann, H.E.: Psychopharmacological approaches to the organic brain syndrome. *Comprehens. Psychiat. 24*, 412–430 (1983).

Meyer, J.S., Welch, K.M.A., Deshmukh, V.D., Perez, F.I., Jacob, R.H., Haufrect, D.B., Mathew, N.T., and Morrell, R.M.: Neurotransmitter precursor amino acids in the treatment of multi-infarct dementia and Alzheimer's disease. *J. Am. Geriatric Soc. 25*, 289–298 (1977).

Murphy, E.: The prognosis of depression in old age. *Br. J. Psychiatry 142*, 111–119 (1983).

Olsen, E.J., Hank, J., and Jarvik, L.F.: Gerovital-H-3: A clinical trial as an antidepressant. *J. Gerontology 33*, 514–520 (1978).

Pfeiffer, E.: A short portable mental status questionnaire for the assessment of organic brain deficit in elderly patients. *J. Am. Geriatric Soc. 23*, 433–441 (1975).

Schmidt, C.W. Jr.: Psychiatric problems of the aged. *J. Am. Geriatric Soc. 22*, 355–359 (1974).

Smith, J.S., and Kiloh, L.G.: The investigation of dementia: results in 200 consecutive admissions. *Lancet I*, 824–827 (1981).

Task Force, National Institute on Aging. Senility reconsidered. Treatment possibilities for mental impairment in the elderly. *J.A.M.A. 244*, 259–263 (1980).

Thompson, T.L. II, Moran, M.G., and Nies, A.S.: Psychotropic drug use in the elderly. *New Engl. J. Med. 308*, 134–138, 194–199 (1983).

Wells, C.E.: Chronic brain disease: An overview. *Am. J. Psychiatry 135*, 1–12 (1978).

Wells, C.E.: Pseudodementia. *Am. J. Psychiatry 136*, 895–900 (1979).

Whitlock, F.A., and Evans, L.E.J.: Drugs and depression. *Drugs 15*, 53–71 (1978).

Yesavage, J.A., Tinklenberg, J.R., Hollister, L.E., and Berger, P.A.: Vasodilators in senile dementias. A review of the literature. *Arch. Gen. Psychiatry 36*, 220–223 (1979).

Yoshikawa, M., Hirai, S., Aizawa, T., Kuroiwa, Y., Goto, F., Soltue, I., Iida, M., Toyokura, Y., Yamamura, H., and Iwasaki, Y.: A dose– response study with dihydroergotoxine mesylate in cerebrovascular disease. *J. Am. Geriatric Soc. 31*, 1–7 (1983).

Chapter 26

Considerations for Treating the Elderly with Psychotropic Medications

William E. Fann and Bruce W. Richman

Summary

Elderly people are at high risk for encountering the type, frequency, and severity of stresses that can lead to psychiatric disturbance. When they seek the assistance of the medical profession for relief of their psychiatric distress they enter still another arena in which they are at higher risk than younger cohorts for adverse experiences. Because old people often suffer multiple ailments for which they may be prescribed a number of medications by a number of physicians, the possibility of untoward drug interactions increases accordingly. Deficits in organ function common to old age can affect the ability of the aged body to absorb, distribute, metabolize, and excrete medications with the same efficiency and at the same rate as a younger body. Increased retention may require modification of dosage, frequency, and concomitant medications. Some practical considerations can augment the psychiatrist's pharmacologic expertise in providing effective treatment to the elderly.

The elderly are a population at high risk for development of psychiatric disorders. They typically face an unprecedented series of losses, including loss through death of contemporary friends, family, or spouses, loss of income at retirement, loss of sensory acuity, and loss of robust physical health. For many, these losses can constitute intolerable stressors. The response to such massive stresses can be neurotic, affective, or even psychotic, and can require psychiatric intervention. If that intervention requires psychotropic medication, the elderly are thrown into yet another high-risk pool, first because the psychotropic medication they are prescribed must interact, possibly adversely, with medications they have been prescribed for the physical ailments common to old age, and because altered metabolism and compromised organ function will increase their sensitivities to the actions, especially deleterious side actions, of their medication. International studies (Hurwitz, 1969; Williamson and Chapin, 1980; Learoyd, 1972; Achong, Bayne, Gershon, and Golshian, 1978) have shown that 12–25% of psychiatric hospitalizations among the elderly are precipitated by adverse reactions to medications prescribed for the psychiatric condition. The most commonly prescribed medications for treatment of anxiety disorders, affective disorders, and psychoses are, respectively, the benzodiazepine compounds, tricyclic antidepressants, and neuroleptics. The range of side effects prominent among these compounds includes confusion, lethargy, syncope, euphoria, dysphoria, dry mouth, urinary retention, blurred vision, drowsiness, difficulty concentrating, hypotension, parkinsonism, akathisia, agitation, cardiovascular changes, and tardive dyskinesia. Clearly, this is a very formidable array of discomforts to be imposed upon an individual who did not feel well upon first being presented for medical attention and who may question whether the psychic distress which brought him or her to care was easier to tolerate than the therapy. It is not uncommon for the situation to become even worse when a physician sees agitation, confusion, or depression in a patient for whom he or she has prescribed a psychotropic medication, fails to realize that the symptom is a drug side effect, and prescribes more of the offending agent or yet another potentially discomforting medication. Many of these perils of medical intervention are not limited to old people, but old people are generally less equipped than younger people to adjust to the assaults of medication upon the body and mind (Table 26-1). Seldom does even the most distressed organism recognize as welcome curatives the chemicals which well-trained and well-meaning physicians prescribe, despite their ultimate benefits. The body reacts to medications as intruding foreign substances which must be eliminated from the system, and young bodies as well as old bodies absorb, distribute, metabolize, and excrete medications accordingly. The rate at which this elimination process occurs can differ markedly from the young to the old, however, with the elderly usually retaining the foreign compound longer. With increased retention, actual drug levels in the body can build up as subsequent doses are administered, and, while a younger patient may, for example, have excreted the morning dose by the time an evening medication dose is administered, an older patient may still have enough of the morning medication active internally to create, in effect, an overdose when the evening medication is added. The biological mechanisms involved in slowing of the drug elimination process can be complex, and attention will be directed to some of these mechanisms here.

Table 26-1. Some systemic functions which have been observed to decline with age

1.	Albumin/globulin ratio
2.	Basal metabolic rate
3.	Cardiac index
4.	Hepatic enzyme activity
5.	Maximal breathing capacity
6.	Nerve conduction velocity
7.	Standard cell water
8.	Standard glomerular filtration rate
9.	Standard renal plasma flow
10.	Vital capacity

Absorption

The oral route is the most commonly used avenue for getting medication into the patient's body. Age-related changes in the GI tract may contribute to alterations in the rate and the manner in which the medication is absorbed into the blood stream from the GI tract (Shader, Greenblatt, Harmatz, Franke, and Koch-Weser, 1977; Garattini, Marcucci, Marselli, and Mussini, 1973). Gastric pH rises, meaning that the environment of the stomach becomes less acid as the individual ages. This change in pH may alter the ionization of the medication. Drugs are usually classified as lipid soluble (i.e., remaining in the un-ionized state), which usually results in their increased absorption through stomach and intestinal walls. The water-soluble (ionized) compounds may show a reduced absorption through the gut wall. Weak acids such as aspirin and barbiturates are more likely to ionize in the more alkaline environment, which might reduce the rate at which they are being absorbed. The rate of intestinal blood flow decreases in the elderly, suggesting that drugs which are absorbed through the GI tract wall may not be distributed to other parts of the body as rapidly as they might otherwise be (Van Praag, 1977; Hollister, 1979). The number of absorbing cells in the GI tract is also reduced, and drugs which are actively taken up by these cells are absorbed at a reduced rate. The gastric emptying process may be slower in the older person, due to decreased motility of the intestinal tract, resulting in decreased peristaltic movement of the GI tract. Diminished motility delays the absorption, but probably does not affect the overall quantity of medication absorbed. Complicating this problem, most commonly prescribed psychotropic medications have strong atropine-like effects and block GI tract muscarinic receptor sites, further diminishing gastrointestinal tract motility (Fann, Wheless, and Richman, 1976). Many psychotropic agents possess antimuscarinic effects as well, and may present an additional aggravating factor. The number of duodenal diverticulae increase with age. These small out-pouchings of the GI tract wall are, in terms of absorption, metabolically inactive, and portions of the medication dose finding their way into these out-pouchings would, in effect, be sequestered and not available for immediate absorption.

Distribution

Once in the bloodstream the medication becomes distributed throughout the body. Since the body mass of an elderly person is often smaller than the average younger adult because metabolically active tissue is commonly lost in aging, the medication is effectively being distributed in a smaller vessel, in a smaller fluid mass, resulting in a higher concentration in the body for any given dose. Fat replaces much of the metabolically active tissue of the body, and probably further impairs metabolism and excretion of the medication (Ramsey and Tucker, 1981).

Much of the medication transported in blood is protein-bound, leaving only a small percentage of the total amount in blood as free compound available for action at the target site. Plasma albumin falls in the older person, reducing the organism's ability to bind the medication to the protein, thereby leaving a larger fraction of the total blood concentration free. A small increase in the percentage of free compartments results in a large increase in the percentage of free drug, finally resulting in increased effective dosage (Ritschel, 1976; Smith and Rawlins, 1973). Many drugs such as phenothiazines, tricyclic antidepressants, phenylbutazone, salicylates, phenytoin, sulfonamides, and warfarin are highly protein bound.

Metabolism

The liver enzymes which metabolize the drug, that is, render the lipid-soluble drugs more water soluble so that they may be excreted by the kidney, are also reduced in old people. This diminution in the ability of hepatic enzymes to metabolize the drugs may lead to higher blood levels than desired or expected of the administered compound. This effect is variable, but should be anticipated by the physician as he or she monitors the elderly patient's response to medication (Van Praag, 1977; Nies, Robinson, Friedman, Green, Cooper, Ravaris, and Ives, 1977). If profound side effects occur, or if the drug effects ordinarily considered therapeutic occur in exaggerated form, it may be the result of inefficient drug metabolism by the individual patient. Should such signs develop, medication dosage and frequency should be adjusted to compensate for slowed metabolic rates.

After a distribution equilibrium for a drug in serum occurs, the half-life of this drug (the so-called elimination or beta half-life) is prolonged in the elderly. This means that once the medication has been absorbed and distributed through the body it stays around longer. These changes are attributable to alterations in the rate of transformation of the drugs by the liver. Benzodiazepines are probably the most widely and intensively studied psychotropic medications in the elderly (Klotz, Avant, Hyoumpa, Schenker, and Wilkinson, 1975; Greenblatt, Harmatz, and Shader, 1978). These agents have been shown to vary in their pharmacokinetics in the elderly according to how extensively they must be transformed by the liver prior to excretion by the kidney. Medications such as chlordiazepoxide (Librium) and diazepam (Valium) are broken down initially into active metabolites and the half-life of these compounds increases markedly with age. Oxazepam (Serax), which resembles the metabolites of chlordiazepoxide and diazepam, requires no further metabolism before it is excreted, and shows little or no change in half-life in the elderly. Because of its short half-life, oxazepam would be less likely to accumulate and reach inordinately high serum levels in old people. For that reason it is often recommended as the anxiolytic of choice for the elderly patient.

Propranolol, a beta-blocking antiarrhythmic widely used in cardiac patients, is also reputed to have antianxiety properties and is often prescribed for that purpose (Pitts and Allen, 1979). This treatment approach is especially prominent in persons with strong cardiac components to their anxiety or who have mitral valve prolapse associated with panic disorders. Propranolol's transformation in the liver is also affected by age, and side effects associated with higher doses can mimic psychiatric symptoms such as depression, confusion, or hallucinations. The prescribing physician should accordingly begin the dose at lower levels in the elderly patient. Many other psychotropic medications such as chlorpromazine (Thorazine), thioridazine (Mellaril), haloperidol (Haldol), and the tricyclic antidepressants have been studied relative to their specific action in the elderly. With the possible exception of haloperidol, these medications are not efficiently metabolized and excreted by elderly people (Hicks and Davis, 1980).

Excretion

Once the medication is in the bloodstream the kidneys begin to excrete it. Excretion processes through saliva, perspiration, and bile have little effect upon psychotropic medications and are secondary routes with most other medications. The ability of the kidney to excrete drugs is determined by the amount of blood flowing to the kidney, the ability of the glomeruli to filter, and the ability of the tubular cells to perform their function of reabsorption. One measure of the kidney's ability to remove substances from the blood is the creatinine clearance, which has been shown to decrease approximately 30% in men between the years of 30 and 80 (Rowe, Andres, Tobin, Norris, and Shock, 1976). It is also known that the glomerular filtration rate drops in older people. This factor is important in prescribing lithium since this ion is eliminated by the kidney and changes in renal function will affect the ability of the body to excrete it. Since lithium has a rather narrow therapeutic range, a small decrement in the ability of the kidney to eliminate the compound may result in an unanticipated toxic build-up of lithium blood levels. Many psychotropic drugs are conjugated to glucuronides so that they may be eliminated by the kidney. A sufficient decrease in renal function may allow a buildup of the medication in question despite normal metabolism and conjugation by the liver.

Some Other Considerations

Many aspects of medication prescription to the elderly require very little knowledge of complex pharmacologic actions but a lot of thought about some of the practical limitations which old people must deal with. For example, childproof medication bottles now commonly used by pharmacists can also be "elderly proof" when instructions are too complicated or when weak and painful arthritic fingers cannot perform the multiple simultaneous maneuvers often required to open these bottles. The result can be missed medication doses. The physician can help by ordering a conventional screw or snap-top bottle on the medication prescription blank. A complex dosing schedule can often defeat itself if the elderly patient's diminished memory cannot retain it. The patient can forget to take one or several doses, or even forget that a dose has been taken and take another. Because the elderly are often prescribed several medications simultaneously, they may confuse the dosage and schedule of the green tablets for those of the red capsules, again resulting in too much of one and too little of the other. The physician can help by introducing the patient to the inexpensive medication trays now available and showing him how to organize a week's supply of each prescribed medication in the tray's daily compartments. The patient can thereby be easily reminded of whether the day's pills have been taken. Dosing instructions should be as simple as possible and schedules arranged around daily events such as meals and bedtime that can serve as reminders, rather than at fixed hours or open multiples such as "four times a day."

The physician should be aware of the possibility of unexpected medication interactions. Old people with a variety of ailments often see more than one physician, and they do not always realize the importance of informing one doctor of what the other is doing or what medications have been prescribed. Particularly when the elderly patients have felt the need to see a psychiatrist for the first time in their lives, they may be embarrassed about telling their internists about it, or about the "nerve medicine" the psychiatrist has prescribed. The careful physician will inquire closely about what other ailments the new patient is being treated for, and obtain the patient's permission to contact the other physician or physicians to coordinate care. The elderly are big consumers of over-the-counter drugs and they may not think that there is a reason to advise their physician about them, or even consider them real medications. Of course, the patient who has prescribed her- or himself a laxative, a gel antacid, or a sleep aid can confound some of the most exquisite pharmacologic wisdom of physicians who are unaware of what their own prescriptions are interacting with. Again, the careful physician will remind the patient to include OTCs in the report of current medications. The bathroom medicine cabinet is another source of unhappy surprises for the prescribing physician. Elderly patients typically have household medicine chests full of old prescriptions, some of which they cannot remember being told to stop taking, or what they were for in the first place. The physician should instruct the patient to throw away all obsolete prescriptions, thereby eliminating another source of occult drug interactions.

The type of preparation to be used can be an important element of medication compliance among old people. Some will be unable to swallow a pill and require a capsule or liquid concentrate. When alternative preparations are not routinely available, the physician may have to ask the pharmacist to powder a tablet (they really do still use those mortars and pestles) and fill a gelatin capsule with the compound. The physician will find it easier than the patient to deal with chain-store pharmacists on such requests, and can do so by writing the instruction on the prescription. If the medication route is relatively unusual, such as by suppository or the newly developed epidermal preparations, the prescribing physician's instructions should be clear, unambiguous, and given more than once. Asking the patient to repeat the instructions to the physician is a good way to insure that they have been heard, understood, and remembered.

Medication side effects which can be relatively innocuous in younger people can be of major importance when they occur in old people. A dry mouth occurring secondary to tricyclic antidepressant medication may be an annoyance to an otherwise healthy young person; in an old person it can make dentures so uncomfortable that the patient's nourishment may be affected or he or she stops taking the medication. The side effect can be anticipated, and a nonsystemic saliva-substitute mouth rinse can be prescribed when the tricyclic is started. Similarly, urinary hesitation or urinary retention which sometimes accompanies therapy with strong anticholinergic agents, such as tricyclics and antiparkinsonians, is more likely to occur in patients with prostatic hypertrophy (i.e., in elderly males), and to be more severe when it does occur, even to the extent that delirium can ensue when retention is unreported and untreated. The physician cannot afford to let personal attitudes toward what side effects are routine and worth the benefits of therapy in younger patients prevail without modification of treatment of the elderly.

In making the elderly patient an informed partner in the treatment of the ailment, the physician should define the objectives of the therapy, clearly stating the expected therapeutic effects as well as the profile of expectable side effects. The expected duration of therapy with any and all of the medications administered should be discussed at the outset. Physician failure to specify the duration of therapy creates patient misunderstandings about when to stop taking one medication and start another, and is a major cause of the phenomenon of polypharmacy so often seen in the older patient. The result is increased potential and actual adverse drug interactions, discomfort to the patient, reduced compliance with the medication regimen, and therapeutic failure.

References

Achong, M.R., Bayne, J.D.R., Gershon, L.W., and Golshian, S.: Prescribing of psychoactive drugs for chronically ill elderly patients. *Can. Med. Assoc. J. 118*, 1503–1508 (1978).

Fann, W.E., Wheless, J.C., and Richman, B.W.: Treating the aged with psychotropic drugs. *The Gerontologist 16*(4), 322–328 (1976).

Garattini, S., Marcucci, F., Marselli, P.L., and Mussini, S.: The significance of measuring blood levels of benzodiazepines. In Davies, D.S., and Prichard, B.N.C. (Eds.), Biological Effects of Drugs in Relation to Their Plasma Concentration. Baltimore: University Park, 1973.

Greenblatt, D.J., Harmatz, J.S., and Shader, R.I.: Factors influencing diazepam pharmacokinetics: Age, sex, and liver disease. *Int. J. Clin. Pharmacol. 16*, 177–179 (1978).

Hicks, R., and Davis, J.M.: Pharmacokinetics in geriatric psychopharmacology. In Eisdorfer, C., and Fann, W.E. (Eds.), *Psychopharmacology of Aging*. New York: Spectrum, 1980.

Hollister, L.E.: Psychotherapeutic drugs. In Levenson, A.J. (Ed.), *Neuropsychiatric Side Effects of Drugs in the Elderly*. New York: Raven, 1979.

Hurwitz, N.: Predisposing factors in adverse reactions to drugs. *Br. Med. J. 1*, 536–539 (1969).

Klotz, U., Avant, G.R., Hoyumpa, A., Schenker, S., and Wilkinson, G.R.: The effects of age and liver disease in the disposition and elimination of diazepam in adult man. *J. Clin. Invest. 55*, 347–359 (1975).

Learoyd, B.M.: Psychotropic drug use and the elderly. *Med. J. Aust. 1*, 1131–1133 (1972).

Nies, A., Robinson, D.S., Friedman, M.J., Green, R., Cooper, T.B., Ravaris, C.L., and Ives, J.O.: Relationship between age and tricyclic antidepressant plasma levels. *Am. J. Psychiatry 134*(7), 790–793 (1977).

Pitts, F.N., and Allen, R.E.: Biochemical induction of anxiety. In Fann, W.E., Karacan, I., Pokorny, A.D., and Williams, R.L. (Eds.), *Phenomenology and Treatment of Anxiety*. New York: Spectrum, 1979.

Ramsey, L.E., and Tucker, G.T.: Drugs and the elderly. *Br. Med. J. 282*, 125–127 (1981).

Ritschel, W.A.: Pharmacokinetic approach to drug dosing in the aged. *J. Am. Geriatric Soc. 24*, 344–354 (1976).

Rowe, J.W., Andres, R., Tobin, J.D., Norris, A.H., and Shock, N.W.: The effect of age on creatinine clearance in men: A cross-sectional and longitudinal study. *J. Gerontol. 31*, 155–163 (1976).

Shader, R.I., Greenblatt, D.J., Harmatz, J.S., Franke, K., and Koch-Wester, J.: Absorption and disposition of chlordiazepoxide in young and elderly male volunteers. *J. Clin. Pharmacol. 17*, 709–718 (1977).

Smith, S.E., and Rawlins, M.D.: Drug metabolism: general principles. In *Variability in Human Drug Response*. London: Butterworths, 1973.

Van Praag, H.M.: Psychotropic drugs in the aged. *Comp. Psychiatry 18*, 429–441 (1977).

Williamson, J., and Chapin, J.M.: Adverse reactions to prescribed drugs in the elderly: A multicenter investigation. *Age and Aging 9*, 73–80 (1980).

Chapter 27

Rationale for the Use of Therapeutic Agents in Affective Disorders (AD) and Senile Dementia of the Alzheimer Type (SDAT)

Carl G. Gottfries

Summary

Several studies have focused on the role of the metabolism of acetylcholine and the monoamines in the pathophysiology of AD/SDAT.

Different methods have been tried to activate the cholinergic system in the brain. By giving different forms of precursors the synthesis of ACh has been stimulated. Also by giving enzyme inhibitors, the breakdown of ACh has been inhibited, and by giving receptor agonists cholinergic functioning has been activated. The effect of this treatment has, however, been very marginal.

Treatment models in which one tries to substitute monoamines have also been adapted in the care of demented patients. The positive effect of levodopa treatment in parkinsonism is well known and as there is reduced activity of DA in the brains of patients with AD/SDAT, the same treatment has been offered to demented patients. Again, however, the effect of the treatment has been marginal or negative. DA agonists have also been used but the experience with this kind of drug is still very limited and convincing positive effects are as yet not shown.

Investigations have been made in which an attempt has been made to substitute in the 5-HT system. These investigations are of special interest as malabsorption of tryptophan has been suspected in some subgroups of senile dementia. Experience is, however, still limited and no conclusion can be drawn.

From a theoretical point of view it would be of interest to use drugs that down-regulate the activity in the NA system. Biochemical findings indicate an increased speed of turnover in the locus ceruleus. Such investigations have not been made.

Alaproclate is a drug which selectively blocks the reuptake of 5-HT, and in preliminary investigations this drug has given positive results in the treatment of organic symptoms. In brains from patients with AD/SDAT there is an increased activity of MAO-B. Although the increase is not considered to be of biological importance the use of MAO inhibitors would be of interest in the treatment of dementia disorders. Such investigations are as yet not made.

Hydergine, a drug that has long been used in the treatment of organic brain syndromes, has gained new interest as its mode of action is reconsidered. The drug seems not only to influence cerebral blood flow, but also neurotransmitter function in the brain. A stimulating effect on DA and 5-HT functioning, and a blockade of NA activity is reported. This pattern of action is of great interest.

Some neuropeptides, such as somatostatin, ACTH analogues and vasopressin have attracted attention. Experience with these peptides in man is still limited. Although the effect on dementia syndromes does not seem to be dramatic, it is of great interest to further investigate the therapeutic value of these drugs. The nootropic agent piracetam has also created interest in the treatment of organic brain disorders. The drug has not been shown to be of value in severely demented patients, but in mild organic brain syndromes effects have been reported, although the findings are not consistent.

Introduction and Diagnostic Aspects

Old-age dementias can be divided into those due to disturbances in cerebral blood flow and those due to a primary degenerative process. Dementia caused by disturbed cerebral blood flow is called "multi-infarction dementia." It was formally assumed that arteriosclerotic narrowing of the brain vessels was the primary pathology responsible for cerebral ischemia, which gave rise to the dementia syndrome. Today it is assumed that infarctions of the brain are the necessary pathology for dementia to appear. This may be an oversimplification.

The most important group of primary degenerative diseases of the brain is the one with onset at the age of 65 and above called senile dementia (Fig. 27-1). If the onset of the dementia process occurs earlier it is called presenile dementia. The latter group includes several forms of which Alzheimer's disease (AD) is one. In the beginning of this century Alzheimer (1907) described the neuropathological lesions occurring in this disease. Later on the same lesions were also found in patients with senile dementia and therefore this group is called senile dementia of the Alzheimer type (SDAT). This group is often combined with AD to a group

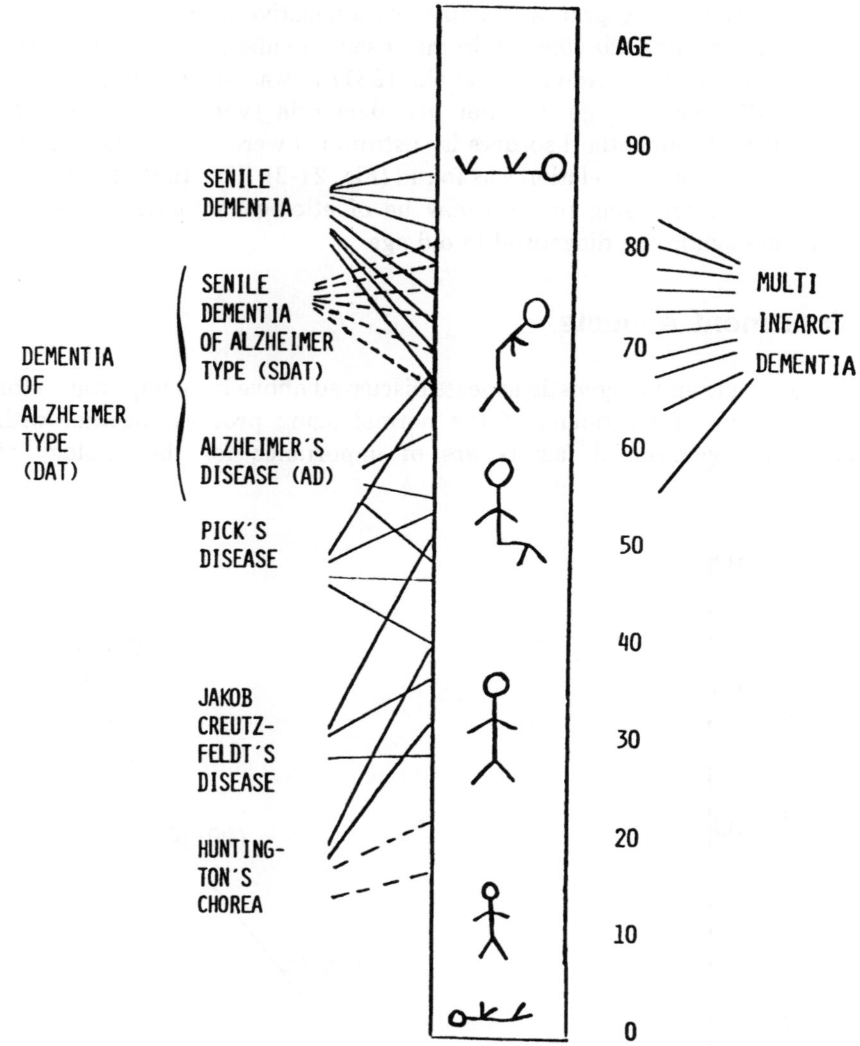

Figure 27-1. A diagrammatic representation of the age of onset of the most common dementia disorders of human beings.

called dementia of the Alzheimer type (AD/SDAT). The grouping of AD and SDAT together may cause problems. It can be assumed that AD is a homogenous group while SDAT is a more heterogenous group. It is evident from biochemical research that there are great similarities between the biochemical changes in normal aging and in senile dementia. From a clinical point of view it is difficult to distinguish normal aging from senile dementia. It can be assumed that the biochemical changes caused by the normal aging process together with negative psychosocial factors may cause a dementia-like syndrome (pseudodementia). In an epidemiologic investigation (Adolfsson et al., 1981) it was shown that 3.7% of people 65 years of age or older had dementia syndromes. When the frequency of dementia disorders in institutions were correlated to age a highly significant correlation was found (Fig. 27-2). This finding indicates that the normal aging process may be of etiologic importance for the dementia syndrome diagnosed in old age.

Treatment Aspects

The etiologic and diagnostic aspects discussed above have importance for the strategy of treatment. If the normal aging process together with negative psychosocial factors are of importance for the etiology of

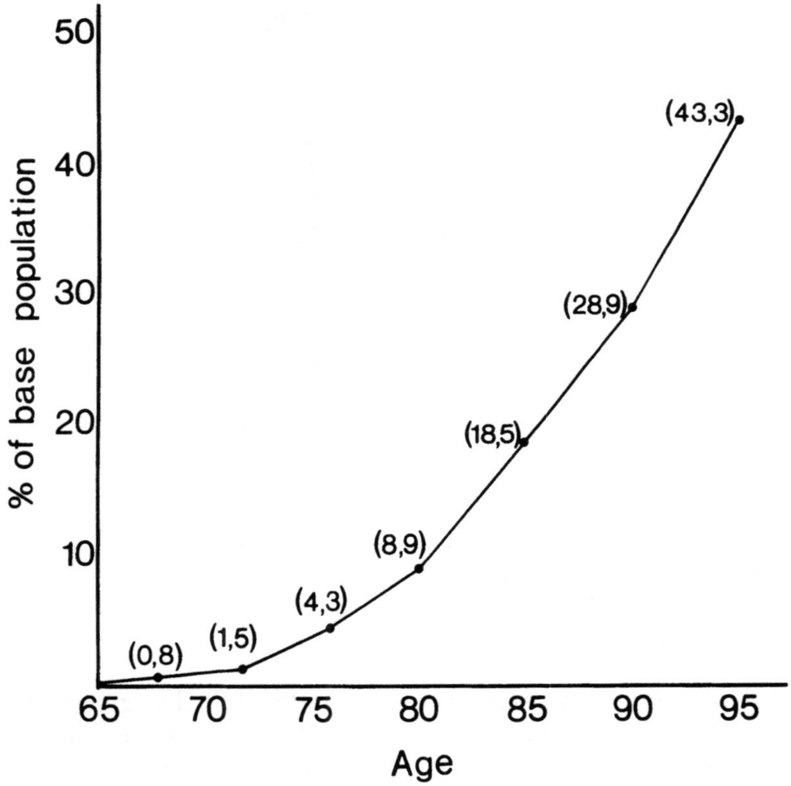

Figure 27-2. Frequency of demented institutionalized individuals expressed as percent of total population of 65 years of age or older in a Swedish county. 3523 institutionalized individuals were investigated. Total population 65 years of age or older was 33,838.

dementia syndromes seen in older age the treatment, especially the prophylactic treatment, must include mental activation. This treatment does not, of course, exclude pharmacologic treatment. Although the aging process is considered "normal," pharmacologic treatment may very well be possible and may improve the situation of the aged.

During the last decades there has been interesting research on AD/SDAT, giving clues as to its pharmacologic treatment. The cholinergic system has been singled out as the possible primary locus of memory impairment related to AD/SDAT. However, it seems unlikely that in a disease with such widespread degeneration as AD/SDAT only one transmitter system should be disturbed. Data have also been collected indicating that monoamine transmitters and neuropeptides are disturbed as well.

Before going into details about biochemical disturbances, I would like to emphasize that it is evident for the clinician that patients with AD/SDAT not only are intellectually impaired but also have emotional and motor-functioning impairment. One could say that these patients have an "intellectual dementia" as well as an "emotional dementia" and a "motor-functioning dementia." It is also evident that it is mainly the emotional disturbance that causes the suffering of the patient and brings the patient to the institution. In textbooks usually the intellectual impairment is stressed, but when interpreting the biochemical findings in AD/SDAT the other symptoms must be kept in mind.

In Figure 27-3 the biochemical findings made in AD/SDAT are summarized. The findings are compared to those made in normal aging and in parkinson's disease. As is evident from this figure there are biochemical similarities not only between normal aging and AD/SDAT but also between normal aging, AD/SDAT, and Parkinson's disease. As there is in Parkinson's disease a treatment model in which the failing dopaminergic system is supported by giving L-dopa, this treatment model has also been applied in the treatment of AD/SDAT.

Drugs Affecting the Acetylcholinergic Neurotransmitter System

A reduced activity in choline acetyltransferas (CAT) is reported from several groups (for review see Corkin, 1981) in AD/SDAT. Animal and human studies using substances affecting the cholinergic neurotransmitter system show that this system is of importance for memory functions. It has been shown in the rat that there is an increase of acetylcholine (ACh) brain levels after administration of choline (Wurtman, Hirsch, and Growdon, 1977). Various choline salts have been used in the treatment of humans. The natural dietary source of choline in man is lecithin, which has also been used as a precursor to stimulate ACh

		A	AD/SDAT	PD
AcH	CAT	↓	↓ ↓	
	CHE	↓	↓ ↓	
	RECEPTORS	↓		
5-HT	5-HT	↓	↓ ↓	↓ ↓
	5-HIAA	↓	↓	↓ ↓
	RECEPTORS			
	MAO	↑	↑ ↑	
NA	NA	↓	↓ ↓	↓
	MHPG		↑	
	DBH		↓	
DA	DA	↓	↓ ↓	↓ ↓ ↓
	HVA	↓	↓ ↓	↓ ↓ ↓
	RECEPTORS			↓ ↑
	DDC	↓	↓ ↓	↓ ↓
	TH	↓	↓ ↓	↓ ↓
GABA	GAD	↓	↓	
	GABA		↓	↓
	RECEPTORS			↓
	SOMATOSTATIN		↓	↓ ↓
	SUBSTANCE P		↓	

Figure 27-3. Biochemical changes in normal aging (A), dementia of Alzheimer type (AD/SDAT), and Parkinson's disease (PD).

synthesis. It is also possible to influence ACh metabolism by giving physostigmine which inhibits the breakdown of the neurotransmitter. Giving postsynaptic receptor agonists such as arecoline is another way to activate cholinergic functioning in man. All of these pharmacologic tools have been used in treatment trials in patients with AD/SDAT. The result is rather disappointing (for review see Corkin, 1981, and Gottfries, 1983). Treatment with precursors has in some investigations given a slight improvement which is not considered of clinical importance. The treatment with physostigmine and arecoline has given somewhat better results, but again this treatment cannot be used clinically. If the treatment model is correct, still more effective treatment is needed to increase the activity in the ACh system in patients with AD/SDAT.

Drugs Affecting the Monoaminergic Neurotransmitter Systems

As is obvious from Figure 27-3 there are reduced concentrations of dopamine (DA), noradrenaline (NA), and 5-hydroxytryptamine (5-HT). The activity in these systems can, from a theoretical point of view, be influenced with drugs that act on presynaptic, synaptic, and postsynaptic levels. Some data indicate that the DA system is of importance not only for motor functioning but also for intellectual functioning (Gottfries, 1981). It seems that DA metabolism in putamen is of importance for motor functioning, while DA metabolism in the caudate nucleus is of importance for intellectual functioning (Winblad, 1983). A beneficial effect of levodopa and the DA-receptor agonists bromocriptine and lisuride may be assumed. Some investigations have been made (for review see Gottfries, 1983). Again, the results of these treatment trials are disappointing. In some investigations a slight improvement of intellectual functions have been seen but this effect is of no clinical importance.

Substitution of the disturbed serotonergic system in AD/SDAT has also been discussed, especially in view of findings concerning tryptophan malabsorption, which according to some investigators (Lehmann et al., 1981) is a risk in SDAT patients. No convincing effect of tryptophan treatment in AD/SDAT, however, has been proven (Gottfries, 1983).

As is evident from Figures 27-3 and 27-4, there are reduced levels of NA in patients with AD/SDAT. However, the end metabolite 3-methoxy-4-hydroxyphenylglycol (MHPG) is significantly increased. It is known that there is a reduced number of NA neurons in the locus ceruleus in patients with AD/SDAT (Bondareff, Mountjoy, and Roth, 1981) which possibly is reflected by the reduced concentrations of NA. The increased concentrations of MHPG may indicate an increased speed of turnover in the remaining NA neurons. The increased activity in the NA system may explain some of the symptoms seen in AD/SDAT. For instance, the symptoms of stress intolerance, aggressiveness, and irritability may be related to this biochemical disturbance. Thus it would be of interest to study the effects of drugs that down-regulate the activity in the NA system. Such investigations have not been made.

As is evident from Figures 27-3 and 27-5, an increased activity of MAO-B in old-aged and a still higher increase in patients with AD/SDAT is found (Adolfsson et al., 1980; Gottfries et al., 1983). The biological importance of this increased enzyme activity is uncertain. When MAO inhibitors are used in the treatment of depression, MAO activity has to be inhibited up to 90% before there is any clinical effect; therefore a slight increase in MAO activity may perhaps not have any biological importance. Yet it would be of interest to try MAO inhibitors in the treatment of AD/

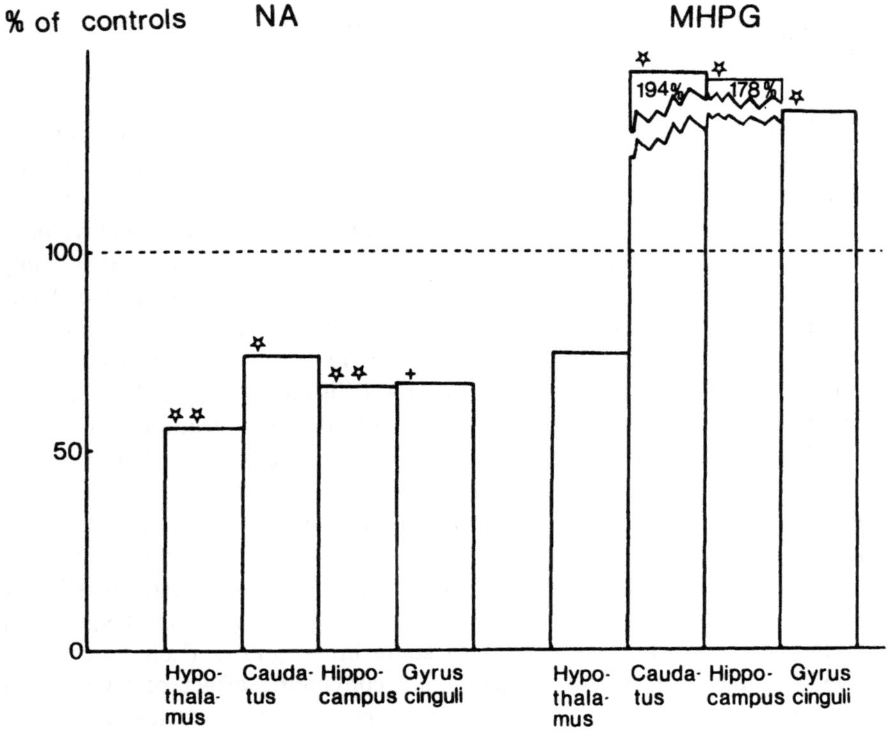

Figure 27-4. The reduced mean levels of noradrenaline (NA) and the increased mean levels of 3-methoxy-4-hydroxyphenylglycol (MHPG) in patients with AD/SDAT ($n = 14$). The levels are expressed in percent of the means from an age-matched control material ($n = 16$).

SDAT. Selective MAO inhibitors are available and MAO-A as well as MAO-B inhibitors can be used clinically.

Alaproclate is a drug which has a selective effect on the reuptake of 5-HT in the synaptic cleft. Besides, the drug also seems to have a regional effect in the brain; 5-HT-metabolism is especially influenced in the hippocampus and the hypothalamus (Ögren, Lindberg, and Hall, 1980). In a clinical investigation by Bergman et al. (1983), it was found that this drug was well tolerated by old and demented patients. In this pilot study there also seemed to be a beneficial effect on dementia symptoms. It was mainly emotional symptoms that were improved. A controlled investigation with this drug is in progress at the University of Göteborg.

The effect of hydergine has been reinvestigated. The clinical effect in the treatment of organic brain syndromes with this drug may not be due to the effect of the drug on cerebral blood flow but to the effect on neuronal metabolism. Several different actions have been suggested which in terms of neurotransmitter activity means that the hydergine mainly induces a

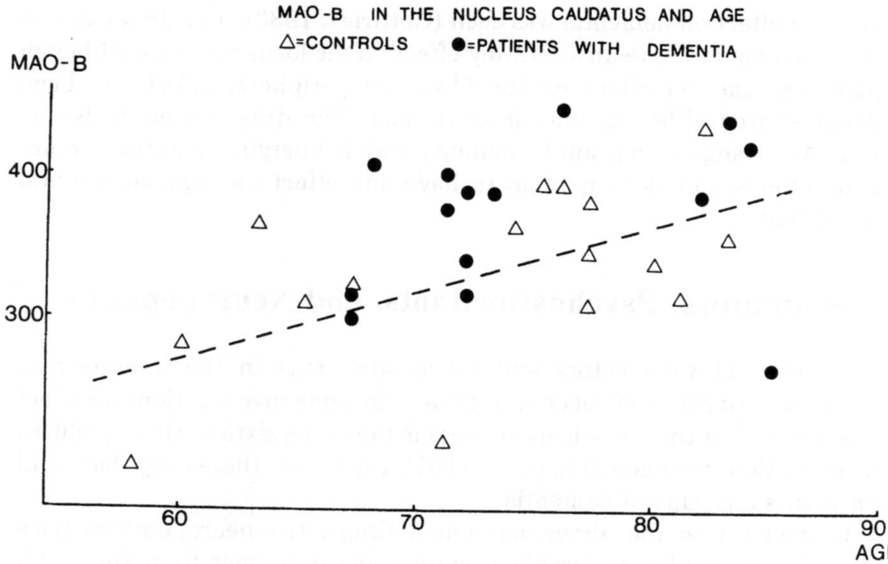

Figure 27-5. The activity of MAO-B in the nucleus caudatus (nkat per gww) plotted against age. The dotted line is the linear regression for 16 controls (△). The circles (●) are 14 patients with dementia of the Alzheimer type (AD/SDAT).

blockade of central alpha-adrenergic and stimulation of both dopaminergic and serotoninergic receptor sites (Loew, Van Deusen, and Meier-Ruge, 1978). As is obvious from Figure 27-3 the type of action of hydergine is of interest in treatment of AD/SDAT. In this disease a reduced activity in the 5-HT and DA system and an increased speed of turnover in the NA system may be assumed. In fact, hydergine has been used for many years and is one of the most commonly used drugs for institutionalized populations (for review see Zawadski, Glazer, and Lurie, 1978, and Reisberg, Ferris, and Gershon, 1981). The variables that improved significantly with hydergine were mental alertness, orientation, confusion, recent memory, depression, emotional ability, anxiety, fear, motivation, initiative, agitation, vertigo, and locomotion. In some studies improvement was considered to be of practical importance but it has never been reported as impressive.

Hydergine is called a nootropic drug, which means that the drug has an effect on the metabolism of the neuron. Another drug which belongs to this group is piracetam. This drug increases the tolerance to brain anoxia in animals. It also improves memory function in animal experiments and reduces amnesia after electroshock therapy. Piracetam has been tested on elderly psychiatric patients. In some investigations improvements have been recorded, but there are also investigations in which no significant positive effect on dementia was seen (Gottfries, 1983). The drug has also been assumed to have an activating effect on the locus ceruleus. Although piracetam has an effect on the CNS, no peripheral effect has been demonstrated either in animals or in man. The drug has no analgesic, sedative, tranquilizing, antihistaminic, anticholinergic, or antiserotoninergic effects, nor does it seem to have any effect on regional cerebral blood flow.

Vasodilators, Psychostimulants, and Neuropeptides

The effect of vasodilators and psychostimulants in the treatment of dementia disorders has been questioned. In some investigations an effect was shown, but the investigations were made in the sixties. More qualified investigations are needed to better clarify the effects these drugs have and on what subgroups of dementia.

In contrast to the above-mentioned drugs, the neuropeptides have recently attracted considerable attention. As can be seen from Figure 27-3 there are reduced levels of somatostatin and substance P in brains from patients with AD/SDAT. The brain proteins ACTH and vasopressin have been shown to influence the learning process. The same effect has been proven of some ACTH analogues. However, the effect of ACTH in man seems to be the result of a nonspecific effect on arousal systems.

A great deal of evidence has accumulated supporting the physiologic role of vasopressin in the learning and memory processes (de Wied et al., 1976). A therapeutic effect of lysine-vasopressin on memory in patients with senile dementia has been reported (Delwaide, Devoitille, and Ylieff, 1980). Some preliminary results have suggested that patients with AD performed better in learning and recall tasks after treatment with the synthetic vasopressin analogue DDAVP (Weingartner et al., 1981). In spite of the limited number of patients treated with neuropeptides the data support the hypothesis that some of these drugs act on the central nervous system in man and further investigations are necessary to determine if the drugs can be used as therapeutic agents in patients with cognitive impairment.

Conclusions

The biochemical research showing disturbed neurotransmitter function in brains from patients with AD/SDAT has given clues to treatment. Many efforts have been made to substitute or activate failing neurotransmitter functioning. The results, however, have been rather disappointing. In the author's opinion, we are still on a very naive level in the treatment of dementia disorders. First, better diagnostic methods are needed to define homogenous groups of dementias. Second, better instruments are needed to evaluate the effects of drugs in patients. Many of the rating scales in present use have focused on intellectual disturbances. Drugs that influence emotional symptoms cannot be evaluated with these instruments. Third, in AD/SDAT it is not possible to single out one neurotransmitter system as the possible primary locus of impairment. Etiologic factors of importance for the disease must be searched out beyond the neurotransmitter level. Still, the disturbed neurotransmitter function may have pathogenetic importance. The neurotransmitters, however, are certainly very much integrated and balance each other and therefore the treatment of only one system may not give rise to positive effect. For instance, treatment with dopamine receptor agonists causes confusion, which may be due to increased activity in the DA system overbalancing the activity in the ACh system. Thus combined treatments may be necessary to improve the mental activity of the patients. The ideal would be that by studying the clinical picture and/or by making CSF investigations, it would be possible to map out the disturbances in the patient and then introduce a treatment tailor-made for that patient.

References

Adolfsson, R., Gottfries, C.G., Oreland, L., Wiberg, Å., and Winblad, B.: Increased activity of brain and platelet monoamine oxidase in dementia of Alzheimer type. *Life Sci. 27*, 1029 (1980).

Adolfsson, R., Gottfries, C.G., Nyström, L., and Winblad, B.: Prevalence of dementia disorders in institutionalized Swedish old people. *Acta Psychiat. Scand. 63*, 225 (1981).

Alzheimer, A.: Ueber eine eigenartige Erkrankung der Hirnrinde. Cbl. *Nervenheilk Psychiat. 18*, 177 (1907). Cited in Torack, R., In Wells, C. (Ed.), Dementia. Philadelphia: F.A. Davis, 1971.

Bergman, I., Brâne, G., Gottfries, C.G., Jostell, K.G., Karlsson, I., and Svennerholm, L.: Alaproclate: A pharmacokinetic and biochemical study in patients with dementia of Alzheimer type. *Psychopharmacology 80*, 279 (1983).

Bondareff, W., Mountjoy, C.Q., and Roth, M.: Selective loss of neurons of origin of adrenergic projection to cerebral cortex (nucleus locus coeruleus) in senile dementia. *Lancet I*, 783 (1981).

Corkin, S.: Aceteylcholine, aging and Alzheimer's disease. Implications for treatment. *Trends NeuroSci. 4*, 287 (1981).

Delwaide, P.J., Devoitille, J.M., and Ylieff, M.: Acute effect of drugs upon memory of patients with senile dementia. *Acta Psychiat. Belg. 80*, 748 (1980).

De Wied, D., Van Wimersma Greidanus, T.B., Bohus, B., Urban, I., and Gispen, W.H.: Vasopressin and memory consolidation. *Progr. Brain Res. 45*, 181 (1976).

Gottfries, C.G.: Levels of monoamines, monoamine metabolites, and activity in related enzyme systems correlated to normal aging and in patients with dementia of Alzheimer type. In Corsini, G.L., and Gessa, G.I. (Eds.), Apomorphine and Other Dopaminomimetics, Vol. 2, pp. 243–249. New York: Raven, 1981.

Gottfries, C.G.: Dementia. In Hippius, H., and Winokur, G. (Eds.), Psychopharmacology 1. Part II: Clinical Psychopharmacology, pp. 271–285. Amsterdam, Excerpta Medica (1983).

Gottfries, C.G., Adolfsson, R., Aquilonius, S.M., Carlsson, A., Eckernäs, S.Å., Nordberg, A., Oreland, L., Svennerholm, L., Wiberg, Å., and Winblad, B.: Biochemical changes in dementia disorders of Alzheimer type (AD/SDAT). *Neurobiology of Aging* 4:261–271 (1983).

Lehmann, J., Persson, S., Wålinder, J., and Wallin, L.: Tryptophan malabsorption in dementia. Improvement in certain cases after tryptophan therapy as indicated by mental behaviour and blood analysis. A pilot study. *Acta Psychiatr. Scand. 64*, 123 (1981).

Loew, D.M., Van Deusen, E.B., and Meier-Ruge, W.: Effect on the central nervous system. In Berde, B., and Schild, H.O. (Eds.), Ergot alkaloids and related compounds. Handbook of experimental pharmacology, Vol. 49, pp. 421–531. New York: Springer-Verlag, 1978.

Ögren, S.O., Lindberg, U., and Hall, H.: Effects of Alaproclate on the 5-HT uptake mechanism in vivo: Evidence for regional selectivity. Abstract, 12th CINP Congress, Göteborg, Sweden, 22–26 June 1980.

Reisberg, B., Ferris, S.H., and Gershon, S.: An overview of pharmacologic treatment of cognitive decline in the aged. *Am. J. Psychiat. 138*, 593 (1981).

Weingartner, H., Gold, P., Ballenger, J.C., Smallberg, S.A., Summers, R., Rubinow, D.R., Post, R.M., and Goodwin, F.K.: Effects of vasopressin on human memory functions. *Science 211*, 601 (1981).

Winblad, B.: Personal communications (1983).

Wurtman, R.J., Hirsch, M.J., and Growdon, I.H.: Lecithin consumption raises serum-free choline levels. *Lancet II*, 68 (1977).

Zawadski, R.T., Glazer, G.B., and Lurie, E.: Psychotropic drug use among institutionalized and noninstitutionalized medicaid aged in California. *J. Gerontol. 33*, 824 (1978).

Chapter 28

Prospects for the Development of Safer Antipsychotic Agents for the Treatment of the Elderly

John M. Kane

Summary

Treatment of psychoses in the elderly is complicated by effects of aging on drug absorption, metabolism, and toxicity. Not all of the effects are well understood and considerable research remains to be done to improve the safety and efficacy of antipsychotic drugs in the elderly.

Neurological side effects, particularly tardive dyskinesia (TD) remain a serious problem. The incidence, prevalence, persistence, and severity of TD all appear to be substantially greater in the elderly, even allowing for the presence of some cases of spontaneous dyskinesias in older-patient populations.

The possibilities for developing or identifying safer antipsychotic drugs and the clinical strategies needed to test them are discussed.

The treatment of psychosis in the elderly can be a complex problem involving interaction of physical illness, impaired cognitive functioning, and psychopathology. Planning treatment strategies, preventing or identifying adverse drug reactions, and defining the limits of therapeutic impact become much more difficult.

Behavioral disorders in the elderly may result from preexisting schizophrenia; late-onset paraphrenia; preexisting or late-onset affective disorder with or without psychotic features; or delirium or a variety of dementias, particularly senile dementia of the Alzheimer's type or multi-infarct dementia.

Neuroleptic drugs remain a major treatment for severe behavioral disturbances occurring in these conditions and estimates suggest that neuroleptic drugs are prescribed four times more frequently than other psychopharmacologic agents in the elderly (Prien et al., 1975). The potential for adverse reactions however, is substantially increased in elderly populations and the need for treatments with a superior benefit-to-risk ratio is quite apparent.

Unfortunately, there are a paucity of well-controlled psychopharmacologic investigations in the elderly and less is known regarding basic questions such as neuroleptic dosage requirements, time course of response, indications for long-term treatment, etc.

Some basic considerations regarding the effects of age on pharmacokinetics are necessary to any discussion of neuroleptic treatment. Absorption may be affected by the activity of the intestine, its blood flow, and the characteristics of the drug. It does not appear that absorption of neuroleptics is significantly reduced in the elderly, but there remains a lack of systematic studies. As Cooper and Robinson (1981) suggest, the extent to which drug metabolism may occur in the gastrointestinal (GI) lumen or intestinal wall, and possibly be affected by microflora in the GI tract, could be especially an important consideration in the elderly, since delayed gastric emptying, decreased intestinal blood flow, and diminished intestinal motility are more likely. In addition, anticholinergic agents (e.g., antiparkinsonian drugs and some neuroleptics) may further inhibit gastric emptying and intestinal activity, thereby accentuating these effects. Distribution may be altered due to change in body composition, in plasma protein, and in blood flow. For highly lipid-soluble drugs such as neuroleptics the fact that body fat tends to increase with age leads to increased drug accumulation in the body. In addition, these drugs are highly protein-bound and when circulating plasma albumin is reduced with age, more unbound drug will be available. The rate of drug elimination from blood may also be decreased in the elderly, although this is not uniformly true for all drugs. Some reports on elderly patients indicate an increase in steady-state plasma levels on a milligram/kilogram dosage schedule. The data available, however, do not allow for complete pharmacokinetic analysis. As suggested by Cooper and Robinson (1981), the reduction in hepatic blood flow and liver mass may reduce intrinsic clearance, but this may be offset to some extent by increased hepatic microsomal enzyme induction, especially in chronically treated patients. Other factors to be considered are reduced renal blood flow, possible diminution in the integrity of the blood/brain barrier, and age-related changes in the sensitivity or number of specific receptor sites. [For a more detailed review of these issues see Cooper and Robinson (1981) and Friedel (1978)].

Elderly patients are not only more prone to a variety of drug side effects, but are also much more likely to have concomitant medical illnesses and to be receiving a variety of medications. All of these factors complicate the assessment, prevention, and treatment of adverse reactions.

Neuroleptic agents can produce a variety of side effects: neurological, ocular, hematologic, dermatologic, hepatic, endocrine, and cardiovascular. It is beyond the scope of this review to discuss all of these possible adverse effects and we have chosen to focus on the neurological side effects since these may represent the most frequent clinically significant adverse effects.

Antipsychotic drugs result in a variety of adverse effects on the autonomic nervous system, including blockade of alpha receptors and muscarinic cholinergic receptors.

Postural hypotension is a not infrequent and potentially serious effect in elderly patients. In general, however, the seriousness and potential impact of this effect can be minimized by patient education and careful clinical management. Most anticholinergic side effects are not clinically significant. However, increased intraocular pressure, urinary retention, and paralytic illness can occur and the anticholinergic potency of the neuroleptic should be considered (as well as that of other drugs the patient may be receiving) in planning psychopharmacologic treatment.

The neurological side effect which remains a major concern in the long-term use of neuroleptics, particularly in the elderly, is tardive dyskinesia (TD). The condition is made more serious by the fact that no proven safe and effective treatments are available and the fact that the condition in its more severe forms may be socially and physically disabling. There are no pathognemonic signs or symptoms for the diagnosis of TD. It is not a diagnosis which can be made simply on the basis of a rating-scale score or a physical examination, particularly in the elderly patient. These procedures may indicate a high index of suspicion or a "presumptive" diagnosis, but additional steps are necessary to rule out other possible etiologies and to implicate to the extent possible neuroleptics in the etiology. TD should be a diagnosis reserved for a condition occurring in neuroleptic-treated patients characterized by a variable mixture of orofacial dyskinesia, tics, facial grimacing, truncal or axial muscle involvement, chorea, athetosis, and dystonias. In addition, speech and respiration may also be affected.

Several books and major review articles have appeared in recent years discussing prevalence, incidence, risk factors, treatment, and etiologic hypotheses (Baldessarini et al. 1980; Fann et al. 1980; Jeste and Wyatt, 1981; Kane and Smith, 1982).

There is general consensus that age is a major risk factor in increasing the prevalence of tardive dyskinesia (far less is known regarding incidence). However, the diagnosis of TD in the elderly is complicated by the potential role of other neuromedical conditions producing or contributing to the development of abnormal involuntary movements.

There have been reports of "spontaneous dyskinesias" occurring in elderly populations, but the prevalence of this has varied enormously (Kane and Smith, 1982). Highest rates are reported in institutionalized elderly individuals who may also be suffering from a variety of neuromedical conditions.

A few reports have focused on healthy elderly individuals in the community. Kane et al. (1982a) reported on 127 individuals (average age 72) with no history of neuroleptic exposure or significant neuromedical illness, among whom 4% had abnormal involuntary movements. In a second series (Lieberman et al., 1984) 400 similar individuals (average age 73) were examined, yielding a prevalence of 1.2%.

Klawans and Barr (1982) reported on patients between the ages of 50 and 79 without any history of neuroleptic exposure or known CNS disease and who were referred for neurologic evaluation not involving movement disorders (e.g., migraine, back pain, etc.). The prevalence of abnormal involuntary movements was 0.8% between 50 and 59 years of age, 6% between 60 and 69 years of age, and 7.8% between 70 and 79 years of age.

Varga et al. (1982) reported a somewhat higher prevalence (10%) in a sample of 365 elderly individuals, many of whom (236) were patients in nursing homes.

Our own survey of individuals in a chronic medical care facility found a significantly higher (7.3%) prevalence among institutionalized individuals without exposure to neuroleptics as compared to the healthy community sample (Lieberman et al., 1984). However, the former were on the average 10 years older. Among neuroleptic-treated elderly individuals, the prevalence rates are extremely high. Incidence figures are not generally available; however, our survey of elderly individuals in a chronic care medical facility who had received neuroleptics (mean age of first treatment 83) suggest an incidence of 16.5% after 1 year of neuroleptic exposure in contrast to an incidence of 4% after 1 year in younger (mean age 29) neuroleptic-treated psychiatric patients (Lieberman et al., 1984; Kane et al., 1982b, 1983).

Not only do elderly individuals appear more vulnerable to developing TD, but the cases which do occur are both more severe and more persistent (Smith and Baldessarini, 1980). (Both of these factors would lead to an increase in point prevalence estimates in older populations.)

In general, data from these studies suggest that spontaneous dyskinesias do occur in the elderly but not to a degree that could fully account for the high prevalence of presumptive TD observed in neuroleptic-treated elderly patients. These findings certainly underscore the importance of attempting a careful differential diagnosis and assessing to the extent possible the direct causal relationship between drug exposure and onset of movements. In addition, we cannot emphasize enough the importance of careful examination prior to the initiation of neuroleptic treatment to determine the presence or absence of preexisting movement disorders.

The question as to why elderly individuals are at greater risk for the development of this condition remains largely unanswered, as does the larger question of the pathophysiology of TD in general.

Several observations have suggested that TD may result from a state of relative dopaminergic hyperactivity. For example, the condition tends to first become apparent or worsen upon withdrawal of neuroleptic medication. Given the putative mechanism of action of neuroleptics being the blockade of dopamine receptors, this serves to implicate this system. In addition, tardive dyskinesia can resemble the dyskinesias produced by dopamine agonists or L-dopa in patients with Parkinson's disease. The administration of dopamine agonists or L-dopa has also been observed to exacerbate tardive dyskinesia (though not consistently). The fact that tardive dyskinesia can be reduced or entirely suppressed by the administration of dopamine-receptor blockers (neuroleptics) or dopamine-depleting agents (reserpine, tetrabenazine, alpha-methyl-*p*-tyrosine) provides additional evidence to support this hypothesis.

Anticholinergic drugs generally tend to exacerbate or have little effect on tardive dyskinesia, whereas in Parkinson's disease these drugs have a therapeutic effect. These observations taken together have suggested that the parkinsonian state and tardive dyskinesia may reflect opposite ends of the same spectrum (Parkinson's disease resulting from a deficit of dopamine in nigro-striatal dopaminergic tracts, as opposed to tardive dyskinesia which may be associated with nigro-striatal dopaminergic hyperactivity).

Numerous animal studies have been carried out which support the hypothesis of a postsynaptic dopamine receptor hypersensitivity occurring in animals following chronic neuroleptic treatment. Unfortunately, there is relatively little parallel evidence in humans.

Neuroleptic-treated monkeys have been reported to develop choreoathetosis and oral dyskinesias which in some cases have persisted after cessation of treatment (Gunne and Barany, 1976; Gunne, 1983). These models may prove to be very useful in increasing our understanding of the disorder and could provide an opportunity to assess treatment strategies as well as identify antipsychotic agents which might be free of this risk.

Some animal model investigations have suggested that elderly animals may be more vulnerable to the development of dopamine-receptor hypersensitivity; however, many questions remain as to the actual mechanism involved in this phenomenon and to ultimate relevance to the human condition (Tanner and Domino, 1977; Smith and Leelavathi, 1980; Campbell and Baldessarini, 1981).

There is little doubt that neuronal loss occurs with age in various brain areas, including the nigro-striatal system. In addition, neuronal plasticity or the efficiency of compensatory mechanisms may be reduced in the elderly. Peripheral factors such as altered pharmacokinetics, increased production of toxic metabolites, and/or reduced efficiency of the blood/brain barrier may also be factors.

Since there are no proven safe and effective treatments for TD, prevention remains a major goal. Given the evidence implicating advanced age as a risk factor, preventive strategies in this population become even more crucial. Several steps in this regard should be taken. First of all, avoiding the use of neuroleptics unless there are no suitable alternatives and until neuroleptics prove to be effective. Second, the use of the lowest effective dose for the briefest possible period should be attempted. Though extensive literature reviews do not indicate a clear-cut dose–response relationship it does appear that such a relationship may exist during the early years of treatment for some patients and we would suggest that this effect may be even more important in the elderly population, among whom the condition appears to develop much more rapidly. At present, however, there are no prospective studies of tardive dyskinesia development in elderly populations, nor are there studies which could help in better defining minimum effective dosage requirements for either acute or prolonged treatment.

Third is the development of new compounds (and more extensive study of available compounds) to identify effective "antipsychotic" agents which carry less or preferably no risk of tardive dyskinesia.

There are reports in the literature of behavioral and biochemical evidence suggesting regional differences in the extrapyramidal and limbic effects of "typical" neuroleptics and those "atypical" antipsychotic agents (e.g., clozapine, thioridazine, molindone, and sulpiride) with less tendency to produce acute neurological side effects (Costall and Naylor, 1975; Sayers et al., 1975; Smith and Davis, 1976; Gianutsos and Moore, 1977; Scatton, 1977; Waldmeir and Maitre, 1976).

The present literature is not entirely consistent and the atypical drugs may be more atypical in one experimental paradigm than another (Borison et al., 1981; Reynolds et al., 1982; White et al., 1983). These findings do, however, support the possibility that agents which are effective antipsychotics may be demonstrably different in their propensities to effect specific neurochemical systems. The hope is that the development of tardive dyskinesia could be prevented if drugs could be identified which are selectively antipsychotic rather than being both antipsychotic and neurotoxic.

The problem, however, remains the clinical validation of the hypothesis implied in these findings. Given the uncertain relevance of many animal models to the clinical condition, the ultimate test remains the results of controlled, long-term clinical trials. Epidemiologically it remains quite difficult to determine the incidence and course of TD associated with specific antipsychotic agents. Several methodological problems require attention in drawing any conclusions from existing data. Examples include the fact that patients are not randomly assigned to antipsychotic agents;

that compliance, bioavailability, and blood levels may be important factors to control or at least analyze; and that age, sex, concomitant medications, and illness being treated may all have an impact on the vulnerability to develop TD.

In order to establish whether or not a particular agent is relatively free of the risk of TD a prospective, random assignment trial would be necessary. Obviously, such an undertaking is potentially enormous. It may be that in particularly high-risk groups such as the elderly an appropriately designed trial could discriminate between drugs fairly rapidly. Until such trials are carried out, it will be difficult to establish compounds as being truly "safe."

References

Baldessarini, R.J., Cole, J.O., Davis, J.M., Gardos, G., Preskorn, S.H., Simpson, G.M., and Tarsy, D.: Tardive dyskinesia: A Task Force Report of the American Psychiatric Association. Washington, D.C.: American Psychiatric Association, 1980.

Borison, R.L., Fields, J.Z., and Diamond, B.I.: Site-specific blockade of dopamine receptors by neuroleptic agents in human brain. *Neuropharmacology 20*, 1321–1322 (1981).

Campbell, A., and Baldessarini, R.J.: Effects of maturation and aging on behavioral responses to haloperidol in the rat. *Psychopharmacology* (Berlin) *73*, 219–222 (1981).

Cooper, T.B., and Robinson, D.S.: Pharmacokinetics of neuroleptic drugs in the aged. In Raskin, A., Robinson, D.S., and Levine, J. (Eds.), Age and the Pharmacology of Psychoactive Drugs, pp. 181–189. New York: Elsevier, 1981.

Costall, B., and Naylor, R.J.: Detection of the neuroleptic properties of clozapine, sulpiride and thioridazine. *Psychopharmacologia 43*, 69–75 (1975).

Fann, W.E., Smith, R.C., Davis, J.M., and Domino, E.F. (Eds.), Tardive Dyskinesia: Research and Treatment. New York: Spectrum Publications, 1980.

Friedel, R.O.: Pharmacokinetics in the geropsychiatric patient. In Lipton, M.A., DiMascio, A., and Killam, K.F. (Eds.), Psychopharmacology: A Generation of Progress. New York: Raven, 1978.

Gianutsos, G., and Moore, K.E.: Dopaminergic supersensitivity in striatum and olfactory tubercle following chronic administration of haloperidol or clozapine. *Life Sci. 20*, 1585–1592 (1977).

Gunne, L.M.: Studies on the pathophysiology of persistent neuroleptic-induced dyskinesia. Paper presented at American College of Neuropsychopharmacology, San Juan, Puerto Rico, Dec. 12–16, 1983 (unpublished).

Gunne, L.M., and Barany, S.: Haloperidol-induced tardive dyskinesia in monkeys. *Psychopharmacology 50*, 237–340 (1976).

Jeste, D.V., and Wyatt, R.J.: Understanding and Treating Tardive Dyskinesia. New York: Guilford, 1982.

Kane, J.M., Rifkin, A., Woerner, M., Reardon, G., Sarantakos, S., Schiebel, D., and Ramos-Lorenzi, J.: Low dose neuroeptics in the treatment of outpatient schizophrenics: I. Relapse rates: preliminary results. *Arch. Gen. Psychiatry 40*, 893–896 (1983).

Kane, J.M., and Smith, J.M.: Tardive dyskinesia: Prevalence and risk factors 1959–1979. *Arch. Gen. Psychiatry 39*, 473–481 (1982).

Kane, J.M., Weinhold, P., Kinon, B., Wegner, J., and Leader, M.L.: Prevalence of abnormal involuntary movements (spontaneous dyskinesias) in the normal elderly. *Psychopharmacology* 77, 105–108 (1982a).

Kane, J.M., Woerner, M., Weinhold, P., Wegner, J., and Kinon, B.: A prospective study of tardive dyskinesia development: Preliminary results. *J. Clin. Psychopharmacology* 2, 345–349 (1982b).

Kane, J.M., Woerner, M., Weinhold, P., Wegner, J., and Kinon, B.: Incidence of tardive dyskinesia: Five year data from a prospective study. *Psychopharm. Bull.* (in press). 20:39–40.

Klawans, H.L., and Barr, A.: Prevalence of spontaneous lingual–facial–buccal dyskinesias in the elderly. *Neurology 32*, 558–559 (1982).

Lieberman, J., Kane, J.M., Woerner, M., and Weinhold, P.: Prevalence of tardive dyskinesia in elderly patients. *Psychopharm. Bull.* 20:22–26 (1984).

Prien, R.F., Haber, P.A., and Caffey, E.M.: The use of psychoactive drugs in elderly patients with psychiatric disorders. *J. Am. Geriatric Soc. 23*, 104–112 (1975).

Reynolds, G.P., Cowey, L., Rossor, M.N., and Iversen, L.L.: Thioridazine is not specific for limbic dopamine receptors. *Lancet 2*, 499–500 (1982).

Sayers, A.C., Burki, H.R., Ruch, W., and Asper, H.: Neuroleptic-induced hypersensitivity of striatal dopamine receptors in the rat as a model of tardive dyskinesia. Effects of clozapine, haloperidol, loxapine, and chlorpromazine. *Psychopharmacologia 41*, 97–104 (1975).

Scatton, B.: Differential regional development of tolerance to increased dopamine turnover upon repeated neuroleptic administration. *Eur. J. Pharmacol. 46*, 363–369 (1977).

Smith, J.M., and Baldessarini, R.J.: Changes in prevalence, severity and recovery in tardive dyskinesia with age. *Arch. Gen. Psychiatry 37*, 1368–1373 (1980).

Smith, R.C., and Davis, J.M.: Behavioral evidence for supersensitivity after chronic administration of haloperidol, clozapine, and thioridazine. *Life Sci. 19*, 725–732 (1976).

Smith, R.C., and Leelavathi, D.E.: Behavioral and biochemical effects of chronic neuroleptic drugs: Interaction with age. In Fann, W.E., Smith, R.C., Davis, J.M. et al. (Eds.), Tardive Dyskinesia: Research & Treatment. New York: SP Medical and Scientific Books, 1980.

Tanner, R.H., and Domino, E.F.: Exaggerated response to (+) amphetamine in geriatric gerbils. *Gerontology 23*, 165–173 (1977).

Varga, B., Sugarman, A.A., Varga, V., Zomorodo, A., and Zomorodi, W.: Prevalence of spontaneous oral dyskinesia in the elderly. *Am. J. Psychiatry 139*, 329–331 (1982).

Waldmeir, P.C., and Maitre, L.: Clozapine: reduction of the initial dopamine turnover increase by repeated treatment. *Eur. J. Pharmacol. 38*, 197–203 (1976).

White, F.J., and Wang, R.Y.: Differential effects of classical and atypical antipsychotic drugs on A 9 and A 10 dopamine neurons. *Science 221*, 1054–1057 (1983).

Chapter 29

Prospects for Safer Psychopharmacologic Treatment of Affective Disorders in the Elderly

Charles A. Shamoian

Summary

With our present pharmaceutical and somatic modalities of intervention a very high percentage of elderly depressives may be effectively treated. Although a wide variety of side effects have been associated with the use of antidepressants such as TCAs, these may be minimized by (1) an understanding of the drug's affinities for specific receptors; (2) a knowledge of the physiologic changes associated with normal and pathological aging which effect the pharmacokinetics of the TCA; (3) appropriate sampling of plasma levels; and (4) avoiding drug–drug interactions.

The future holds great promise for the development of new antidepressants that will be more specific and have fewer side effects. As the specificity of antidepressants is increased, the greater will be the opportunities for understanding the biological underpinnings of depression in the elderly who so often challenge our diagnostic and clinical abilities.

Affective disorders and specifically depression are common in the elderly. Depending upon the study severe depressive symptomatology requiring psychiatric intervention has been reported in 5–20% of the elderly. However, the more accurate estimate is thought to be 15% (Blazer, 1982). In absolute numbers, approximately 6 million elderly are today needlessly suffering from depression. Twenty percent of the depressed elderly will receive psychiatric treatment, whereas the remaining 80% will not. Reasons for the latter are multidetermined. A major factor is that many elderly and their families, as is the case with some medical professionals, view depression as a normal component of this phase of the life cycle. This is unfortunate since approximately 70–80% of the elderly depressives vigorously and appropriately treated will show a therapeutic response to our present pharmaceutical and somatic (electroconvulsive therapy) interventions. The 20–30% who are nonresponders may remain clinically depressed or assume a course of chronicity. One of our future tasks in geropsychiatry is to comprehensively study phenomenologically, biologically, and pharmacologically this heterogenous group of nonresponders.

Assessment of the Depressed Elderly

Prior to institution of treatment, the depressed elderly require a comprehensive multidisciplinary assessment including medical, neurological, and psychiatric evaluations. Of importance is an in-depth history of all pharmacologic agents, prescribed and nonprescribed, currently being used. The elderly are known to share and to hoard drugs and to ingest outdated medications. Over-the-counter preparations are a favorite, inexpensive source of self-medication. Many of the prescribed medications are depressogenic. These include the more commonly prescribed drugs such as reserpine, propanolol, alphamethyl dopa, clonidine, hydralazine, indomethacin, and L-dopa (Hollister, 1981). Also, a variety of medical diseases are known to be associated with depression and include, to mention only a few, hepatitis, rheumatoid arthritis, systemic lupus, parkinsonism, carcinoma of the head of the pancreas, focal lesions of the nondominant lobe of the brain, diabetes, and hypothyroidism (Hollister, 1981). The contribution of prescribed medications and that of concomitant medical illnesses to the depression must be evaluated. Discontinuation of any unnecessary medications and/or substitution for the depressogenic drugs are the first steps in providing safe and proper pharmacologic treatment of the depressed elderly.

With the ensuing physiologic changes of normal aging, a variety of pharmacokinetic parameters are effected to such a degree that the elderly do not require the high oral doses of psychopharmacologicals as younger aged individuals. There are changes in absorption, transportation, distribution, metabolism, and excretion (Hollister, 1981). Of importance is the half-life of the drugs, which are usually greater in the elderly. Since achieving the steady state in the elderly takes longer, numerous frequent changes in dosages may lead to excessively high plasma levels and subsequent unwanted side effects.

Since the elderly have multiple chronic medical illnesses, a better understanding of the pharmacokinetic changes induced by pathological states is needed. This is highlighted, for example, by the state of malnutrition which is not uncommon in the elderly. Normally, 90–95% of a circulating tricyclic antidepressant is bound to albumin and not available for pharmacologic action. In the cachectic elderly, albumin synthesis may be decreased and may result in a higher percentage of free, active drug (Hollister, 1981).

Treatment Modalities

Three major types of intervention are available for the treatment of depression. These are psychotherapy and electroconvulsant and psychopharmacologic therapies. Of these, psychotherapy is probably the most underrated and underutilized modality of treatment in the elderly. Psychotherapy should be considered as the modality of treatment in situational reactions, depressive neuroses, bereavement, and the beginning stages of senile dementia—Alzheimers type. Prescribing medications in the major depressive disorders does not preclude using "supportive" psychotherapy concomitantly.

Electroconvulsive therapy (ECT) is a relatively safe and effective modality of treatment and is the treatment of choice in the psychotically depressed patient who is suicidal, cachectic, and dehydrated. ECT is also indicated in patients with medical illnesses contraindicating the use of psychopharmacologicals, a history of nonresponsiveness to pharmacologic intervention, and serious complications secondary to psychopharmacologicals negating their use. Elderly patients should not be receiving psychopharmacologicals when undergoing ECT treatment.

Psychopharmacologic treatment of affective disorders and specifically depression consists of the following categories of agents: tricyclic antidepressants (TCAs), second-generation antidepressants, monoamine oxidase inhibitors, lithium, and the stimulants. These have been used in the United States during the past 30 years. Although the introduction of these pharmacologic agents catalyzed our understanding and treatment of depression, they have not unequivocally fulfilled our initial hopes and expectations. However, they have provided heuristic models for the current thinking about neurotransmitters, biochemical substrates, and affective disorders.

The focus of this paper is on the TCAs and the second-generation antidepressants; however, a few comments about the other antidepressants are indicated.

The monoamine oxidase inhibitors have been used successfully for the treatment of "atypical" depression (Hollister, 1981). The use of these antidepressants in the elderly requires frequent monitoring and close supervision. Lithium is effective in the bipolar patient, but its efficacy as an antidepressant during the acute state of a unipolar depression is still equivocal. The use of lithium in the elderly who are on low-salt diets, salt-free diets, or diuretics requires frequent monitoring, not only of lithium levels but also of the mental status. The elderly require much smaller oral doses of the salt to achieve comparable therapeutic serum lithium levels. Toxicity can ensue very quickly.

The stimulants as exemplified by methylphenidate have been reported anecdotally to be effective in elderly depressives. However, the efficacy of this class of drugs is still equivocal and a double-blind study in the elderly is urgently required to resolve this issue. The use of stimulants may be associated with suppression of the appetite, addiction, and a rebound depression (Hollister, 1981).

Tricyclic Antidepressants

The use of TCAs in elderly depressives is frequently associated with numerous unwanted side effects and, at times, serious adverse effects (Hollister, 1981). These include, to mention only a few, the many anticholinergic side effects, cardiotoxicity, orthostatic hypotension, sedation, and mental confusion (Richelson, 1982; Cassem, 1982; Cole, 1983a, 1983b). Also of major concern to the clinician has been the relatively slow onset of clinical response to an effective TCA. This delay is noted in the presence of immediate pharmacologic–biochemical changes (Richelson, 1982, 1983). Simplistically, these observations would suggest that these drugs are not acting at the critical steps or sites. Animal studies have shown chronic pharmacological dosing changes to be quite different from those of acute single doses, which have in fact been the foundation for the currently popular hypotheses of affective disorders (Richelson, 1982).

The availability of antidepressants which are relatively free of major side effects is mandatory for providing safe treatment of elderly depressives. With the recent development of isolating various central nervous system neurotransmitter receptors and assaying the affinity of antidepressants for the various receptors, the TCAs are thought to act on multiple systems probably concomitantly (Richelson, 1982, 1983). For example, amitriptyline has been reported to have an affinity for the adrenergic, muscarinic, and histaminic receptors (Richelson, 1982). Multiple receptor affinities have been demonstrated for the vast majority of currently available antidepressants excluding lithium, the monoamine oxidase inhibitors, and the stimulants (Table 29-1).

Familiarity with the drugs' in vitro affinities for specific receptors may predict the in vivo side effects (Table 29-2). The antidepressant which is a potent muscarinic antagonist will probably induce urinary retention, blurred vision, dry mouth, etc., whereas the drug which is an $alpha_1$ adrenergic receptor blocker may result in orthostatic hypotension, which occurs very commonly with most of these drugs in the elderly. Inter-

Table 29-1. Antidepressant affinities for selected receptors (adapted and modified from Richelson, *J. Clin. Psychiatry 43*, 4, 1982; *44*, 4, 1983. Reprinted with permission)

Muscarinic Receptor		Serotonin Receptor		$Alpha_1$ Adrenergic Receptor		Histamine H_1 Receptor	
Amitriptyline	Highest	Doxepin	Highest	Doxepin	Highest	Doxepin	Highest
Protriptyline	→	Amitriptyline	→	Trimipramine	→	Trimipramine	→
Trimipramine		Trimipramine		Amitriptyline		Amitriptyline	
Doxepin		Nortriptyline		Trazadone		Nortriptyline	
Imipramine		Imipramine		Nortriptyline		Imipramine	
Nortriptyline		Protriptyline		Imipramine		Protriptyline	
Desipramine		Desipramine		Protriptyline		Trazadone	
Trazadone	Lowest		Lowest	Desipramine	Lowest	Desipramine	Lowest

Table 29-2. Some clinical consequences of receptor blockade by antidepressants (modified from Richelson, *J. Clin. Psychiatry 44,* 4, 1983. Reprinted with permission.)

Receptor Blocked:	Possible Clinical Effects:
Muscarinic	Blurred vision
	Dry mouth
	Constipation
	Urinary retention
	Sinus tachycardia
	Cognitive dysfunction
Histamine H_1	Drowsiness
	Sedation
	Weight gain
	Hypotension
$Alpha_1$ adrenergic	Dizziness
	Postural hypotension
	Reflex tachycardia
$Alpha_2$ adrenergic	Blockade of antihypertensive effect of drugs

estingly, nortriptyline, which is an $alpha_1$ adrenergic receptor blocker to the same degree as imipramine, does not appear to cause significant postural hypotension (Thayssen et al., 1981). Nortriptyline within the therapeutic window plasma-concentration range has also been reported as not inducing significant orthostatic hypotension in the elderly (Young et al., 1982).

These in vitro systems provide the opportunity for the development of relatively specific drugs which bind to one neurotransmitter receptor and not to multiple systems. The prototype of this was thought to be Trazadone which appears to be a pure serotoninergic drug relatively free of anticholinergic side effects. Other antidepressants recently added to our pharmaceutical armamentarium, such as maprotiline, trimipramine, and amoxapine, however, have not been reported to be devoid of unwanted side effects (Richelson, 1982, 1983; Cole, 1983). Interestingly, amoxapine, which is a metabolite of the antipsychotic, loxapine, is a dopamine-blocking agent and may be the drug of choice for psychotic depressions (Cole, 1983a).

The greater the specificity of an effective antidepressant, the greater our opportunities for understanding the biological underpinnings of depression.

Benzodiazepines as Antidepressants

Many of the newer antidepressants are not structurally tricyclics. Some are uni-, bi-, and tetracyclics. Recently another nontricyclic drug, alprazolam, has been recommended as an antidepressant. Feighner (1983) studied this triazolobenzodiazepine in 723 depressed outpatients in a 6-week double-blind comparison with imipramine and placebo. Alprazolam was found to be as effective as imipramine and relatively free of anticholinergic side effects (Feighner, 1983). Subsequently, in an open study alprazolam was reported to be an effective antidepressant in severely depressed inpatients (Feighner, 1983). This latter study should be replicated in a double-blind design in geriatric patients. These are exciting findings and offer great hope for the treatment of elderly depressives, hopefully without inducing severe cardiovascular problems, and may open new vistas to our understanding of depression.

TCA Plasma Levels

With the development of sensitive techniques for assaying minute plasma concentrations of antidepressants, the hope has been that plasma levels of TCAs would be correlated with clinical response and adverse side effects. However, this has not been unequivocally reported (Feighner, 1982). Of all the TCAs nortriptyline is the only secondary amine which has been shown consistently to manifest a correlation between plasma concentrations and therapeutic response (Friedel, 1982). The inverted-U curve with a positive therapeutic response between 50–150 ng/ml, referred to as the therapeutic window, was first described by Asberg et al., (1971). Recent studies have suggested that a therapeutic window with similar plasma concentrations of nortriptyline also exists in the elderly (Young et al., 1982). Thus if the elderly depressive is to respond to this TCA, a therapeutic response should be achieved within 50–150 ng/ml. However, this picture is now complicated by the presence of an active metabolite of nortriptyline, 10-hydroxynortriptyline. Recent data by Young et al. (1983) suggest that the ratio of 10-OH-NT/NT in the elderly is approximately 2.5 times that in younger patients. The clinical importance of this in the aged is currently being investigated (Young, 1984).

Imipramine is the only other TCA which has unequivocally a relatively clear relationship between plasma levels and clinical therapeutic response (Friedel, 1982). This relationship, unlike that of nortriptyline, is sigmoid in nature with a therapeutic clinical effect occurring at and above 200 ng/ml of imipramine plus desipramine. The relationship between plasma levels and response for the other TCA has also been studied (Friedel, 1982). However, sufficient data for these drugs is lacking to draw firm conclusions. This also applies to the newer drugs such as the tetracyclic maprotiline (Friedel, 1982; Miller et al., 1977).

If TCA plasma levels in general do not correlate with therapeutic response, then are they of any use in clinical situations? Plasma level determinations may be useful for those elderly patients who are receiving adequate oral doses but are not clinically responding. This is especially important with the use of nortriptyline, where the therapeutic window has been clearly established. Thus if the plasma level is above 150 ng/ml then decreasing the oral dose to achieve plasma levels within the therapeutic window may result in a clinical response (Kragh-Sorensen et al., 1976). Also, those patients who have been maintained at therapeutic levels or presumably at adequate levels for at least 3 weeks without a clinical response may then be changed to an antidepressant of a different class. To be noted is that the elderly will generally achieve higher TCA plasma levels than younger aged patients (Nies et al., 1977).

Many patients who do not respond to TCAs may not be taking their medications as prescribed or not ingesting the medication at all. Plasma level determinations may help identify these noncompliant patients. Compliance of the elderly, who are usually on multiple medications, will decay as the frequency of dosing and number of tablets is increased (Blackwell, 1982). The elderly often are on a variety of prescribed and nonprescribed medications and, at any one time, may be ingesting many different drugs, not including alcohol. The possibility of drug–drug interactions are thus enhanced.

Interactions between antidepressants and antipsychotics have been documented (Siris et al., 1982). Antipsychotic medications such as haloperidol may augment the plasma levels of TCAs by decreasing the rate of metabolism of the TCA. Such combinations are often used in the treatment of delusional depression. Similar effects have been reported with the concomitant use of TCAs and stimulants such as methylphenidate. However, alcohol, barbiturates, and other nonbenzodiazepine hypnotics may result in decreased plasma levels by accelerating the metabolism of the TCA (Friedel, 1982). Under these conditions a therapeutic response may be difficult to achieve, especially in those elderly patients who are extremely sensitive to these drugs and who develop side effects at very low oral dosages.

References

Asberg, M., Cronholm, B., Sjoquist, F., et al.: Relationship between plasma levels and therapeutic effect of nortriptyline. *Br. Med. J. 3*, 331–334 (1971).

Blackwell, B.: Antidepressant drugs: side effects and compliance. *J. Clin. Psychiatry 43*, 14–18 (1982).

Blazer, D.: Depression in Late Life, 1st ed., Ch. 2. St. Louis: C.V. Mosby, 1982.

Cassem, N.: Cardiovascular effects of antidepressants. *J. Clin. Psychiatry 43*, 22–28 (1982).

Cole, J.: New antidepressant drugs. *McLean Hospital Journal 8*, 62–77 (1983a).

Cole, J.O., Branconnier, R., Solomon, M., and Dessain, E.: Tricyclic use in the cognitively impaired elderly. *J. Clin. Psychiatry 44*, 14–19 (1983b).

Feighner, J.P.: Open label study of alprazolam in severely depressed inpatients. *J. Clin. Psychiatry 44*, 332–334 (1983).

Friedel, R.O.: The relationship of therapeutic response to antidepressant plasma levels: An update. *J. Clin. Psychiatry 43*, 37–42 (1982).

Hollister, L.E.: General principles of psychotherapeutic drug use in the aged. In Crook, T., and Cohen, G. (Eds.), Physician's Handbook on Psychotherapeutic Drug Use in the Aged, 1st ed., Ch. 1, Mark Powley Associates, Inc. New Canaan, Conn.: 1981.

Kragh-Sorensen, P., Hansen, C.E., Baastrup, P.C., et al.: Self-inhibiting action of nortriptyline's antidepressive effect at high plasma levels. *Psychopharmacologia 42*, 305–312 (1976).

Miller, P.I., Beaumont, G., Seldrup, J., et al.: Efficacy, side effects, plasma and blood levels of maprotiline. *J. Int. Med. Res. 5*(Suppl. 4), 101–111 (1977).

Nies, A., Robinson, D.S., Friedman, M.J., Green, R., et al.: Relationship between age and tricyclic antidepressant plasma levels. *Am. J. Psychiatry 134*, 790–793 (1977).

Richelson, E.: Pharmacology of antidepressants in use in the United States. *J. Clin. Psychiatry 43*, 4–13 (1982).

Richelson, E.: Are receptor studies useful for clinical practice? *J. Clin. Psychiatry 44*, 4–9 (1983).

Siris, S.G., Cooper, T.B., Rifkin, A.E., et al.: Plasma imipramine concentrations in patients receiving concomitant fluphenazine decanoate. *Am. J. Psychiatry 139*, 104–106 (1982).

Thayssen, P., Bjerre, M., Kragh-Sorensen, P., et al.: Cardiovascular effects of imipramine and nortriptyline in elderly patients. *Psychopharmacology 74*, 360–364 (1981).

Young, R.C., Manley, M.W., Shamoian, C.A., and Kutt, H.: Therapeutic Response to Nortriptyline in the Elderly. Proceedings of American Psychiatric Association, 135th Annual Meeting, Toronto, 1982, p. 210. Washington, D.C.: APA, 1982.

Young, R.C., Alexopoulos, G.S., Manley, M.W., Shamoian, C.A., et al.: Plasma 10-hydroxynortriptyline in elderly depressives. *Cl. Pharm. Ther. 35*,540–544 (1984a)

Young, R.C., Alexopoulos, G.S., Shamoian, C.A., et al.: Heart failure and plasma 10-hydroxynortriptyline. *Am. J. Psychiatry 141*, 3 (1984b).

Part IX

Dihydroergotoxine Mesylate (Hydergine)

Chapter 30

Hydergine: Interaction with Neurotransmitter Systems in the Central Nervous System

Rudolf Markstein

Summary

Hydergine (co-dergocrine, ergoloid mesylates, dihydroergotoxine) is an ergot preparation shown to be of value in the treatment of senile mental impairment.

In experimental animals, Hydergine induces behaviors suggesting an influence on monoaminergic systems. Results from biochemical in vitro studies indicate that Hydergine has multiple effects and interacts directly with α-adrenoceptors, dopamine (DA), and serotonin (5-HT) receptor subtypes. In rat cerebral cortex slices, it blocks noradrenaline (NA)-induced cyclic adenosine monophosphate (cAMP) formation and facilitates evoked NA release. This indicates antagonistic effects at α_1- and α_2-adrenoceptors. Furthermore, Hydergine has mixed agonistic/antagonistic effects at postsynaptic DA receptors, stimulating adenylate cyclase and inhibiting action-potential-evoked acetylcholine release in the rat striatum. Also, at presynaptic DA receptors inhibiting evoked DA release in the rat striatum, Hydergine has mixed agonistic/antagonistic effects.

Moreover, Hydergine was found to have mixed agonistic/antagonistic effects on 5-HT receptors involved in stimulating adenylate cyclase activity in homogenates of rat hippocampus. In slices of rat hippocampus, Hydergine enhanced electrically evoked acetylcholine release. Based on these findings, it is suggested that Hydergine can counteract and prevent disturbances in the interplay between various transmitter systems in the central nervous system.

Introduction

Aging is associated with an increasing incidence of degenerative brain diseases such as Parkinon's disease and senile dementia of Alzheimer's type. But also in the absence of such brain diseases, various symptoms of impaired brain functions are frequently observed with progressing age. Behavioral changes, instability of mood, and cognitive deficits make it more and more difficult for affected elderly people to cope with everyday life. With the increase in life expectancy in many parts of the world, a possibility for a symptomatic pharmacotherapy of such age-related brain dysfunction will became a problem of growing sociological, medical, and economic importance.

Postmortem investigations in humans have shown losses in neurotransmitter synthetic enzymes, and alterations in the content of various putative neurotransmitters and their appropriate receptors with age (McGeer, 1981; McGeer and McGeer, 1976). In particular, central monoaminergic systems appear to be damaged during the aging process. Age-related decreases in the activity of tyrosine hydroxylase (McGeer and McGeer, 1976) and the contents of dopamine, noradrenaline, and serotonin and their metabolites have been detected in several brain areas (Gottfries, 1982; Adolfsson et al., 1979; Carlsson, 1978; Carlsson et al., 1979; Pradhan, 1980).

However, the reported changes in the monoaminergic systems are not uniform throughout the brain. Moreover, the changes of the contents of the different monoamines and their metabolites are not always comparable. For instance, in the caudate nucleus, there is a parallel decrease of dopamine and its metabolite homovanillic acid (HVA), whereas in the cerebral cortex and in the hippocampus, the content of noradrenaline is decreased but that of its main metabolite 4-hydroxy-3-methoxyphenylethylglycol (MOPEG) is increased (Carlsson et al., 1979). This suggests that the activity of the nigro-striatal dopaminergic pathway is decreased, whereas that of noradrenergic pathways innervating the cerebral cortex and the hippocampus is increased.

Since in the CNS the various transmitter systems are mutually interdependent as is schemactically illustrated in Figure 30-1, we can speculate that age-related brain disturbances may not only result from neurotransmitter losses but also from imbalances between the relative activity states of various transmitter systems. Monoamines such as noradrenaline, dopamine, and serotonin have been found to participate in the regulation of complex brain functions which are thought to require coordinate cooperation of various neuronal subsystems in the brain (e.g., motor control, mood, sleep, learning, and memory).

Histochemical, immunohistochemical, and electrophysiologic techniques have shown that monoamines have a widespread distribution throughout the brain (Nieuwenhuys et al., 1978) and it has been suggested

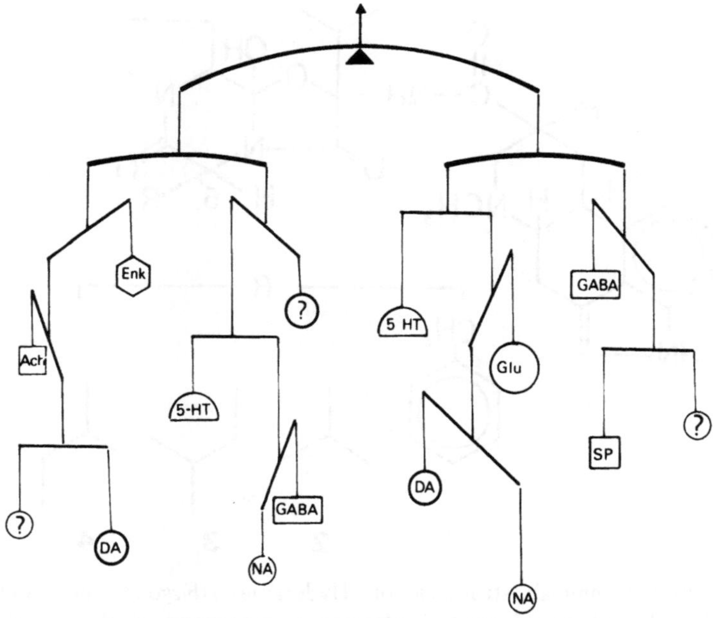

Figure 30-1. Neurotransmitter mobile in the CNS. The indicated relationships are not necessarily real but serve only as a hypothetical model to illustrate the interdependence of various transmitter systems in the CNS.

that they do not act as conventional neurotransmitters, but more as modulators of neuronal responsiveness to inhibitory and excitatory synaptic inputs of conventional transmitter systems (Woodward et al., 1979; Azmitia, 1978; Anden et al., 1969; Reader et al. 1979). Thus, monoamines such as noradrenaline, dopamine, and serotonin appear to be of particular importance for the coordination of interneuronal communications. Disturbances in monoaminergic systems might therefore result in various disorders of complex brain functions.

For that reason, it is suggested that a drug which could interfere with several monoaminergic systems in a dualistic way might have beneficial effects in senile mental impairment. Hydergine (co-dergocrine, ergoloid mesylates, dihydroergotoxine, Fig. 30-2) is an ergot preparation which has been shown to be of therapeutic value in the elderly with senile mental impairment (Venn, 1978; Loew and Weil, 1982). Biochemical and behavioral studies indicate that Hydergine interacts with at least three monoaminergic transmitter systems. Using membrane fractions from rat and bovine brain, Hydergine has been reported to displace radioligands labelling dopaminergic, α-adrenergic, and serotoninergic receptor sites. In contrast, radioligands labelling β-adrenergic, histaminergic, or cholinergic receptors are not displaced (Table 30-1).

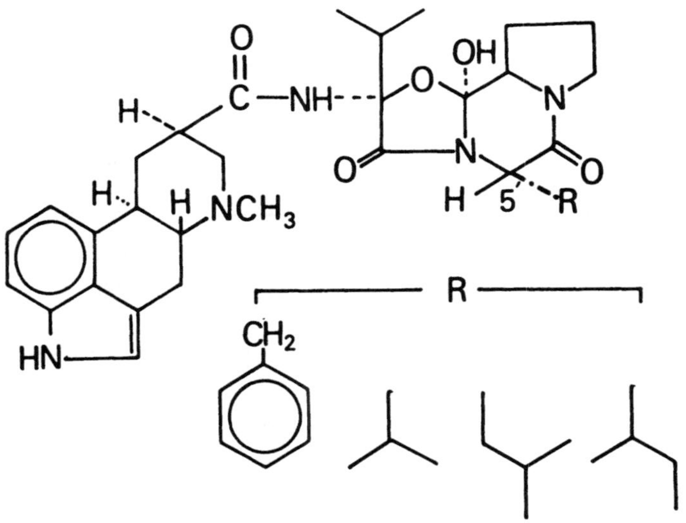

Figure 30-2. Chemical structure of Hydergine (Ergolid mesylates, Codergocrine, Dihydroergotoxine). Hydergine is composed of the mesylates of dihydroergocristine (1), dihydroergocornine (2), dihydro-α-ergokryptine (3), and dihydro-β-ergokryptine (4) in the proportions 3:3:2:1.

Receptor binding studies usually have the disadvantage of not providing clear information about drug effects exerted at the receptor site (e.g., whether the drug mimics or blocks transmitter actions). Thus, tests allowing the measurement of a specific response following drug receptor interactions provide more detailed information. In the following section, experimental findings with Hydergine in functional in vitro and in vivo tests are described which indicate that this drug has direct effects on dopaminergic, serotoninergic, and α-adrenergic receptors.

Effects of Hydergine in Dopaminergic Systems

There is evidence that the various physiologic and behavioral effects of dopamine are mediated by distinct types of dopamine receptors (Cools and Van Rossum, 1980; Beart, 1982). Based on biochemical criteria, dopamine receptors have been subdivided into D_1 and D_2 subtypes (Kebabian and Calne, 1979). By definition, D_1 receptors stimulate an adenylate cyclase and are activated by dopamine at micromolar concentrations. In contrast, D_2 receptors are activated by dopamine at nanomolar concentrations and inhibit adenylate cyclase or are not linked to that enzyme. In the striatum, D_1 receptors occur postsynaptically (Garau et al., 1978). In contrast, D_2 receptors occur both on dopaminergic

Table 30-1. Radioligand binding studies with Hydergine

Receptor	Preparation	Radioligand	Affinity measure (nM)	Reference
$Alpha_1$	Rat brain membranes	^{3}H-WB 4101	$K_i = 5.7$	Markstein et al. (1983)
		^{3}H-WB 4101	$K_i = 6.7$	Goldstein et al. (1978)
$Alpha_2$	Rat brain membranes	^{3}H-Clonidine	$K_i = 4.7$	Markstein et al. (1983)
		^{3}H-Rauwolscine	$K_i = 2.0$	Markstein et al. (1983)
Dopamine	Bovine striatal membranes	^{3}H-Dopamine	$K_i = 63.2$	Goldstein et al. (1978)
		^{3}H-Haloperidol	$K_i = 3.0$	Goldstein et al. (1978)
		^{3}H-Sprioperidol	$IC_{50} = 7.0$	Closse et al. (1980)
		^{3}H-Bromokryptine	$IC_{50} = 3.3$	Closse et al. (1980)
Serotonin	Rat brain membranes	^{3}H-Serotonin	$IC_{50} = 60$	Markstein et al. (1980)
Beta	Rat brain membranes	^{3}H-Alprenolol	$IC_{50} = 1000$	Bürki et al. (1978)
$Histamine_1$	Rat brain membranes	^{3}H-Mepyramine	$IC_{50} = 10000$	Loew and Vigouret (1982)
Acetylcholine	Rat brain membranes	^{3}H-QNB	$IC_{50} = 10000$	Loeu and Vigouret (1982)

terminals and postsynaptically on cholinergic interneurones, where they regulate in an inhibitory manner evoked release of dopamine and acetylcholine, respectively (Starke et al., 1978; Stoof et al., 1979; Helmreich et al., 1982).

In homogenates of rat striatum, Hydergine alone stimulates dopamine-sensitive adenylate cyclase, indicating agonistic effects at D_1 receptors (Markstein, 1983a). However, Hydergine had a lower EC_{50} value and induced a lower maximal stimulation of dopamine-sensitive adenylate

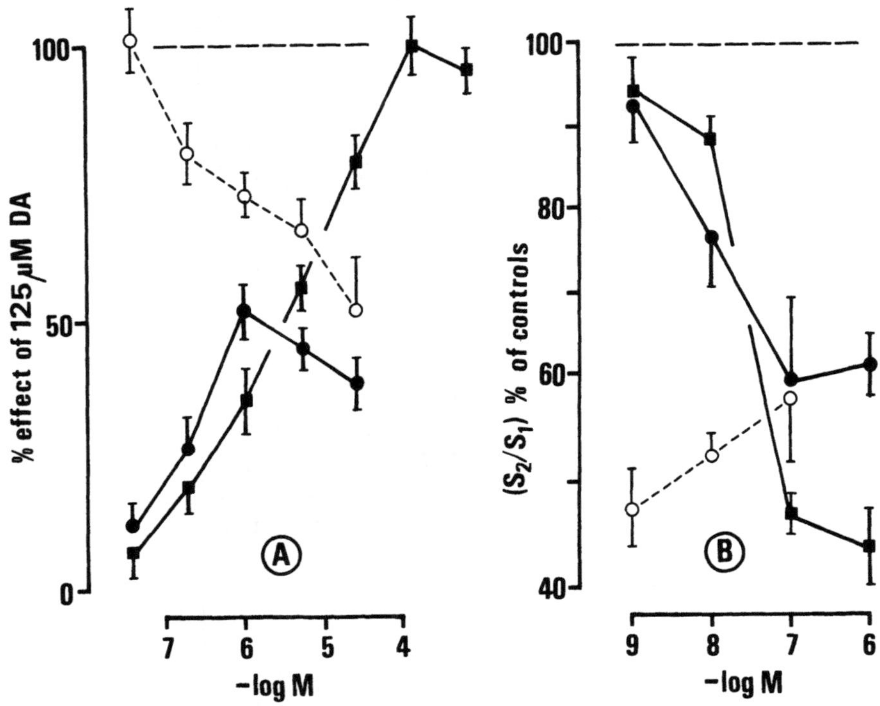

Figure 30-3.A. Effect of various concentrations of dopamine (-■-) and Hydergine alone (-●-) and Hydergine in combination with 125 μM dopamine (○) on cyclic AMP formation in homogenates of rat striatum (test for postsynaptic dopamine receptor; D_1 type). Results are expressed as percentage of the maximal stimulation elicited by 125 μM dopamine. Means ± S.E.M. of at least three experiments. B. Effect of various concentrations of apomorphine (-■-) and Hydergine alone (-●-) and Hydergine in combination with 0.1 μM apomorphine (-○-) on electrically-evoked tritium overflow from [^{3}H]choline-prelabelled rat striatal slices (test for postsynaptic dopamine receptor; D_2 type). [^{3}H]choline-prelabelled rat striatal slices were superfused and stimulated electrically for 2 min in the absence of drugs (S_1) and 75 min later in the presence of drugs (S_2). Drug effects are expressed as percentage of the ratios of evoked tritium overflow by S_2 to that evoked by S_1 (S_2/S_1) in control experimental. Means ± S.E.M. of at least three experiments (Markstein, 1983a).

cyclase than did dopamine, and was also able to reduce the stimulating effect of a high concentration of dopamine (Figure 30-3A).

This suggests that at D_1 receptors, Hydergine has mixed agonist/antagonistic properties. In the absence of dopamine, it acts as an agonist, and in the presence of high concentrations of dopamine as an antagonist.

Inhibition of evoked dopamine or acetylcholine release from striatal slices is mediated by presynaptic and postsynaptic D_2 receptors, respectively (Helmreich et al., 1982). Hydergine alone, similar to apomorphine,

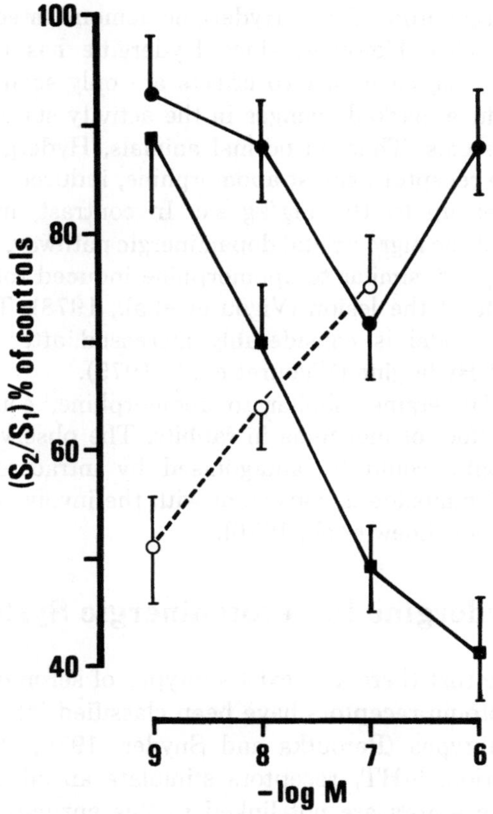

Figure 30-4. Effect of various concentrations of apomorphine (-■-) and Hydergine alone (-●-) and Hydergine in combination with 0.1 μM apomorphine (-○-) on electrically-evoked tritium overflow from [^{3}H]dopamine-prelabelled rat striatal slices (test for presynaptic dopamine receptor, D_2 type). [^{3}H]dopamine-prelabelled rat striatal slices were superfused and stimulated electrically for 2 min in the absence of drugs (S_1) and 75 min later in the presence of drugs (S_2). Drug effects are expressed as percentage of the ratios of evoked tritium overflow by S_2 to that evoked by S_1 (S_2/S_1) in control experiments. Means ± S.E.M. of at least three experiments.

inhibits electrically evoked dopamine and acetylcholine release from rat striatal slices at nanomolar concentrations, indicating agonistic effects at D_2 receptors. Here again Hydergine had a smaller maximal effect than apomorphine, and counteracted the effect of a high concentration of the latter (Figures 30-3B and 30-4). This suggests that also at presynaptic and postsynaptic D_2 receptors, Hydergine has mixed agonist/antagonist properties.

Thus, Hydergine in dopaminergic systems might be able to compensate for a transmitter deficit, but also counteract at the same time an overactivity in another brain region, thereby stabilizing dopaminergic tone in the CNS.

The dopaminergic properties of Hydergine demonstrated in vitro could also be seen in vivo. However, since Hydergine has mixed agonist/antagonist properties, clear in vivo effects are only seen after manipulations which induce marked changes in the activity state of the central dopaminergic systems. Thus, in normal animals, Hydergine, unlike the potent dopamine receptor agonist apomorphine, induced no stereotyped behavior in doses up to 100 mg/kg s.c. In contrast, in rats with an unilateral lesion of the nigrostriatal dopaminergic pathway, Hydergine in a dose of 30 mg/kg s.c. similar to apomorphine induced rotations contralateral to the side of the lesion (Vigouret et al., 1978). The number of turnings in this model is considerably increased after repeated oral administration of Hydergine (Vigouret et al., 1979).

Furthermore, Hydergine, similar to apomorphine, counteracted the antinociceptive effect of morphine in rabbits. The observation that this effect of Hydergine could be antagonised by intracerebroventricular administration of pimozide is consistent with the involvement of central dopamine receptors (Loew et al., 1976).

Effects of Hydergine in Serotoninergic Systems

There is evidence that there also exist subtypes of serontonin receptors. In the CNS, serotonin receptors have been classified into $5\text{-}HT_1$ and $5\text{-}HT_2$ receptor subtypes (Peroutka and Snyder, 1979; Peroutka et al., 1979). By definition, $5\text{-}HT_1$ receptors stimulate an adenylate cyclase, whereas $5\text{-}HT_2$ receptors are not linked to this enzyme. Presently, no functional in vitro model is available to measure responses mediated by $5\text{-}HT_2$ receptors in the CNS.

In homogenates of rat hippocampus, both dopamine and serotonin stimulate adenylate cyclase activity, suggesting the presence of D_1 and $5\text{-}HT_1$ receptors. In the presence of the selective D_1 receptor antagonist bulbocapnine, the activity of the dopamine-sensitive adenylate cyclase was nearly abolished, whereas that one of the serotonin-sensitive adenylate cyclase remained unaffected.

In the presence of bulbocapnine, Hydergine stimulated the serotonin-sensitive adenylate cyclase in homogenates of rat hippocampus to a smaller degree than serotonin, but was also able to antagonise the stimulating effect of a high concentration of the latter (Figure 30-5). This suggests that Hydergine also has mixed agonist/antagonist properties at 5-HT_1 receptors in the hippocampus.

Serotonin-agonistic effects of Hydergine have also been reported from animal studies. In cats, whose central serotonin stores have been depleted by reserpine, repetitive electric potentials can be recorded from brain regions such as pons, lateral geniculate, body and occipital cortex. It has been suggested that these so-called PGO waves are triggered by a central pacemaker which is under an inhibitory serotoninergic control (Jouvet, 1972). In this model, Hydergine, similar to the serotonin precursor 5-hydroxytryptophan, reduced the number of PGO waves in a dose-dependent manner. This effect could be antagonised by the serotonin receptor antagonist methiothepin, providing evidence for the involvement of central serotonin receptors (Züger et al., 1978).

Furthermore, Hydergine has been reported to decrease serotonin turnover in the rat brain cortex (Bürki et al., 1978), probably by activating presynaptic serotonin autoreceptors (Engel et al., 1983).

Effects of Hydergine in Noradrenergic Systems

It is generally accepted that the physiologic effects of noradrenaline are mediated by α- and β-adrenergic receptors. Ligand binding studies indicate that Hydergine has affinity to α-adrenoceptors, but not to β-adrenoceptors. Based on pharmacologic differences, α-adrenoceptors in the periphery have been subdivided into α_1 and α_2 types (Berthelsen and Pettinger, 1977). The same α-adrenoceptor subtypes appear to be present also in the CNS (U'Prichard et al., 1977). Results from ligand-binding studies following surgical noradrenergic denervation suggest that in the rat cortex, α_1-adrenoceptors occur on postsynaptic elements, whereas α_2-adrenoceptors are located both on noradrenergic terminals and on postsynaptic elements (Morris et al., 1981). In slices of rat brain cortex, α_1-adrenoceptors have been shown to be involved in mediating noradrenaline-induced cyclic AMP formation (Daly et al., 1981), whereas presynaptic α_2-adrenoceptors appear to regulate evoked noradrenaline release from nerve terminals in an inhibitory manner (Starke, 1977). In rat cerebral cortex slices, Hydergine alone had no measurable effect on cyclic AMP formation, but antagonized the stimulating effect of noradrenaline in a way typical for a noncompetitive antagonist (Markstein and Wagner, 1978). Moreover, Hydergine facilitated electrically evoked noradrenaline release from rat cerebral occipital cortex slices and this effect could be antagonized by the selective α_2-adrenoceptor agonist clonidine in a

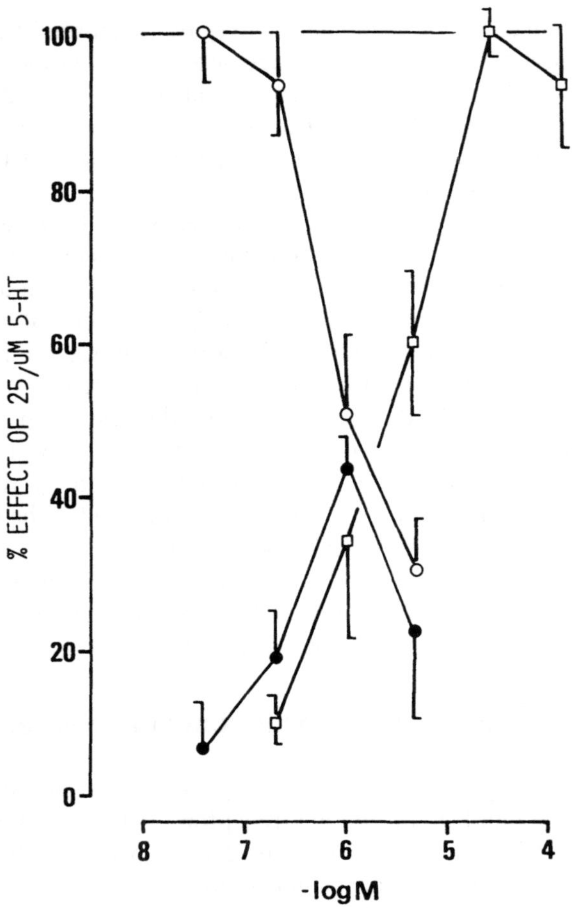

Figure 30-5. Effect of various concentrations of serotonin (-□-) and Hydergine alone (-●-) and Hydergine in combination with 25 μM serotonin (-○-) on cyclic AMP formation in homogenates of rat hippocampus in the presence of 10 μM Bulbocapnine ($5\text{-}HT_1$ receptor test). Results are expressed as percentage of the maximal stimulation elicited by 25 μM serotonin in the presence of 10 μM Bulbocapnine. Means ± S.E.M. of three experiments.

competitive manner (Figure 30-6A) (Markstein et al., 1983). This suggests that Hydergine is also an antagonist at α_2-adrenoceptors. The affinity measures of Hydergine to α_1- and α_2-adrenoceptors estimated in the functional tests suggest that Hydergine has a higher affinity to α_2-adrenoceptors (Figures 30-6A,B).

Drug effects on central α-adrenoceptors in vivo are not so easy to demonstrate since there is no specific behavior mediated by noradrenaline. However, Olpe and Steinmann (1982) recently reported that after

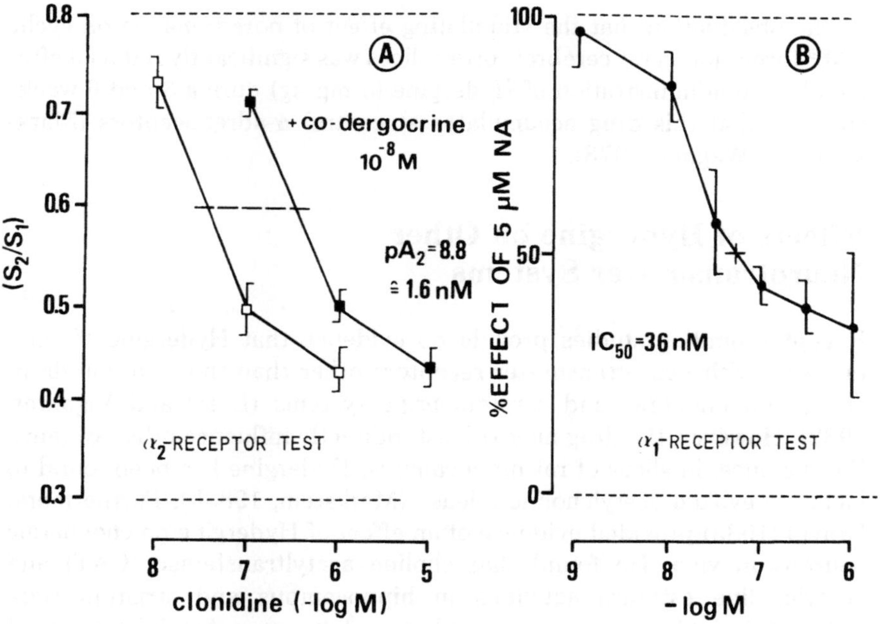

Figure 30-6.A. Effect of clonidine alone (-□-) and in combination with 10^{-8} M Co-dergocrine (Hydergine) (-■-) on electrically-evoked tritium overflow from [^{3}H]noradrenaline-prelabelled rat cerebral occipital cortex slices (test for presynaptic α-adrenoceptors, α_2-type). [^{3}H]noradrenaline-prelabelled rat cerebral occipital cortex slices were superfused and stimulated electrically for 2 min in the absence of drugs (S_1) and 75 min later in the presence of drugs. Results are ratios of tritium overflow evoked by S_2 to that evoked by S_1 (S_2/S_1). The pA_2-value was calculated from the shift of the concentration response curve of clonidine induced by a fixed concentration of Hydergine, according to Schild (1949). B. Effect of various concentrations of Hydergine on noradrenaline-induced cyclic AMP formation in slices of rat cerebral occipital cortex slices (test for antagonistic effects at postsynaptic α-adrenoceptors, α_1-type). IC_{50}-value corresponds to the drug concentration where the stimulating effect of 5 μM noradrenaline was inhibited by 50%.

intraperitoneal administration of Hydergine in doses from 0.3–10 mg/kg, increases of the firing rate of locus coeruleus neurons are seen. It was suggested that this effect of Hydergine is due to its antagonistic effects at soma-dendritic α-adrenoceptors which regulate the firing rate of noradrenergic neurons in an inhibitory manner. Furthermore, at high parenteral doses, Hydergine increased noradrenaline turnover in the rat brain stem, which is consistent with its antagonistic effects at presynaptic α_2-adrenoceptors (Bürki et al., 1978).

The observation that the stimulating effect of noradrenaline on cyclic AMP formation in rat cerebral cortex slices was significantly reduced after a daily oral administration of Hydergine (3 mg/kg) during 3 and 6 weeks suggests that this drug accumulates at central α-adrenoceptors (Markstein and Wagner, 1978).

Effects of Hydergine on Other Neurotransmitter Systems

Receptor binding studies provide no evidence that Hydergine directly interacts with neurotransmitter receptors other than those in noradrenergic, dopaminergic, and serotoninergic systems (Loew and Vigouret, 1982). However, the drug may at least indirectly influence other systems. For instance, in slices of rat hippocampus, Hydergine has been found to facilitate evoked acetylcholine release (Markstein, 1983b). Furthermore, Dravid (1983) provided evidence of an effect of Hydergine on cholinergic neurons in vivo. He found that choline acetyltransferase (CAT) and acetylcholine esterase activities in hippocampus and striatum were reduced in old rats as compared to adult rats. Administration of Hydergine in a daily oral dose of 3 mg/kg over 4 weeks significantly increased CAT activity in old animals in both brain regions to levels almost identical to adult control rats, whereas in adult animals, no change of CAT activity was found. These results indicate that Hydergine may also indirectly affect cholinergic systems.

Conclusion

The presented pharmacologic data show that Hydergine has multiple effects on various subtypes of monoaminergic receptors. At dopaminergic and serotoninergic receptor subtypes, it has mixed agonistic/antagonistic properties. Hydergine might therefore be able to compensate for a deficit of dopamine or serotonin in one brain region and, at the same time, counteract an overactivity of the same transmitter system in other brain regions. The noradrenergic system could be affected in a similar way, however, by a different mechanism of action. Thus, Hydergine increases evoked noradrenaline release from nerve terminals by blocking presynaptic α_2-adrenoceptors, but at the same time by blocking postsynaptic α_1-adrenoceptors in a noncompetitive manner sets a ceiling effect to the noradrenergic stimulation. Hydergine appears therefore to be able to restore the balance in the interplay between the different monoaminergic systems. Furthermore, Hydergine appears also to indirectly influence cholinergic systems. In analogy to a chemical buffer system, Hydergine could therefore be understood to act as a synaptic buffer system which could be the basis of its therapeutic effects in senile mental impairment.

References

Adolfsson, R., Gottfries, C.G,. Roos, B.E., and Winblad, B.: Post-mortem distribution of dopamine and homovanillic acid in human brain, variations related to age, and a review of the literature. *J. Neural. Transm. 45*, 81–105 (1979).

Anden, N.E., Carlsson, A., and Häggendal, J.: Adrenergic mechanisms. *Ann. Rev. Pharmacol. 9*, 119–134 (1969).

Azmitia, E.C.: The serotonin-producing neurons of the midbrain median and dorsal raphe nuclei. In Handbook of Psychopharmacology, Vol. 9, pp. 233–314. New York, Plenum, 1978.

Beart, P.: Multiple dopamine receptors—new vistas. *Trends in Pharmacol. Sci. 5*, 100–102 (1982).

Berthelsen, S., and Pettinger, W.A.: A functional basis for classification of α-adrenergic receptors. *Life Sci. 21*, 595–606 (1977).

Bürki, H.R., Asper, H., Ruch, W., and Züger, P.E.: Bromocriptine, dihydroergotoxine, methysergide, d-LSD, CF 25-397 and 29-712: Effects on the metabolism of the biogenic amines in the brain of the rat. *Psychopharmacology 57*, 227–237 (1978).

Carlsson, A.: Age-dependent changes in central dopaminergic and other monoaminergic systems. *Adv. Exp. Med. Bio. 113*, 1–13 (1978).

Carlsson, A., Adolfson, R., Aquilonius, S.M., Gottfries, C.G., Orland, L., Svennerholm, L., and Winblad, B.: Biogenic amines in human brain in normal aging, senile dementia and chronic alcoholism. In Ergot Compounds and Brain Function: Neuroendocrine and Neuropsychiatric Aspects, pp. 295–304. New York: Raven, 1979.

Closse, A., Frick, W., Hauser, D., and Sauter, A.: Characterisation of ^{3}H-bromocriptine binding to calf caudate membranes. In Psychopharmacology and Biochemistry of Neurotransmitter Receptors, pp. 463–474. New York: Elsevier/North Holland, 1980.

Cools, A.R., and Van Rossum, J.M.: Multiple receptors for brain dopamine in behavior regulation: Concept of dopamine-E and dopamine-J receptors. *Life Sci. 27*, 1237–1253 (1980).

Daly, J.W., Padgett, W., Creveling, C.R., Cantacuzene, D., and Kirch, K.L.: Cyclic AMP generating systems: Regional differences in activation by adrenergic receptors in rat brain. *J. Neurosci. 1*, 49–59 (1981).

Dravid, A.R.: Deficits in cholinergic enzymes and muscarinic receptors in the hippocampus and striatum of senescent rats. Effect of chronic Hydergine treatment. *Arch. Int. Pharmacodyn. Ther. 264*, 195–202 (1983).

Engel, G., Göthert, M., Müller-Schweinitzer, E., Schlicker, E., Sistonen, L., and Stadler, P.A.: Evidence for common pharmacological properties of [^{3}H]5-hydroxytryptamine binding sites, presynaptic 5-hydroxytryptamine autoreceptors in CNS and inhibitor presynaptic 5-hydroxytryptamine receptors on sympathetic nerves. *Naunyn-Schmiedeberg's Arch. Pharmacol. 324*, 116–124 (1983).

Garau, L., Govani, S., Stefanini, E., Trabucchi, M., and Spano, P.F.: Dopamine receptors: Pharmacological and anatomical evidences indicate that two distinct dopamine receptor populations are present in rat striatum. *Life Sci.* *23*, 1745–1750 (1978).

Goldstein, M., Lew, J.Y., Hata, F., and Lieberman, A.: Binding interactions of ergot alkaloids with monoaminergic receptors in the brain. *Gerontology* *24* (Suppl. 1), 76–85 (1978).

Gottfries, C.G.: The metabolism of some neurotransmitters in aging and dementia disorders. *Gerontology* *28* (Suppl. 2), 11–19 (1982).

Helmreich, J., Reimann, W., Hertting, G., and Starke, K.: Are presynaptic dopamine autoreceptors and postsynaptic dopamine receptors in the rabbit caudate nucleus pharmacologically different? *Neuroscience* *7*, 1559–1566 (1982).

Jouvet, J.: The role of monoamines and acetylcholine containing neurons in the regulation of the sleep–waking cycle. *Erg. Physiol.* *64*, 166–307 (1972).

Kebabian, J.W., and Calne, D.B.: Multiple receptors for dopamine. *Nature* *277*, 93–96 (1979).

Loew, D., Vigouret, J.M., and Jaton, A.L.: Neuropharmacological investigations with two ergot alkaloids, Hydergine and bromocriptine. *Postgrad. Med. J.* *52* (Suppl. 1), 40–46 (1976).

Loew, D.M., and Vigouret, J.M.: Neuropharmakologische Charakterisierung von Dihydroergotoxin (Hydergin). In Mutterkornalkaloide heute, pp. 69–79. Stuttgart: Georg Thieme, 1982.

Loew, D., and Weil, C.: Hydergine® in senile mental impairment. *Gerontology* *28*, 54–74 (1982).

Markstein, R., and Wagner, H.: Effect of dihydroergotoxine on cyclic AMP generating systems in rat cerebral cortex slices. *Gerontology* *24* (Suppl. 1), 94–105 (1978).

Markstein, R.: Dopamine receptor profile of Co-dergocrine (Hydergine®) and its components. *European J. Pharmacol.* *86*, 145–155 (1983a).

Markstein, R.: Co-dergocrine has multiple effects on monoaminergic neurotransmission. *Fed. Proc.* *42*, 496 (1983b).

Markstein, R., Closse, A., and Frick, W.: Interaction of ergot alkaloids and their combination (Co-dergocrine) with α-adrenoceptors in the CNS. *European J. Pharmacol.* *93*, 156–169 (1983).

McGeer, E.G., and McGeer, P.L.: Neurotransmitter metabolism in the aging brain. In Neurobiology of Aging, pp. 389–403. New York: Raven, 1976.

McGeer, E.G.: Neurotransmitter systems in aging and senile dementia. *Progr. Neuro-Psychopharmacol.* *5*, 435–445 (1981).

Morris, M.J., Elkozi, J.L., Dausse, J.P., and Meyer, P.: α_1- and α_2-adrenoceptors in rat cerebral cortex. Effect of lobotomy. *Naunyn-Schmiedeberg's Arch. Pharmacol.* *316*, 424 (1981).

Nieuwenhuys, R., Voogd, J., and Van Huijzen, Chr.: The Human Central Nervous System. Berlin: Springer-Verlag, 1978.

Olpe, H.R., and Steinmann, M.W.: The effect of vincamine, Hydergine and piracetom on the firing rate of Locus coeruleus neurons. *Behav. Neural. Biol.* *33*, 249–251 (1982).

Peroutka, S.J., and Snyder, S.H.: Multiple serotonin receptors: Differential binding of [^{3}H]serotonin, [^{3}H]lysergic acid diethylamide and [^{3}H]spiroperidol. *Molec. Pharmacol. 16*, 687–699 (1979).

Peroutka, S.J., Lebowitz, R.M., and Snyder, S.H.: Two distinct central serotonin receptors with different physiological functions. *Science 212*, 827–829 (1979).

Pradhan, S.N.: Central neurotransmitter and aging. *Life Sci. 26*, 1643–1656 (1980).

Reader, T.A., Ferron, A., Descanies, L., and Jasper, H.H.: Modulatory role of biogenic amines in the cerebral cortex. Microiontophoretic studies. *Brain Res. 160*, 217–229 (1979).

Schild, H.O.: pA and competitive drug antagonism. *Br. J. Pharmacol. 4*, 277–280 (1949).

Starke, K.: Regulation of noradrenaline release by presynaptic receptor systems. *Rev. Physiol. Biochem. Pharmacol.* 77, 1–124 (1977).

Starke, K., Reimann, W., Zumstein, A., and Hertting, G.: Effect of dopamine agonists and antagonists on release of dopamine in the rabbit caudate nucleus in vitro. *Naunyn-Schmiedeberg's Arch. Pharmacol. 305*, 27–36 (1978).

Stoof, J.C., Thieme, R.E., Vrijmoed-De Vries, M.C., and Mulder, A.H.: In vitro acetylcholine release from rat caudate nucleus as a new model for testing drugs with dopamine receptor activity. *Naunyn-Schmiedeberg's Arch. Pharmacol. 309*, 119–124 (1979).

U'Prichard, D.C., Greenberg, D.A., and Snyder, S.H.: Binding characteristics of a radiolabelled agonist and antagonist at central nervous system. Alpha-noradrenergic receptors. *Mol. Pharmacol. 27*, 454–473 (1977).

Venn, R.D.: Clinical pharmacology of ergot alkaloids in senile cerebral insufficiency. In Ergot Alkaloids and Related Compounds, pp. 533–566. New York: Springer-Verlag, 1978.

Vigouret, J.M., Bürki, H.R., Jaton, A.L., Züger, P.E., and Loew, D.M.: Neurochemical and neuropharmacological investigations with four ergot derivatives: Bromocriptine, dihydroergotoxine, CF 25-397 and CM 29-712. *Pharmacology 16* (Suppl. 1), 156–173 (1978).

Vigouret, J.M., Jaton, A.L., and Loew, D.: Increased sensitivity after repeated administration of ergot derivatives in rats. *Experientia 35*, 953 (1979).

Woodward, C., Moises, H.C., Waterhouse, P.D., Hoffer, B., and Freedman, R.: Modulatory actions of norepinephrine in the central nervous system. *Fed. Proc. 38*, 2109–2116 (1979).

Züger, P.E., Vigouret, J.M., and Loew, D.M.: Inhibition of reserpine-induced PGO-waves in the cat by ergot derivatives. *Experientia 34*, 637–639 (1978).

Chapter 31

Implications of Long-Term Study of Hydergine in Elderly Patients with Chronic Senile Cerebral Insufficiency

S. Chierichetti, D. Cucinotta, and V. Santini

Summary

A total of 559 patients entered a multicenter double-blind trial to compare the effects of Hydergine and placebo in long-term (1 year) treatment of chronic senile cerebral insufficiency (CSCI). A battery of tests (SCAG, Geriatric Rating Scales, NUDS, Nowlis, Birren, digit-symbol substitution, digit-span, Toulouse-Pieron) was used before starting treatment to select the patients, and was done again after 1, 3, 6, and 12 months of treatment with placebo or Hydergine, 1.5 mg, t.i.d. p.o. Data from 388 patients who completed 6 months of treatment and from 204 patients who completed 1 year of treatment show that after the first month both placebo- and Hydergine-treated patients improved but, at 6 months and 1 year only patients on Hydergine had improved and patients on placebo had worsened. Thus the usefulness of Hydergine in the treatment of mild-to-moderate CSCI has been confirmed.

Progress in medical science during the past 40 years has significantly increased average human life expectancy and, of course, the number of individuals who now reach geriatric status. Thus, all populations are getting older, and this fact has increased the problems of aging, which are often problems of the aging brain.

The deterioration of mental functioning with age is one of the greatest problems facing the world at the present time, and it will increase considerably in the future (Lloyd, Brocklehurst, Palmer, 1978; Rabins, Mace, and Lucas, 1982).

The most realistic goal, at least for the moment, is to reduce the clinical manifestations of decline not only of the "pathologically" aged brain but also of the "normal" aged brain (Zarifian, 1982). Thus the hope for the immediate future is to preserve mental, cognitive, and neurological functions, so that the elderly may remain self-sufficient in the late life.

The management of these people, and particularly of those who have experienced mild-to-moderate deterioration of cerebral functions, variously defined as chronic brain failure (Isaacs, Caird, 1976), organic brain syndrome (Gaitz, Varner, Overall, 1977), and chronic senile cerebral insufficiency (CSCI) (Venn, 1978; Lazzari et al., 1983), must consist of multiple interventions (Table 31-1).

The principal and apparently simplest tool of this type of care should be pharmacotherapy, but at present no drug reverses the aging process, nor is it likely that such a medication will be discovered in the near future (Yesavage, Westphal, and Rush, 1981).

There are, however, some drugs that may be useful, even if they are effective in treating only some symptoms of older patients who have CSCI.

We believe that, for these patients and also for persons undergoing normal aging of the brain, specific medical intervention is not only justified but necessary (Zarifian, 1982) and should be based on the use of specific drugs (e.g., Hydergine) that act on the pathogenic factors, particularly on the imbalance of neurotransmitters and neuropeptides (Gottfries, 1982). In a large number of controlled clinical trials of Hydergine, many patients with CSCI have shown improvement and good tolerance of the drug (Banen, 1972; Bazo, 1973; Ditch, Kelly, and Resnick, 1971; Gerin, 1969; Jennings, 1972; McConnachie, 1973; Rehman, 1973; Rosen, 1975), probably as a result of multiple effects. The drug interacts directly with 1- and 2-adrenoceptors, dopamine, and serotonin-receptor subtypes, with a clear dopaminergic mechanism of action and the possibility that it plays a predominant role in the equilibrium between various transmitters in the central nervous system (CNS) (Spano et al., 1983; Fuxe et al., 1983; Hruska et al., 1983; Fanchamps, 1983; Exton-Smith et al., 1983).

Another suggested pharmacodynamic effect of this drug is an increased firing rate of neurons in the locus ceruleus (Gottfries, 1982).

Nevertheless, the use of Hydergine is still controversial. We therefore conducted another long-term, double-blind study to evaluate the results and implications of this therapy in a large group of selected elderly patients suffering from mild to moderate CSCI. Fifty centers throughout Italy were asked to take part in the study; those that accepted were

Table 31-1. Multiple and global interventions for the patients with chronic senile cerebral insufficiency

Complete clinical evaluation and psychological approach

↑

Financial and social intervention ← Patients suffering from C.S.C.I. need → Aids and environmental adaptation

↓

Global Medical Care

1. For associated problems (infections and cardiovascular, respiratory, genitourinary, endocrine, metabolic, haematologic, muscoloskeletal disease, etc.)
2. For dehydration and electrolyte disturbances
3. Against recumbency and prolonged immobilisation
4. For psychic disturbances (i.e., anxiety, depression, etc.)
5. Aimed at neuronal functioning and cerebral metabolic improvement, based on timely and specific therapeutic intervention

required to treat at least 10 patients for 1 year. The data obtained from preliminary observations after 1, 3, and 6 months of therapy have been published (Lazzari et al., 1983), but we now wish to report and discuss the results after 1 year of treatment.

Materials and Methods

The protocol of this study and the criteria for patient selection were defined in discussion with all the invited centers during four regional meetings in Italy before the trial began. It was carried out in accordance with the ethical and scientific principles of the Declaration of Helsinki, and with consideration of the possibility of improving the quality of later life.

Patients were not included if they (a) had severe concomitant hepatic, renal, or cardiac illness; (b) had a psychotic disease or recent, and not yet stabilized, central vascular or traumatic accidents; (c) had tremors, involuntary movements, blindness, deafness, or other physical disabilities that could interfere with the execution of the tests; or (d) were undergoing treatment involving any drug that might interfere at the CNS level.

The main criterion for admission to the study was a score of 3–5 on 7 of the 18 items on the Sandoz Clinical Assessment Geriatric rating scale (SCAG). The seven items were confusion, impaired alertness, reduced recent memory, disorientation, anxiety, depressed mood, and emotional lability.

The patients were screened for 10 days before starting treatment. After a washout period during which patients were not allowed to take any CNS-active drugs, the patients took a battery of tests (Table 31-2) to evaluate their basal profiles. The rationale for choosing these tests was as follows:

1. The SCAG scale can be considered a valid instrument in the light of the most recent literature and as demonstrated by its wide use. It is evident now that the scale provides a reliable and valid method for assessing psychopathology in elderly patients (Hamilton, 1982).
2. The GRS measures the response of patients to their environment.
3. The NUDS offers a detailed behavior description.
4. The Nowlis mood adjective checklist has good factorial validity.
5. The Mental Status Evaluation explores short- and long-term memory and spatiotemporal orientation.
6. The digit-symbol substitution test is the most age-sensitive instrument and its results are influenced significantly by motor persistence, sustained attention, and response speed, but not by learning (Lezak, 1976).
7. The digit-span subtest indicates short-term memory and/or attention.
8. The Tolouse–Pieron test is frequently used for the elderly as a task of attention and concentration and indicates the patient's mental status.

Patients were assigned randomly to treatment with Hydergine, 1.5 mg three times per day, or an indistinguishable placebo three times per day.

Table 31-2. Battery of rating scales and psychometric tests

1. Sandoz Clinical Assessment Geriatric Rating Scale (SCAG).
2. Geriatric Rating Scales (Bronx State Hospital).
3. Northwestern University Disability Scales (NUDS).
4. A Simplification of the Nowlis Mood Adjective Checklist.
5. Mental status evaluation (after Birren).
6. Digit-symbol Association Subtest from the WAIS.
7. Digit-span Subtest from the WAIS (digit forward and backward).
8. Toulouse-Pieron Test.

After the trial started in January 1981, data were collected monthly during the first 6 month period and bimonthly during the second 6 month period. An assistant of the Sandoz Medical Department in Italy visited all centers monthly to solve any research problems and to collect the patients' forms.

By August 31, 1982, 559 patients had entered the study and 458 were still under treatment; 101 had dropped out. Of those in the study, 388 were treated for 6 months (195 with Hydergine, 193 with placebo) and 204 were treated for 1 year (111 with Hydergine, 93 with placebo).

Statistical Analysis

Data collected from 388 patients who completed 6 months treatment and from 204 patients who completed 1 year of treatment were analyzed statistically. Student's t-test for paired data was used to compare the post-treatment mean value with the pretreatment mean value of the SCAG score after 1 month of treatment. At 3, 6, and 12 months, the mean values of scores obtained with SCAG and other tests by the placebo and Hydergine groups were compared with Student's t-test. The statistical analysis was undertaken to attempt to answer three main questions: Did Hydergine-treated patients improve more than placebo patients on any specific symptom or function? Did they deteriorate less than the placebo group? Were the results different than one expected simply from a general placebo effect?

Results

The number of patients under treatment obviously decreased over time, but of the 204 who reached the end point of 1 year, 111 were treated with Hydergine.

Considering the main characteristics of the patient sample, it is possible to see that the two groups (Hydergine and placebo) were homogeneous on all variables taken into account (Table 31-3).

From basal values on the rating scales, we can describe the "average patient" of the elderly research population as having (a) a mild-to-moderate degree of CSCI, according to the SCAG score and clinical assessment on admission; (b) a fairly good degree of self-sufficiency, as assessed by the geriatric rating scale; (c) moderate degrees of mental deterioration, with marked deficits in initiative, cooperation, sociability, motivation, and indifference to surroundings. During the trial these patients presented some modifications of their clinical picture, which were documented by the variation of the findings of tests and rating scales. The data are reported below.

Table 31-3. Main characteristics of patients who completed 6 months and 1 year of treatment with placebo or Hydergene, 1.5 mg t.i.d.

	6 months		1 year	
	PL	HYG	PL	HYG
No. of patients (m/f)	193 (82/111)	195 (73/122)	93 (37/56)	111 (38/73)
Inpatients/outpatients	123/70	121/74	55/38	58/53
Mean age (SD)	75.9 (7.8)	76 (7.5)	76 (7.9)	75.8 (6.9)
Educational level (%) elementary/medium/higher	78/15/7	79/16/5	78/16/6	79/15/6
Economic conditions (%) insuff./suff./good	13/74/14	14/74/12	14/70/16	14/71/15
Intellectual level (%) bad/fair/good	25/65/10	26/63/11	10/61/30	12/71/27
Concomitant illness (No.): 0/1/2	30/107/56	28/104/63	13/49/31	17/57/37
Concomitant chronic therapy (No.): 0/1/2	48/93/52	39/100/56	22/41/30	21/54/36

Sandoz Clinical Assessment Geriatric Rating Scale (SCAG)

The 18 items of the SCAG scale were analyzed by the cluster procedure of Gaitz et al. (1977):

a. Agitation/irritability (items: emotional lability, irritability, bothersomeness, hostility, uncooperativeness);
b. Cognitive dysfunction (items: confusion, reduced recent memory, reduced mental alertness, disorientation, reduced self-care);
c. Mood depression (items: anxiety, mood depression, fatigue, anorexia, dizziness);
d. Withdrawal (items: lack of motivation, indifference to surroundings, lack of initiative, unsociability).

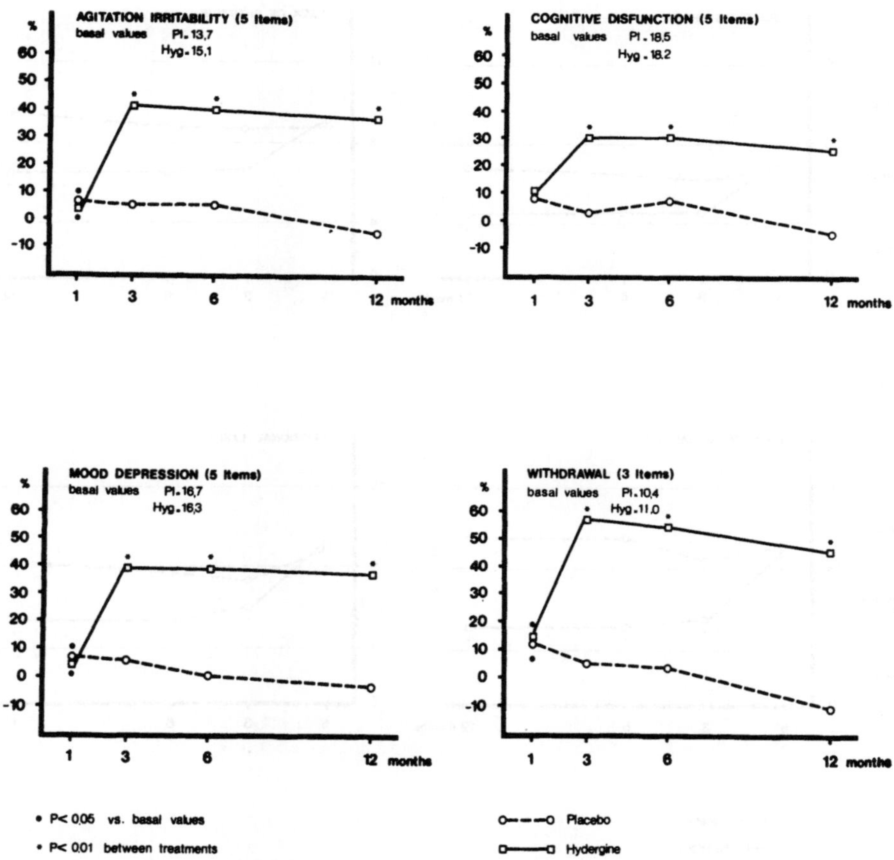

Figure 31-1. Mean percentage increases (+) or decreases (−) from basal values for SCAG items, clustered into four factors after 1, 3, 6, and 12 months of treatment with placebo or Hydergine, 1.5 mg t.i.d.

All factors, except cognitive dysfunction (Figure 31-1), showed improvement in both groups at 1 month after admission. From the third month up to 1 year, however, the factors for patients treated with placebo were unchanged or became worse, while patients treated with Hydergine had improved by 30% at 12 months on the cognitive dysfunction factor, and by 57% at 3 months on the withdrawal factor.

Geriatric Rating Scale

Scores on the geriatric rating scales by Hydergine-treated patients (Figure 31-2) also improved by the end of the third month of treatment. The patients' lack of initiative, lack of sociability, and emotional lability were

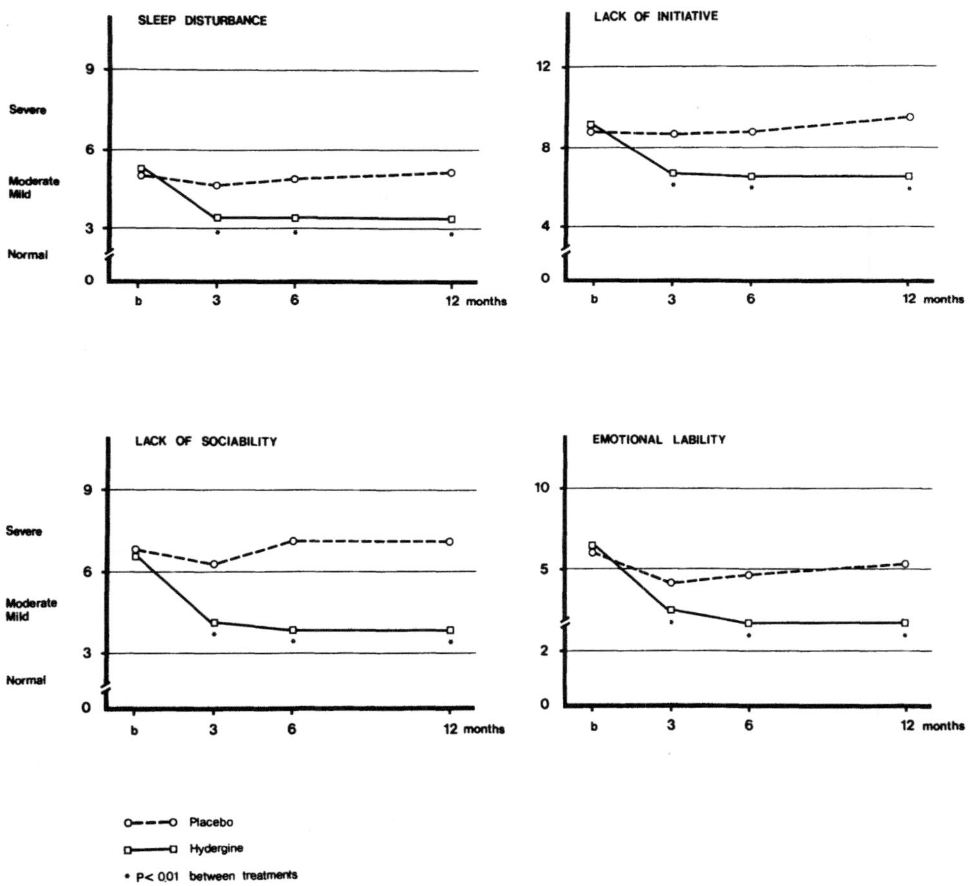

Figure 31-2. Mean raw scores for items of the geriatric rating scales before (b) and after 3, 6, and 12 months of treatment with placebo or Hydergine, 1.5 mg t.i.d.

especially improved, and we observed a shift from severe to mild-to-moderate status that is the normal condition for a patient population like ours.

Mental Status (Birren) Test

On the Birren test (Figure 31-3), significant improvement was seen in the Hydergine group in retention and in space–time orientation, from poor to good. Not clinically important, although statistically significant, were improvements in both remote and recent memory.

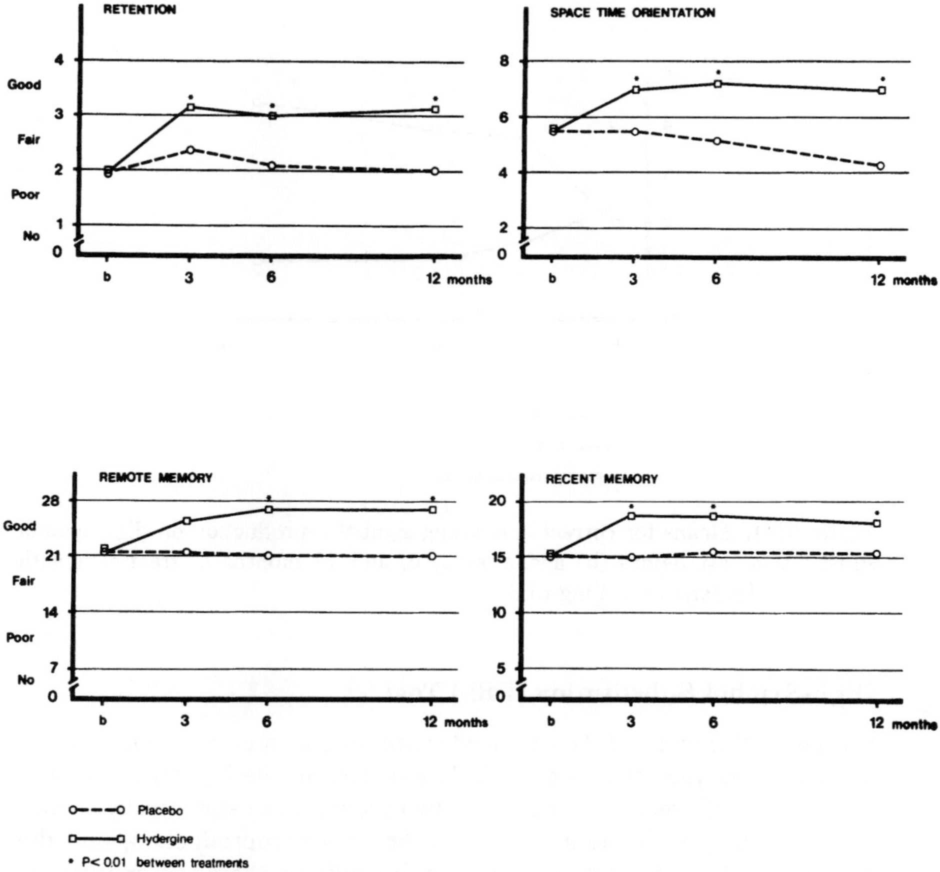

Figure 31-3. Mean raw scores for items of the Birren test before (b) and after 3, 6, and 12 months of treatment with placebo or Hydergine, 1.5 mg t.i.d.

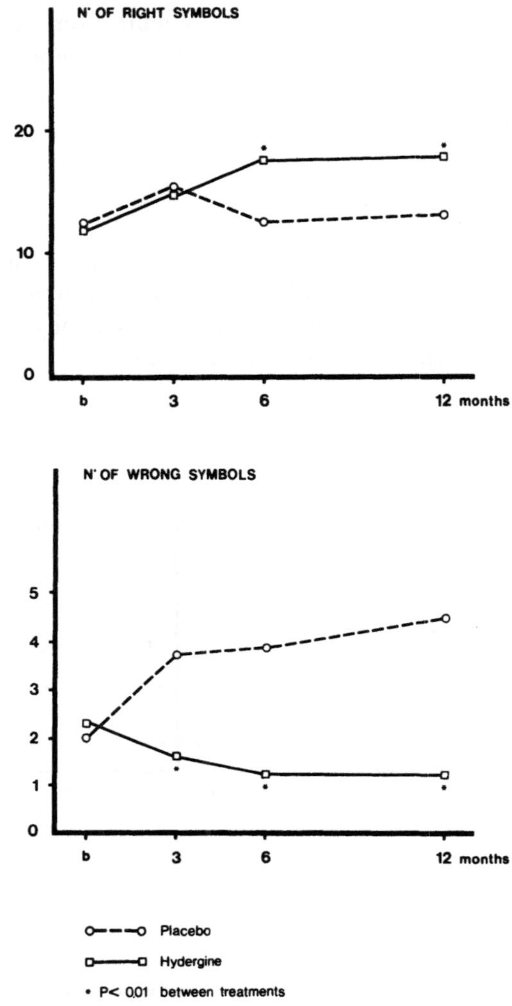

Figure 31-4. Means for correct and wrong symbol reproduction on digit-symbol substitution test before (b) and after 3, 6, and 12 months of treatment with placebo or Hydergine, 1.5 mg t.i.d.

Digit-Symbol Substitution (DSS) Test

On the DSS (Figure 31-4) increased reproduction of correct symbols and decreased copying of wrong symbols was seen in the Hydergine-treated group. The differences between the two groups were statistically significant beginning with the sixth month for correct reproduction, and the third month for incorrect reproduction. In addition, there was an increase

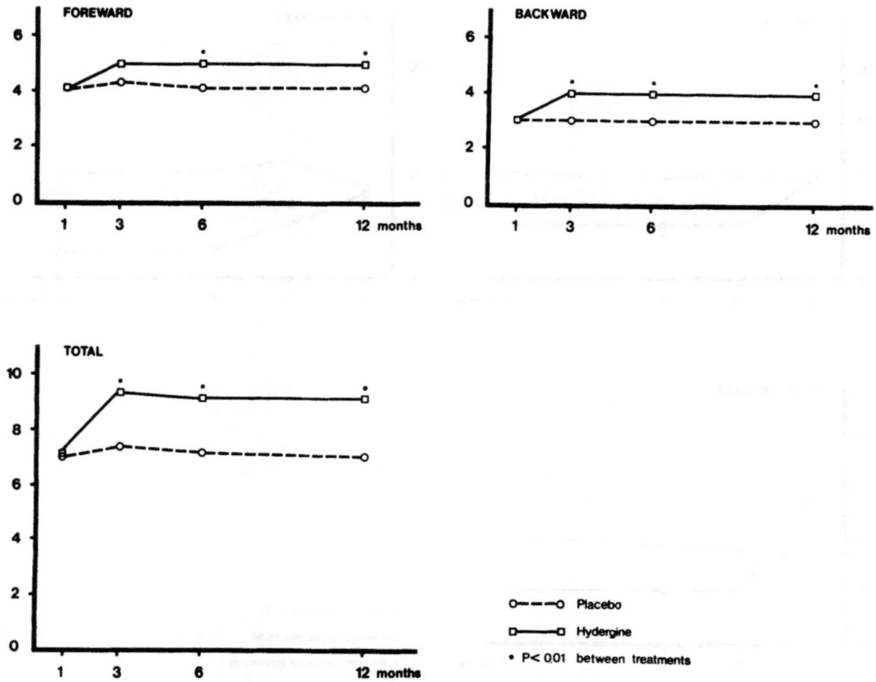

Figure 31-5. Mean forward, backward, and total digit span before (b) and after 3, 6, and 12 months of treatment with placebo or Hydergine, 1.5 mg t.i.d.

(not statistically significant) in the number of patients who performed the test within 2 minutes.

Digit-Span Test

Patients treated with Hydergine improved more than did those taking placebo in both forward and backward repetition of digits (Figure 31-5). The differences between the two groups were statistically significant from the sixth month for forward repetition and the third month for backward repetition.

Toulouse-Pieron Test

With the Toulouse-Pieron test (Figure 31-6), by the third month of treatment, patients on Hydergine required less time to perform the test, and made fewer mistakes and fewer omissions. In addition, as an indication of increased initiative, the percentage of patients who per-

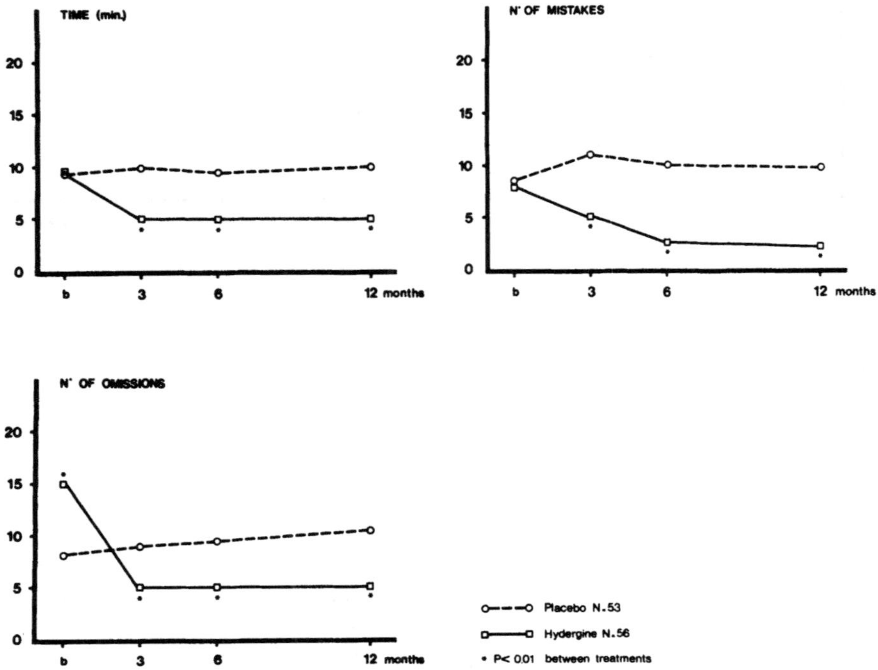

Figure 31-6. Mean time required to perform Toulouse-Pieron test, mean number of mistakes, and omissions before (b) and after 3, 6, and 12 months of treatment with placebo or Hydergine, 1.5 mg t.i.d.

formed the test was significantly higher after treatment with Hydergine than was the case for the placebo group.

Overall Clinical Judgment

The physicians' and relatives' overall clinical assessments of patients scored as "improved," "unchanged," or "worsened" agree well with the results of all tests (Figure 31-7). Physicians and relatives both found that Hydergine was better able than placebo to cause improvement and that the placebo-treated patients often deteriorated more than those taking Hydergine. In addition, it is clear that more relatives than physicians were able to differentiate between Hydergine- and placebo-treated patients. This is not really surprising and is probably due to the fact that relatives know the patients better than physicians, and perhaps relatives have more faith in treatment.

Dropouts

The causes for patients' dropping out of the study are summarized in Table 31-4. Only three patients in the Hydergine group dropped out

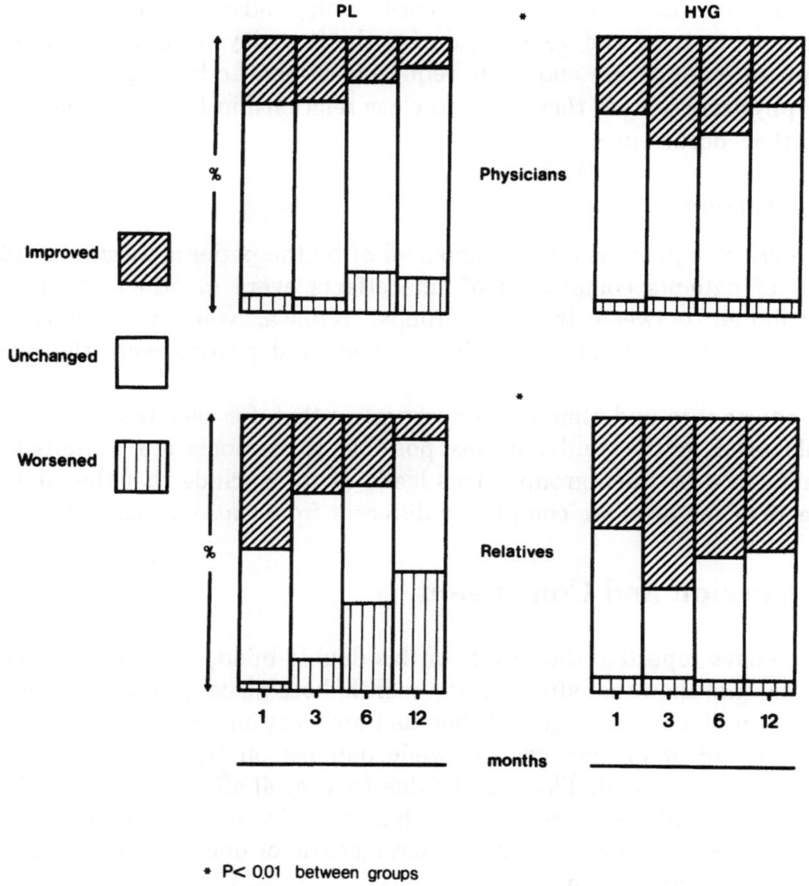

Figure 31-7. Mean percentage of overall clinical assessments by physicians and relatives as improved, unchanged, or deteriorated after 1, 3, 6, and 12 months of treatment with placebo or Hydergine, 1.5 mg t.i.d.

Table 31-4. Causes for dropout of patients treated with placebo or Hydergene, 1.5 mg t.i.d.

	Total	HYG	PL
Intercurrent illness	24	13	11
Exitus	23	14	9
Lack of activity	18	3	15
Refusal to continue	33	15	18
Side effects	3	3	—
Total	101 (18%)	48	53

because of side effects, which were mainly adverse gastrointestinal reactions (nausea and vomiting during the first days of administration). They were not severe enough to require treatment to be stopped and, as the physician stated, there was no clear relationship between treatment and their occurrence.

Side Effects

Side effects spontaneously complained of by the patients were rare (10–15% of patients complained of side effects every month) and equally distributed between the two groups. Nausea, vomiting, orthostatic hypotension, gastrointestinal disturbances, and pruritis were the main ones.

Important to underline is the observation that, for each test and rating scale used in the study, it was possible to demonstrate a statistical significance between groups. This leads us to conclude that the clinical effects of the drug are completely different from those of placebo.

Discussion and Conclusion

As we have reported, the results of this double-blind, placebo-controlled clinical trial show that after the first month, both placebo- and Hydergine-treated patients improved but that, as time went on, patients on placebo deteriorated or did not change, while patients on Hydergine improved (Lazzari et al., 1983). This may be due to a recall effect that, in the first part of the study, was present in both groups. As the trial continued, the progressive mental deterioration characteristic of dementia was reduced in the Hydergine group.

Some of the SCAG scores shifted the clinical assessments from "severe" to "normal." Lack of sociability, emotional lability, and initiative were influenced remarkably in the Hydergine-treated group.

The positive results on the SCAG scale are consistent with those of other tests, such as those for long- and short-term memory, the digit-symbol substitution test, digit span, Toulouse-Pieron, and space–time orientation. As an index of improved initiative and attention, there was a considerable increase in the percentage of patients treated with Hydergine whose performance on the digit-symbol substitution and Tolouse-Pieron tests improved.

Relatives and physicians noticed improvement in overall clinical condition and less deterioration in patients in the Hydergine-treated group, compared to those in the placebo group. Patients in the placebo group did not improve and, in fact, deteriorated more severely.

Therefore, the usefulness of Hydergine in the treatment of mild-to-moderate CSCI can be confirmed.

The findings reported here allow us to affirm that the drug is not fast acting and provokes clinically detectable effects after some months. Hydergine administration improves the main manifestations of CSCI, so that behavior and performance tend to conform to those normal for the patient's age. The drug is, therefore, useful for increasing self-sufficiency and for offering the possibility of rehabilitation, reactivation, and social reintegration of the elderly who may have seemed unmotivated toward rehabilitation because of age-specific changes in their cognitive functions (Hesse and Campion, 1983).

In the single patient, alteration in sensitivity to medication could be secondary to a variability in absorption, transport, metabolism, storage, and/or excretion that occur frequently as a consequence of aging.

In long-term treatment with Hydergine, attention to compliance factors is also crucial to obtaining the best possible results. The patient's understanding about prescription instructions and his or her ability to ingest the drug at prescribed times are essential to the success of the therapy. Because of this, great emphasis in treating patients suffering from CSCI must be given to educating the patient's family and all persons who take care of them.

Care of geriatric patients with CSCI must primarily take into account the necessity to modify their environmental and social conditions to gather some social, financial, or psychological support (Passeri and Cucinotta, 1981a,b, 1982). Dietary advice should be tailored to individual needs. These patients' global clinical picture may also be modified by a complete rehabilitation program, as well as by treatment of the dysfunction caused by extracerebral and cerebral illnesses with medication such as Hydergine.

Avoiding any discussion about the etiology of CSCI and theoretical consideration of the action of Hydergine, the results of this clinical study suggest that the drug has a greater effectiveness than placebo and may counteract the progressive evolution of primary dementias.

These results support the suggestion that pharmacotherapy of primary dementias may be successful, provided the distinct type of dementia is treated with an appropriate drug, the dementia is not chronic and severe, and drug treatment can be carried out over a period of weeks.

Therapeutic nihilism in regard to primary dementia is no longer justified (Hoyer et al., 1982). In late life, even if "the end is at hand," we may conclude that there is always some possibility of slowing the deterioration of the elderly person's quality of life.

In the light of our findings, we affirm that Hydergine will be useful for timely treatment of patients suffering from chronic senile cerebral insufficiency.

References

Banen, D.M.: An ergot preparation (Hydergine) for relief of symptoms of cerebrovascular insufficiency. *J. Am. Geriatr. Soc. 20*, 22–24 (1972).

Bazo, A.J.: An ergot alkaloid preparation (Hydergine) versus papaverine in treating common complaints of the aged: Double-blind study. *J. Am. Geriatr. Soc. 21*, 63–71 (1973).

Ditch, M., Kelly, F.J., and Resnick, O.: An ergot preparation (Hydergine) in the treatment of cerebrovascular disorders in the geriatric patient. Double-blind study. *J. Am. Geriatr. Soc. 19*, 208–217 (1971).

Exton-Smith, A.N., Piper, M., Phillips, M., and Simpson, J.: Clinical experiences with ergot alkaloids. In Agnoli, A., Crepaldi, G., Spano, P.F., and Trabucchi, M. (Eds.), Aging Brain and Ergot Alkaloids, Vol. 23, pp. 323–328. New York: Raven, 1983.

Fanchamps, A.: Dihydroergotoxine in senile cerebral insufficiency. In Agnoli, A., Crepaldi, G., Spano, P.F., and Trabucchi, M. (Eds.), Aging Brain and Ergot Alkaloids, Vol. 23, pp. 311–322. New York: Raven, 1983.

Fuxe, K., Agnati, L.F., Kohler, C., Ogren, S.O., Andersson, K., Benfenati, F., Calza, L., and Cimino, M.: Ergot drugs and cholecystokinin peptides as modulators of dopamine synapses in the brain. In Agnoli, A., Crepaldi, G., Spano, P.F., and Trabucchi, M. (Eds.), Aging Brain and Ergot Alkaloids, Vol. 23, pp. 179–201. New York: Raven, 1983.

Gaitz, C.M., Varner, R.V., and Overall, J.E.: Pharmacotherapy for organic brain syndrome in late life. Evaluation of an ergot derivative versus placebo. *Arch. Gen. Psychiatry 34*, 839–844 (1977).

Gerin, J.: Symptomatic treatment of cerebrovascular insufficiency with Hydergine. *Current Therapeutic Research 11*, 539–546 (1969).

Gottfries, C.G.: The metabolism of some neurotransmitters in aging and dementia disorders. *Gerontology 28* (Suppl. 2), 11–19 (1982).

Hamilton, M.: Use of rating scales in geriatric patients. *Gerontology 28* (Suppl. 2), 42–48 (1982).

Hesse, K.A., and Campion, E.W.: Motivating the geriatric patient for rehabilitation. *J. Am. Geriatr. Soc. 31* (10), 586–589 (1983).

Hoyer, S., OesterReich, K., and Wagner, O.: Pharmacotherapy of primary dementias in "energy transduction and neurotransmission." Proceedings of special point meeting of the European Society for Neurochemistry and the World Federation of Neurology, Rome, 1982, pp. 150–157.

Hruska, R.E., Weir, R., Pitman, K.T., and Silbergeld, E.K.: Ergot derivatives are potent drugs at CNS aminergic receptors: Correlations to behavior and aging. In Agnoli, A., Crepaldi, G., Spano, P.F., and Trabucchi, M. (Eds.), Aging Brain and Ergot Alkaloids, Vol. 23, pp. 215–226. New York: Raven, 1983.

Isaacs, B., and Caird, F.I.: Brain failure. A contribution to the terminology of mental abnormality in old age. *Age Ageing 5*, 241–244 (1976).

Jennings, W.G.: An ergot alkaloid preparation (Hydergine) versus placebo for treatment of symptoms of cerebrovascular insufficiency: Double-blind study. *J. Am. Geriatr. Soc. 20*, 407–412 (1972).

Lazzari, R., Franzese, A., Chierichetti, S.M., Vibelli, C., Rudelli, G., Passeri, M., and Cucinotta, D.: Multicenter double-blind placebo-controlled long-term clinical trial of Hydergine in chronic senile cerebral insufficiency: An interim report. In Agnoli, A., Crepaldi, G., Spano, P.F., and Trabucchi, M. (Eds.), Aging Brain and Ergot Alkaloids, Vol. 23, pp. 347–371. New York: Raven, 1983.

Lezak M.D.: Neuropsychological Assessment. New York: Oxford University Press, 1976.

Lloyd Evans, S., Brocklehurst, J.C., and Palmer, M.K.: Assessment of drug therapy in chronic brain failure. *Gerontology 24*, 304–311 (1978).

McConnachie, R.W.: A clinical trial comparing Hydergine with placebo in the treatment of cerebrovascular insufficiency in elderly patients. *Current Medical Research Opinion 1*, 463–468 (1973).

Passeri, M., and Cucinotta, D.: Principles and methods of evaluating mental disorders in the aged and the modification following drug administration. In The Aging Brain—Neurological and Mental Disturbances, p. 275. New York: Plenum, 1981a.

Passeri, M., and Cucinotta, D.: Aspetti clinico therapeutici dell'insufficienza cerebrale cronica senile. *Rassegna Clinica Scientifica 58*, 18 (1982).

Passeri, M., and Cucinotta, D.: Possibilita' di prevenzione e di terapia della encefalopatia chronica senile. *Giorn. Geront. 29*, 703–713 (1981b).

Rabins, P.V., Mace, N.L., and Lucas, M.J.: The impacts of dementia on the family. *JAMA 248*(3), 333 (1982).

Rehman, S.A.: Two trials comparing Hydergine with placebo in the treatment of patients suffering from cerebrovascular insufficiency. *Current Medical Research Opinion 1*, 465–462 (1973).

Rosen, H.J.: Mental decline in the elderly: Pharmacotherapy (ergot alkaloids versus papaverine). *J. Am. Geriatr. Soc. 23*, 169–174 (1975).

Spano, P.F., Govoni, S., Uzumaki, H., Bosio, A., Memo, M., Lucchi, L., Carruba, M., and Trabucchi, M.: Stimulation of D_2-dopamine receptors by dopaminergic ergot alkaloids: Studies on the mechanism of action. In Agnoli, A., Crepaldi, G., Spano, P.F., and Trabucchi, M. (Eds.), Aging Brain and Ergot Alkaloids, Vol. 23, pp. 165–177. New York, Raven, 1983.

Venn, R.D.: Clinical Pharmacology of Ergot Alkaloids in Senile Cerebral Insufficiency: Ergot Alkaloids and Related Compounds, Ch. 7, p. 533. New York: Springer-Verlag, 1978.

Yesavage, J.A., Westphal, J., and Rush, L.: Senile dementia: Combined pharmacologic and psychologic treatment. *J. Am. Geriatr. Soc. 29*, 4–164 (1981).

Zarifian, E.: Classification of disorders and therapeutics of the aging brain. *Gerontology 28* (Suppl. 2), 1–4 (1982).

Chapter 32

Determinants of Successful Aging: Findings from a Study with Ergoloid Mesylates (Hydergine)

René Spiegel, Susan Köberle, and Fritz Huber

Summary

A long-term double-blind comparison between Hydergine, 4.5 mg per day and placebo, including 148 healthy pensioners of both sexes, was analyzed after 3 years of study. Based on medical and psychological assessment criteria, 52 subjects were considered to have successfully aged, and 45 to have poorly aged over this time span. The remaining subjects had either withdrawn from the study or could not be allocated to one of the two groups. A retrospective analysis of possible predictor variables yielded two statistically significant and meaningful predictors: a diagnosis of hypertension at baseline, and treatment with Hydergine. Hypertensive subjects were less likely to age with success, while treatment with Hydergine was found to be significantly associated with successful aging in our sample. The study is still ongoing.

Introduction

The expression "successful aging" is occasionally found in the gerontological literature. Although it is not a technical term, different authors have very similar views on the subject: Lehr (1977) speaks of "getting older in a state of psychophysical well-being." L. Jarvik (1975) expressed successful aging in terms of an index containing "physical and mental vigour as judged by medical examination, physical appearance, and psychiatric and psychological evaluations." Several investigations have shown well-being in the elderly to be highly correlated with subjectively assessed health (Larson, 1978; Lazarus and DeLongis, 1983). Factors which appear to favor successful aging are continuing intellectual and, if possible, physical activity, social contacts, and a certain degree of challenge or tension in daily life (Jarvik, 1975; Lehr, 1977; Busse and Maddox, 1980), a high intellectual level (Siegler and Botwinick, 1979) and, last but not least, the lack of economic concern (Larson, 1978; Busse and Maddox, 1980).

The most reliable statements about determinants of successful aging are derived from longitudinal investigations such as the Duke studies (Palmore, 1970, 1974) and the Bonn longitudinal studies (Thomae, 1976), which ran for between 7 and 21 years. Only retrospectively can elements be isolated that were present at a certain time and can at a later time be correlated with relevant aspects of successful aging. An investigation of our own was started in 1976 and, despite some differences from the Duke and Bonn studies, provided an opportunity to search for further factors which also made contributions to successful aging (see Spiegel, Huber, and Köberle, 1983).

Materials and Methods

This investigation is taking place in Basel and poses two general questions: First, it is devoted to medical, physiological and psychological aspects of the aging process, the possible interaction and the prognostic significance of these aspects. Second, we are investigating whether regular application of a drug, in this case ergoloid mesylates (Hydergine), has a preventive effect on some of the undesired physical and mental concomitants of aging.

The subjects (Table 32-1) are former employees of Sandoz Ltd. in Basel and their spouses who, in 1976 and 1978, were invited to volunteer for a gerontological investigation. In return for their participation they receive regular medical checkups every year and a brief examination every 3 months. Any abnormality detected on these occasions is communicated to the subject's personal physician but, with the exception of dietary counseling, there is no therapy involved in our study.

Table 32-1. Description of sample

Numer of Ss	148
Females: males	64:84
Age	$\bar{x} = 63$ (52–72) years
Criteria for exclusion	Early retirement due to disease or invalidity Severe physical or mental disease

Numerous medical parameters, corresponding roughly to the initial medical workup in a Swiss hospital, are assessed every year (Table 32-2). In addition, EEG and polygraphic sleep studies are carried out but are not reported here. Psychometric tests include a shortened version of Wechsler's Intelligence Scale and the Colored Progressive Matrices by Raven. The Maudsley Personality Inventory is also filled out, so that every yearly checkup lasts about 4 hours. Each 3-monthly visit lasts about 1½ hours.

Since the investigation is also concerned with the possible prophylactic effect of long-term Hydergine administration, it was necessary to divide the subject sample into two equivalent groups, one to be treated with Hydergine (3 × 1.5 mg/day orally), the other with a similar-tasting placebo. As shown in Table 32-3, the two groups resulting from a meticulous matching procedure were similar initially in the most relevant parameters. Subjects had been informed that some of them would be treated with an inactive preparation; they were assured, however, that they would be switched individually to the active preparation if symptoms emerged which were considered responsive to Hydergine. The study is being carried out double blind. Treatment compliance is checked by pill counting and by questioning the subjects. In addition, plasma samples taken at regular intervals have recently been assayed for the presence of Hydergine.

The most important findings after 3 years of study have recently been reported (Spiegel et al., 1983). Regardless of whether they were in the Hydergine or the placebo group, many subjects felt better after 3 years than at the outset of the study and also showed objective improvements, both medically and psychologically, in comparison with baseline values. Moreover, Hydergine displayed favorable effects on several parameters, in

Table 32-2. Parameters investigated

Medical history & status (ca. 250 items) ECG Laboratory (ca. 40 items) Clinical EEG	1 × per year
Computer-analyzed EEG	2 × per year
Wechsler Adult Intelligence Scale (abridged version)	1 × per year
Colored Progressive Matrices (Raven)	4 × per year
Maudsley Personality Inventory (MPI)	1 × per year
Polygraphic sleep recordings (with a subsample of Ss)	Years 0, 3, 6

Table 32-3. Baseline values of hydergine and placebo subjects

	Hydergine	Placebo
Number of Ss	75	73
Females	33	31
Males	42	42
Age (years)	63 (52–72)	63 (56–71)
Body-mass index	26.5 (18.9–42.9)	26.4 (19.6–37.3)
Systolic blood pressure mm Hg	131 (80–200)	131 (98–165)
Diastolic blood pressure mm Hg	77 (55–125)	76 (55–105)
Intelligence (Raven Test)	29 (22–36)	28 (17–35)

particular on cardiovascular measures, cholesterol, subjective symptoms, and psychometric test scores.

In the present context, there is particular interest in those parameters which, for the study period of up to 3 years, can predict successful or poor aging in a statistically valid way. In order to ascertain such factors, we defined successful or poor aging, as suggested by Jarvik, Lehr, and other authors, and in terms of the parameters of our study. These were, first of all, death during the study period, regardless of cause, and severe diseases leading to withdrawal from the study, both obviously indicators of poor aging (Figure 32-1). According to these two criteria, 26 of the 148 subjects have aged poorly; 8 other subjects withdrew from the investigation for nonmedical reasons and are not considered in the following report. The remaining 114 subjects were then assessed according to medical and psychometric criteria (Table 32-4) which may be seen as indicators of successful or poor aging. A sum score was formed from these criteria which, theoretically, could vary between about −10 and +12 points.

Subjects with a sum score of 0 and less were considered successfully aged, while those with a sum score of 3 and more were included in the poorly aged group and added to those who had died or dropped out for medical reasons. Forty-two subjects from the central part of the distribution (i.e., with a sum score of 1 and 2) were excluded so that two extreme groups of 52 and 45 subjects, representing successfully and poorly aged individuals, resulted. These two groups were then compared in terms of a large number of variables which had been recorded at baseline and which are potential predictors of successful or poor aging (Table 32-5). Naturally, this large number of comparisons involves a

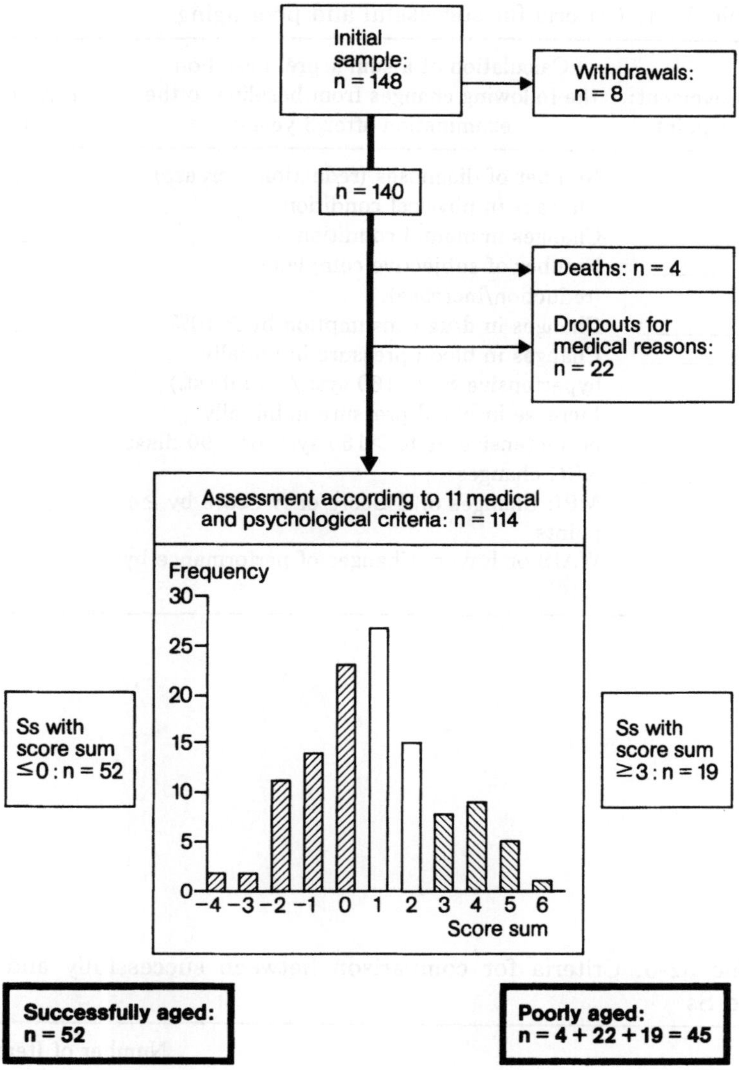

Figure 32-1. Selection of successfully and poorly aged subjects: Subjects who had died or dropped out for medical reasons (n = 4 + 22) were included in the poorly aged group. The shaded areas represent poorly aged subjects with a sum score of 3 and more (right) and successfully aged subjects with a sum score of 0 and less (left).

Table 32-4. Criteria for successful and poor aging

Improvement: −1 point	Calculation of a sum score, based on the following changes from baseline to the examination after 3 years:	Deterioration: +1 point
______	Number of diagnoses (reduction/increase)	______
______	Changes in physical condition	______
______	Changes in mental condition	______
______	Number of subjective complaints (reduction/increase)	______
______	Changes in drug consumption by ≥ 10%	______
______	Changes in blood pressure in initially hypertensive Ss (>160 syst./>90 diast.)	______
	Increase in blood pressure in initially normotensive Ss to >160 syst. or >90 diast.	______
______	ECG changes	______
______	MPI: Changes of *E*-Score or *N*-Score by ≥4 points	______
______	WAIS or Raven: Changes of performance by ≥10%	______

Table 32-5. Criteria for comparison between successfully and poorly aged Ss

	Number of Items
Sex, age, body-mass index	3
Diagnoses	8
Number of these main diagnoses	1
Number of further diagnoses, general state of health, mental state, amount of stress	4
Systolic an diastolic blood pressure, ECG abnormalities	3
Subjective physical complaints	14
Laboratory	12
Psychometric tests	4
Drug: Hydergine or placebo	1

danger of finding spuriously significant results; however, we considered the procedure useful in an exploratory sense.

Results

The following items indicated statistically significant differences between the two groups:

1. The diagnosis of hypertension at baseline was less frequent in successfully aged subjects ($p = 0.026$, chi-square test).
2. The complaint of vertigo at baseline was more frequent in successfully aged subjects ($p = 0.042$, chi-square test).
3. The extraversion score of the MPI at baseline was lower in successfully aged subjects ($p = 0.042$, t test).
4. Subjects belonging to the Hydergine group were found to be successfully aging more frequently than those in the placebo group ($p = 0.032$, chi-square test).

Discussion

The prognostic value of some of these items does not come as a great surprise, while for others an interpretation appears more difficult. Thus, the finding that hypertensive subjects were less frequently found among the successfully aging ones is not unexpected, since hypertension has repeatedly been described as a risk factor for several diseases and symptoms (Colandrea et al., 1970; Kannet et al., 1980). The finding that successfully aging subjects complained more frequently about vertigo is more difficult to understand since vertigo may be indicative of a number of potentially dangerous diseases. However, analysis of this paradoxical finding reveals that the complaint of vertigo was quite common at the outset of the study and disappeared in a sizable number of subjects over the years. This may have contributed in a proportion of cases to their being included in the successful group because changes from baseline were used for defining successful aging. A similar mechanism may have been operating in case of the MPI extraversion score, which was found to be lower in successfully aged subjects.

Of significance is the finding that subjects belonging to the Hydergine group aged more successfully overall than those being treated with placebo for 3 years. Differences in favor of the Hydergine group had already been found when the analysis was based on individual criteria (Spiegel et al., 1983). It is of importance that, of the 48 subjects who had been in the Hydergine group and included in the present analysis, only 17 (i.e., 35%) were aging unsuccessfully, compared with 28 of 49 (i.e. 57%) in the placebo group (Figure 32-2). This result becomes even more

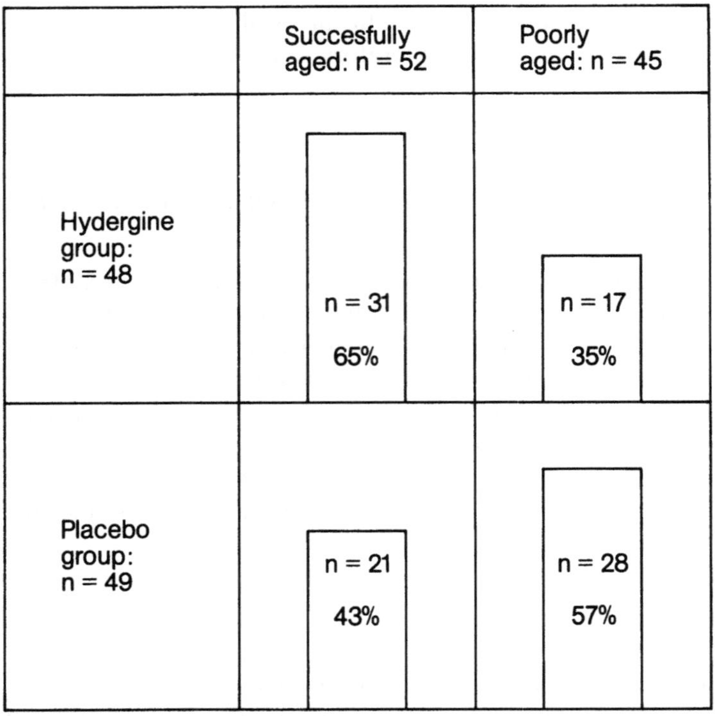

Figure 32-2. Hydergine and successful vs. poor aging.

impressing if one considers that, of the 17 poorly aged subjects in the Hydergine group, one had never taken the drug (as revealed in the recent determination of drug plasma levels and subsequent questioning) and 5 had dropped out of the study owing to diseases which did not involve cardiovascular or CNS function. On the other hand, treatment with Hydergine was no guarantee for successful aging, and the placebo group also contained a considerable number of subjects who, according to our criteria, aged successfully.

Of interest in the light of the aforementioned findings of other long-term studies is the fact that the intelligence tests used were useless as predictors. Thus, we could not confirm that more intelligent subjects aged more successfully on the whole than less intelligent ones; however, one must admit that a time span of 3 years is probably not long enough in this respect and that our sample was more homogeneous both socially and economically than the subjects in the Duke studies (Siegler and Botwinick, 1979). It will in any case be interesting to reanalyze our findings with regard to potential predictors after more years of study. In addition to the Maudsley Personality Inventory, which so far has yielded paradoxical data, the results of a questionnaire providing information about social contact and other activities of our subjects will also be available. The prognostic significance of the quantitatively analyzed EEG and of polygraphic sleep recordings which are carried out with a subsample will also be considered at that time.

For the moment the following conclusions can be drawn from our investigation:

1. A clinical diagnosis of hypertension, in otherwise healthy elderly subjects, is prognostically unfavorable, even for a comparatively short time span of 3 years.
2. Permanent treatment with Hydergine (ergoloid mesylates), 3 × 1.5 mg/day and over 3 years, significantly increases the chances of successful aging in elderly healthy persons.

Acknowledgment

We are grateful to Ms. Marianne Schweingruber who helped us with the statistical analysis of the data.

References

Busse, E.W., and Maddox, G.L.: Final Report—The Duke Longitudinal Studies, an Integrated Investigation of Aging & the Aged, 1955–1980. Durham, N.C.: Center for the Study of Aging and Human Development, 1980.

Colandrea, M.A., Friedman, G.D., Nichaman, M.Z., and Lynd, C.N.: Systolic hypertension in the elderly. *Circulation 41*, 239–245 (1970).

Jarvik, L.F.: Thoughts on the psychobiology of aging. *Am. Psychol. 30*, 576–583 (1975).

Kannel, W.B., Sorlie, P., Castelli, W.P., and McGee, D.: Blood pressure and survival after myocardial infarction: The Framingham study. *Am. J. Card. 45*, 326–330 (1980).

Larson, R.: Thirty years of research on the subjective well-being of older Americans. *J. Gerontol. 33*, 109–125 (1978).

Lazarus, R.S., and DeLongis, A.: Psychological stress and coping in aging. *Am. Psychol. 38*, 245–254 (1983).

Lehr, U.: Die Vorbereitung auf das Alter—nicht nur ein medizinisches Problem. *Triangel 16*, 93–103 (1977).

Palmore, E. (Ed.): Normal Aging. Durham, N.C.: Duke University Press, 1970.

Palmore, E. (Ed.): Normal Aging II. Durham, N.C.: Duke University Press, 1974.

Siegler, I.C., and Botwinick, J.: A long-term longitudinal study of intellectual ability of older adults: The matter of selective subject attrition. *J. Gerontol. 34*, 242–245 (1979).

Spiegel, R., Huber, F., and Köberle, S.: A controlled long-term study with ergoloid mesylates (Hydergine) in healthy, elderly volunteers: Results after three years. *J. Am. Ger. Soc. 31*, 549–555 (1983).

Thomae, H.: Patterns of Aging: Findings from the Bonn Longitudinal Study of Aging. Basel: Karger, 1976.

Chapter 33

Differential Patient Response to Ergoloid Mesylates According to Current Etiopathic Notions of Dementia

Jack M. Singer, Herman B. Hamot, and John R. Patin

Summary

Data obtained from 1165 patients treated from 3 to 12 months in 21 double-blind studies with ergoloid mesylates (Hydergine, Sandoz) reveal a differential patient response based upon current etiopathic notions of dementia. Patients who were classified as having degenerative/idiopathic dementia derived the most benefit from ergoloid mesylates following 3 months of treatment.

Patients presumed to have multi-infarct dementia based on historical evidence of at least one cerebrovascular accident were also improved significantly with ergoloid mesylates but somewhat less on an overall symptom-by-symptom basis. Patients with evidence of cardiopulmonary dysfunction demonstrated less consistent improvement. Ergoloid mesylates had no demonstratable effect on specific target symptoms of dementia associated with systemic/metabolic or neurological disease. Less consistent results emerged from analyses for the 6 and 12 month evaluations compared to the 3 month assessment period.

Introduction

Among the numerous methodological problems encountered in evaluating any therapeutic agent in the elderly is the tendency to utilize a nonspecific diagnosis such as organic brain syndrome in characterizing patients entered into clinical trials (Prien, 1972). Physicians commonly attribute the varied cognitive, emotional, and social problems of the elderly to chronic brain disease without regard to specific etiology. It has been widely assumed that many of the symptoms associated with aging have been caused by arteriosclerotic cerebrovascular disease. There is, however, considerable evidence that refutes this contention (Wells, 1978a; Seltzer and Sherwin, 1978; Paulson and Perrine, 1968).

Attempts at distinguishing chronic brain disorders based on clinical–pathological data have provided an impetus for modifying traditional diagnostic methods (Tomlinson, Blessed, and Roth, 1970). It has been suggested that the term cerebral vascular insufficiency be restricted only to conditions manifested by focal neurological signs (Obrist, 1972). The terms multi-infarct dementia (MID) and primary degenerative dementia have been distinguished on the basis of pathology, clinical findings, and patient history (Fisher, 1968; Hachinski and Lassen, 1974). Both the presenile and senile forms of Alzheimer's disease (SDAT) can be considered on the basis of similar pathology to be synonymous with idiopathic/degenerative dementia (Blessed, Tomlinson, and Roth, 1968). This has resulted in various refinements in the psychiatric nomenclature and are reflected in the American Psychiatric Association's DSM III classification which delineates only progressive idiopathic dementia and multi-infarct dementia as senile, non-drug-induced forms of organic mental disorder (Spitzer, 1980).

While these disorders are generally considered irreversible, it has been estimated that approximately 15% of patients with symptoms of dementia will have reversible conditions, and that another 20–25% will require specific therapeutic intervention (Wells, 1977). There are numerous medical conditions and chronic disease states including endocrine, cardiovascular, systemic, metabolic, and neurological disorders which give rise to the dementia syndrome (Wells, 1978b). It thus becomes critical to consider seriously such conditions in the evaluation of any elderly patient with symptoms of organic brain disease.

Over the past 15 years, ergoloid mesylates has been extensively evaluated in clinical studies in the United States and abroad for the treatment of symptoms associated with "cerebrovascular insufficiency", "cerebral arteriosclerosis", "senile deterioration," and "organic brain syndrome" (Bazo, 1973; Rosen, 1975; Rehman, 1973; McConnachie, 1973; Thibault, 1974; Banen, 1972; Rao and Norris, 1972; Jennings, 1972; Triboletti and Ferri, 1969; Ditch, Kelly, and Resnick, 1971; Gerin, 1969; Roubicek, Geiger, and Abt, 1972; Nelson, 1975; Einspruch, 1976; Hollister, 1955; Popkin, 1956; Gaitz, Varner, and Overall, 1977). The use of such descriptive labels without the application of more precise diagnostic inclusion criteria has caused some criticism of these investigations (Hughes, Williams, and Currier, 1976).

With the available evidence suggesting a rather limited role of arteriosclerosis in the pathogenesis of dementia, an attempt was made to define the differential response of patients to treatment with ergoloid mesylates more appropriately in accord with current etiologic concepts. Concomitant illness and chronic disease states possibly contributing to or accounting for clinical symptomology were considered along with the other current notions of senescent cerebral dysfunction.

Materials and Methods

Study Design

A retrospective analysis from 15 double-blind ergoloid mesylates vs. placebo comparative studies and 6 ergoloid mesylates vs. papaverine* studies were undertaken. Under general supervision of a psychiatrist, four nurse-clinicians reviewed all case report forms, patient records containing pertinent medical history, and results of physical examinations. X-ray and laboratory reports were examined in detail when available. Patients with concurrent medical illness, history of significant disease states, or other psychiatric illness were identified and classified into separate predetermined operational categories (Table 33-1). These are consistent with current nosological concepts regarding dementia and were considered on an a priori basis to be representative of the overall patient sample. This contrasts with diagnostic nomenclature employed during the actual conduct of these studies such as senility (not further defined), cerebrovascular insufficiency, cerebral arteriosclerosis with trauma, etc. Where more than one secondary diagnosis was available, patients were assigned to that category considered most probably responsible for the presenting clinical symptoms. Where no history of cerebrovascular accident or history of neurological or medical disease could be identified as playing at least a possible etiological role, patients were presumed to be most likely suffering from idiopathic/degenerative dementia. In order to eliminate potential sources of bias, personnel involved in the reclassification project were kept unaware of study drug assignment.

Patient Sample

The 1165 valid patients from 21 double-blind studies were included in the reanalysis. The duration of the various studies and the number of patients in each treatment group are set forth in Table 33-2. Ages ranged from 65 to 133 with a median of about 81 years. Although most were residents of

*Half of these 6 studies employed papaverine hydrochloride as the active control, while the other half used its slow-release variant Pavabid®. Hereafter, the term papaverine will refer to both groups as the response characteristics for both forms were not significantly different.

Table 33-1. Revised diagnostic classification of 1165 patients from 21 studies with ergoloid mesylates

Multi-infarct Dementia	Major Sensory Deficits
Old CVA	Total blindness
New CVA	Total deafness
Hemiparesis	
Hemiplegia	Endocrine Disorders
Cerebral Thrombosis	
Paralysis	Thyroidectomy
Stroke	Hypothyroid
Aphasia	Hyperthyroid
	Parathyroid
Neurological Disorders	Pituitary
Parkinson's disease	Systemic/Metabolic Disorders
Huntington's chorea	
Subdural hemorrhage	Kidney disease, uremia
Epilepsy	Chronic urinary tract infection
Seisures	Addison's disease
Multiple sclerosis	Glumerulonephritis
Trauma—unknown	Lupus erythematosus
Trauma—known	Anemia
Infection CNS	Pernicious anemia
Hydrocephalus	Vitamin deficiencies
Cardiopulmonary Decompensation	Alcohol Related
Congestive heart failure	Cirrhosis
Atrial fibrillation	Alcoholic
Premature ventricular contractions	Korsakoff's syndrome
Severe heart enlargement (X-ray)	
Emphysema	Syphilis
Chronic lung disease	
Chronic bronchitis	
Idiopathic/Degenerative Dementia (SDAT)	

nursing homes, out-patients predominated in two studies. Nearly 70% were female. Patients suffering from psychosis, posttraumatic brain damage, postinfective brain disease, or cerebral neoplasm were excluded. All patients exhibited symptoms of cognitive, emotional, and behavioral impairment. Some patients had, in addition, secondary medical or psychiatric conditions which were classified in accordance with conventional diagnostic standards. Patients underwent physical examinations together with vital sign recordings and laboratory evaluations prior to and

Table 33-2. Double-blind studies

	Duration of Study	No. of Studies	No. of Patients	
			Erg. Mesyl.	Control
Ergoloid mesylates vs. placebo	3 months	8	187	190
Ergoloid mesylates vs. papaverine HCl or Pavabid	3 months	6	152	144
Ergoloid mesylates vs. placebo	6 months	3	60	67
Ergoloid mesylates vs. placebo	12 months	4	187	178

at the conclusion of the respective study periods. Concomitant medications likely to cloud activity of the test agents were prohibited during the course of these studies. A 2 or 3 week washout period was enforced during which all psychoactive medications such as tranquilizers, antidepressants, vasodilators, and CNS stimulants were discontinued. The regimen for all patients receiving ergoloid mesylates was 1 mg t.i.d.

The clinical efficacy for all patients was measured by use of the SCAG (Sandoz Clinical Assessment Geriatric) Scale which contains 18 specific cognitive, behavioral, affective, and somatic items as well as a 19th global item requiring the examiner to provide an overall impression of patient status independent of assessments rendered for the other individual symptoms. Each item carried a 7 point rating schedule, from 1 indicating lack of symptom or normal function to 7 referring to the most severe manifestation (Venn, 1983). The scale has been widely employed in studies throughout the world and its sensitivity, reliability, and validity thoroughly documented (Shader, Harmatz, and Salzman, 1974; Maurer et al., 1982; Venn, 1980) so that it has been approved for use in research on senile dementia by the drug regulatory bodies of both the United States (Guy, 1976) and West Germany (CIPS, 1981). Comparative efficacy between treatments for each individual study had been assessed by application of the Student's t test (or its variants) for each item and factor of the SCAG. With reclassification of patients according to the new current nosology, the number of patients for individual studies per diagnostic class was significantly reduced.

Statistical Procedures

The statistical model employed for this reanalysis was the $2 \times k$ factorial design where 2 indicates two test agents and k the number of investigators. As most of the comparative drug effects in each of the studies tended to favor ergoloid mesylates treatment groups over the controls on a rather consistent basis, significant drug × investigator interaction did not inhibit pooling the data across all patients within a diagnostic subset (Scheffe, 1959). Also, since the number of patients in each of the $2 \times k$ cells was unequal, the unweighted mean across all investigators was taken as the unbiased estimate of relative drug effect in accordance with the methods developed by Yates (1934) and Searle, Speed, and Henderson (1981). Hence, the results reported here do not give greater weight to investigators with greater numbers of patients.

The efficacy comparisons (Tables 33-4 through 33–6) contain in parentheses the fraction of studies with raw scores favoring the ergoloid mesylates-treated groups. Earlier forms of the SCAG included some items not incorporated in the final version and not all items were evaluated in each of the 21 studies. Similarly, not all investigators had patients who fit into the new diagnostic categories. Therefore, these fractions will vary accordingly. Only five of the new diagnostic categories had an aggregate number of patients sufficient for analysis by the procedures described above. Data from investigators with fewer than four patients per treatment group for a given category were also excluded from this analysis. Hence, this reanalysis covers about 80% of the overall patient sample.

Results

The average age of the 1165 patients was 80.1 years (range, 60–133). There were 365 males and 800 females who were distributed according to the diagnoses presented in Table 33-3. Two hundred and six patients (17.7%) presented evidence of at least one cerebrovascular accident and were regarded as probably having multi-infarct dementia. One hundred and twenty-six patients (10.8%) displayed evidence of metabolic/systemic disorders which possibly contributed to the clinical condition, while 110 patients (9.4%) had some history suggestive of cardiopulmonary decompensation. Six hundred and four patients (51.8%) could not be excluded on the basis of other significant medical conditions and were therefore designated as likely having idiopathic progressive dementia. No differences in demographic features were characteristic of the diagnostic subsets.

A factor analysis of the pre-trial SCAG ratings for the 1165 patients yielded five factors (Hamot, Patin, and Singer, 1984): *cognitive dysfunction* (impaired mental alertness, confusion, impaired recent memory, and disorientation); *interpersonal relationships* (uncooperativeness, irritability, bothersomeness, and hostility); *affective* (emotional lability, depression,

Table 33-3. Background data by diagnostic category for 1165 patients

	Idiopathic/Degenerative $N = 604$ (51.8%)			
Male	162	(26.8%)		
Female	442	(73.2%)	Mean age 80.7 years	(60–133)
	Multi-Infarct Dementia $N = 206$ (17.7%)			
Male	78	(37.9%)		
Female	128	(62.1%)	Mean age 78.1 years	(60–96)
	Primary Neurological Disorders $N = 66$ (5.7%)			
Male	22	(33.3%)		
Female	44	(66.7%)	Mean age 77.8 years	(60–95)
	Systemic/Metabolic Disorders $N = 126$ (10.8%)			
Male	31	(24.6%)		
Female	95	(75.4%)	Mean age 82.6 years	(60–99)
	Endocrine Disorders $N = 28$ (2.4%)			
Male	9	(32.1%)		
Female	19	(67.9%)	Mean age 74.3 years	(60–88)
	Alcohol Related $N = 10$ (.9%)			
Male	6	(60.0%)		
Female	4	(40.0%)	Mean age 72.5 years	(61–89)
	Syphilis $N = 6$ (.5%)			
Male	2	(33.3%)		
Female	4	(66.7%)	Mean age 76.2 years	(61–89)
	Cardiopulmonary Decompensation $N = 110$ (9.4%)			
Male	51	(46.4%)		
Female	59	(53.6%)	Mean age 81.1 years	(62–99)
	Major Sensory Deficits $N = 9$ (.8%)			
Male	4	(44.4%)		
Female	5	(55.6%)	Mean age 82.2 years	(73–90)
	Total $N = 1165$ Patients			
Male	365	(31.3%)		
Female	800	(68.7%)	Mean age 80.1 years	(60–133)

and anxiety); *apathy* (lack of motivation/initiative, indifference to surroundings, unsociability, and impaired self-care); and *somatic functioning* (lack of appetite or anorexia, dizziness, and fatigue). The criterion of drug effect for each patient was defined as the factor score obtained by aggregating the SCAG ratings for all items comprising the factor divided by the number of items in the factor. This report focuses attention on seven indices of drug effect: the results for the five factors, the average of the ratings for all of the specific SCAG items, which is here called *total pathology*, and the global *overall impression* of patient status. Hamot, Patin, and Singer, (1984) demonstrated that analyses limited to the five factors capture at least 65% of the entire SCAG information while being free of redundancies arising from analyses for the individual items.

Baseline clinical pathology as assessed by the SCAG revealed some differences among groups. Impaired self-care was significantly greater in the MID patients, while overall clinical symptomatology was more severe in the endocrine group. Thirty-seven percent of the patient sample had been previously treated with some psychotropic agent, but no important differences among diagnostic subsets were observed.

The mean differences in drug response at the 3 month evaluation according to diagnostic categories is found in Table 33-4 for the ergoloid mesylates–placebo studies. Positive entries indicate that the unweighted mean differences favor the ergoloid mesylates-treated group, while negative entries indicate superiority of the comparative agent. For the idiopathic/degenerative dementia patients, the significant superiority of the ergoloid mesylates treatment is noted in all SCAG factors: interpersonal relationships, cognitive dysfunction, affective symptoms, apathy, and somatic functioning, as well as total pathology and overall impression. Similarly, ergoloid mesylates was superior to placebo for the factors of cognitive dysfunction, affective symptoms, apathy, somatic functioning, total pathology, and overall impression in multi-infarct dementia patients.

Patients with evidence of cardiopulmonary decompensation demonstrate significant ($p < 0.05$) improvement for affective symptoms, somatic functioning, total pathology, and overall impression, each favoring ergoloid mesylates over placebo. Patients with systemic/metabolic and neurological disorders register no significant differences between treatments for any SCAG factor notwithstanding the fact that the global item overall impression shows significant gains for the ergoloid mesylates-treated group compared to placebo.

Double-blind data covering 6 and 12 months were too few to merit statistical analyses for each diagnostic subset except for the idiopathic/degenerative and multi-infarct dementia classes. At 6 months of treatment, idiopathic/degenerative dementia patients demonstrated significant improvement in the areas of cognitive dysfunction, affective symptoms, somatic function, total pathology, and overall impression for the ergoloid

Table 33-4. Comparison of results across different diagnostic classes by third treatment month, ergoloid mesylates vs. placebo

Factor	Mean Differences[1]				
	Idiopath/Degen. ($N = 439$)	MID ($N = 130$)	Systemic/ Metabolic ($N = 81$)	Cardiopulmonary Decompensation ($N = 42$)	Neurological ($N = 22$)
Interpersonal relationships	0.30***	0.17	−0.03	0.42	−0.29
	(9/14)	(5/9)	(2/6)	(3/4)	(0/2)
Cognitive dysfunction	0.50***	0.51**	0.31	0.30	0.39
	(12/13)	(7/8)	(4/6)	(3/4)	(2/2)
Affective	0.47***	0.43**	−0.20	0.61*	0.03
	(12/14)	(8/9)	(2/6)	(3/4)	(2/2)
Apathy	0.31***	0.33*	0.07	0.28	0.17
	(9/14)	(8/9)	(3/6)	(3/4)	(2/2)
Somatic functioning	0.39***	0.41**	0.03	0.63*	0.11
	(11/14)	(9/9)	(4/6)	(2/4)	(2/2)
Total pathology	0.38***	0.38***	0.04	0.44*	0.08
	(12/14)	(8/9)	(2/6)	(3/4)	(2/2)
Overall impression	0.61***	0.92***	0.09	0.55*	0.96*
	(12/14)	(9/9)	(4/6)	(3/4)	(2/2)

[1]Positive differences indicate superiority for ergoloid mesylates.

*$P < 0.05$; **$P < 0.01$; ***$P < 0.001$.

mesylates-treated group over placebo. In multi-infarct dementia patients only the investigator's overall impression favors ergoloid mesylates compared to placebo after 6 months of treatment. After 12 months of treatment significant improvement was observed in the areas of cognitive dysfunction as well as in the overall impression for ergoloid mesylates-treated multiple-infarct dementia patients. Only the overall impression favored ergoloid mesylates in the idiopathic/degenerative dementia group (Table 33-5).

In ergoloid mesylates vs. papaverine studies, similar results are obtained following three months of treatment in the idiopathic/degenerative and multi-infarct dementia groups (Table 33-6): the five factors, total pathology, and overall impression all favor ergoloid mesylates compared to papaverine. (There were too few patients in the other diagnostic groups to merit formal comparisons between these two active agents.)

Table 33-5. Comparison of results for the 6 and 12 months of treatment for the idiopathic/degenerative and multi-infarct dementia groups, ergoloid mesylates vs. placebo

	Mean Differences[1]			
	6 months		12 months	
Factor	Idiopath/ Degen. ($N = 218$)	MID ($N = 59$)	Idiopath/ Degen. ($N = 218$)	MID ($N = 59$)
Interpersonal relationships	0.16 (5/7)	0.10 (3/4)	0.03 (2.4)	0.30 (3/3)
Cognitive dysfunction	0.29* (6/7)	0.20 (2/4)	0.19 (3/4)	0.92* (2/3)
Affective	0.35** (6/7)	0.11 (3/4)	0.16 (2/4)	0.18 (1/3)
Apathy	0.06 (4/7)	0.23 (3/4)	0.18 (3/4)	0.77* (3/3)
Somatic functioning	0.25* (5/7)	0.12 (4/4)	0.06 (2/4)	0.32 (3/3)
Total pathology	0.22* (4/7)	0.15 (2/4)	0.13 (2/4)	0.50* (3/3)
Overall impression	0.54** (6/7)	0.79** (4/4)	0.70** (4/4)	1.80*** (3/3)

[1]Positive differences indicate superiority for ergoloid mesylates.
*$P < 0.05$; **$P < 0.01$; ***$P < 0.001$.

Table 33-6. Comparison of results for the idiopathic degenerative and multi-infarct dementia groups by third treatment month, ergoloid mesylates vs. papaverine

	Mean Differences[1]	
Factor	Idiopath/Degen. ($N = 160$)	MID ($N = 42$)
Interpersonal relationships	0.57*** (5/6)	0.04 (1/2)
Cognitive dysfunction	0.60** (5/6)	0.91*** (3/3)
Affective	0.76*** (5/6)	0.95*** (3/3)
Apathy	0.66*** (5/6)	0.86*** (3/3)
Somatic functioning	0.51*** (5/5)	0.51* (3/3)
Total pathology	0.55*** (5/6)	0.67*** (3/3)
Overall impression	0.51** (5/6)	0.98** (3/3)

[1]Positive differences indicate superiority for ergoloid mesylates.
*$P < 0.05$; **$P < 0.01$; ***$P < 0.001$.

Discussion

All 1165 patients in a data bank consisting of 21 comparative studies with ergoloid mesylates originally given the nonspecific diagnoses of cerebrovascular insufficiency, organ brain syndrome, or cerebral arteriosclerosis were reclassified according to currently accepted nomenclature. The data for these patients were then reanalyzed according to their redefined diagnoses and response to treatment with ergoloid mesylates determined. Certain problems are associated with this kind of retrospective classification, which of necessity was based on a number of assumptions. Approximately 30% of the patients in this survey had evidence of concurrent disease or history of chronic medical illness. This figure is consistent with estimates for the incidence of reversible dementias (Hachinski and Lassen, 1974). While physical conditions commonly present with a variety of psychiatric symptoms, the extent to which such disorders might contribute to the overall dementia syndrome has been questioned (Hall et al., 1978; Roth, 1971). An acute exacerbation of symptoms due to medical illness which can be manifested by frank delirum or confusional episodes may often be superimposed on a chronic progressive brain syndrome and confound the clinical assessment.

It is therefore difficult in such an analysis to precisely designate a predominant illness or to assess the impact of one coexisting disorder on another. Consideration of distinct categories of patients with various chronic medical problems may then serve to underestimate the true incidence of idiopathic/degenerative dementia in this patient sample. No particular attention was paid to certain common disease states such as diabetes, since clinical symptoms possibly attributable to this illness would most likely result from poor metabolic control, or from a vascular complication, whereby patients would be classified elsewhere.

Data based upon autopsied specimens from patients with diagnosed dementia point out the relative etiologic importance of Alzheimer's disease compared to arteriosclerosis (Tomlinson, Blessed, and Roth, 1970). Yet the two forms may coexist and potentiate each other in the causation of clinical symptoms (Roth, 1976). Data obtained from four series of patients with organic brain syndrome who were completely worked up clinically also suggest a higher prevalence of progressive idiopathic dementia than arteriosclerosis (Wells, 1978a; Seltzer and Sherwin, 1978). Noteworthy is the fact that in the series of 222 patients discussed by Wells, 51% of the patients were diagnosed as having atrophy of unknown cause associated with dementia. The data presented in this analysis are therefore highly consistent with both the pathological and clinical surveys in the literature. These comparisons speak to the question of what may be considered as a rather arbitrary classification of patients, in that careful prospective neurological workups including CAT scans were not performed at the time of these clinical investigations.

It is often impossible on clinical grounds or even through psychometric testing to distinguish the "early" or "mild" dementias with insidious, progressive onset from the nonprogressive forms of intellectual and emotional impairment of later life (Arie, 1973). Patients with early illness may complain of affective or somatic symptoms with only minimal organic deficits (Post, 1961). One might assume that some patients in this sample had symptoms which could be considered benign and static in course, but who were nevertheless classified as having progressive dementia. Similarly, those patients with pseudodementia could not be identified by the procedures employed in this analysis (Post, 1975).

There were no substantial differences observed in baseline SCAG symptomatology among the various diagnostic groups which underscore further the difficulty for the practicing physician to establish a definitive etiology on the basis of clinical symptoms alone. This serves, in addition, to further emphasize the necessity of a comprehensive dementia workup in patients suspected of organic brain disease. Notwithstanding these critical methodological issues, analyses of results from these studies do, in fact, reveal highly significant statistical differences between ergoloid mesylates and placebo-treated patients with degenerative/idiopathic and multi-infarct dementia in the key areas of cognitive, affective, and behavioral functioning. The ergoloid mesylates–papaverine studies confirm these results.

The results for these retrospective analyses may also provide hints on the limitations of the SCAG as a valid instrument for measuring changes in symptom severity for diagnostic classes other than idiopathic degenerative and multi-infarct dementias. The chief characteristic distinguishing superior response to ergoloid mesylates among the reclassified groups is that patients with idiopathic/degenerative and multi-infarct dementia tend to obtain improvement in cognitive function whereas such gains were not achieved by the groups demarcated by systemic/metabolic diseases, cardiopulmonary decompensation, or neurological disorders. For two of the latter groups, however, the results for the global overall impression significantly favored ergoloid mesylates over placebo (Table 33-4), suggesting improved patient response not associated with specific SCAG symptoms. Although some work has been done on validating the SCAG as an appropriate instrument for assessing patient pretrial status for the other diagnostic classes (Patin, Hamot, and Singer, 1984), additional research is required to demonstrate whether this instrument is sensitive to changes in clinical status for patients falling into such categories. On the basis of the results reported here and elsewhere (Hamot, Patin, and Singer, 1984; Patin, Hamot, and Singer, 1984), the SCAG appears to be a reliable, sensitive, and valid instrument for use in evaluating drug effects in multi-infarct dementia as well as meriting continued use in idiopathic/degenerative dementia.

On the basis of the above analysis, it would appear that a trial of ergoloid mesylates is warranted for the treatment of patients with symptoms of mild-to-moderate dementia associated with progressive idiopathic disease or cerebrovascular accidents. Because of the difficulty in distinguishing early dementia from more static intellectual decline in the elderly, one might consider using ergoloid mesylates in all elderly patients with cognitive impairment accompanied by affective, somatic, or behavioral symptoms of nonpsychotic proportion, and in whom the possibility of reversible conditions due to medical, neurological, or psychiatric illness have been ruled out.

References

Airie, T.: Dementia in the elderly, diagnosis and assessment. *Br. Med. J. 4*, 540–543 (1973).

Banen, D.M.: An ergot preparation (Hydergine) for relief of symptoms of cerebrovascular insufficiency. *J. Am. Geriatrics Society 20*, 22–24 (1972).

Bazo, A.J.: An ergot alkaloid preparation (Hydergine) vs. papaverine in treating common complaints of the aged: double-blind study. *J. Am. Geriatrics Society 21*, 63–71 (1973).

Blessed, G., Tomlinson, B., and Roth, M.: The association between quantitative measures of dementia and of senile change in the cerebral grey matter of elderly subjects. *Br. J. Psychiat. 114*, 797–811 (1968).

CIPS (Collegium Internationel Psychiatriae Scalarum): Internationale Skalen fur Psychiatrie. Beltz Test Gmb H. Wenheim, Germany, 1981.

Ditch, M., Kelly, E.J., and Resnick, O.: An ergot preparation (Hydergine) in the treatment of cerebrovascular insufficiency in the geriatric outpatient: double-blind study. *J. Am. Geriatric Society 19*, 208–217 (1971).

Einspruch, B.C.: Helping to make the final years meaningful for the elderly residents of nursing homes. *Diseases of the Nervous System 37*, 439–442 (1976).

Fisher, C.M.: Dementia in cerebrovascular disease. In Toole, J.F., Gilberg, R.G., and Whisnant, J.P. (Eds.), Cerebral Vascular Diseases, Sixth Congress, pp. 103–134. New York: Grune & Stratton, 1968.

Gaitz, C.M., Varner, R.V., and Overall, J.E.: Pharmacotherapy for organic brain syndrome in late life—evaluation of an ergot derivative vs. placebo. *Arch. Gen. Psychiat. 34*, 839–845 (1977).

Gerin, J.: Symptomatic treatment of cerebrovascular insufficiency with Hydergine. *Current Therapeutic Research 11*, 539–545 (1969).

Guy, W.: ECDEU Assessment Manual for Psychopharmacology (revised), pp. 568–571. Rockville, Md.: U.S. Department of Health, Education and Welfare, 1976.

Hachinski, V.C., and Lassen, M.: Multi-infarct dementia: A cause of mental deterioration in the elderly. *Lancet 2*, 207–299 (1974).

Hall, R., Popkin, M., Devaul, R., Faillace, L., and Stickney, F.: Physical illness presenting as psychiatric disease. *Arch. Gen. Psychiat. 35*, 1315–1320 (1978).

Hamot, H.B., Patin, J.R., and Singer, J.M.: Factor structure of the Sandoz Clinical Assessment—Geriatric (SCAG) Scale. *Psychopharm. Bull. 20*, 142–150 (1984).

Hollister, L.E.: Combined hydrogenerated alkaloids of ergot in senile and arteriosclerotic psychoses. *Diseases of the Nervous System 16*, 259 (1955).

Hughes, J., Williams, J., and Currier, R.: An ergot alkaloid preparation (Hydergine) in the treatment of dementia: Critical review of the clinical literature. *J. Am. Geriatric Society 24*, 490–497 (1976).

Jennings, W.G.: An ergot alkaloid preparation (Hydergine) vs. placebo for treatment of symptoms of cerebrovascular insufficiency: double-blind study. *J. Am. Geriatrics Society 20*, 407–412 (1972).

Maurer, W., Ferner, U., Patin, J., and Hamot, H.B.: Sandoz Clinical Assessment Scale (SCAG): eine transkulturelle factorenalytische study. *Z. Gerontal. 15*, 26–30 (1982).

McConnachie, R.W.: A clinical trial comparing "Hydergine" with placebo in the treatment of cerebrovascular insufficienty in elderly patients. *Current Medical Research Opinion 1*, 463–468 (1973).

Nelson, J.J.: Relieving select symptoms of the elderly. *Geriatrics 30*, 133–142 (1975).

Obrist, W.D.: Cerebral physiology of the aged: Influence of circulatory disorders. In Gaitz, C.M. (Ed.), Aging and the Brain, pp. 117–133. New York: Plenum, 1972.

Patin, J.R., Hamot, H.B., and Singer, J.M.: Replicated evidence on the construct validity of the SCAG (Sandoz Clinical Assessment—Geriatric) scale. *Prog. Neuropsychopharmacol. Biol. Psychiat.* 8(2):293–306, 1984.

Paulson, G.W., and Perrine, G.: Cerebral vascular disease in mental hospitals. In Toole, J.F., Siebert, R.G., and Wishnant, J.P. (Eds.): Cerebral Vascular Diseases, Sixth Congress, pp. 237–241. New York: Grune & Stratton, 1968.

Popkin, R.J.: The hydrogenated alkaloids of ergot (Hydergine) in geriatrics follow-up study. *Am. Pract. Dig. Treat. 7*, 1594–1597 (1956).

Post, F.: Dementia, depression and pseudodementia. In Benson, D.F., and Blumer, D. (Eds.), Psychiatric Aspects of Neurological Disease, pp. 99–120. New York: Grune & Stratton, 1975.

Post, L.G.: Pseudo-dementia. *Acta Psychiatrica Scand. 37*, 336–351 (1961).

Prien, R.: Chronic organic brain syndrome. Washington, D.C.: Veterans Administration, Dept. of Medicine and Surgery (1972).

Rao, E.B., and Norris, J.R.: A double-blind investigation of Hydergine in the treatment of cerebrovascular insufficiency in the elderly. *John Hopkins Medical J. 130*, 317–324 (1972).

Rehman, S.A.: Two trials comprising "Hydergine" with placebo in the treatment of patients suffering from cerebrovascular insufficiency. *Current Medical Research Opinion 1*, 456–462 (1973).

Rosen, H.J.: Mental decline in the elderly: Pharmacotherapy (ergot alkaloids vs. papaverine). *J. Am. Geriatrics Society 23*, 169–174 (1975).

Roth, M.: Classification and etiology in mental disorders of old age: Some recent developments. In Kay, D.W.K., and Walk, A. (Eds.): Recent Developments in Psychogeriatrics. *Br. J. Psychiat.*, Special Publication No. 6, pp. 1–18, 1971.

Roth, M.: Psychiatric disorders of later life. *Psychiat. Annals 6*, 417–444 (1976).

Roubicek, J., Geiger, C., and Abt, K.: An ergot alkaloid preparation (Hydergine) in geriatric therapy. *J. Am. Geriatric Society 20*, 222–229 (1972).

Scheffe, H.: The Analysis of Variance, pp. 112–119. New York: John Wiley and Sons, 1959.

Searle, S.R., Speed, F.M., and Henderson, H.V.: Some computational and model equivalences in analysis of variance of unequal-subclass-numbers data. *Am. Stat. 35*, 16–33 (1981).

Seltzer, B., and Sherwin, I.: "Organic brain syndromes," an empirical study and critical review. *Am. J. Psychiat. 135*, 13–21 (1978).

Shader, R.I., Harmatz, J.S., and Salzman, C.: A new scale for clinical assessment in geriatric populations: Sandoz Clinicial Assessment Geriatric (SCAG). *J. Am. Geriatric Society 22*, 107–113 (1974).

Spitzer, R.L. (Ed.): DSM-III, Diagnostic and Statistical Manual of Mental Disorders, 3rd ed. Washington, D.C.: Am. Psychiatric Assn. 1980.

Thibault, A.: A double-blind evaluation of "Hydergine" and placebo in the treatment of patients with organic brain syndrome and cerebral arteriosclerosis in a nursing home. *Current Medical Research Opinion 2*, 482–487 (1974).

Tomlinson, B.E., Blessed, G., and Roth, M.: Observation on the brains of demented old people. *J. Neurological Sci. 11*, 205–242 (1970).

Triboletti, F., and Ferri, H.: Hydergine for treatment of symptoms of cerebrovascular insufficiency. *Current Therapeutic Research 11*, 609–620 (1969).

Venn, R.D.: Review of clinical studies with ergots in gerontology. In Goldstein, M., Calne, D.B., Lieberman, A., and Thorner, M.O. (Eds.), Ergot Compounds and Brain Function, pp. 363–377. New York: Raven, 1980.

Venn, R.D.: The Sandoz Clinical Assessment Geriatrics (SCAG) Scale, a general purpose psychogeriatric rating scale. *Gerontology 29*, 185–198 (1983).

Wells, C.E.: Diagnostic evaluation and treatment in dementia. In Wells, C.E. (Ed.), Dementia, 2nd ed., pp. 247–276. Philadelphia: F.A. Davis Co., 1977.

Wells, C.E.: Chronic brain disease. *Am. J. Psychiat. 135*, 1–12 (1978a).

Wells, C.E.: Geriatric organic psychosis. *Psychiat. Annals 8*, 466–478 (1978b).

Yates, F.: The analysis of multiple classification with unequal numbers in the difference classes. *J. Am. Stat. Assn. 29*, 51–66 (1934).

Chapter 34

A Dose–Response Study of Dihydroergotoxine (DHET) Mesylate for Cerebrovascular Disturbances

Fumio Eto and Masaki Yoshikawa

Summary

The efficacy of and tolerance of patients to a higher than usual dose of dihydroergotoxine mesylate (Hydergine) were investigated to examine the optimal dose by means of multicentric double-blind method. Utility ratings of subjective and psychiatric symptoms in a group of patients impaired by cerebrovascular disorders showed that daily doses of 6 mg were significantly better than 3 mg daily doses. The results confirm that despite the complexity of neurohumoral transmitter mechanisms in the brain, the drug has a relatively simple dose-dependent efficacy in the range of therapeutic dosages for many subjective and psychiatric symptoms of patients with cerebrovascular disorders. In addition, a preliminary study measured levels of cyclic nucleotides in the lumbar cerebrospinal fluid in aged demented patients who were given Hydergine.

A major problem in treating patients suffering from "dementia" is to define exactly the condition being treated. Dementia is a clinical syndrome that affects behavior and global intellectual performances. Senile dementia should, in the strict sense, be discriminated from cerebrovascular dementia, but major or minor cerebral infarctions frequently are combined with primary degenerative processes in the aging brain.

The therapeutic efficacy of dihydroergotoxine mesylate (Hydergine) in senile cerebrovascular insufficiency has been documented in many controlled comparisons with placebo and comparable drugs. In a double-blind multicentric comparative study of Hydergine and cinnarizine, Hydergine was found to have a favorable effect on various symptoms of cerebrovascular disturbances (Yoshikawa, 1977). In addition, we recently investigated the efficacy of and tolerance of patients to a higher than usual Hydergine dose to examine the optimal dose by means of the multicentric double-blind method. In Japan, the daily standard dose of Hydergine is 3 mg although a pilot study comparing 3 to 6 mg doses indicates that more pronounced therapeutic effects might be achieved with higher doses (Yesavage, 1979). I shall report the results of this study and also mention a preliminary study of cyclic nucleotide levels in the lumbar cerebrospinal fluid (CSF) of aged patients with dementia. The latter study sought to learn whether or not cyclic nucleotides levels in CSF may help to index general brain function.

Materials and Methods

Researchers in 68 hospitals and rehabilitation centers throughout Japan participated in this investigation. Sixteen facilities are in the metropolitan Tokyo area. The 550 patients included 361 men and 189 women who were referred to the study by clinical neurologists and general practitioners. The majority of patients, 476, suffered from sequelae of cerebral infarction that included cerebral thrombosis, cerebral emoblism, and so-called cerebral arteriosclerosis. The remainder had experienced cerebral or subarachnoid hemorrhages and other cerebrovascular disturbances. Excluded were patients with severe cardiac, hepatic, renal, and cerebral disturbances and, in particular, patients who had recently had a seizure. We also excluded patients who were receiving cerebral and peripheral vasodilators, stimulants of brain metabolism other than Hydergine, psychoneurotropic drugs, adrenocortical hormones, and ACTH. If the patients were being treated with minor tranquilizers and/or antihypertensive drugs before beginning the study, their physicians were instructed not to alter the dosages of these drugs during the Hydergine study.

The patients were placed randomly into two groups. One group received one 1 mg sublingual tablet of Hydergine, plus one placebo tablet, three times per day; the placebo tablets resembled the 2 mg Hydergine tablets used by the other group. Three times per day, the second group received one 2 mg tablet of Hydergine, plus a placebo tablet that resembled the 1 mg Hydergine sublingual tablets used by the first group (Figure 34-1). As the effects of 3 mg of Hydergine versus placebo have been well documented, ethical considerations precluded the use of a third group receiving placebo exclusively. The randomed and double-blind distribution of drugs was supervised by two "controllers" who were not actively engaged in the study of patients. All drugs were dispensed in

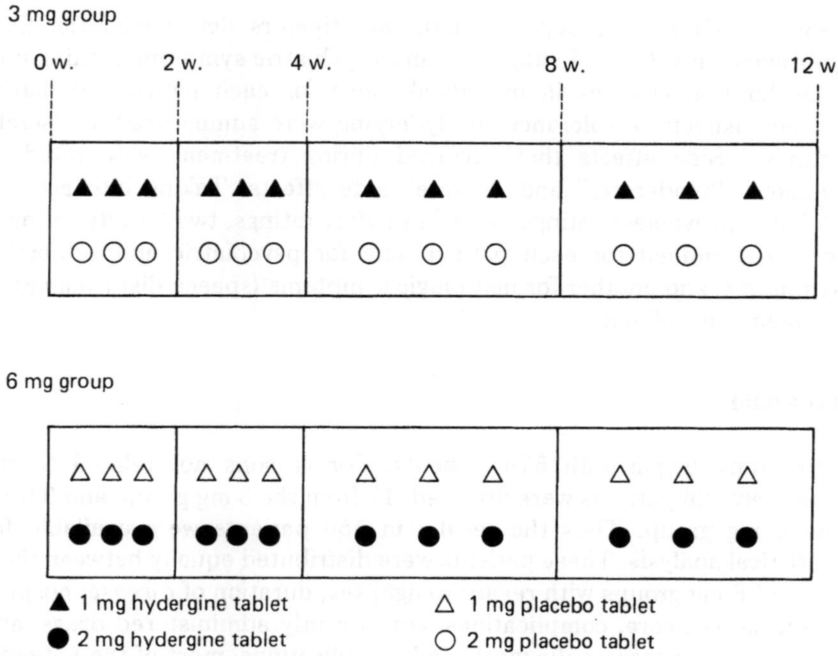

Figure 34-1. Prescription design.

numbered and sealed packages; the randomization list remained in the controller's hands. Duration of treatment for all patients was 12 weeks.

The clinical condition of the patients at the beginning of the investigation and the changes during the 12 weeks of treatment were assessed by a rating system. We distinguished psychiatric and subjective symptoms, assessing them at the beginning of the study (week 0) and 2, 4, 8, and 12 weeks after Hydergine treatment had begun. A four-point scale (severe, moderate, minor, and none) was used for grading individual symptoms. The individual symptom profiles that resulted from this procedure were then summarized as "severity ratings." All changes in individual symptoms that occurred after 2, 4, 8, and 12 weeks of treatment were summarized into an "improvement rating" ranging from +3 to −2 (+3 meaning clear-cut, clinically relevant improvement, −2 meaning relevant deterioration). Like severity scores, improvement ratings were summarized as "global improvement ratings" of psychiatric and neurologic symptoms. These global ratings were the basis for statistical comparisons between the two treatment groups.

To ensure that the conversion of individual symptoms into global severity and improvement scores was done in all centers according to the same principles, a group of senior investigators determined the final improvement ratings of subjective and psychiatric symptoms, taking into consideration changes in individual items for each patient. Similarly, various aspects of tolerance to Hydergine were summarized as "safety ratings." Side effects that occurred during treatment were rated as "minor," "moderate," and "severe" side effects. Taking into account global improvement ratings as well as safety ratings, two "utility ratings" were determined for each patient, one for psychiatric and subjective symptoms, and another for neurologic symptoms (speech disturbances or problems in walking).

Results

The study began with 576 patients. For reasons not related to the treatment, 26 patients were dropped, 17 from the 3 mg group, and 9 from the 6 mg group. Thus the results in 550 patients were available for statistical analysis. These patients were distributed equally between the 3 mg and 6 mg groups with regard to age, sex, duration of disease, hospital or outpatient care, complications, concurrently administered drugs, and diagnosis. Concerning diagnosis and complications, most of the patients, 86% of the 3 mg group and 87% of the 6 mg group, suffered from sequelae of cerebral infarction. Hypertension was a most prevalent complication, and diabetes mellitus was not rare in both groups. With regard to diagnosis and complications, however, the distribution was not significantly different between the two groups (Table 34-1).

Table 34-2 shows a statistical analysis of final global improvement ratings (FGIR) with regard to subjective and psychiatric symptoms. Almost one-half of the patients in the 6 mg group experienced moderate-to-marked improvement, compared to 18% in the 3 mg group, a statistically significant difference. The frequency of at least moderate improvement was significantly higher in all subgroups of the 6 mg group, except for patients who had had subarachnoid hermorrhages, whose number was too small to allow statistical analysis. The difference between the 3 mg and 6 mg groups almost disappeared when the number of patients with slight improvement or better was compared. Using this milder criterion, a tendency in favor of the 6 mg group remained, but the statistically significant difference was much smaller than in the first analysis, which compared patients according to moderate improvement or better. Another analysis, which took into account the presence or absence of target symptoms in patients at the beginning of the study, showed that the higher Hydergine dose was particularly more effective in patients who suffered from heavy-headedness, sleep disturbances of various kinds, problems of concentration, loss of vigor, memory disturbances, and giddiness. Again, when a milder criterion (slight improvement or better)

Table 34-1. Background characteristics of the patients

Item	DEM 3 mg	DEM 6 mg	Notation
Sex			
Male	179	182	$\chi^2 = 0.102$
Female	91	98	NS
Age			
<40	27	23	
41–59	60	64	$\chi^2 = 1.485$
60–69	104	100	df = 4
70–79	67	79	NS
>80	12	14	
Average ± SD	63.5 ± 10.14	64.2 ± 10.22	t = 0.854 NS
Duration of disease			
<6 months	62	74	
6 months–1 year	30	41	$\chi^2 = 3.850$
1–3 years	80	80	df = 3
>3 years	86	72	NS
unknown	12	13	
average ± SD	2.4 ± 2.38	2.1 ± 2.50	t = 1.283 NS
Hospital or outpatient			
hospitalized	82	84	$\chi^2 = 0.008$
outpatients	188	196	NS
Diagnosis			
cerebral infarction	233	243	
cerebral thrombosis	161	171	
cerebral embolism	15	15	
so-called cerebral arteriosclerosis	47	49	$\chi^2 = 1.567$
unable to distinguish thrombosis/embolism	10	8	df = 6
cerebral hemorrhage	26	23	NS
subarachnoid hemorrhage	3	2	
other cerebrovascular disturbances	8	12	
Complications			
no	69	91	$\chi^2 = 3.213$
yes	201	189	NS
hypertension	130	133	
diabetes	8	8	
hypertension + diabetes	25	20	
hypertension + diabetes + other	2	3	
hypertension + other	18	12	
diabetes + other	0	1	
other	18	12	

NS = no significant difference; df = degree of freedom.

Table 34-2. Final global improvement ratings

	Moderate Improvement		Slight Improvement		No Change or Worse
Hydergine Dose	No. Patients	Percent	No. Patients	Percent	No. Patients
Subjective and psychiatric symptoms					
3 mg	46	17.9	199	77.4	58
6 mg	132	48.9	232	85.9	38
Neurologic symptoms					
3 mg	19	9.3	88	42.7	117
6 mg	45	20.7	112	51.6	105

was applied, differences between the 3 mg and 6 mg groups were less pronounced.

With regard to FGIR of neurologic symptoms, improvements were not as marked as in the case of subjective and psychiatric symptoms. Yet moderate improvement occurred in 9.3% of patients in the 3 mg group, compared with 20.7% of patients in the 6 mg group. The difference is significant at the 0.01 level (χ^2 test). When percentages of patients with slight improvement or better were compared, a tendency in favor of the 6 mg group remained (Table 34-2).

Comparing incidence of side effects, we found that no serious side effects had occurred in either group. Minor side effects were experienced by 10.2% of patients in the 3 mg group and 11.3% in the 6 mg group.

Table 34-3 shows utility ratings for subjective and psychiatric symp-

Table 34-3. Utility ratings

	Useful or Better		Slightly Useful or Better		Useless or Worse
Hydergine Dose	No. Patients	Percent	No. Patients	Percent	No. Patients
Subjective and psychiatric symptoms					
3 mg	50	18.9	196	74.0	69
6 mg	139	50.5	227	82.5	48
Neurologic symptoms					
3 mg	21	10.2	86	42.0	119
6 mg	47	21.7	112	51.6	105

toms, taking into account the FGIRs of subjective and psychiatric symptoms and overall safety ratings. In the 3 mg group, the medication was rated at least "useful" for 18.9% of the patients, compared to 50.5% of patients in the 6 mg group. The difference is significant at the 0.001 level (χ^2 test). If one compares the numbers of patients for whom the medication was rated at least "slightly useful," the difference between the two groups is again less pronounced. When the chi-square test was applied to useful or better ratings in treatment for subjective and psychiatric symptoms, the 6 mg dose was found to be significantly superior. When the groups were divided into "slightly useful" or better and "useless" or worse subgroups, the difference between the 3 mg and 6 mg groups was no longer significant.

Measurement of Cyclic Nucleotide Levels in CSF

Sixty patients, 28 women and 32 males, were included in a study of the concentrations of cyclic 3′,5′-monophosphate (cAMP) and cyclic guanosine 3′,5′-monophosphate (cGMP) in lumbar CSF. The patients were classified into four categories. Group 1 included 23 patients who had primary degenerative dementia, mostly senile dementia of the Alzheimer type. Group 2 included 19 patients who had cerebrovascular disorders with or without dementia. In the third group were 10 patients who had no neurological disorders, while the fourth group included 8 patients who had miscellaneous neurological disorders. Our methods for measuring cyclic nucleotides by competitive protein-binding assay and radioimmunoassay were described in detail elsewhere (Eto, 1979).

The results are shown in Table 34-4. Mean values of cAMP concentrations in the lumbar CSF of Groups 2 and 3 were significantly higher than those in Group 1. There was no significant correlations between age and concentrations of cyclic nucleotides in lumbar CSF. CSF pressure, cell count, and protein concentration had no effect on cAMP and cGMP levels, according to statistical analysis of correlation coefficients in the whole series. Conclusively, patients with dementia caused by either a primary degenerative or cerebrovascular process had significantly lower lumber CSF concentrations of cAMP compared to patients without dementia who might have other neurological disorders. This finding, as well as that of other investigators (Fleischer, 1977) suggests that the decreased cAMP level in CSF might reflect a remarkably hypoactive state of the central nervous system, such as dementia.

Since Hydergine is a useful drug for treating patients who have cerebrovascular disturbances, and has been described by some authors as useful in treating patients for dementia, we often prescribe Hydergine to demented patients.

Table 34-4. Subjects and results

Group	No. Patients	Average Age	cAMP in CSF (pmole/ml)	cGMP in CSF (pmole/ml)
1. Presenile dementia (≦65 yrs.): Ia	7	60.7	8.92 ± 3.67	2.42 ± 1.72
Senile dementia (>65 yrs.): Ib	16	73.0	9.75 ± 2.96	2.50 ± 1.56
subtotal	23	69.2	9.50 ± 3.13	2.47 ± 1.57
2. CVD with dementia :IIa	9	64.2	10.11 ± 2.86	2.30 ± 1.14
without dementia :IIb	10	65.9	15.82 ± 5.46	2.73 ± 1.86
subtotal	19	65.1	13.11 ± 5.21**	2.52 ± 1.54
3. Control	10	58.4	15.99 ± 5.41***	2.90 ± 0.88
4. Other neurological diseases*	8	55.2	11.65 ± 3.89	2.06 ± 0.89

*Group 4 included 2 patients with Parkinsonism; 2 with spinocerebellar degenerations; 2 with myasthenia gravis; 1 with intracranial tumor; and 1 with epilepsy.

Difference from Group 1: **$p < 0.01$; ***$p < 0.0001$ (Student's t test).

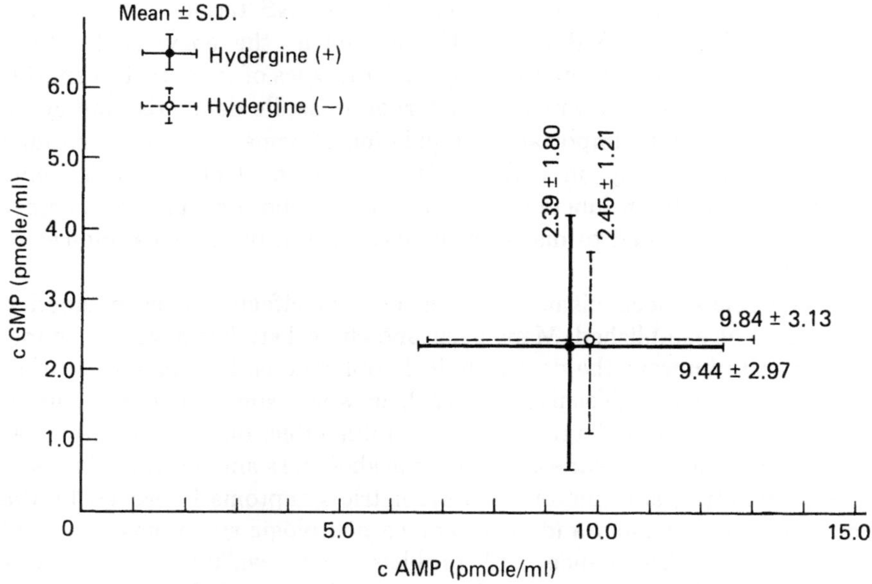

Figure 34-2. Concentrations of cyclic AMP and cyclic GMP in lumbar CSF of demented patients who were taking Hydergine (n = 13) or not (n = 19). The statistical significant difference was observed between both groups.

Figure 34-2 shows cAMP and cGMP levels in the lumbar CSF of demented patients who were taking Hydergine (n = 13) or not (n = 19). The levels did not differ between patients treated with Hydergine and those without it. Changes in cyclic nucleotide levels in lumbar CSF were examined in 6 demented patients after they had taken Hydergine for more than 2 weeks. We found that the administration of Hydergine did not affect cyclic nucleotides levels in CSF of these patients.

Discussion

Hydergine is an ergot alkaloid derivative that acts on such biogenic amines as noradrenaline, adrenaline, dopamine, and serotonin, which are a part of ergoline, the essential constituent of ergot alkaloid. The compound probably improves neuronal function by modifying energy turnover and the mechanism of sodium and potassium ATPase by blocking catecholamine transmission. Hydergine may also have a vasodilating effect but to produce this, the drug may have to be given for a long time. Trials with Hydergine—and it is one of the most extensively studied substances—have shown it to be superior to placebo, if not by much.

Measurement of cyclic nucleotides in the cerebrospinal fluid may provide valuable information concerning certain alterations of central nervous system tissues because mammalian CNS tissues contain large amounts of cyclic AMP and GMP, as well as the enzymes for their synthesis and degradation. Recently, several types of synaptic transmitter function have been shown to be disturbed in senile dementia, and cyclic nucleotides may be important in regulation of some synaptic membrane functions. Our study on CSF levels of cyclic nucleotides, which may reflect general brain function, was preliminary and inconclusive. Further study will be needed to discover clinically useful biochemical indices of brain failure.

Hydergine's mechanisms of action and its effects on brain function remain to be established. Many basic and clinical studies have been done, however, to improve the drug's clinical applications. In Japan, the earlier double-blind study (Yoshikawa, 1977), in which similar patients participated, found that Hydergine had a favorable effect on such symptoms as dizziness, heavy-headedness, stiffness in shoulders and neck, weakness of the extremities, and numbness. Psychiatric symptoms improved by the drug included memory and vigor; among neurologic symptoms improved were speech disturbance and problems with walking. As previous investigation had been done with a 3 mg daily dose of Hydergine, and in view of the experiences of researchers in other countries, we raised the question of whether or not higher doses might induce still more pronounced improvements and still be tolerated. Several difficulties could be foreseen in our attempt to find differences between two doses of the clinically active drugs in heterogenous patient groups. We decided, therefore, to include a large number of patients, which required a multicentric trial and refinement of the assessment system for subjective and objective symptoms.

The results show convincing that the effects of Hydergine on psychiatric, subjective, and neurologic symptoms in patients with cerebrovascular disease are considerably more favorable when a higher dose is used. In all symptom categories, results in the 6 mg group were superior to those in the 3 mg group. The differences between the 3 mg and 6 mg groups were much clearer when stricter criteria were used, that is, when patients with clear-cut improvement in different symptom areas were considered rather than patients who showed at least slight improvement. This suggests that a majority of patients will improve slightly with a daily 3 mg dose of Hydergine, whereas the percentage of patients who improve moderately or more rises considerably when a daily 6 mg dose is used. A daily 3 mg dose may therefore be insufficient for some patients who have cerebrovascular disease, and clinically relevant improvement may be obtained by more patients if the dose is increased to 6 mg per day.

At the same time, a detailed and strict analysis of side effects and dropouts provided no hint that the higher efficacy of an increased daily dose is nullified by more frequent or more severe side effects. In neither the 3 mg nor the 6 mg group were there patients with clinically significant side effects or with symptoms that could be attributed to Hydergine rather than to the disease. We believe, therefore, that a daily 6 mg Hydergine dose is more suitable for treating patients who have various symptoms caused by cerebrovascular disorders.

References

Eto, F., Okano, K., Yoshikawa, M., and Hirai, S.: Concentration of cyclic nucleotides in the cerebrospinal fluid of aged patients with dementia. *Clin. Neurol. 19*, 22–26 (1979) (in Japanese).

Fleischer, A.S., Rudman, D.R., Fresh, C.B., and Tindall, G.T.: Concentration of 3′5′ cyclic adenosine monophosphate in ventricular CSF of patients following severe head trauma. *J. Neurosurg. 47*, 517–524 (1977).

Yesavage, J.A., Hollister, L., and Burain, E.: Dihydroergotoxine: 6 mg versus 3 mg dosage in the treatment of senile dementia. Preliminary report. *J. Am. Geriatr. Soc. 27*, 80–82 (1979).

Yoshikawa, M., Hirai, S., Aizawa, T., et al.: The efficacy of Hydergine in cerebrovascular diseases—investigations by the double blind method. *Igaku no Ayumi 100*, 836 (1977) (in Japanese).

Part X

Psychiatric Treatment in the Future

Chapter 35

The Mental Health Professional in a Preventive Role

Eric Pfeiffer

Summary

The author predicts that mental health professionals will add a major prevention role to their current diagnostic and therapeutic role. Preventive techniques differ markedly from treatment techniques in a number of important ways: preventive services can best be offered to groups of individuals, even very large groups; motivational factors differ markedly; and measurement of impact requires different types of statistical techniques. Nevertheless the author predicts that by the year 2000 care of the chronically ill and chronically well will assume an importance equal to that of the care of the acutely and the dramatically ill. The author anticipates that the benefits derived from prevention will far outweigh the benefits derived from treatment and/or rehabilitation.

On Making Predictions

Those who control the future are best able to predict it. Since none of us here do, we likely will not even come close to hitting the mark with our predictions. We bring to our task little more than the light of a single candle: the farther we are removed from that minute source of light, the dimmer our vision. The farther we seek to project into the future, the greater the risk of being overtaken by the unforeseen or the unforeseeable.

Yet we are all here trying to focus our paltry vision on what lies ahead, both immediately and in the intermediate future. Our motivations in doing so are varied; we wish to assure our own safety and well-being in the future, and to assure the safety and well-being of special groups, like the aged. These first two types of motivation are relatively noble ones, but there can also be less noble motivations for predicting the future such as the profit motive, the motive to gain advantage over others, or whatever ego gratification there is in making predictions which might just possibly turn out to be right. Undoubtedly, however, there is a great deal of interest in predicting the future and surely the devil could profit handsomely from selling to the highest bidder a copy of tomorrow's Wall Street Journal on any corner. In addition, attempting to peer into the future can be a game, a game which incidently we have all been recruited to, more or less willingly, by the organizers of this volume.

Predicting the Future as Agenda Setting

But I would now like to focus on another aspect of prediction making which I think has perhaps the greatest merit. I believe that a prediction can also function as an agenda for the future. Predictions can function positively in holding out for us trophic images of a desired outcome (as in the science fiction writer's projection of space travel and other spectacles and spectaculars) but it can also function negatively as in an Orwell's *1984*, which seeks to warn us off an undesirable course or outcome.

I want to make one further general point about predictions before going on to my special topic of predictions about preventive aspects of mental health services. It is much easier to be right about *what* is going to happen than *when* or *where* it is going to happen. 1984 already exists in certain totalitarian governments, for instance. To illustrate further, in 1975 I made ten predictions about things that might happen relevant to health care and the elderly by the year 2025. One of these predictions has already come true (the prediction that mandatory retirement would itself be retired) while two others are partially fulfilled (the prediction that spending on health care services would exceed 10% of the gross national product and an expansion of life expectancy towards 90 years of age). Since that time we have gone from a life expectancy of approximately 70 years to a life expectancy of 74 years, well on our way to 90 years of age. Thus while some of these predictions are being fulfilled "ahead of schedule," others may not happen in my lifetime, which I predicted would end in line with my prediction of a life expectancy of 90 years of age, in the year 2025.

A Single Major Relatively Comprehensive Prediction About Preventive Services

On the basis of current observations, of some briefly observed trends (3–4 year trends), and of using predictions for agenda setting, I would like to make the following prediction concerning preventive services for the elderly by the year 2000:

Care of the chronically ill and the chronically well will assume an importance equal to that of the care of the acutely and dramatically ill by the year 2000!

What do I mean?

I mean that psychiatry, and other medical fields as well, will be deeply involved in preventive care and in chronic care, including psychological care of the chronically physically and mentally disabled.

Why do I believe this?

We see currently emerging trends towards all kinds and types of self-help, self-care, holistic care, health food stores, health fads, wellness services, wellness institutes, vitamin supplements, life extension books, and life extension clinics, as well as longevity research and longevity research foundations headed by nonagenarians, Noble Laureates, and the beautiful people. A growing number of people, as they grow older, are getting sick and tired of being sick and retired in their old age. They won't stand for it.

A second currently emerging trend comes from the government. There is now emerging a trend toward the rhetoric of prevention. In my mind rhetoric preceeds action. Prevention is viewed by some as a fiscal panacea at all levels of government. The Department of Health and Human Services has an office of health promotion and disease prevention. Even in the previous administration several documents appeared which focused on prevention. Current authorizing language relating to the Veterans Administration and several requests for proposals from HCVA, NIMH, and other HHS or related agencies include "prevention" as a prominent part of the headlines.

Yet how much do we really know today? Painfully little. Painfully little, in any case that can be supported by "hard facts" but a few things can be cited.

> Regular exercise clearly improves self-image and mood at all adult ages, with findings better documented for men than for women. These findings are far more impressive than any documented improvements in survivors for myocardial infarction and other physical outcomes.

Weigh reduction lowers high blood pressure, thereby reducing the risk of stroke and of multi-infarct dementia, regardless of whether used alone or in conjunction with other antihypertensive measures.

Excessive use of alcohol is a serious risk to older patients in terms of a number of adverse health outcomes (falls, confusion, poor nutrition, dementia).

Smoking.

Caloric undernutrition may be associated with some modest degree of life extensions. It should be noted, however, that caloric restriction which can bring about this affect will not supply adequate amounts of vitamins and minerals and these must be supplemented programmatically.

Well, that is not yet a whole lot to go on. What about the mental health arena specifically? We are on even less firm ground here. But a few positive findings, as yet poorly documented, have emerged:

Peer support groups are of undoubted value to persons facing chronic illess, death, or chronic pain, in either themselves or in their nearest relatives. I said of "undoubted" value deliberately, and did not say of proven value. There is a difference.

Having a spouse is of undoubted survival value. Remaining life expectancy of the married exceeds by several years that of persons who are single, widowed, divorced, or separated. The mediating factors are not fully understood, but the facts are quite dramatic.

There are other data as well which point to the positive value of belonging to some common group that supports its members. These groups may be quite varied, such as family groups, religious groups, interest groups, minority groups, even such peer groups such as the Mafia.

Definition of Prevention

Before going too far afield into the arena of specific preventive mental health efforts, let me pause to focus on the nature of preventive efforts in general. I will offer you two relatively cynical definitions of what constitutes prevention. One of these says, A preventive service is a service for which you cannot get reimbursement. A second, equally cynical definition is, A preventive service is one which we do not yet know how to deliver.

Regrettably, there is more truth than poetry in both of these definitions. Our reimbursement mechanisms clearly favor an illness orientation. Our skill in demonstrating the efficacy of preventive efforts, as well as the statistical appreciation of the possible effectiveness of preventive efforts, leaves much to be desired. Also, the motivational factors involved in prevention contrast sharply with those involved in acute care. A broken leg demands fixing. We hardly need to persuade anyone of this. A gradual decimation of social roles and of meaningful activities, or the gradual accumulation of bodily toxins, make only a small and silent plea for intervention and can easily be ignored. Accordingly it may be well to focus for a few moments on the characteristics of preventive services, and on how they differ from treatment type of interventions.

Characteristics of Preventive Services

1. Preventive service can best be applied to groups of individuals rather than to single individual patients. There are several advantages in this in that the cost per person of a preventive service tends to be quite small, as contrasted with treatment services which can be quite high. In addition, group participation tends to provide some of the motivational incentives for participating in preventive activities which is otherwise not present.
2. Preventive services make use primarily of educational or behavioral changes involving some positive action to be taken on the part of the participating individual rather than the taking of some medication prescribed by a health provider. To comment on this, I will simply remind the reader that the original meaning of the term doctor is not "healer" but is, in fact, "teacher," from the Latin word *docere* which defines the physician as a health educator.
3. Preventive services are not intended to allay some present suffering but rather to guard against some future calamity, requiring investment of current motivational capital.
4. Documenting the benefits of any preventive strategy requires large samples of participating individuals and highly sophisticated statistical techniques.
5. Cost–benefit analyses are even more difficult to conduct on preventive services than they are on treatment services.
6. In the absence of quick and easy documentation, unfortunately *hope* and *hype*, fads and fantasies, often far outpace scientific knowledge in the area of prevention. The risk of this is that it may give legitimate preventive efforts a bad name and leave the "consumer" or participant in possible preventive services at a loss of which of various available preventive strategies to pursue.

Yet let there be no doubt about it. We have gotten to where we are not on the basis of heroic one-on-one treatment of individual patients, but on the basis of group-applied measures, insights, and procedures, such as vaccination, sterile childbirth, antibiotics, clean water supplies, etc.

There is little doubt in my mind that sooner or later (and I am not at all certain about the time dimension involved), preventive measures in the mental health arena will make a far greater difference to the mental well-being to the populations of older persons than will one-on-one psychotherapy, drug therapy, or any other individually focused form of therapy.

Some Specifics

It is tempting to take this opportunity to lay before you a full range of possible and desirable mental health initiatives of a preventive nature. I will not resist this temptation entirely. I am constrained, however, not so much by time as I am by a lack of detailed knowledge. I will therefore confine myself to sketching out a few headlines, rather than full programs of preventive activities. Reminding the reader, however, of the agenda-setting nature of predictions, I feel that these sketchy programs will constitute trophic incentives for their more complete development and refinement. This brief catalogue of suggested preventive services will be quite diverse in its nature, quite incomplete, and does not constitute a sequential priorities list. Since we have been asked to address preventive services in the mental health arena by the year 2000, we have some 17 years left to fill in the details.

Nine Predictions

1. The development of mental health checkups in middle life, which will evaluate the individual's major areas of psychological functioning, including work performance and work satisfaction, family life and family satisfaction, leisure activities, stress-handling capacities and major crises and their resolution, interpersonal skills, especially one-on-one interpersonal skills of the I–thou type, and plans for retirement preparation.
2. The inclusion of a brief cognitive examination as a routine part of all physical examinations for persons over age 65 or, for men, over age 60.
3. Periodic comprehensive assessment, including mental health assessment, of all persons over age 75. Such assessment would include assessment of physical health, mental health, social resources, economic resources, and self-care capacity for the activities of independent daily living.
4. Development of educational programs for older persons, utilizing our emptying classrooms to teach older persons how to cope with aging,

how to prepare the next generation of life left to live after retirement, and an understanding of the values and risks of social and health services to the elderly.
5. The publication and widespread dissemination of an authoritative guidebook or guidebooks on how to adapt to old age, a sort of Dr. Benjamin Spock for old people.
6. A developing focus on the nature and the importance of the inner life of older persons, emphasizing their participation in fantasy, creativity, sexuality, close interpersonal relationships, and so on.
7. A frank recognition of the excoriating effect of social disconnectiveness, and programs aimed at effectively reconnecting socially isolated individuals with other persons in similar need on an intergenerational level.
8. The development of relatively side-effect-free medication for the treatment of such disorders and depression, hypertension, Alzheimer's disease, and related disorders.
9. Attention to the avoidance of age segregation and age group scapegoating or antagonisms, through the pursuit of national policies that are fair to the aged as well as to other voting and nonvoting segments of the population.

I will stop here. I have given us all more than enough to do. I hope to be able to elaborate on these predictions and programs over the next 17 years and strongly invite discussion of these proposals. I would welcome from the reader any additional suggestions and proposals of what can and should be done along preventive lines in the mental health arena. I have no illusions about how easy or how difficult any of these programs are to achieve. My interest is in furthering this agenda as far as it can be taken. In football terms, I want to take what the defense will give us. To put it another way, programs will be incremental, but there may be sudden breakdowns in the defense against preventive measures, and for those times, we need to be prepared for the game plan. We need to know what to do.

Chapter 36

Concepts of Depression in the Elderly: Signposts to Future Mental Health Needs

Barry J. Gurland, David E. Wilder, and John Copeland

Summary

A broad and reliable diagnosis of "pervasive depression" was used in the U.S.–U.K. Geriatric Community Study. The great majority of these cases were judged to be in need of psychiatric intervention and were heavy users of health services, but interventions for their psychiatric problems were mostly from medical practitioners.

In setting the goals of the system of services directed at the needs of the older population for the prevention or relief of mental health problems, we should clarify at least the two following issues:

1. What mental health conditions should be the main concern for prevention and treatment?
2. In what clinical settings and with what personnel should be concentrate therapeutic efforts for these mental health conditions?

The conventional classification of the mental health conditions of old age may not be a suitable guide to planning appropriate mental health services. Each domain of mental health problems must be carefully examined in order to determine what definition of a mental health problem best reflects the need for services. After this decision is made one can examine these implications for manpower and training that arise from the nature of the problem and the contexts in which it occurs.

This paper will pursue these issues with respect to depression in the elderly. An argument will be advanced that the concept of depression that is currently attracting most attention is too narrow to be useful as a signpost to improving mental health services for the elderly. In particular, this paper will seek to show that preoccupation with a narrow concept of depression can lead the health care professions to look in the wrong places for the elderly client with mental health problems.

In order to bolster these arguments with empirical data we will refer to the United States–United Kingdom Cross-National Geriatric Community Study (Gurland et al., 1983). The principal aims of this study were to compare New York City and London for the prevalence of psychiatric impairments in the community elderly, the associated medical and social problems, the services and supports received, and the outcome of the psychiatric and other health impairments over a followup period of 1 year.

Data was gathered from randomly drawn samples of persons 65 years of age and older throughout the two cities. However, for the present purposes mainly the data gathered in New York will be considered. Subjects were examined in their homes by project staff trained in the administration of a reliable and systemtic semistructured interview, the Comprehensive Assessment and Referral Evaluation (CARE).

There were 445 completed interviews in New York and 396 in London. Psychiatrists interviewed all cases in London and a random one-half of cases in New York and made a clinical diagnosis according to the International Classification of Diseases, 9th edition, where appropriate. In addition, a diagnosis according to operational criteria specifically developed for classifying mental disorders in the community elderly was applied after review of the extensive systematic information and a narrative summary on each patient. The reliability and validity of these operational diagnoses has been published (Gurland et al., 1983; Gurland et al., 1982).

The concepts of depression that can be examined with these data include two main types that vary principally in their breadth. The narrow concept is embodied in the psychiatric diagnosis of manic-depressive disorders (International Classification of Diseases, 9th edition) which corresponds closely to the DSM III category of major depression. The criteria for these diagnoses are found in their respective nomenclatures. It is these relatively narrow concepts which have attracted most professional interest in recent years. By way of contrast, the broad concept of depression termed "pervasive depression" was developed and applied to the data on this study in the expectation that it would prove useful as an indicator of need for intervention. The criteria for this new category are shown in Table 36-1. The operational criteria for pervasive depression can be simply and reliably applied; they do not rely upon the presence of somatic symptoms which might require complex judgements about their source (i.e., whether they are physical or psychiatric in nature). Inter-

Table 36-1. Criteria for diagnosis of prevasive depression

At least one from two of following sets:
Depression lasts whole day or longer
Cries or feels like crying, often
Depression is bothersome and not easily shaken off
Future looks bleak or unbearable
Can't stop worrying—worry is disproportionate to cause
Looks depressed through much of interview
Not taken into consideration
Depression lasts only a few hours—can snap out of it
Occasional low days
Worried about specific problem—can turn mind to other things
Cries only when a particular event or situation is discussed
Future looks empty

disciplinary reliability between psychiatrists and nonpsychiatrists is satisfactory (Gurland et al., 1983).

Pervasive depression is intended to include the categories of depression meeting criteria for DSM III diagnoses (major depression, dysthymic reaction, atypical depression, and adjustment reaction) as well as other states or traits of depression which are persistent from day to day and pervade the person's current life. Pervasive depression does not include such transient or limited negative mood as depression lasting only a few hours (i.e., subject can snap out of it); occasional low days; worry about specific problems (i.e., subjects can turn their minds to other things); or crying only when a particular event or situation is discussed.

In order to examine the conditions lying outside of even the broad concept of pervasive depression, we have also defined two other groups which will appear in some of the following illustrations: *latent depression*, a group identified by statistical procedures (latent class analysis) as having an excessive degree of depression, yet who do not meet the criteria for pervasive depression; and *other*, those subjects who are none of the above and also showed no signs of dementia nor an unusual degree of cognitive impairment.

Since some of the data that follow were based upon judgements made by interviewers, it is necessary to emphasize that interviews, ratings, and judgements were by psychiatrists for all the subjects in London and one-half the subjects in New York; the remainder of subjects in New York were interviewed by social scientists with clinical experience.

The proportion of pervasive depressives who were judged to have definite psychiatric symptoms is shown in Figure 36-1. Definite psy-

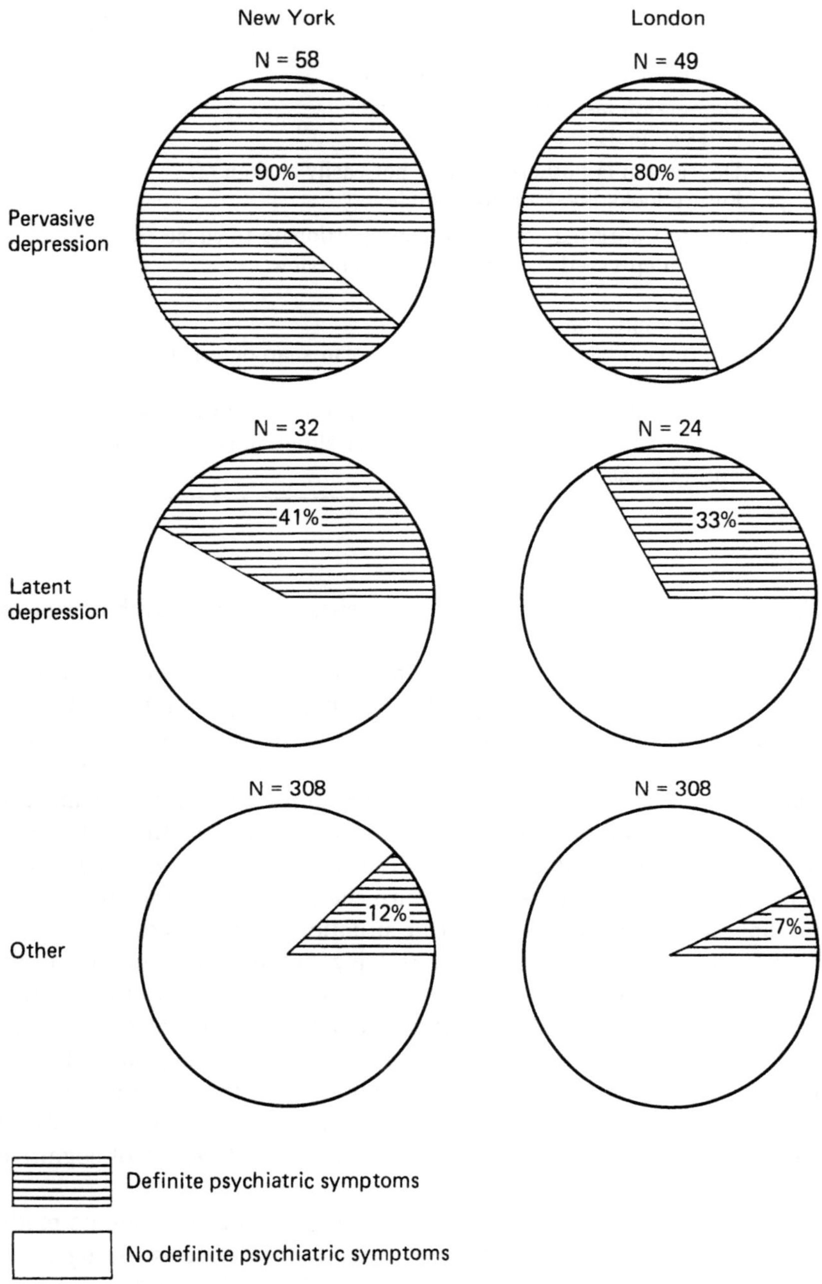

Figure 36-1. Proportions of community elderly in New York and London samples with pervasive depression, latent depression, and other.

chiatric symptoms comprised the two worst categories of a four-level anchored global scale completed by the interviewer after the extensive semistructured CARE interview. A variety of symptoms are included in the anchoring descriptions of these two categories such as deep depression, marked anxiety, obvious withdrawal, self-deprecation, clear-cut agitation, or suicidal ideation. The proportion of the cognitively intact community elderly rated as having definite psychiatric symptoms was 25.1% in New York and 17.8% in London. The vast majority of pervasive depressives in both cities are judged to be have definite symptoms, but less than one-half of the latent depressives are so judged (most are judged to be mild or negligible in severity). Very few of the "other" group are judged to have definite symptoms (one should bear in mind that subjects with cognitive impairment have been eliminated).

Figure 36-2 shows what proportion of the community elderly with definite psychiatric symptoms are included in the group diagnosed as having pervasive depression. A little over one-half of those subjects who have severe psychiatric symptoms have pervasive depressions. (It should again be remembered that the elderly with cognitive impairment have been removed from the sample, leaving only the cognitively intact). The latent depressions account for only 12–13% of the subjects with definite psychiatric symptoms.

Thus, the concept of pervasive depression is (1) sufficiently narrow that it mostly excludes other than definite psychiatric syndromes; (2) sufficiently broad that it captures about one-half of definite functional psychiatric syndromes in the community elderly (though it is by no means a catchall); and (3) sharply different from latent depressions in the proportions of the respective groups which have definite psychiatric syndromes and also in the proportion of definite functional psychiatric syndromes in the community elderly for which they respectively account.

Further evidence of the health service implications of the diagnosis of pervasive depression is shown (in Figure 36-3) by the proportion who were judged to have a need for a major or crucial intervention for their psychiatric problems (such as counseling, prescription drugs, hospitalization, or diagnostic procedures). The majority of pervasive depressions were judged to be cases by these tokens, while less than one-half of the latent depressions and negligible proportions of the other category were judged to be cases. These results are in accord with the view that pervasive depression is a concept which appropriately reflects a need for services to relieve a mental health condition.

The relative prevalence rates of the narrow and broad concepts of depression were determined in the samples of New York and London community elderly. Prevalence figures given refer to all elderly residing in the community (i.e., the cognitively impaired elderly have not been removed from the sample). Pervasive depressives are in the region of 12–13% (over a period of 1 month); they include the manic-depressive–

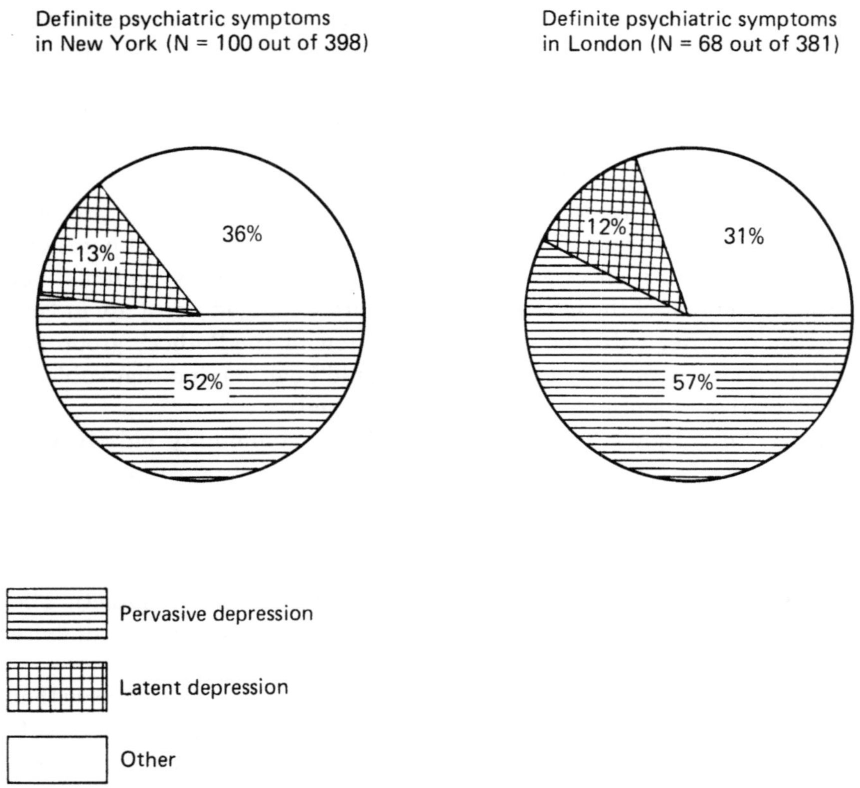

Figure 36-2. Proportions of community elderly in New York and London samples with psychiatric symptoms of depression.

group, but are many times greater in numbers (fivefold in New York and ninefold in London).

Discussion

The data presented in this chapter show the importance of the concept and diagnosis of pervasive depression from a clinical and public health perspective. Pervasive depression is a broader concept than that of manic-depression or major depression and is consequently much more prevalent among the elderly; yet, as we have shown, its breadth does not diminish its health services relevance. The clinical and public health relevance of pervasive depression has been shown by the high proportion who are judged to have definite psychiatric symptoms and to need intervention for their psychiatric problems.

Despite the relevance of pervasive depression as an indicator of the need for intervention only about one-half of this group in the New York community sample were noted to have received a major or crucial

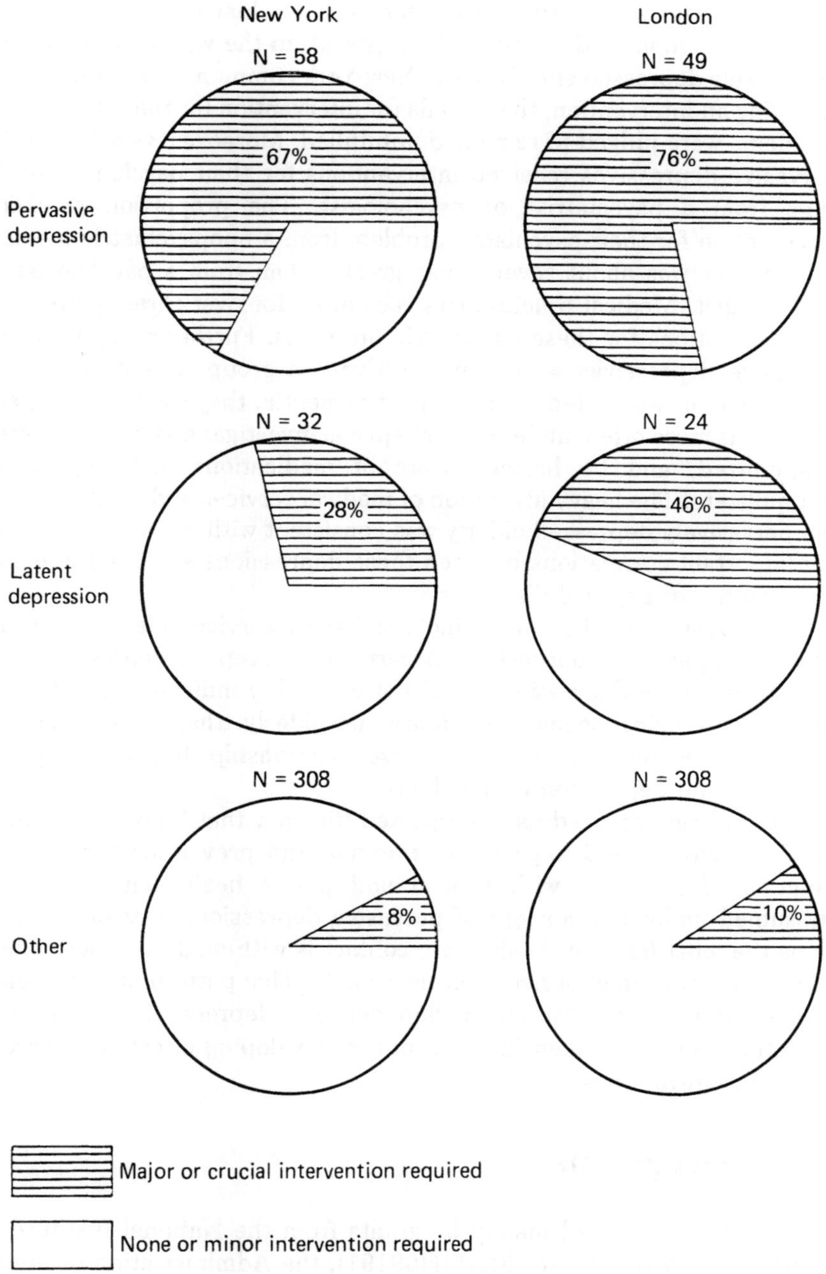

Figure 36-3. Proportions of sample populations in New York and London who were judged to have a need for psychiatric intervention.

intervention (as previously defined) for their psychiatric problems during the previous month (Gurland et al., in press). In the vast majority of the pervasively depressed elderly in the New York community, whether or not receiving an intervention, their needs for intervention for their psychiatric problems were judged to remained unfulfilled. Moreover, very few of the pervasive depressives received interventions for their psychiatric problems from a psychiatrist or psychologist. The proportion receiving intervention for their psychiatric problem from a nonpsychiatric medical practitioner was about seven times greater than from a psychiatrist or psychologist. Medical practitioners accounted for over three-quarters of all interventions for these psychiatric problems. Furthermore, when the pervasive depressives were compared with a group who were neither depressed nor warranted a diagnosis of dementia, they were found to see physicians more often, undergo more special investigations, be more often hospitalized, and be heavier users of medications including minor tranquilizers. The heavy utilization of medical services and treatments by the pervasively depressed elderly was consistent with other data indicating important correlations between these depressions and the frequency and severity of physical disorders.

These results further underline the health service relevance of the concept of pervasive depression. A narrower concept of depression than that of pervasive depression would not as readily indicate the nature of the health-seeking behavior of depressed elderly, their accessibility in medical care settings, and the close relationship between physical disorders and depression in the elderly.

The findings reported have supported the view that there is an urgent need to increase and improve intervention and prevention for a broad range of depressions with clinical and public health importance as subsumed under the concept of pervasive depression. In these depressions the most frequent health care contact is with medical practitioners rather than with mental health professionals. This pattern of health care contact and the substantial overlap between depression and physical conditions must be taken into account in developing effective interventions and preventions.

Acknowledgments

This study was funded mainly by grants from the National Institute of Mental Health (Grant No. 5R1MH09191), the Administration on Aging (Grant No. 93-P-57467), by the New York State Office of Mental Health, and the Department of Health and Social Security, London.

The names of the investigating teams are listed in *Mind and Mood of Aging: The Mental Health Problems of the Community Elderly in New York and London*. New York: Haworth Press, 1983.

References

Gurland, B., Copeland, J., Kelleher, M., Kuriansky, J., Sharpe, L., and Dean, L.: The mind and mood of aging: The mental health problems of the community elderly in New York and London. New York: Haworth Press, 1983.

Gurland, B., Dean, L., Copeland, J.R.M., Gurland, R., and Golden, R.: Criteria for the diagnosis of dementia in the community elderly. *Gerontologist* *22*(2), 180–186 (1982).

Gurland, B., Golden, R., Lantigua, R., and Dean, L.: Overlap between physical conditions and depression in the elderly: A key to improvement in service delivery. In Nayer, D. (Ed.), The Patient & Those Who Care: The Mental Health Aspects of Long Term Physical Illness. Watson Publishers International (in press).

Chapter 37

Psychiatric Treatments for the Aged: 2000 and Beyond

Kenneth Z. Altshuler

Summary

The aged of the future are children of the 1940s and 1950s. Raised on Freud and used to making their presence felt, they will recognize their mental health needs and press for proper services. This alone should partially remediate today's problem whereby 3–5% of the aged receive service, while 25% require it. Another ground for optimism is that psychological treatments have been shown to work. Already there is general agreement about modifications for psychotherapy with the elderly. Newer, codified therapies are being refined and tested, and these too must soon be honed for use in geriatrics. In psychopharmacology, we are witnessing a chemical dissection of the brain. The results will doubtlessly bring still better success with depression, and relief of anxiety and agitation rather than suppression. Whether the new techniques of molecular biology will rid us of the specter of Alzheimer's disease early in the next century is problematic. If they do not, it will be the courts' responsibility to resolve, in the uniquely principled and public fashion characteristic of our judiciary, questions of when there is a right to die and under what conditions enabling death is either allowed or required.

Forecasting the future is always risky. Assumptions, by definition, are uncertain, and the precise dimensions of the future are inscrutable. The forecaster can only comfort him- or herself with the ideas that forecasts are remembered inversely in proportion to how far ahead they look, and that 20–50 years is a large enough margin to excuse mistakes. With these disclaimers in mind, let us turn to the task. It is to review our concerns; to look at what treatments we have and will have, and whether they will be available to, and sought out by, those in need; and to clarify what options exist (pleasant or otherwise), should treatment(s) be insufficient.

We all know the figures that embody our concerns: The year 2030 will bring us 60 million Americans over 65. Five percent will be institutionalized, if the current picture continues; and 15% will require institutionalization at some time. Twenty-five percent or more will require mental health services of some kind, and about 3–5% receive them (Butler, 1975; Siegel, 1980). Whether what is received matches what is needed even in this 3–5% no one knows. The cost of health care this year reached 10% of the Gross National Product. The greater proportion of it is spent on the elderly, who are a far smaller proportion of the population than they soon will be. Society as a whole is worried about the current expense, and both scared and resentful of projected costs if they remain uncontrolled. Poverty is a major problem confronting the aged as their dollar buys less and less. Alzheimer's disease is the most intractable medical–psychiatric entity facing us in the aged population; the specter of millions of decaying citizens, warehoused without hope and vegetating until death, has made discussion of euthanasia acceptable where once it was beyond the pale of ethical possibility (Gaylin, 1974; Kahn, 1975).

Four other factors need to be entered into the ledger to complete the page: First, despite the vastness of the problems—now and into the future—no solutions are in sight, and no one really knows what to do. Second, whatever the solutions are to be, we are dramatically short of personnel to implement them. No meeting on aging in the last 20 years has failed to bemoan the fact that the elderly are the outcasts of society, and I am sure that there will be a continuation of exhortations for more interest and better training. Third, and a special subset related to the second, is that despite increasing expressions of concern, mental health professionals expressly have ignored the aged and preferred to concentrate their expertise and resources elsewhere. And fourth, elderly people—even in need—have been about as loathe to seek services that are labeled psychiatric or mental as society and the professions have been to provide them.

Now is there any room for optimism in all this? Putting what I just said together in writing this a few months ago, I was surprised to find myself answering, "yes." I am still surprised, but still find myself responding with the same "yes" answer.

Let us look at the last issue first: Elderly people are not eager to come for psychiatric help or help that is labeled mental health. A number of studies show they avoid it (Kahn, 1975; Butler and Lewis, 1977; Riley and Foner, 1968). They are seldom self-referred to emergency rooms, but instead are brought by others; they feel such illness is stigmatizing, more than their younger counterparts; they judge—or rationalize—that psychotherapy is baloney rather than helpful, and surely do not seek it out or see it as a matter of status to be "in shrinkage," as current vogue has labeled our therapeutic relationship. Reflecting these attitudes, 25 years ago when I first started a psychiatric program in a home for the aged, both the medical and administrative directors were fearful about whether the residents would be willing to talk to me. And for our own part, many professionals have not forgotten (or have clung to) Freud's dictum that the mid-forties were about the upper limit for fruitful psychotherapeutic work (Freud, 1924).

It is strange how even those of us in the field (or in related fields) can be blinded by our own anxieties and believe the rationalization they lead us to. At the time, the concerns of my medical director worried me; I was younger and assumed authority to be knowledgeable. But over a period of nearly 20 years, and while the place itself grew from a 100 bed old age home to a 760 bed geriatric center, no one ever refused to see me. A principle I adopted, that I would still recommend to anyone working with the aged in an institutional setting, is to visit the patient where he or she lives. If you wait—or hide—in your office, you will not see the patients because they are, in truth, reluctant to come. Second, you would not see the patient anyway because you would see someone with his best foot forward and anxieties increased by the artificial setting. Visiting patients where they are is more comfortable for patients; it is on their own turf. It is also more revealing since you can see more of patients, their important possessions, and their evident and unadorned levels of function. And finally, it is more personal: your visit dignifies the patient; it satisfies and gives him or her opportunity to share with you, and it is therefore often supportive and therapeutic in itself.

In case any of you are about to embark on such a venture—working with the elderly in an institution—I want to reassure you. When I knocked on the door and identified myself, I would occasionally be greeted with "What do you want? Do you think I'm crazy?" or even "Go away! I'm not crazy." But with a little reassurance, the door always opened. And once inside no visit was unpleasant. Al Goldfarb, who died a few years ago, was one of the pioneers in psychotherapy with the aged. He was a good friend, and his friendship as well as what more he could have contributed will be sorely missed. But he was right when he called attention to the potential transferences that any resident has toward any authority in a home or institutional setting. The positive regard with which doctors and other professionals are held—even "shrinks"—is a strong force for eliciting helpful change (Goldfarb, 1955).

I want to comment more about treatment of psychiatric illness of the aged, but first let us take a moment to correct a concern I think grows out of a failure of historical perspective. The aged we have been working with 20 or 10 years ago, or even nearer in time, are 70–80 years or more of age. That means most of them were born and reared before, or near, the turn of the century. Their lack of psychiatric interest or psychological mindedness is a product of attitudes ingrained in those years. Recall that much of medicine itself was then quackery. Late into the last century surgeons were transmogrified from barbers, and medicine was taught as much in the preceptorial mode as in the university. In 1893, Johns Hopkins became the first university to claim that medicine was a postgraduate course of study, and undergraduate training was prerequisite. It was only after 1910 that medical education in this country was made uniform and included basic science and organized clinical instructional experience. Ehrlich developed antisyphilitic medication in 1910, but antibiotics—our first mass weapon against infectious diseases—did not appear until the 1930s (Starr, 1982). Persons raised in the "good old days," therefore, had little reason to have faith in doctors, and in us "alienists" least of all.

We are at a vastly different point now. The aged we will be concerned with in 2000 and beyond derive from the baby boom after World War II. This huge bolus has been the center of our nation's concern as it has moved through the population. Many who read these words are a part of it. You have been raised in what has been called "The Age of the Child," so centered have been the adults on you. You have been a major force in the economy, and all marketing efforts have been aimed at you: we sold you Barbie and Ken dolls when you were little, makeup and pimple aids through puberty, disposable diapers in your 20s and 30s, and we will sell you hair colorings, spectacles, and hearing aids in the next several decades. These—you—are the aged we will be talking about. This is the generation raised on Freud, on Modern Child Rearing for Psychological Health, on debates about penis envy, women's liberation, the anti-establishment social and liberal protests of the 1970s. You are more educated than any generation hitherto, less restricted in outlook, and used to making yourselves heard and felt. I have no doubt that you will force involvement upon the government or whatever agencies need to be approached and that (far from avoiding it) your psychological mindedness will cause you to demand and get attention to the psychological and psychosocial needs of individuals, as well as those more narrowly defined as medical. More than anything else, I think these facts are reasons for an optimistic outlook for the future.

Turning to treatments themselves, I believe there is also room for optimism. We have now the strictly psychological treatments and psychopharmacological ones. The future will refine these and add new weapons at the level of molecular genetics. We have come a long way in recognizing the psychological issues that confront the aged and in helping to deal with them. Grotjahn and Meerlo in the 50s were the first to affirm that psychoanalytic principles, or even psychoanalysis itself, could be usefully applied to problems of the elderly (Grotjahn, 1951; Grotjahn, 1955; Meerloo, 1953; Meerloo, 1955). Freud, as usual, had been misunderstood, since he never said the aged should not be helped or that analytic principles would not be useful in understanding the issues that engaged them; he said only that psychoanalysis itself was unlikely to be of much use. And in fact, after the initial flurry of rediscovery, psychoanalysis per se has not had much currency in psychotherapeutic work with the aged. But Goldfarb used the psychodynamic principles of analysis to codify an approach to the elderly (Goldfarb, 1956; Goldfarb and Turner, 1953). He saw them as concerned with loss: psychological losses, losses of social role, financial losses, and physical ones. He said that people with such preoccupations feel weak or damaged, as well as sad or outraged, and are increasingly prone to transferential relationships with persons regarded as powerful. From this he deduced the idea that brief contacts with a therapist could cause the illusion of an alliance to flourish, and that a patient's sense of being able to rely on or command the allegiance of a powerful physician was a powerful aid to restitution and better function. Others have extended this work and added to it (Wolf, 1970; Verwoerdt, 1976; Verwoerdt, 1969; Pitt, 1974; Lewis and Butler, 1974; Weinberg, 1975). All stress limited goals and empathic understanding, the need for active interchange, support, and touching as well as demonstration. Dr. Pfeiffer (Chapter 35) has contributed five principles in modification of psychotherapies for work with the aged, which parallel and further codify this approach (Pfeiffer, 1971; Pfeiffer, 1976). But the important thing is that a hopeful view of such psychotherapeutic work has supplanted a hopeless one. And all who have worked with or reported research series in psychotherapy with the aged agree that it can succeed. Baekeland and Lundwall (1975), in a review of studies that correlated age with treatment dropout, concluded that the elderly are more likely to stick with treatment than are younger patients. Bourestrom (1970) suggests that older patients may derive the greatest benefit from socioenvironmental treatments. And there is even evidence that older, long-term, chronic schizophrenics burn out their disease and can ultimately recover (Bridge, Cannon, and Wyatt, 1978).

This enthusiasm for psychotherapeutic work with the aged must be tempered by the fact that to this point there has been more opinion than demonstration. I know of only one controlled and comparative study of psychotherapy with elderly patients (Godbole, 1974). The outcome was positive, and despite the study's methodological flaws, that fact is encouraging. But we are now in an era of formalization of treatment approach and of new methods of studying outcome. Manuals exist for cognitive therapy, interpersonal therapy, and even psychodynamic therapy (Beck et al. 1979; Klerman et al., in press; Strupp, in press; Luborsky, in press). Some of these treatments are being tested nationally in a series of the depressed (DuRubeis, Hollon, Evans, et al., 1982). It is only a matter of time before trials are extended to elderly populations.

I also believe, however, that the idea that human relationships can be helpful to those who are isolated, weakened, and lonely stands de facto.

Demonstration of it is demonstration of the obvious, and therefore trivial. Moreover, I think the distinction aimed at, between supportive and insightful treatments with the aged, is mislabeled. All treatments include support, and what should be considered instead is a distinction between levels of insight. To help anyone, you can provide sympathy and empathy, and the illusion of alliance; you can also actually do something: guide, suggest, or alter the environment, or you can offer increased self-awareness. Knowing the roots and genesis of his Oedipus complex may not be necessary for an elderly patient, but if he stumbles because he steps on his own toes, no amount of support or sympathy can replace the greater self-awareness that would help him walk a firmer and straighter path. I predict that the problem-focused manuals, with emphasis on areas of difficulty and techniques to help navigate them, will help in this connection. This is a substantial change which we can hope for in the future for psychotherapy of aged individuals.

Even greater advances can be expected in clinical diagnosis and psychopharmacologic treatments. We have already begun to separate the pseudodementia of depression from true dementia on clinical grounds (Wells, 1979). The former is eminently treatable. Such biological tests as the Dexamethasone Suppression test, the Reduced REM Latency test, and the TRH tests are also being investigated. Controversy continues about their utility as yet, and I believe that these three at least will have less than clear predictive power (Rush et al., 1983). But they are only a first wave, and other discoveries, more solid as trait or state indicators with which to direct treatment, will surely follow.

Similarly, we can expect enormous progress in pharmacology. We can already successfully treat 80% of depressions medically. Not only new tricyclic antidepressants, but new classes or families are being discovered. Tetracyclics are available; alprazolam (Xanax) is a benzodiazapine derivative that has antidepressant effects; and trazadone (Desyrel) inhibits serotonin uptake almost purely, rather than both serotonin and norepinephrine, and is effective in depressions. Zimelidine and bupropion are other new and different medications either tested or already available (Branconnier et al., 1983; Feighner, 1983).

The explosion of pharmacologic tools heralds more than an increase in our therapeutic armamentarium. What it amounts to is the possibility of a chemical dissection of the brain, and I believe it will yield a thoroughgoing understanding of the biochemistry and physiology of depression in the next 20 years. What this means in terms of the elderly, where depression increases in frequency with each decade, and so many of whom suffer from it, can barely be imagined.

We are also making rapid progress in the pharmacologic understanding of anxiety. The discovery of benzodiazepine receptors was a first step (Braestrup and Squires, 1978). Defining their structure is another, which will allow modeling of antianxiety agents in terms of how they fit structurally, in addition to how they can compete for binding sites (Costa and Guidotti, 1979). A recent first, and useful animal model of anxiety, based on such understanding at the molecular level has been proposed by Ninan et al. (1982). Such work in pharmacology will increasingly buttress our psychotherapeutic approaches to anxiety (so pervasive among the aged) and augment the relief to be brought. We do not know precisely the physiologic bases of agitation in the confused, but I suspect it carries the physiology of anxiety somewhere in its causal chain. The new agents based on these models will enable us to meet agitation more accurately in the physiological sense than we do now, where we more or less overpower it with neuroleptics.

But what about the confused? A swelling in their ranks is anticipated with dread. The bulge can probably be slowed, though only modestly, by our increasing focus on certain risk factors and the better treatment of others (e.g., smoking, hypertension). But even less than 5% of 60 million is awesome. At this time, diagnosing the dementia of Alzheimer's remains indirect, a matter of excluding other causes. Increased degrees of resolution by improved CAT scans and especially of nuclear magnetic resonance techniques (NMR) will make earlier and cleaner diagnosis possible, probably in the next 10 years.

And then what? We know that Alzheimer's is in some measure or fraction genetic, that it bears a relation to Down's syndrome in physiology, and more recently that acetylcholine and the nucleus basalis of Meynert are involved (Coyle et al., 1983; Heston, 1979). But the illness has been refractory to treatment, and enhancers of metabolism as well as vasodilators and other magic memory agents have all failed so far (Reisberg et al., 1981). There is promise in the new techniques of molecular genetics, which sequence, characterize and create, and may ultimately allow replacement of the genes themselves. If one could rearrange the genetic program that tells neurons when to give up the ghost, Alzheimer's disease perhaps could be preventable. The technology of this field is burgeoning; but the question of whether such godlike interventions will be possible even in the next 50 years clouds my crystal ball: wish interferes with judgment, but the latter I fear is nay.

Failing medical solution, the potential problem of Alzheimer's is enormous. Society will have to attend to it, most likely by the less sanguine alternatives of increasing facilities for custodial care and resolution through the court. Discussion of either alternative is unpleasant and threatens to mar what has so far been a generally upbeat approach. Increased custodial and more active care will be provided. The government, through the Veterans Administration, is already building a series of nursing homes throughout the country. While not so labeled, I believe this program is in preparation for the increase in the ranks of the elderly. It is also a step towards modeling a socialized system for such care.

The courts too have begun to face the issues involved. And when courts get involved in questions of withholding treatment and allowing death, they do so at the urgings of society.

There are a few things that make our legal system uniquely able to deal with these kinds of problems (Baron, 1981; Levinson, 1981). First of all, judicial decisions are principled. That does not mean only that they are ethical, but rather than decisions embody a principle that can be extended to other, similar situations. Modifications are also possible, to fit circumstances that vary, by means of the adversarial process. That decisions are made under adversarial conditions is a second strength of our judicial system. It means that lawyers, advocates of opposing views, marshal arguments and precedents, and compel the judiciary to see the situation from many viewpoints and with all possibilities laid out. The third strength is that all judgments are public; the judge must write an opinion, frame its bases, and review the lines of thought and points of law involved in making the decision—and all of this is then under the critical eye of public scrutiny.

Issues of voluntary death were raised in 1978 in the Sakewicz decision, which first made the distinction between life-saving measures and those that were merely life prolonging. Later the courts hinted that even life-saving measures might be refusable on the basis of invasion of bodily integrity (Lane vs. Candura, Hall vs. Myers). Through subsequent reworking of cases, the early requirement that decisions to allow death required judicial endorsement seems to have been withdrawn and left to the family and physician (in re Dinnerstein); and freedom from liability is hinted at—though not affirmed—if the doctor's judgment is "in good faith" and "not unreasonable by medical standards" (in re Earle N. Spring). Courts have discussed the possibility that relatives can judge what an incompetent patient would decide were he or she competent, and have acknowledged that quality of life and bankruptcy by costs of care are factors that merit consideration (Baron, 1981).

The courts have not caught up with the ethicists yet. They have still to deal with Gaylin's suggestion that removal of life support systems should be seen as mandatory rather than allowable at times (Gaylin, 1974), and to grapple fully with questions of personhood, a life worth living, and active vs. passive measures to enable life to end. But over the next few decades these issues will be before the courts and their elements ground fine in the judicial mill. Doctors can define what kind of life is present and if it can be maintained. The judiciary must balance the interests of individuals and families against those of a moral society at large, and decide under what circumstances life can or should be ended.

Any overview is limited in scope by the constraints of space and time allotted. I have chosen to discuss whether the elderly of 2000 and beyond will seek and get the help they will require, some of the means that will develop to provide it, and some of the problems to be resolved in balancing finite resources, life in the human mold, and expanding need. In conclusion, I want to note also that I believe the personnel resources will be available: the doctor glut will grow, and there is an excess also of psychologists and social workers which will follow the market as it grows in turn. Whether the care will be as excellent in quality as we might hope is a subject for another discussion, but I think that is not so likely. On balance, the diagnostic picture as I see it is guardedly optimistic.

References

Baekeland, F., and Lundwall, L.: Dropping out of treatment: A critical review. *Psychol. Bull. 82*, 738 (1975).

Baron, C.H.: Termination of life support systems in the elderly: To die before the gods please: Legal issues surrounding euthanasia and the elderly. *J. Geriat. Psychiatry 14*, 45 (1981).

Beck, A.T. et al.: Cognitive Therapy of Depression. New York: Guilford Press, 1979.

Bourestrom, N.C.: Evaluation of mental health programs for the aged. *Aging & Human Development 1*, 187 (1970).

Braestrup, C., and Squires, R.F.: Brain specific benzodiazapine receptors. *Brit. J. Psychiatry 133*, 249 (1978).

Branconnier, R.J., et al.: Clinical pharmacology of buproprion and imipramine in elderly depressions. *J. Clin. Psychiatry 44*, 130 (1983).

Bridge, T.P., Cannon, H.E., and Wyatt, J.D.: Burned-out schizophrenia: Evidence for age effects on schizophrenic symptomatology. *J. Gerontology 33*, 835–839 (1978).

Butler, R.N.: Psychiatry and the elderly. *Am. J. Psychiat. 132*, 893 (1975).

Butler, R.N., and Lewis, M.I.: Aging & Mental Health: Positive Psychosocial Approaches, 2nd ed. St. Louis: Mosby, 1977.

Costa, E., and Guidotti, A.: Molecular mechanisms in the receptor action of benzodiazapines. *An. Rev. Pharmacol. Toxicol. 19*, 531 (1979).

Coyle, J.T., Price, D.L., and DeLong, M.R.: Alzheimer's disease: A disorder of cholinergic innervation. *Science 219*, 1184–1190 (1983).

DeRubeis, R.J., Hollon, S.D., Evans, M.D., et al.: Can systems of psychotherapy be discriminated? A systematic investigation of cognitive therapy and interpersonal therapy. *J. Consult. Clin. Psychol. 50*, 744 (1982).

Feighner, J.P.: "Second- and third-generation antidepressants: A clinical overview." In Zales, M.R. (Ed.), Affective and Schizophrenic Disorders. New York: Brunner/Mazel, 1983.

Freud, S.: On psychotherapy. In Collected Papers, Vol. 1, p. 249. London: Hogarth, 1924.

Gaylin, W.: Harvesting the dead. *Harpers*, Sept. 23, 1974.

Godbole, A., and Verinis, J.S.: Brief psychotherapy in the treatment of emotional disorders in physically ill geriatric patients. *Gerontologist 14*, 143 (1974).

Goldfarb, A.I.: Psychotherapy of aged persons. IV: One aspect of the psychodynamics of the therapeutic situation with aged patients. *Psychoanalytic Rev. 42*, 180 (1955).

Goldfarb, A.I.: Psychotherapy of the aged: The use and value of an adaptational frame of reference. *Psychoanalytic Rev. 43*, 68 (1956).

Goldfarb, A.I., and Turner, H.: Psychotherapy of the aged. II: Utilization and effectiveness of "brief" therapy. *Am. J. Psychiatry 109*, 916 (1953).

Grotjahn, M.: Some analytic observations about the process of growing old. In Rogheim, G. (Ed.), Psychoanalysis & Social Science, Vol. 3. New York: International Universities Press, 1951.

Grotjahn, M.: Analytic psychotherapy with the elderly. *Psychoanalytic Rev. 42*, 419 (1955).

Heston, L.L.: Alzheimer's disease and senile dementia: Genetic relationship to Down's syndrome and haematologic cancer. In Katzman, R. (Ed.), Congenital and Acquired Cognitive Disorders. New York: Raven, 1979.

Kahn, R.L.: The mental health system and the future aged. *Gerontologist 15*, 24 (1975).

Klerman, G.L., et al.: Manual for Short-Term Interpersonal Therapy (ITP) of Depression. New York: Basic Books (in press).

Levinson, A.J.R.: Termination of life support systems in the elderly: Ethical issues. *J. Geriat. Psychiatry 14*, 71 (1981).

Lewis, M.I., and Butler, R.N.: Life review therapy: Putting memories to work in individual and group psychotherapy. *Geriatrics 29*, 165 (1974).

Luborsky, L.: Principles of Psychoanalytic Psychotherapy: A Manual for Supportive–Expressive Treatment. New York: Basic Books (in press).

Meerloo, J.A.M.: Contribution of psychoanalysis to the problem of the aged. In Heiman, M. (Ed.), Psychoanalysis & Social Work. New York: International Universities Press, 1953.

Meerloo, J.A.M.: Psychotherapy with elderly people. *Geriatarics 10*, 583 (1955).

Ninan, P.T., Insel, T.M., Cohen, R.M., Cook, J.M., Skolnick, P., and Paul, S.M.: Benzodiazepine receptor-mediated experimental "anxiety" in primates. *Science 218*, 1332–1334 (1982).

Pfeiffer, E.: Psychotherapy with elderly patients. *Postgrad. Med. 50*, 254 (1971).

Pfeiffer, E.: Psychotherapy with elderly patients. In Bellak, L., and Karaser, T.B. (Eds.), Geriatric Psychiatry. New York: Grune & Stratton, 1976.

Pitt, B.: Psychogeriatrics. London: Churchill-Livingston, 1974.

Reisberg, B., Ferris, S.H., and Gershon, S.: An overview of pharmacologic treatment of cognitive decline in the aged. *Am. J. Psychiatry 138*, 593 (1981).

Riley, M.W., and Foner, A.: Aging and Society, Vol. 1. New York: Russell Sage Foundation, 1968.

Rush, A.J., Schlesser, M., Fulton, C., and Allen, M.: The biologic bases of psychiatric disorders. In Rosenberg, R. (Ed.), Clinical Neurosciences. London: Churchill-Livingston, 1983.

Siegel, J.S.: Recent and prospective demographic trends for the elderly population and some implications for health care. In Haynes, S.G., and Feinleib, M. (Eds.), Second Conference on the Epidemiology of Aging. Washington, D.C.: U.S. Government Printing Office, 1980.

Starr, P.: The Social Transformation of American Medicine. New York: Basic Books, 1982.

Strupp, H.R.: Time Limited Dynamic Psychotherapy: A Treatment Manual. New York: Basic Books (in press).

Verwoerdt, A.: Training in geropsychiatry. In Busse, E.W., and Pfeiffer, E. (Eds.), Behavior and Adaptation in Late Life. Boston: Little, Brown & Co., 1969.

Verwoerdt, A.: Clinical Geropsychiatry. Baltimore: Williams & Wilkins, 1976.

Weinberg, J.: Geriatric psychiatry. In Freedman, A.M., Kaplan, H.I., and Sadock, B.J. (Eds.), Comprehensive Textbook of Psychiatry—II. Baltimore: Williams & Wilkins, 1975.

Wells, C.E.: Pseudodementia. *Am. J. Psychiatry 136*, 895 (1979).

Wolff, K.: The Emotional Rehabilitation of the Geriatric Patient. Springfield, Ill.: Thomas, 1970.

Chapter 38

Aging and Mental Retardation: An International Perspective

Gunnar Dybwad

Summary

In 1953 when the World Health Organization called together for the first time an expert committee on mental retardation, the chosen topic for that conference and the subsequent publication was (using British terminology) "The Mentally Subnormal Child." Scant attention was given to the problem of the adult person; the approach was, as in most countries, overwhelmingly child oriented.

Three decades later a marked shift in focus is evident. The development of comprehensive programs in early intervention and advances in special education, with increasing emphasis on integration, have brought tremendous advances to retarded children in preparing them for adult life.

There is now not only increasing recognition that new, imaginative ways must be found to deal with occupational, recreational, residential, and personal needs of adult persons with mental retardation and their families, but a markedly lengthening lifespan of these individuals has now focused attention on their eventual needs as senior citizens.

The first international conference of significance in the field of mental retardation was the meeting of a Joint Expert Committee convened by the World Health Organization in Geneva in 1953, with participation from the United Nations, the International Labor Organization, and UNESCO. The name of the Committee reflected its charge: Joint Expert Committee on the Mentally Subnormal Child, and reflected also the then prevalent view that mental retardation was a problem associated with childhood.

Subsequently WHO (1954) published a report on the Committee's work. The 46 page booklet with the title *The Mentally Subnormal Child* was for more than a decade the authoritative international reference. It had one brief section on adolescents and young adults, but nothing at all was said about problems these individuals might encounter in later life.

A few years later the Canadian Film Board produced a full-length educational film on the subject of mental retardation. Its title, *Eternal Children*, reemphasized this view, as did Pearl Buck's (1950) widely read book about her daughter, *The Child Who Never Grew*.

In 1950 a national voluntary organization had been established in the United States, the National Association for Retarded Children (a name which was kept for the next 20 years when it became the National Association for Retarded Citizens). In England, France, New Zealand, and Sweden similar organizations were created in the early 1950s whose names included the word children. It is fair to say that throughout the 1950s and beyond, mental retardation was considered a child-related problem (Dybwad, 1973).

In 1960 the Woods School Spring Conference, held in Boston, broke new ground by choosing as its theme: "Outlook for the Adult Retarded." In an address on "developing patterns for aid to aging retarded and their families," the keynote speaker stated:

> . . . We are confronted with a vary rapid increase in the life span of the mentally retarded, but if we look for documentation by statistics, we have to be content with information that is limited to the institutional population.

He spoke of the beginning recognition that the older person with mental retardation was entitled to adult status:

> . . . This new insight, stemming largely from the more progressive work in community facilities for the retarded, reflects a rejection of the old cliché which termed a twenty year old Mongoloid with an I.Q. of 40 as a "child at heart." Today we recognize that such a person is an adult with a severe mental handicap, but one who may well be capable of performing tasks of reasoning and of expressing feelings considerably beyond those of the child whose mental age he presumably possesses (Dybwad, 1960a).

Later in that year, at the 1960 Golden Anniversary White House Conference on Children and Youth, a call was made for greater attention to the legal status of the mentally retarded child and adult, particularly with reference to the degree of legal protection required as related to the degree of the mental handicap (Dybwad, 1960b).

This theme was picked up by the Task Force on Law of President Kennedy's Panel on Mental Retardation (1964) and was further developed in a Symposium on the Legislative Aspects of Mental Retardation called together in Stockholm in June 1967 by the International League of

Societies for the Mentally Handicapped, an organization that spearheaded internationally the movement of parents of children with mental retardation. The published *Conclusions* of the Stockholm Symposium included the following statement:

> The Symposium considered that no examination of the legislative aspects of the problem of mental retardation would be complete without general consideration being given to the basic rights of the mentally retarded, not only from the standpoint of their collective rights and those of their families, but also from that of the individual rights of the retarded person as a human being (International League, 1967).

This was followed by an enumeration of general and special rights such as the right to choose a place to live, to dispose of property, to vote, to marry, and by principles which would govern modification or denial of such rights where this was indicated for compelling reasons.

One year later the League rephrased the Symposium's findings on individual rights into a formal Declaration which was adopted by the League's General Assembly, meeting in Jerusalem in its Fourth World Congress.

In the meantime, the World Health Organization had called together in 1967 another Expert Committee whose report, *Organization of Services for the Mentally Retarded*, documents the tremendous change that had occurred in the field in the intervening 14 years since the first Expert Committee's deliberations. Let me quote from the section on "Support of retarded adults in the community":

> Some fifteen years ago, the mentally retarded adult was looked upon as a child incapable of taking responsibility. Important changes have occurred in recent years since research and experience have shown that moderately and even severely retarded adults can perform useful work in a realistic job situation . . . Finding suitable employment opportunities for the retarded (and at the same time giving them an opportunity to contribute to the national economy) remains an urgent task for industry, commerce, and agriculture. Government agencies should set a good example by accepting mentally retarded men and women in suitable service positions.
>
> As increasing numbers of these adults take up work in the community, under sheltered or independent conditions, the need arises for development of hostels, boarding houses, and clubs to provide partial support in dealing with the problems of everyday living. In line with the move to retain the retarded in the community, several authorities are using a variety of existing residential facilities for the general population rather than building new residential institutions for retarded adults. At the same time, increasing emphasis is being laid on the provision of continued support for retarded adults through outpatient facilities of the mental health and general health services and appropriate social welfare agencies.
>
> The Committee considered that, in general, the care of mentally retarded old persons, whose numbers are increasing, is best organized as part of the general geriatric services (World Health Organization, 1968).

Needless to say, this pronouncement from WHO's Expert Committee stimulated, and indeed, necessitated a rethinking of the problem of mental retardation on the part of governments, the professions, and the consumer organizations. But infinitely greater was the impact of the next development on the international scene, the adoption by the General Assembly of the United Nations, in December 1971, of the Declaration on the Rights of Mentally Retarded Persons, adapted with few changes from the League's Declaration of 1968. By referring in the Preamble of the Declaration to the Universal Declaration of Human Rights which it had passed in 1948 as a "common standard of achievement for all people and all nations," the U.N. gave recognition and dignity to persons with mental retardation who previously had been so largely excluded from society and indeed, from the human family (United Nations, 1971).

In a report commissioned by the United Nations, Richard Sterner (1976), leader of the Swedish parent movement, wrote:

> . . . it is difficult to believe that there is any country where the principles expressed in the Declaration have been fully implemented, even though there has been progress in most parts of the world, with a pioneering development in economically less advanced countries, and an increase, more or less rapid, in provisions, services and resources for the mentally retarded in industrialized countries. This makes the Declaration all the more important as a programme for action.

To consider a Declaration of the United Nations as a program for action in our own country may at first appear implausible, considering the increasingly negative attitude in the United States toward the United Nations. However, the Declaration was specifically endorsed by the President's Committee on Mental Retardation, has been widely used by governmental and voluntary agencies as a guideline for action, and already in 1972 was cited by Judge Johnson of the federal bench as substantiating new trends in the field of mental retardation (Wyatt vs. Stickney, 1974).

There is no question that the Declaration has significantly contributed to make the decade of the 1970s in many countries, including ours, a time of recognition of the adult person with mental retardation, and what we can observe now, again on a broad international basis, is a widening of this emphasis to include the challenge of the aging person.

Foreseeing this development, the International League of Societies for Persons with Mental Handicap at its 1978 World Congress in Vienna established a Task Group on Aging and Mental Retardation under the chairmanship of Ingeborg Thomae, a pioneer in the German parent movement. She and her husband, Professor Hans Thomae, director of the Psychological Institute, University of Bonn, were personally confronted with the challenge of planning for the future (and that meant the aging) of their adult son with mental retardation. Fortuitously, Professor Thomae was the organizing and program chairman of the 12th International

Congress of Gerontology which met in Hamburg in July 1981, and he arranged for a full session on "The Aging Mentally Retarded." Additionally, Mrs. Thomae was instrumental in having the Faculty of Education at the University of Cologne hold a three-day workshop on the same topic for an invited international group. The Proceedings of these meetings are available so far only in German. It is with great sorrow that I must report that Mrs. Thomae died last month after a long illness; we hope to publish some of these papers in English in a volumn dedicated to her memory.

I would like to share with you at this point some of the concluding paragraphs of the paper she gave at the Cologne Workshop.

> ... To remain in the parental house or in the family apartment must be recognized, in any realistic look into the future, as one additional possible living arrangement for the aging person who is handicapped. Because of the increasing life expectancy and the constantly growing number of persons with mental retardation, it will be less and less feasible for the existing and planned residences to meet the local needs ... Therefore it probably cannot be avoided within the foreseeable future that those older persons, for whom the domestic situation makes it feasible, will remain at home, probably beyond the death of their parents. It should be obvious that this cannot be done without considerable support and a well arranged network of social services. In addition, much learning must take place to prepare the retarded persons themselves as well as their parents, brothers and sisters and other relatives for this new situation ...
>
> To grow old is human fate. It confronts our handicapped sons and daughters just as it confronts us. We can prepare ourselves for this, and we *must* prepare our children for it. Once we parents learn to understand that our handicapped children are no more our "property" than are our non-handicapped children, that someday we must let them go so they can live their own lives, then we are helping them best—and ourselves—to manage the road into the future.
>
> The earlier we learn this and pass it on to our sons and daughters, the better we prepare them for their lives without us. This would also make it conceivable that they could continue to live—in appropriate form—in the parental home, perhaps with one or more companions, and that *our* home can then become *their* own home. It should in any case be tried (Thomae, 1983).

I am glad to report that this unusual scheme proposed by Mrs. Thomae is now under active consideration by a few families in this country.

But what about international developments in general for this aging client group? Concrete activities proceed at a rather slow rate, in part because of the unfavorable economic condition, but at least there seems to be increasing agreement on some basic principles. There is the principle of normalization, which suggests the creation of life environments for these clients as close as possible to what is generally accepted in the community; the principle of the least restrictive alternative, which implies that clients should not be unnecessarily confined or restrained in their freedom of movement and activities; the principle of individuality, which emphasizes personhood, privacy and the dignity of risk; the principle of integration in all significant life experiences; and finally, emphasis on the developmental potential, meaning that everyone should have room to learn and grow.

In various countries questions are raised about the extent to which elderly persons with mental retardation could be accommodated by existing programs in the geriatric field, as suggested by the 1967 WHO Committee cited earlier. However, such planning has not progressed very far. Programs most frequently observed relate to residential needs, whether for those who no longer can or should live in their parental home or for those leaving the large institutions which are being phased down. Opinions differ strongly. In some countries it is felt that persons who have spent 20, 30, or 40 years in institutions should remain there, while others point to experiences showing that after decades in institutions even aged retarded persons find a more satisfying life in the community. Some institution residents understandably do not wish to leave their friends, and a few thoughtful administrators have arranged for such people to move out as a group, either to one community residence or to apartments in close proximity.

In some countries administrators feel that small living units are uneconomical. In England, for instance, many of the hostels opened since 1971 are larger even than the recommended 24 places. In any case, planning living space for aging retarded people is an urgent task in most of the industrial countries.

A complicating factor in the planning process is the problem of projecting future needs, both quantitatively (How many people will need such services?), and qualitatively (What levels of care and supervision will be required in the various residences?).

The situation is more complicated when it comes to day programs. Should there be an earlier retirement age? What kind of activities are appropriate for the elderly handicapped person? Opinions differ widely, and few programs have been initiated.

Even less has been done in the area of recreation and leisure time in general, most likely because so little is known of what range of programs would be enjoyed by these people.

Perhaps there is some advantage in this delayed response to a newly recognized need because it does provide time to ask the aged clients what it is they, individually and collectively, would like to see develop. After all, "growing old in dignity" should imply an opportunity, if not a right, to make choices and decisions concerning one's daily living.

In conclusion, I would like to report on two studies which seem to me of particular note. The first was undertaken by Betty Anglin, a Canadian journalist and mother of an adult son with mental retardation, and a member of the International League's Task Group on Aging and Mental Handicap. Realizing that there was almost no information available in

Canada which she could contribute to the Task Group, she decided to get her own information. She began with some preliminary communications with the 10 Provincial governments, and with interviews conducted by a team of 8 volunteers with 80 delegates to the Annual Conference of the Canadian Association for the Mentally Retarded in Vancouver, B.C. The delegates included parents and professionals having a special interest in older people who are retarded, and also included adult members of People First, a self-help advocacy group of persons who are mentally handicapped. Mrs. Anglin reports:

> Three points of particular interest became clear through these early inquiries: (1) More and more people who are retarded and over age 50 are coming to the attention of governments, agencies and Associations for the Mentally Retarded often for the first time even though some have lived in the community all their lives; (2) Older residents of institutions are returning to their homes and local communities; (3) The need is clear for appropriate organizations to be aware of this "new" area of service demand, to become acquainted with existing programs for senior citizens into which some who are retarded may fit and to begin to develop special services as required (Anglin, 1981).

With help from the professional staff of the Metro Toronto AMR and with funding from "Help the Aged," an international voluntary organization formed in England in 1962, Mrs. Anglin proceeded to undertake a study on the needs of elderly retarded people in Metro Toronto. The study involved 28 adults and their family or staff members, but only 21 adults with handicap and 27 family and staff respondents were actually interviewed with a questionnaire having respectively 99 and 118 items.

The report of this study contains a brief but highly informative vignette of each of the persons with handicap studied, and summarizes the findings in six chapters dealing with residential accommodation, work, recreation and leisure, nutrition and health, aging and dying, guardianship, and the search for an "ideal living situation."

As an activist in the parent movement, Mrs. Anglin addresses her recommendations to the local mental retardation associations as follows:

> The Associations for the Mentally Retarded [must] recognize the special needs of people over age 50 who are retarded and advocate for services to meet these special needs, some of which are defined below:
>
> 1. For those living at home: (a) Homemaker support to help elderly parents develop more confidence in a son's or daughter's ability to assist about the home and to participate in outside social and recreational pursuits, including occasional weekends in community residences designed to give both parents and offspring a holiday. (b) Literature and discussion groups to update parents and siblings on current thinking in the field of retardation, available services and the need to plan for the future of the family member who is retarded.
> 2. Home management support to teach elderly parents and residential counsellors how to deal with difficult behavior changes likely to

accompany aging, so that these may be modified before they break up a home or force an abrupt change of living situation.

3. Opportunities to cultivate friendships among peers (a two-way process which does not occur naturally for people who have become used to taking what others give) through discussion groups, social events, exchange weekend visits (home-to-residence and residence-to-residence). Such experiences can be of great assistance in choosing compatible companions for any move toward more independent living.
4. Opportunities to expand friendships and acquaintances beyond peer groups through Citizen Advocacy programs, church and other volunteer groups likely to generate invitations out to dinner, special events, cottage weekends, etc., thus developing broader human supports that can prove invaluable when parents die or other dislocations occur.
5. Education for aging: (a) What it means to grow older, how to avoid premature aging through proper diet and exercise, how to prepare for the loss of friends and relatives and the importance of developing more friendships. (b) How to get along in different living situations from community residences to homes for senior citizens by developing social and self-sufficiency skills and participating in community activities.
6. Consideration that some of the foregoing developmental opportunities be integrated into the daily ARC Industries program recognizing that this occupies the greater part of workers' lives, that this is their chief point of contact with other people and that aging and retirement require preparation.
7. Develop a variety of living situations for seniors who are retarded including apartment complex, small homelike residences, boarding homes, regular senior citizen homes, etc.
8. Interpret persons who are aging and retarded to generic agencies to encourage their inclusion in regular community recreation, education, health and residential services.
9. Include retardation in gerontology courses and include gerontology in mental retardation counsellor courses. Select experienced counsellors with special interest in aging and mental retardation to take advanced courses in gerontology.
10. Develop guardianship alternatives so that parents may plan with confidence for the offspring's future, with particular emphasis on the establishment of knowledgeable agencies to assume legal guardianship of the person. (Anglin, 1981; reprinted by permission of the author and publisher.)

The other study was undertaken in 1981 in England by the Campaign for Mentally Handicapped People, one of the most outstanding advocacy agencies that has come to my attention in my international travels. I know of no other organization which has produced over 10 years, on a veritable shoestring budget, such consistently valuable material—critiques of governmental reports, informational bulletins, and studies, or, as they say, enquiry papers.

This study does not address itself directly to persons with mental retardation, but rather to "Older Parents with a Mentally Handicapped Person Living at Home." Their number is now steadily increasing, but few programs are in existence to deal with their often acute and indeed disasterous problems. The reason for this lack of planning is obvious: Until the recent dramatic lengthening of the lifespan of persons with mental retardation forced itself on the attention of government, private agencies and consumer groups, it was assumed that, as before, the parents were more than likely to outlive their handicapped son or daughter.

Since the aim of the CMH study was to look in depth at the mentally handicapped person and his or her family in a number of settings, at the life within the (nuclear) family, at the family's contacts with the outside world, and at the use the families made of service provisions, the research plan called for detailed interviews (average length 2 hours) with 16 families having parents over 60 years of age. Significantly, only 13 of the selected families could be interviewed because in three cases death intervened—an indication of the high-risk nature of these family situations.

The published study, available from the Campaign for Mentally Handicapped People in London, provides a wealth of sensitive material depicting the day-to-day problems encountered by such families. The following are some selected items from the final section entitled Practical Recommendations:

> The establishment of parents' groups would provide a focus for discussion with parents on the need to prepare the mentally handicapped person (and the family) for the change from parental home to a home elsewhere, and the desirability of this happening before the parents die. The emphasis should be on mutual support and on helping parents face and assess their own feelings about the mentally handicapped person leaving home . . .
>
> Planning for the future needs of the mentally handicapped person should not start at the point where parental support is terminated through illness or death. Preparation for such a major life crisis must start long before that. This means, for example, making regular periods of short-term residential care available so that the handicapped person becomes used to living away from home. These periods of short-term care should be well organized and geared to increasing independence and general survival skills away from the family . . .
>
> Planning for the future needs of handicapped people should be worked out and implemented on an individual basis. Each person should have an individual plan which sets out what is likely to happen to them over the next one, two and five years. It is important not to try to fit mentally handicapped people into existing facilities if they are inappropriate. Individual plans should result in individual programmes. Plans should, for example, be sensitive to such issues as the importance of people remaining within their own communities . . .
>
> Future residential accommodation for the mentally handicapped person should concentrate on the use of ordinary housing offering varying degrees of care and support according to individual needs and which can be varied as individual circumstances change. Homes should be as unrestrictive as possible; they should be small and non-institutional in character.
>
> If mentally handicapped people are to become more fully integrated into the life of the local community, they must have greater opportunities to mix and meet with non-handicapped people of their own age. For example, there

> should be less emphasis on the use of 'special' leisure facilities such as clubs at training centres, and more encouragement to use ordinary leisure opportunities. (Campaign for Mentally Handicapped People, 1981)

The last major project Mrs. Thomae directed for the International League's Task Group was publication of a position paper on *Ageing and Mental Handicap*, coauthored by her and Thomas Fryers, Professor of Community Medicine at the University of Manchester, England, and translated into several languages. Its concluding paragraphs summarize well the challenge that has to be met worldwide:

> The increasing need for services for aging mentally handicapped persons has not yet been generally or adequately recognized. We can, therefore, expect a large gap in the near future between the demand for services and those available, unless action is taken with some urgency. This is true not only because of their different characteristics. Future generations should not have to experience the same institutionalized processes of socialization into apathy, passivity and docility. Many younger people are achieving a degree of independence and competence in living not expected from previous generations of people with mental handicap. These mentally and physically more active persons will need, as they grow older, new kinds of service; and several alternatives for accommodation and care will need to be developed.
>
> The change in age structure of the general population is already recognized as a major challenge in developed communities. What needs to be recognized is that aging mentally handicapped persons have the same rights to a satisfactory quality of life as the rest of the aging population. (Thomae and Fryers, 1982)

References

Anglin, B.: They Never Asked For Help: A Study of the Needs of Elderly Retarded People in Metro Toronto. Maple, Ontario: Belsten, 1981.

Buck, P.: The Child Who Never Grew. New York: John Day, 1950.

Campaign for Mentally Handicapped People: Living for the Present: Older Parents With A Mentally Handicapped Person Living At Home, pp. 35–36. London: CHM, 1981.

Dybwad, G.: Developing patterns for aid to the aging retarded and their families. In Woods School Conference Outlook for the Adult Retarded, pp. 24–25. Langhorne, PA.: The Woods School, 1960a.

Dybwad, G.: Trends and issues in mental retardation. In 1960 White House Conference on Children and Youth, Children and Youth in the 1960s, p. 269. Washington D.C., The White House Conference, 1960.

Dybwad, R.: The International Scene: Patterns of organization and development in member associations of the International League of Societies for the Mentally Handicapped. *Mental Retardation 11*, 1–4 (1973).

International League of Societies for the Mentally Handicapped: Legislative Aspects of Mental Retardation, pp. 15–16. Brussels: ILSMH (13 rue Forestiere), 1967.

President's Panel on Mental Retardation: Report of the Task Force on Law, pp. 13–27. Washington, D.C.: U.S. Dept. of Health, Education, and Welfare, 1964.

Sterner, R.: Social and Economic Conditions of the Mentally Retarded in Selected Countries, p. 1. Brussels: International League of Societies for the Mentally Handicapped.

Thomae, I., and Fryers, T.: Ageing and Mental Handicap. A Position Paper. Brussels: International League of Societies for Persons with Mental Handicap, 1982.

Thomae, I.: Alte Geistig Behinderte Menschen in der Familie. In Hoffmann, T., Ackermann, K., and Anstötz, C., Altwerden von Menschen mit Geistiger Behinderung, pp. 57–61. Marburg: Bundesvereinigung Lebenshilfe, 1983.

United Nations: Declaration on the Rights of Mentally Retarded Persons, G.A. Res. 2856, 26 U.N. GAOR, Supp. (No. 29), 93–94, U.N. Doc. A/8429, 1971.

World Health Organization: The Mentally Subnormal Child Geneva: W.H.O., 1954.

World Health Organization: Organization of Services for the Mentally Retarded, p. 34. Geneva: W.H.O., 1968.

Wyatt vs. Stickney, 344 F. Supp. 387, 390 n.6, aff'd sub nom. Wyatt v. Aderholt, 503 F. 2nd 1305 (5th Cir. 1974).

Chapter 39

Senile Dementia: Psychological and Behavioral Treatments

Jerome A. Yesavage and Leslie A. Widrow

Summary

Cognitive models of pathology. It is important to continue studying two basic psychological parameters: memory and attention since accurate definition of pathology and measurement of function is necessary for both the diagnosis and treatment evaluation.

Assessment. Although discussion of psychological problems in the dementias often centers on cognitive dysfunction, two major behavioral problems are often associated with such patients: depression and emotional lability.

Psychological retraining and other interventions. Although there is some evidence for clinical effects of cognitive retraining with elderly demented, outcome studies of such therapies have suffered from lack of controls and lack of sophistication of the interventions proposed.

The family. Of major importance is the development of methods of family support which will enable the demented patient to live at home as long as possible without the need for dehumanizing and expensive institutionalization.

Environmental considerations. There is little data on how demented patients respond to environmental manipulations.

This chapter will discuss current knowledge of psychological and behavioral treatments for patients with senile dementias and outline limitations of present research, with an outlook towards what should be learned in the future. There have been many studies of psychological programs for improving cognitive function in the elderly. It is important to realize that not all problems caused by dementia are intellectual. Although we will discuss in detail programs designed to improve cognition in elders with cognitive losses, we will also discuss behavioral, familial, and psychological interventions for other problems, such as assaultive behavior and incontinence.

Cognitive Interventions

Treatments for Community Elders with Memory Complaints

Attempts to improve attention. Several reviews have discussed various impairments of attention with aging (Botwinick, 1978; Thompson, 1980; Craik, 1965; Rabbitt, 1965; Kinsbourne, 1980), including the ability to selectively attend to stimuli, to maintain attention to a particular task, and to resist fatigue in the face of repetitive tasks (Craik, 1965; Rabbitt, 1965; Kinsbourne, 1980). Others have noted that high levels of anxiety impair attention and have suggested that relaxation techniques may reduce anxiety and improve attention (Rimm and Masters, 1974; Spiegel and Spiegel, 1978).

Contrary to these studies, others have found that anxiety reduction techniques, such as deep muscle relaxation, have only limited and perhaps nonspecific effects in the elderly (Labouvie-Vief, 1976; Labouvie-Vief and Gonda, 1976; Zarit et al., 1981b; Treat et al., 1978; Poon et al., 1978; Poon et al., 1980). For example, Labouvie-Vief has shown that a nonspecific problem-solving approach may be as effective as specific training in either anxiety reduction or mnemonics in improving cognitive function in the normal elderly (Labouvie-Vief, 1976; Labouvie-Vief et al., 1976). Zarit included relaxation training in a study of memory complaints in the elderly and found no differences compared to other types of training (Zarit et al., 1981a). Such results may be consistent with suggested cautions in attributing age deficits in memory to attentional dysfunctions. Frederiksen argued that evidence for a general attentional deficit is lacking and cited studies indicating poor correlations among different tests of attention (Frederiksen, 1980). He suggested that validation of the attentional dysfunction theory must await the development of more specific attentional measures.

The effect of training on motivation and arousal must be considered in evaluating techniques such as relaxation training. Since the Yerkes-Dodson law was first proposed (1908), it has been argued that the relationship between motivation and performance is curvilinear, i.e., increases in motivation or arousal have a beneficial effect on performance when motivation is initially low, but tend to disrupt performance when motivation is strong. Many studies have found evidence for this inverted-U relationship between motivation and performance. It has been applied routinely, for example, in studies of test anxiety and achievement motivation (Atkinson and Raynor, 1974). Studies of attempts to modulate anxiety, motivation, and arousal will have to first consider the individual's baseline of such factors to determine appropriate levels for each patient.

Studies of organizational techniques. Several studies of psychological treatments in elderly subjects with normal cognitive decline for their age have shown positive effects from organizational techniques, i.e. mnemonics. Zarit found improvement in affect, ability to do practical memory tasks, and list learning in patients receiving group treatments of mnemonic training (Zarit et al., 1981a; Zarit et al., 1981b). These interventions often involve the use of mnemonic devices based on visual image associations. A typical technique is the method of loci (Robertson-Tchabo et al., 1976), in which the individual first names several loci or locations in a familiar building or setting, such as his or her home. Once these locations have been learned to criterion, the individual forms a visual image association between the first item on the list and the first location in the house. Each subsequent item to be remembered is then associated with the next location in the house. To recall the list, the individual takes a mental "walk" around the house, "stopping" at each location to retrieve the visual image that serves as a retrieval cue for the item to be remembered. This mnemonic not only has a robust effect on the recall of lists but it also helps subjects to retain the original ordering of the lists (Bower, 1972; Roediger, 1980).

Because the elderly have difficulty generating and remembering visual image associations (Mason and Smith, 1977), there is a potential problem with the use of mnemonics in this group. Eysenck, invoking his levels of processing framework (Eysenck, 1974; Craik and Lockhart, 1972), suggests that this difficulty may arise because the elderly do not sufficiently process the material at encoding. Despite this difficulty in forming image associations, positive effects similar to those seen with the loci mnemonic have been noted for paired associate learning using visual imagery in normal elderly individuals (Canestrari, 1968). In addition, recent work has indicated that the elderly can benefit from instruction that leads to more elaborate processing at encoding. An example is the finding that recognition memory for faces can be improved in the elderly, as in younger subjects, if they are asked to judge a person's pleasantness while trying to encode their face (Smith and Winograd, 1978).

Cognitive training in the elderly has been shown to improve intelligence test scores, inductive reasoning, and response speed (Labouvie-Vief et al., 1976); Birkhill and Schaie, 1975; Hoyer et al., 1973; Plemons et al., 1978). A typical study by Willis et al. (1981) examined the effectiveness of cognitive training on measures of fluid intelligence in older adults (Willis et al., 1981). Training involved practice and instructions in a common measure of fluid intelligence, relations within figure patterns. This controlled study indicated that subjects improved fluid intelligence with training, and showed transfer effects to other abilities in which they were not directly trained. These effects persisted for 6 months to the study's end point.

Labouvie-Vief (1976) studied the effect of self-image and societal expectations on memory and other intellectual functions. She found that some of the intellectual decline associated with aging can be modified by social manipulations. Training in which the elderly are encouraged to develop their own strategies for improving performance may be as effective as training in a specific technique such as that proposed by Willis et al. (1981). Evidence for transfer effects and generalizability of skills learned with this approach were observed (Labouvie-Vief et al., 1976).

Recently, a series of studies were completed combining a number of the above approaches and using more recent advances in cognitive theory. In one study, Yesavage, Rose, and Bower (1983) demonstrated that a combination of a standard name–face learning mnemonic (organizational device) with a method designed to increase the elaboration of processing of the mnemonic was more effective than the mnemonic alone. Yesavage et al. (1982, 1983) also showed facilitative effects of combining relaxation training with mnemonic training. These studies have been expanded to cover a number of practical memory problems associated with normal aging.

Thus positive effects have been shown in several studies of cognitive loss associated with normal aging. Many of the studies have used innovative techniques based on current theories of cognitive, educational, and social psychology. The situation is quite different, however, for studies of interventions in the elderly with senile dementia.

Treatments for Elders with Senile Dementias

Reality orientation. There is a 20 year history of psychologic interventions designed to improve cognitive deficits in individuals with senile dementias. Probably the most studied intervention is "reality orientation" which attempts, primarily by repetition and reinforcement of correct responses, to reorient demented nursing home residents. [Workbooks are available for the use of this techique (Cornbleth and Cornbleth, 1977)]. Some controlled studies have indicated that reality orientation can produce reorientation (Cornbleth and Cornbleth, 1977; Citrin and Dixon, 1977). However, others have found that gains decrease rapidly after the classes are discontinued (Harris and Ivory, 1976) and that positive responses may result from nonspecific factors, such as the increased attention given to class members (Barnes, 1974). In addition, reality orientation did not result in measurable improvement in behavior even in those subjects who showed reorientation (Cornbleth and Cornbleth,

1977). Unfortunately, these studies suffer from lack of control of medications, small study group size, use of nonblind raters, and failure to use widely accepted psychometric measures to identify degree of impairment.

Anxiety reduction techniques. Few studies of anxiety reduction techniques in elderly demented subjects have been conducted. One controlled study has indicated benefit from a comprehensive 3-month anxiety reduction program (Weldon and Yesavage, 1982). Three hours of training per week in progressive muscle relaxation techniques and self-hypnosis resulted in moderate behavioral improvement and a substantial reduction in the use of tranquilizing medication in the treatment group. Unfortunately, it is not clear from this study whether the behavioral improvement was a direct result of the training or an indirect result of discontinuation of medication.

Image association techniques. A major gap in our knowledge of treatments for senile dementias is the lack of controlled studies evaluating the use of image association techniques to improve memory. One uncontrolled study indicated that image association techniques were beneficial to brain-injured patients attempting to learn paired associates or to perform a face–name task. These benefits were lost after 1 week (Lewinsohn et al., 1977). Other case report studies indicate longer-term effects of retraining. These studies however, did not control for nonspecific aspects of treatment or for spontaneous remission (Luria et al., 1969; Glasgow et al., 1977).

Combined pharmacologic and psychologic interventions. One study has combined a widely used medication for the treatment of senile dementia with an imagery association technique (Yesavage and King, 1981). Dihydroergotoxine mesylate (DEM, Hydergine) was administered (1 mg p.o. t.i.d.) to 21 moderately demented subjects who also received either supportive psychotherapy or cognitive training using the method of loci in biweekly individual 1 hour sessions for 12 weeks. Subjects receiving DEM plus cognitive psychotherapy improved more than subjects receiving DEM plus supportive psychotherapy, as shown on both a psychometric test of memory and a list-learning task. However, no differences were found between groups on behavioral measures. The fact that cognitive training could not augment even the modest behavioral effect of DEM may argue against its potential as a practical intervention. On the other hand, improvement of function was seen on the task in which the subjects were trained. It may be unreasonable to expect cognitive training in list learning to generalize to overall behavioral improvement without specific effort to relate the training to daily tasks.

Summary of interventions for intellectual decline. Although there is some evidence for clinical effects of cognitive retraining in the elderly demented, outcome studies of such therapies have suffered from both lack of controls and lack of sophistication of the interventions proposed. To date there are no published studies which have used the sophisticated techniques commonly used with less impaired elders with demented subjects.

Additional gaps in our knowledge of the effectiveness of psychological interventions in the elderly with dementia have been enumerated by researchers at the Veteran's Administration Medical Center in Boston (Perlmuter et al., 1980). These investigators have noted that little is known about the effect of individual differences between elderly subjects with memory deficits, and that programs are not tailored to recognize these differences (Treat et al., 1978; Poon et al., 1978).

Another major weakness in these studies has been their concentration on the goal of cognitive improvement, neglecting the usual goals of individual psychotherapy. Hysterical reactions, depression, and anxiety attacks are all target symptoms which can require individual psychotherapy in both the young and old. Yet, there has been little discussion of the use of psychotherapeutic techniques to aid demented elders who may suffer from these problems in addition to their dementia. Verwoerdt (1982) argues that psychotherapy with patients who have senile dementia is an essential part of a comprehensive treatment approach. Yesavage and Karasu (1982) argued that the lack of consideration of individual psychotherapy in even physically normal elderly is often due to "gerontophobic" reactions on the part of the physician. Future research should explore, in a controlled fashion, the role of individual psychotherapy as an adjunct to the treatment of the demented patient.

The roles of affect and motivation in retraining efforts are also poorly understood. It has been well documented that memory complaints are better correlated with depression than with actual degree of cognitive impairment (Kahn et al., 1975; Zarit et al., 1981a; Zelinski et al., 1980). Furthermore, a mood-specific memory effect has been documented (Bower, 1981). Material learned when one is happy is better recalled when happy, and material learned when one is sad is better recalled in that mood state. Finally, poor self-image and societal stereotypes of the aged as having poor memory may contribute to impaired performance (Kinsbourne, 1980). The effects of interventions aimed at improving motivation, self-image, and affect remain to be explored.

Few published studies to date have attempted to combine promising therapies. For example, it would make sense to give preliminary instruction in techniques such as relaxation training to improve concentration or training in visual imagery ability *before* teaching complex mnemonic devices that are based on visual imagery.

There has also been little research into the effects of medications on cognitive training. Medications that have psychostimulant effects might be expected to enhance learning (Weiss and Latiess, 1962) and might make it easier for the elderly to assimilate new techniques. In addition, common psychotropics have state-dependent effects on learning (Reus et al., 1979) which might lead to impairment of learning with changes in medication type and dosage.

In sum, retraining programs for elderly individuals with mild memory loss living in the community are distinguished from programs for patients with senile dementias commonly living in nursing homes. While there are many sophisticated programs for use with the former population, controlled studies with the demented are lacking. Future research in this area should attempt to modify promising programs for the normal elderly for use with the demented, and to further explore the interaction of medications with psychological approaches.

Interventions for Elders with Specific Behavioral Problems

Behavior modification interventions have been used successfully to change a wide variety of behavioral problems associated with demented institutionalized elderly. Three recent reviews discussed these interventions (Patterson and Jackson, 1980; Hussian, 1981; Eisdorfer et al., 1981). The interventions were used to treat a wide range of serious behavioral problems: agitation (Haley, 1983), self-injurous behavior (Mishara et al., 1973), urinary incontinence (Hussian, 1981), and insomnia (Weldon and Yesavage, 1982).

Haley (1983) recently noted several cautions and limitations to these approaches. First, these programs do not work in isolation and are only relatively effective in the context of caring individual relationships with therapists, careful biological assessment, and a supportive and physically adequate environment. They cannot compensate for isolation, medical mismanagement, and decrepit facilities. Second, the term "behavior modification" is highly emotionally charged and may lead to immediate rejection of a program on "humanitarian" grounds. Third, it is necessary to train caretakers, either professionals or families, in how to effectively use behavioral techniques. It is unrealistic to expect one behaviorally trained psychologist to develop, initiate, and maintain an individualized program for large numbers of patients. It is more realistic and cost effective to teach these techniques to groups of caretakers.

The Family and Treatment

The role of the family in the treatment and support of a patient with senile dementia has recently attracted considerable attention (see the *Geron-*

tologist, Feb. 1983, for reviews). It is well known that support from the family is often a crucial factor in determining the level of care and placement necessary for the patient. However, few studies have examined how to maximize the effectiveness of family interactions to the satisfaction of both the patient and family. There are certain themes which deserve considerable attention.

Zarit and associates (1982) found that although training programs for improving cognitive deficits in dementia patients seem to have limited value for the identified patient, groups in the format of mutual problem solving reduced stress over time and ultimately improved memory performance. It was also found that mutual support derived from seeing other families cope with the same problems was of benefit to the family, as was the possibility to "brain-storm" about practical problems. These findings have led Zarit's group to incorporate family support groups using a problem-solving approach into his clinical service.

There has been detailed discussion of how a practical problem-solving approach may be facilitated by teaching families of demented patients certain behavioral techniques shown to be effective in combating specific problems (Haley, 1983). There is an extensive behavior modification literature describing techniques used in an institutional setting to help with particularly difficult problems; For example, urinary incontinence or screaming. It may be that with appropriate guidelines, families can learn to use specific psychological techniques to alleviate these problems.

Of utmost importance is the development of methods of family support which will enable the demented patient to live at home as long as possible without the need for dehumanizing and expensive institutionalization. Research on methods of achieving such goals is in its infancy. Recent reviews of these topics (e.g., Troll, 1979) clearly show there are few cross-sectional studies of families successfully meeting the demands of caring for demented members, and essentially no longitudinal studies. Some basic descriptive work here is clearly indicated.

Examination of several works and programs which are clinically oriented provides a wealth of ideas which should be evaluated in formal research settings. For example, *The 36-Hour Day*, now rapidly becoming a classic book for families with demented members, has several suggestions about behavioral management which should be evaluated for effectiveness and acceptability by families. Others have suggested the use of paradoxical family treatments from the Palo Alto School of family treatment (The Mental Research Institute; see Herr and Weakland, 1979). Others have suggested a number of ways the physician can facilitate positive interactions between the family and the demented elder (Reifler and Wu, 1982). Based upon study of Alzheimer's support groups for patients undergoing reseach in dementia, Steurer and Clark (1982) suggest a number of testable hypotheses about how such groups should be organized. Finally, one is struck by the dearth of material on the use of community-based home care in the United States (Kahn and Tobin, 1982). It is well known clinically that "respite care programs" in which demented patients are hospitalized for a limited period of time allow recuperation of the exhausted family and will prolong the length of time the demented person can stay out of a nursing home. Yet perhaps because "respite care programs" are not documented by well-controlled research, they suffer from a lack of funding (see American Psychiatric Association, Task Force Report on the 1981 White House Conference on Aging).

Psychosocial (Environmental) Aspects of Treatment

As previously discussed, a major effort in psychosocial treatments for patients with dementias is aimed at keeping them with the family and in the community as long as possible. The rationale for delaying institutionalization has been reviewed by Kahn and Tobin (1982), who argue that there is clear evidence that "overdosing" elders with social assistance may lead to elevated mortality and morbidity when such treatments include institutionalization. The few controlled studies that exist show that day care or day hospital programs can effectively reduce the need for hospitalization. Kahn and Tobin identify several aspects of community mental health treatment of elderly that they feel essential to good outcome: (1) early intervention before the family is completely "burnt out" and will have nothing more to do with the patient, (2) keeping intervention to a minimum, with hospitalization only as a last resort, and (3) guarantees that needed services will not vanish once the patient is established in community care services. Virtually no controlled studies of these and other factors which go into a successful community-based program have been undertaken in the United States. Model programs could be started which would provide controlled data on which factors lead to a most productive program.

Despite the goal of community care, institutionalization will become necessary for many patients with severe deficits that require high levels of care. The role of the institutional environment in the treatment of the patient with senile dementia and other geriatric impairments has recently been reviewed (Moos and Lemke, 1983). There is a body of research pertaining to the effects of specialized housing on the elderly. Some research is descriptive, focusing on defining types and characteristics of specialized housing. It has been shown, for example, that compared to general psychiatry wards, demented patient's wards tend to have reduced privacy, few opportunities for activities, and little freedom of movement.

Other studies have considered the relationship between institutional and resident characteristics, Lawton (1982) has developed a widely discussed model of the relationship between people and settings, which may have applications for research on dementia. This model relates "personal competence" and "environmental press" to affective response and adaptive behavior, and argues that positive affect and adaptive behavior result from an appropriate match of environment and personal characteristics.

How to match the environment with the cognitive abilities of patients with dementia remains unclear. One preliminary study (Lawton et al., 1970) suggests that environmental changes will have substantial effects on the behavior of demented patients. Other clinical studies suggest that reorganizing wards along the lines of "token economies" may be effective, but no controlled studies exist (Lawton, 1982). In this area, like in the area of family interventions, hypotheses are formed from a series of clinical observations.

A major set of clinical observations were made at the newly constructed facilities at the Philadelphia Geriatric Center (Lawton, 1982). Although originally planned as a controlled study with random assignment of patients to the new or "ideal" setting versus older facilities, random assignment was not achieved. Nonetheless, some patients were followed and behaviorally rated in the old environment before moving to the new environment, where they were again rated. It was found that although no differences were seen in either mental status decline or loss of physical self-maintenance abilities, in the new setting higher ratings were obtained for positive therapeutic behavior and family visits; lower ratings were obtained for pathological behavior and degree of nursing care needed.

Despite the lack of prior empirical research, many questions remain about the effects of the environment on dementia. Lawton (1982) lists a number of research priorities, and notes two areas which he considers *not* appropriate for research. First, inalienable environmental rights should not be researched, i.e., it need not be proven that demented patients benefit from clean, attractive, and safe environments. Second, Lawton argues that evaluation of small technical changes (e.g., a new door opener) could rapidly dissipate available research resources. The effectiveness of such interventions may be best decided by clinical observations.

There are several basic points which do need to be researched. First, there appears to be little data on the range of behavioral plasticity available in demented patients to respond to environmental manipulations. They seem to respond to manipulations of space, but what about changes in time schedules or social changes? Second, little is known about the effects of sensory deprivation or sensory overload on demented patients. Third, no data is available on how to keep novel environmental interventions from becoming part of the grey background of the ward; for example, the new Reality Orientation board which rapidly becomes dust covered. Fourth, what are the basic problems the demented are having in institutions? These practical organizational problems have not been fully investigated.

Summary of Gaps in Our Knowledge and Future Research Needs

Cognitive models of pathology. Despite the uncertainty about the biological basis of deficits seen in demented patients and patients with normal aging, cognitive psychology has been able to clearly identify the major areas of concern: memory and attention. It is important to continue to study these basic psychological parameters since accurate definition of pathology and measurement of function is necessary for both diagnosis and treatment evaluation (see Table 39-1).

Table 39-1. Knowledge gaps for psychosocial interventions in dementia for future research

Basic Psychological Models of Pathology

Continued need for development of accurate psychometrics and theoretical models to follow treatment effects.

Methods of Assessment and Differential Diagnosis

Need for accurate differential diagnosis of depression and dementia, especially using biological markers.

Psychological Interventions

1. Application of newer ideas of cognitive retraining for the demented.
2. Better matching of patients' individual differences to cognitive retraining program characteristics.
3. Study classical individual psychotherapy techniques with elderly who have appropriate behavioral problems, e.g., hysteria or phobias.
4. Examine effects of psychotropic medications on learning process of psychotherapy.

Family Interventions

1. Study ways of teaching caretakers to use behavioral interventions.
2. Examine types of family support needed to allow demented patients to remain with families as long as possible.
3. Examine modern (e.g., paradoxical) therapeutic techniques in the treatment of families of demented elders.
4. Study best ways to organize dementia family support group therapy.
5. Study ways to organize respite care for families with demented members.

Environmental Interventions

1. Examination of degree of change possible through basic manipulations of environmental space, timetables, and social organization.
2. Study effects of sensory deprivation and overload on the demented.
3. Examine ways to keep environmental changes "novel" enough to continue to effect the desired changes.
4. What is the best "mix" of patients in terms of degree of impairment in a nursing care unit.

Assessment. Although discussion of psychological problems in the dementias often centers on cognitive dysfunction, two other major behavioral problems are often associated with such patients: depression and emotional lability. It is usually not too difficult to assess degree of dementia or emotional lability as long as caretakers or family historians are available. Depression is more problematic to diagnose. Little is known about how to distinguish early dementia from depression. Further research into biological markers of depression and dementia is indicated.

Psychological retraining and other interventions. Although there is some evidence for clinical effects of cognitive retraining in the elderly demented, outcome studies of such therapies have suffered from lack of controls as well as lack of sophistication of the interventions proposed. To date there are no published studies with demented subjects which have used the sophisticated techniques commonly used with less-impaired elders. Little is known about the effect of individual differences in elderly subjects with memory deficits. No attempt to match rehabilitation programs to these differences has been made. Another major gap in these studies has been their concentration on the goal of cognitive improvement, neglecting the usual goals of individual psychotherapy. There has been little discussion of using psychotherapeutic techniques to aid demented elders who may suffer from problems in addition to their dementia. The roles of affect and motivation in retraining efforts are also poorly understood. There has been little research into the effects of medications on cognitive training. Few published studies to date have attempted to combine promising therapies. Finally, we know little about ways of training caretakers to effectively use behavioral techniques.

The family. Of major importance is the development of methods of family support which will enable the demented patient to live at home as long as possible without the need for dehumanizing and expensive institutionalization. Research on methods of achieving such goals is in its infancy, with few cross-sectional studies and essentially no longitudinal studies of families successfully meeting the demands of caring for demented members. Furthermore, modern family treatment techniques remain to be evaluated in families with demented members. Little is known about the best ways to develop support groups for families of patients with dementia. Finally, there is a dearth of material on the use of community-based home care in the United States.

Environmental considerations. There is little data on how demented patients respond to environmental manipulations. Little is known about the effects of sensory deprivation or sensory overload on demented patients. No data is available on how to keep novel environmental interventions from becoming part of the gray background of the ward. Finally, should mildly impaired patients be mixed with those with severe problems or should they be segregated? Low-level descriptive research enumerating these problems has yet to be done.

References

Atkinson, J.W., and Raynor, J.O.: Motivation and Achievement, pp. 193–267. Washington D.C.: V.H. Winston, 1974.

Barnes, J.A.: Effects of reality orientation classroom on memory loss, confusion, and disorientation in geriatric patients. The Gerontologist *14*, 138–142 (1974).

Birkhill, W.R., and Schaie, K.W.: The effects of differential reinforcement of cautiousness in intellectual performance. *J. Geron. 30*, 578–583 (1975).

Botwinick, J.: Aging and Behavior, 2nd ed. New York: Springer-Verlag, 1978.

Bower, G.H.: Mental imagery and associative learning. In Gregg, L. (Ed.), Cognition in Learning and Memory, pp. 51–58. New York: John Wiley and Sons, 1972.

Canestrari, R.E.: Age changes in acquisition. In Talland, G.A. (Ed.), Human Aging and Behavior, pp. 169–188. New York: Academic, 1968.

Citrin, R.S., and Dixon, D.N.: Reality orientation: A milieu therapy used in an institution for the aged. The Gerontologist *17*, 39–43 (1977).

Cornbleth, T., and Cornbleth, C.: Reality Orientation for the Elderly. MS 1539, Journal Supplement Abstract Service. Washington, D.C.: Am. Psychological Association, 1977.

Craik, F.I.M.: The nature of the age decrement in performance on dichotic listening tasks. *Quarterly J. Experimental Psychology 17*, 227–240 (1965).

Craik, F.I.M., and Lockart, R.S.: Levels of processing: A framework for memory research. *J. Verbal Learning and Verbal Behavior 11*, 671–684 (1972).

Eisdorfer, C., and Cohen, D.: The assessment of organic impairment in the aged: In search of a new mental status examination. In Burdock et al. (Eds.), Quantitative Techniques for the Evaluation of Psychiatric Patients. New York: Marcel Dekker, 1981.

Eysenck, M.W.: Age differences in incidental learning. *Developmental Psychology 10*, 936–941 (1974).

Frederiksen, J.R.: Some cautions we might exercise in attributing age deficits in memory to attentional dysfunctions. In Poon, L.W. et al. (Ed.), New Directions in Memory and Aging, pp. 131–134. Hillsdale, NJ.: Laurence Erlbaum Associates, 1980.

Glasgow, R.E., Zeiss, R.A., Barrera, M. Jr., and Lewinsohn, P.M.: Case studies on remediating memory deficits in brain-damaged individuals. *J. Clinical Psychology 33*, 1049–1054 (1977).

Haley, W.E.: Behavioral self management. *Clinical Gerontologist 1(3)*, 45–52 (1983).

Harris, C.S., and Ivory, P.: An outcome evaluation of reality orientation therapy with geriatric patients in a state mental hospital. *The Gerontologist 16*, 496–503 (1976).

Herr, J.J., and Weakland, J.H.: Counseling Elders and their Families. New York: Springer-Verlag, 1979.

Hoyer, W.J., Labouvie-Vief, G., and Baltes, P.B.: Modification of response speed deficits and intellectual performance in the elderly. *Human Development 16*, 233–242 (1973).

Hussian, R.A.: Geriatric Psychology: A Behavioral Perspective. New York: Van Nostrand Reinhold, 1981.

Kahn, R.L., and Tobin, S.S.: Community treatment for aged persons with altered brain function. In Miller, N.E., and Cohen, G.D. (Eds.), Clinical Aspects of Alzheimer's Disease and Senile Dementia, pp. 113–130. New York: Raven, 1982.

Kahn, R.L., Zarit, S.H., Hilbert, N.M., and Niederehe, G.: Memory complaint impairment in the aged. *Archives of General Psychiatry 32*, 1569–1593 (1975).

Kinsbourne, M.: Attentional dysfunctions and the elderly: Theoretical models and research perspectives. In Poon, L.W. et al. (Eds.), New Directions in Memory and Aging, pp. 113–130. Hillsdale, NJ: Laurence Erlbaum Associates, 1980.

Labouvie-Vief, G.: Toward optimizing cognitive competence in later life. *Ed. Geront. 1*, 75–92 (1976).

Labouvie-Vief, G., and Gonda, J.N.: Cognitive strategy training and intellectual performance in the elderly. *J. Geront. 31*, 327–332 (1976).

Lawton, M.P., Liebowitz, B., and Charon, H.: Physical structure and the behavior of senile patients following ward remodeling. *Aging Hum. Devel. 1*, 231–239 (1970).

Lawton, M.P.: Sensory deprivation and the effect of the environment on management of the patient with senile dementia. In Miller, N.E., and Cohen, G.D. (Eds.), Clinical Aspects of Alzheimer's Disease and Senile Dementia (Aging) Vol. 15, pp. 227–251. New York: Raven, 1982.

Lewinsohn, P.M., Danaher, B.G., and Kikel, S.: Visual imagery as a mnemonic: Aid for brain injured persons. *J. Con. and Clinical Psychology 45*, 717–723 (1977).

Luria, A., Naydin, V., Tsvetkova, L., and Vinarskays, E.N.: Restoration of higher cortical function following focal brain. In Bruyn, G., Vinken, P.J. (Eds.), Handbook of Clinical Neurology, pp. 369–380. Amsterdam: North-Holland, 1969.

Mason, S.E., and Smith, A.D.: Imagery in the aged. *Experimental Aging Research 3*, 17–32 (1977).

Mishara, B.L., Robertson, B., and Kastenbaum, R.: Self-injurious behavior in the elderly. *The Gerontologist 13*, 311–314 (1973).

Moos, R.H., and Lemke, S.: Evaluating specialized living environments for older people. In Birren, J.E., and Schaie, K.W. (Eds.), Handbook of Psychology of Aging. New York: Van Nostrand Reinhold, 1983.

Patterson, R.L., and Jackson, G.M.: Behavior modification with the elderly. In Hersen, M., Eisler, R.M., and Miller, P.M. (Eds.), Progress in Behavior Modification. New York: Academic, 1980.

Perlmuter, L.C., and Tenny, Y.J., and Smith, P.A.: The Evaluation and Remediation of Memory Problems in the Aged, *Tech. Rep. 80-02*. Geriatric Research, Educational and Clinical Center, VA Outpatient Clinic, Boston, 1980.

Plemons, J.K., Willis, S.L., and Baltes, P.B.: Modifiability of fluid intelligence in aging: A short-term longitudinal training approach. *J. Gerontology 33*, 224–231 (1978).

Poon, L.W., Fozard, J.L., and Treat, N.J.: From clinical and research findings on memory to intervention programs. *Experimental Aging Research 4*, 235–253 (1978).

Poon, L.W., Walsh-Sweeny, L., and Fozard, J.L.: Memory skill training in the elderly: Salient issues on the use of imagery mnemonics. In Poon, L.W. et al., New Directions in Memory and Aging: Proceedings of the George A. Talland Memorial Conference. Hillsdale, NJ: Laurence Erlbaum Associates, 1980.

Rabbitt, P.: Age-decrement in the ability to ignore irrelevant information. *J. Gerontology 20*, 233–238 (1965).

Reifler, B.V., and Wu, S.: Managing families of the demented elderly. *J. Fam. Pract. 6*, 1051–1056 (1982).

Reus, V.I., Weingartner, H., and Post, R.M.: Clinical implications of state-dependent learning. *Am. J. Psychiatry 136*, 927–931 (1979).

Rimm, D.C., and Master, J.C.: Behavior Therapy Techniques and Empirical Findings. New York: Academic, 1974.

Robertson-Tchabo, E.A., Hausman, C.P., and Arneberg, D.: A classic mnemonic for older learners: A trip that works! *Educational Gerontology 1*, 215–226 (1976).

Roediger, H.L.: The effectiveness of four mnemonics in ordering recall. *J. Experimental Psychology: Human Learn. Mem. 25*, 558–567 (1980).

Smith, A.D., and Winograd, E.: Adult age differences in remembering faces. *Dev. Psychology 14*, 443–444 (1978).

Spiegel, H., and Spiegel, D.: *Trance and treatment: Clinical uses of hypnosis*. New York: Basic Books, 1978.

Steurer, J.L., and Clark, E.O.: Family support groups within a research project on dementia. *Clinical Gerontologist 1*, 87–95 (1982).

Thompson, L.W.: Periodic "lapses" in attentional processes: A possible correlate of memory impairment in the elderly. In Poon et al. (Eds.), New Directions in Memory and Aging, pp. 239–242. Hillsdale, NJ: Laurence Erlbaum Associates, 1980.

Treat, N.J., Poon, L.W., Fozard, J.L., and Popkin, S.J.: Toward applying cognitive skill training to memory problems. *Experimental Aging Research 4*, 305–319 (1978).

Troll, L.E.: Families in Later Life. Belmont, CA: Wadsworth Publishers, 1979.

Verwoerdt, A.: Individual psychotherapy in senile dementia. In Miller, N.E., and Cohen, G.E. (Eds.), Clinical Aspects of Alzheimer's Disease and Senile Dementia, Aging, Vol. 15, pp. 187–208. New York: Raven, 1982.

Weiss, B., and Laties, V.G.: Enhancement of human performance by caffeine and the amphetamines. *Pharmacological Review 14*, 1–36 (1962).

Welden, S.H., and Yesavage, J.A.: Behavioral improvement with relaxation training in dementia. *Clinical Gerontologist* (in press).

Willis, S.L., Blieszner, R., and Baltes, P.B.: Intellectual training research in aging: Modification of per on the fluid ability of figure relations. *J. Educational Psychology 73*, 41–50 (1981).

Yerkes, R.M., and Dodson, J.D.: The relation of strength of stimulus to rapidity of habit formation. *J. Comparative and Neurological Psychology 18*, 459–482 (1908).

Yesavage, J.A., and Karasu, T.B.: Psychotherapy with elderly patients. *Am. J. Psychotherapy 36*, 41–55 (1982).

Yesavage, J.A., and King, R.: Drug treatment of cognitive impairment in the elderly. In Eisdorfer, C. (Ed.), Annual Review of Gerontology and Geriatrics, pp. 199–210. New York: Springer-Verlag, 1981.

Yesavage, J.A., Rose, T.L., and Bower, G.H.: Interactive imagery and affective judgements improve face–name learning in the elderly. *J. Gerontology 38*, 197–203 (1983).

Zarit, S.H., Cole, K.D., and Guider, R.L.: Memory training strategies and subjective complaints of memory in the aged. *The Gerontologist 21*, 158–164 (1981a).

Zarit, S.H., Gallagher, D., and Kramer, N.: The effects of group training on memory and memory complaints. *Educational Gerontology 6*, 11–27 (1981b).

Zarit, S.H., Zarit, J.M., and Reever, K.E.: Memory training for severe memory loss: Effects on senile dementia patients and their families. *The Gerontologist 22*, 373–377 (1982).

Zelinski, E.M., and Thompson, L.W.: Do laboratory tests relate to self-assessment of memory ability in the young and old? In Poon, L.W. et al. (Eds.), New Directions in Memory and Aging, pp. 519–544. Hillsdale, NJ: Laurence Erlbaum Associates, 1980.

Chapter 40

Implications of New Research for Care of Alzheimer's Disease

Marshal F. Folstein and Mary Jane Lucas

Summary

In the future, more care will be needed for Alzheimer's disease because of the expected increase in the elderly population and the development of population screening devices which will detect cases previously unrecognized.

There is little doubt now that Alzheimer's disease is not equally distributed in a population, but that certain families seem to be more vulnerable than others for contracting this illness. Thus, Alzheimer's disease from a familial/genetic point of view is not likely to be a normal consequence of aging.

The implications of new research for the care of Alzheimer's disease patients are derived from the concept that Alzheimer's disease is, in fact, a disease of an elderly population growing in number, and that more of these individuals will be recognized as ill and that their families will demand more care. Furthermore, the kind of care that they receive will differ from the care delivered today for Alzheimer's disease patients.

The most important conceptual advance in the field has been the recognition that Alzheimer's disease is a disease entity. The conceptualization of Alzheimer's disease as a disease entity has led to the creation of methods for the detection, diagnosis, treatment, and further research to discover its prevention. The disease concept conveys the hope that has come through medical and epidemiological success with mental disorders in the past such as syphillis, pellagra, and deficiency states which are now curable if not entirely preventable. In addition to the hope of success, the concept implies that Alzheimer's disease is somehow a mistake of nature rather than an inevitable development such as puberty. As a consequence it seems appropriate to try to correct this error of nature with the methods successful in the past, that is, the clinical methods of diagnosis, treatment, and prognosis based on the advances in basic sciences, and the epidemiologic method of population studies used to discuss preventive measures. From the point of view of service delivery, it also seems appropriate to patients and their families that an individual suffering from a chronic disease similar to other chronic diseases such as cancer or tuberculosis should seek medical care and that medical care should be available. A corollary to this is that appropriate insurance and other reimbursement mechanisms for funding this health care should be available. And finally, following from the idea of Alzheimer's disease as a disease entity, is the idea that appropriate human and financial resources should be devoted to training the physicians and nurses needed to care for the patients and to conduct future research.

The evidence suggesting that Alzheimer's disease is a disease of the elderly springs from epidemiologic, psychological, and genetic studies. Epidemiological studies conducted in Scandanavia and Britain over the last 30 years indicate that only a minority of the elderly individuals develop Alzheimer's disease, even by the age of 85. In a study recently conducted in Baltimore among the elderly who survive to age 85, only 11% meet the diagnostic criteria for Alzheimer's disease. Other studies indicate similar rates (Kay, 1964; Mortimer, Schuman, and French, 1981). Since the disorder only affects a small proportion of individuals even at this advanced stage, it cannot logically be considered to be the normal development in old age.

Although there are documented psychological changes with old age, notably a decrease in mental speed and some loss of recall, psychological studies of Alzheimer's disease indicate that the symptoms are far more than a minor memory loss; they include amnesia, aphasia, and apraxia (Alzheimer, 1907; Sjogven et al., 1952; Constantinidis et al., 1965). These symptoms are qualitatively different than the kinds of nonmemory troubles affecting normal elderly.

Finally, family studies indicate that the relatives of patients with Alzheimer's disease are at least 3–4 times at greater risk than the general population for developing the disease themselves (Folstein and Powell, in press). Our own studies in this area indicate that a population of people in a nursing home who are selected by stringent criteria, which included the presence of classical symptoms of amnesia, aphasia, and apraxia and excluded all individuals with risks for cerebral vascular disease, were much more likely to have affected relatives than controls who did not have these classical symptoms but lived in the same nursing home. In fact, the indexed cases' relatives had a 50% risk of developing Alzheimer's disease by age 85, comparable with the kind of distribution one would expect in an autosomal dominant disorder (Breitner and Folstein, in press).

Further studies in our clinic have indicated that patients with familial Alzheimer's disease account for more than one-half of all patients in a clinic with Alzheimer's. The age of onset of the familial cases ranges between 30 and 90, with average age of onset of 64, and thus this disorder is not limited to only early-onset cases (Powell and Folstein, in press). Early pathological studies suggest that the pathology, as well as the clinical symptoms of the familial cases, are classical.

Since the studies of Williamson, it has been recognized that many patients with Alzheimer's disease are unrecognized as being ill and seldom use health care resources (Williamson et al., 1964). Over the last few years, several screening tests have become available which can be used by nonspecialist clinicians to detect these cases. The Mini-Mental-State Examination is one such test (Folstein, Folstein, and McHugh, 1975). The test consists of a series of questions which assess the patient's orientation, memory, attention, language function, motor skills, and level of consciousness. It is scored and a maximum score is 30 points. Several clinical studies have indicated its high reliability and validity, and a recent community survey indicated that it is a sensitive indicator of Alzheimer's disease in the community. This screening test must be interpreted cautiously, however, because a low score does not indicate a particular diagnosis, but only the need for further evaluation of a cognitive impairment.

Thus, for reasons of new case detection, more elderly individuals will be found who are demented, and from population studies we can expect more elderly individuals in the community; thus the need for more care is inevitable. The kind of care that the patients will receive will be different than the kind of care currently being administered.

Alzheimer's disease patients today are cared for primarily in the community and in nursing homes. Their current level of care is usually intermediate, and not reimbursable for long-term care under Medicare. However, the nature of the symptoms indicate that skilled psychiatric care is required and will need to be required in the future. An appreciation of the communication difficulties of the patients with aphasia and their difficulties using their hands because of apraxia will lead to new forms of rehabilitation designed to maximize function in spite of these disabilities. New facilities will be created that will allow patients more freedom and less required restraints.

The kinds of symptoms that often are the cause of behaviors like agitation, wandering, and violence include depression, delusions, and hallucinations. These symptoms occur in a substantial proportion of patients with Alzheimer's disease and require expert psychiatric management. At this time there are a few clinical trials available to dictate the best treatment, but more research is being conducted in this area.

After the strong data indicating that the disorder is familial is better known, genetic counselling of families of patients with Alzheimer's disease will be frequently requested. At this time counselling should be limited to individual families after complete pedigrees are collected for that family. The maximal risk at this time appears to be 50% by the age of 85 in those families that appear to have clear autosomal distribution of the disorder in the family, as contrasted to the general population rate of 11% at the age of 85. Given the fact that most individuals do not reach this age, the risk to particular family members is usually quite low.

References

Alzheimer, A.: Uber eine eigenartige Erkrankung der Hirnrinde. *Allg. Z. Psychiatr.* Psych.-Gerichtl. Med. 64, 146–148 (1907).

Breitner, J.C.S., and Folstein, M.F.: Familial Alzheimer Dementia: A prevalent disorder with specific clinical features. *Psychological Medicine* (in press).

Constantinidis, J., Garrone, G. et al.: L'incidence familiale des alterations neurobibrillaires corticales d'Alzheimer. *Psychiatr. Neurol. 150*, 235–295 (1965).

Folstein, M.F., Folstein, S.E., and McHugh, P.R.: Mini-mental state: A practical method for grading the cognitive state of patients. *Journal of Psychiatric Research 12*(3), 189–198 (1975).

Folstein, M.F., and Powell, D.: Is Alzheimer Disease inherited? A methodological review. *Integrative Psychiatry* (in press).

Kay, D.W.K., Beamish, P., and Roth, M.: Old age mental disorders in Newcastle Upon Tyne. Part I: A study of prevalence. *British Journal of Psychiatry 110*, 146–158 (1964).

Mortimer, J.A., Schuman, L.M., and French, L.R.: Epidemiology of dementing illness. In Mortimer, J., and Schuman, L. (Eds.), The Epidemiology of Dementia, New York Chapter 1, pp. 3–23. Oxford University Press, 1981.

Powell, D., and Folstein, M.F.: Pedigree study of familial Alzheimer Disease. *Journal of Neurogenetics* (in press).

Sjögren, T. et al.: Morbus Alzheimer and Morbus Pick. *Acta Psychiatr. Scand.* (Suppl.) *82*, 1–152 (1952).

Williamson, J., Stokoe, I.H., et al.: Old people at home: Their unreported needs. *Lancet 1*, 1119–1120 (1964).

Chapter 41

The Future of Psychotherapy and the Elderly

Gene D. Cohen

Summary

The future of psychotherapy for the elderly will inevitably witness tension between two creative forces. On the one hand, there should be refinement of past and present concepts as well as innovation in their application. On the other hand, the search for new principles is a given. In the discussion that follows an attempt is made to portray a background for the future by examining emerging trends and developments. The impact of historical views on psychotherapy for the elderly will be reviewed; the phenomenology of later life as it relates to the older patient will be explored; process and evolving techniques in psychotherapy with the aging will be looked at; the need to pay particular attention to health and behavior considerations in psychotherapeutic approaches with elderly patients will be addressed; and psychodynamic issues in dealing with dementia will also be included.

New directions in a field are determined not just by new information, but by different perspectives on existing knowledge as well. Many of the most notable inventions have been derived not from new principles, but by creative application of existing concepts. The telephone and the light bulb are cases in point. Future directions of psychotherapy for the elderly can similarly be based on expanded perspectives about our present knowledge base, along with new concepts (Cohen, 1980).

Reassessing Historical Views

Misinformation about the place, nature, and efficacy of psychotherapy for the elderly continues to be intermittently revived. Meanwhile, insights about the same, historically, have been intermittently overlooked (Rechtschaffen, 1959; Cohen, 1981; Blum, 1980). The views of Freud and Abraham on this topic illustrate the point.

Freud, in 1905, indicated that

> the age of patients has this much importance in determining their fitness for psycho-analytic treatment, that, on the one hand, near or above the age of 50 the elasticity of the mental processes, on which treatment depends, is as a rule lacking—old people are no longer educable—and, on the other hand, the mass of material to be dealt with would prolong the duration of the treatment indefinitely. (Freud, 1978)

Ironically, Freud wrote this as he was approaching his 50th birthday, a period in his own life marked by elasticity and educability. Ironic, too, is that Freud's view of "the greatest masterpiece of all time" (Jones, 1957) was a work done by an aging playwright in his eighth decade. *Oedipus Rex*, the drama that was probably perceived by Freud as a brilliant literary validation of his concept of the Oedipus complex in his then pioneering psychoanalytic theory, was written by Sophocles at the age of 71. Similarly, Dostoevsky was nearing his 60th birthday when he completed *The Brothers Karamasov*, a narrative Freud referred to as the "greatest novel ever written," dealing with the "same theme" as "Oedipus Rex." Dostoevsky died the next year (Jones, 1957). Perhaps it was the "mass of material," as Freud called it, that these aging authors had to deal with that permitted them, rather than restricted them, to achieve their great efforts, their great insights.

Fifteen years after Freud's reflections on psychoanalysis for the elderly, Karl Abraham expressed a different view in his classic 1919 paper on the "Applicability of Psycho-Analytic Treatment to Patients at an Advanced Age" (Abraham, 1979). Abraham wrote:

> In my psychoanalytic practice I have treated a number of chronic neuroses in persons of over 40 and even 50 years of age. At first it was only after some hesitation that I undertook cases of this kind, But I was more than once urged to make the attempt by patients themselves who had been treated unsuccessfully elsewhere. And I was, moreover, confident that if I could not cure the patients I could at least give them a deeper and better understanding of their trouble than a physician untrained in psychoanalysis could. To my surprise a considerable number of them reacted very favorably to the treatment. I might add that I count some of those cures as among my most successful results.

Despite Abraham's experience and reports, decades of doubts about the role and potential benefit of psychotherapy for older adults persisted. Moreover, there was a tendency to view psychodyamically oriented treatment for the aging in simplistic or limiting terms. Reductionists here might well have benefited from H.L. Mancken's admonition that "for very complicated problem, there is a simple solution; and that simple solutions always fail." Psychotherapy with the elderly—its indication, form, and duration—is no less complicated than psychotherapy with younger adults, and the solutions it seeks no less simple.

Phenomenology and Aging: The Older Person as Patient

An instructive meeting between Sigmund Freud and Sherlock Holmes took place in Nicholas Meyer's narrative *The Seven-Percent Solution*; Meyer suggests early in his book that "the story is true, only the facts have been changed" (Myer, 1982). At one key point both Holmes and Freud are sharing observations about an individual across the room. Finally Holmes pauses in exasperation, turns to Freud, and advises him, "My dear doctor, you look, but you do not see." Such too often has been the case with the clinician looking at the older person as patient—the clinician looks, but too often does not see.

The clinician may not, for example, see the paradoxes that surround the capacity for change and the significance of time in later life (Cohen, 1982a). Somerset Maughm captured these paradoxes when he reflected that "when I was young I was amazed at Plutarch's statement that the elder Cato began at the age of 80 to learn Greek. I am amazed no longer. Old age is ready to undertake tasks that youth shirked because they would take too long (Comfort, 1977). The relevance of Mauhgam's relevation to the potential for psychotherapeutic work with older adults is not difficult to deduce.

The capacity for change in later life has been illustrated from the time of Cato to that of Colonel Sanders. The matter of time, of time left for the older person, continues to become more interesting. It should be recognized that by age 65, one is a survivor with an average life expectancy of almost 15 years for men and almost 19 for women—significant intervals for both life and treatment. And these are only averages, with the number of individuals reaching age 100 continuing to grow. Of comparative note is the fact that in Rome, during the period of the Roman Empire, because of death associated with childbirth, disease, famine, and war, average longevity was only 22 years (Hendricks and Hendricks, 1977). Meanwhile, in contemporary America, at age 65, average longevity is approaching 20 years—a duration, incidentally, more than 3 times the length of most psychoanalyses. These perspectives are clearly important in orienting the therapist to opportunities for psychotherapy with the elderly.

How the therapist views intellectual capacity in later life is obviously another perspective-influencing variable. To begin with, new elderly cohorts continue to be more educated and more articulate. Moreover, the findings show that for the most part those older persons who maintain their general health and remain intellectually active in later life show no significant cognitive decline with aging (Granick and Patterson, 1971). The point is not that changes fail to take place. Older people do not, for example, react to stimuli as quickly. But vocabulary can increase with aging, and this relates to accumulated experience and associated options for action. Severe cognitive impairment in the form of Alzheimer's disease affects about 6% of those over age 65—large in number, but relatively small percentage-wise. On the other hand, memory complaints in the elderly may signal an underlying depression, the complaints representing a form of depressive self-criticism in certain older persons. Keep in mind, too, that misplacing keys or a wallet, or calling one sibling or child by another's name is overlooked at age 30. But after age 50, the same normal forgetfulness may raise eyebrows. While some look but do not see, others misinterpret what they observe when the person is aging.

Whereas memory complaints can be misleading in the elderly, so too can talk about death. Because older persons have a larger number of acquaintances who have died, talk about death or those dying is understandable. But preoccupation about death in those without a terminal illness, especially dread of it or symptomatic anxiety around it, rather than being normal in later life may reflect an underlying depression or a troubled response to serious loss—loss of a loved one, of financial independence, or of self-esteem. To dismiss such concerns about death as normal with aging and not to psychodynamically explore the stress as a symptom could do the patient a severe disservice. Interestingly, concern about death is more typical in the middle years when one often first becomes profoundly aware of his or her mortality, a period in one's life when thoughts about how much time is left replace those about how much time has passed. By later life, though, denial about death once again sets in as a constructive defense mechanism to allow one to procede through life with less anxiety (Cohen, 1982b).

There are other areas, as well, where what one sees with the elderly may elicit different interpretations. Consider, for example, the subject of apparent repetition of ideas, themes, and behaviors in aging individuals. To use a metaphor, one could ask to what extent does such apparent repetition represent a rerun, to what extent an attempted remake? Whereas a rerun might be regarded in the category of reminiscence, a remake attempt could represent new material—an effort with new strategies. We do not make patronizing judgements about film producers or playwrights who attempt remakes of classical myths and stories. Older adults, too, may revisit earlier themes or chapters in their own lives and try them out with a new twist as part of the ongoing process of human growth and development throughout the life cycle. Hence, to the extent one views later life as being mainly in a compensatory mode, exploratory opportunities that can accompany aging might be overlooked.

Related to this discussion is the question: Do the elderly "slow down" or do they "slow up?" The difference may be more than semantic, with slowing down having a pejorative connation, but slowing up suggesting something else. Such concerns relate to analogies between aging and entropy—a continuation of century-old thermodynamic and mechanistic frameworks for viewing psychodynamic phenomena. Even within this mechanistic framework, however, there are alternative analogies that suggest alternative perspectives on changes experienced by the elderly. For example, to move from 19th century engines to 20th century satellites, it can be appreciated that a spaceship early in its course launches into its journey with tremendous thrust and great force as required to get going on its desired course. Eventually it throws off its boosters, and "slows up" its thrust, since less force is necessary to keep its journey on course. The analogy to one's journey through the life-course should be apparent; do we need the same booster strength to keep us on our life course with aging?

As alluded to earlier, the point is not to deny that various losses and declines take place in later life but to separate the course of normal development from the course of various diseases in the elderly. In other words, it is insufficient to look at change per se with aging; one must look at change in the context of resulting new strategies as well as resulting deficits. William Carlos Williams, the physician/poet, has written eloquently on this perspective. In his 60s Williams suffered a stroke, then turned full time to the writing of verse. He wrote about "old age which adds as it takes away (Foy, 1979). From a psychodynmaic vantage point, a disproportionate focus has been directed to what old age "takes away." The clinical literature is replete with well-articulated allusions to later life as a "season of loss" (Pfeiffer, 1976), a "crisis in slow motion" (Berezin, 1963), and in terms of a "depletion hypothesis" (Cath, 1966) or "disengagement theory" (Cumming and Henry, 1961). Clinicians and researchers alike are largely only beginning to look at what old age adds.

To a large extent, up through the present cohort group of elderly we have not had a true opportunity to see what normal aging can be like. This can be attributed to a social climate that has been inordinately stressful in terms of inadequately developed socialization networks for the post-retirement population, sparse high-quality age-oriented activities, housing dilemmas, budgetary problems, transportation difficulties, and so forth. We have not really seen what the true potential for later life is without these external stressors. Moreover, compounding the shortcomings in the social system has been a lack of familiarity with new opportunities for improved illness treatment and prevention. The outcome has been a combination of excessive social stress and illness obscuring opportunities for further inner growth and development as part of normal aging.

Process and Technique in Psychotherapy with Older Patients

Many issues surround process and technique in psychotherapy with the elderly, ranging from questions about transference and countertransference to those on resistance and insight, among others. Berezin reminds us that "transference by definition is unreality; it is unconscious and is not time-oriented. In this sense it is also consistent with the concept of timelessness. In psychotherapy, transference reactions do not follow chronological calendar considerations (Berezin, 1972). Of course, this is not to say that the age of the patient or the age of the therapist has no dynamic impact on transference or countertransference phenomena. The point is that age may or may not make a difference. The therapist may be seen by the older patient as a grandson or granddaughter, son or daughter, sibling or parent. Similarly the therapist may find himself or herself relating to one older person as if the patient were "an elder," to another in a parental mode, and sometimes both ways at different times with the same patient.

What about resistance and insight with the elderly patient? Grotjahn has pointed out that "it looks as if resistance against unpleasant insight is frequently lessened in old age. Demands of reality which in younger people are considered narcissistic threats may finally become acceptable . . . It seems as if, more or less, suddenly resistance is weakened and insight occurs just because it is high time" (Grotjahn, 1955). Indeed, it was a 71 year old who with insight first wrote about Oedipus.

Whereas resistance and insight on the part of the patient influence what will be focused on in psychotherapy, so too does the approach of the therapist as with the use of life review techniques. Butler described the life review approach as a therapeutic use of reminiscing to resolve, reorganize, and reintegrate what is troubling or preoccupying the patient. It is an effort to facilitate the capacity of older people to reconcile or come to better terms with the meaning of their lives (Butler, 1963). Others, however, emphasize that questions of when and for whom to use this technique must be raised, since some older people will look at past life experiences not as they have been, but as they might have been and in the process experience guilt and a profound sense of loss. Weinberg addressed this point when he wrote about "adding insight to injury" (Weinberg, 1976). One is reminded of the admonition against seeking simple solutions for complex problems. One is also reminded of the great variability among older patients as is the case with younger persons.

Health and Behavior with Aging

One of the clinical features distinguishing older patients from younger ones is the greater likelihood of the former to have more than one illness or to be receiving more than one treatment at a time. Furthermore, the elderly are much more likely to have concurrent mental and physical disorders. With the future bringing yet greater numbers of older persons and growing percentages of those at quite advanced ages, knowledge about the interplay of mental and physical phenomena affecting clinical course and treatment with elderly patients will become all the more important. Psychotherapeutic considerations in this area are no exception.

Consider first that psychotherapeutic options may go unrecognized if the course of illness in later life is poorly understood. The concept of exacerbation and remission of illness seems even less well appreciated with mental than with physical disorders. When someone with diabetes or congestive heart failure has a flare-up, family and physican expect that a remission is likely to follow with proper treatment. An aggravation of a psychiatric disturbance, however, is more likely to be reacted to by others with greater impatience and disappointment or a sense of futility. Such reactions can be magnified when the patient is an older person. But the fact remains that mental disorders do remit and do so throughout the life cycle; old age does not break the pattern. Consider further that some serious physical disorders that seem to be getting worse in elderly patients may actually be doing so not for reasons of physiologic decline, but at times because of a covert psychiatric disturbance. This might be reflected in a case of the older patient with congestive heart failure whose health status appears to be deteriorating. On occasion a hidden depression can result in a giving-up feeling in this cardiac patient, leading to passive suicidal behavior in the form of noncompliance in the proper use of medication for the physical disorder. The turnabout toward improved health in this instance would more likely come from psychotherapy than it would from an altered cardiovascular treatment approach. In either case, from a psychodynamic or a physiologic perspective, the decline should not be initially viewed as an inevitable part of aging; otherwise the behavior of the clinician could adversely affect the health of the patient.

The relationship between soma and psyche in terms of their effect on clinical course and psychodynamic phenomena is also illustrated in the following case example:

Case Report: Ms. A., a 78-year-old woman, came on her own to the clinic. She was very angry and demanded to see a psychiatrist. She had found herself getting increasingly angry and annoyed and felt it was time to do something about it. She had also experienced severe deterioration in her vision over the past few years that had not been halted despite extensive opthalmologic intervention and surgery. Not long into the initial interview I, as her therapist, became the object of her anger. The patient said she doubted whether I could do anything about her state of mind and that I was probably incompetent anyway. A few minutes later she said "you have confirmed my expectations—you are inept indeed."

It became apparent that the patient was quickly repeating in this new relationship what happened in other relationships. She would approach someone for help only then to berate them, driving them away. Her severe problems with vision had placed her in the position of needing considerably more help from others, but at the same time they stirred up a long-standing submerged dependency conflict. She had always seen herself as in the driver's seat; she would strive to turn any passive situation into an active one. Despite her age she had several siblings still living, many of whom encouraged her to visit. Her response, though, was, "Who wants a blind lady?" and that she "was not accepting any invitations." Meanwhile she was displaying a tremendous degree of energy, initiative, and resourcefulness, of sorts, in a rather unusual activity. this 78-year-old blind woman took public transportation two nights a week to a course at an inner city university. What was even more unusual was the title of the course: "How to Become a Funeral Parlor Director." She asked me if I knew why she was taking the course. I asked why. She said, "To perform your funeral."

For many people rapid loss of vision can represent both literally and figuratively that the lights are going out, which can symbolize death or dying. This woman had gone through life attempting to turn the passive into the active; her present situation was to be no different. With loss of vision symbolizing a form of death she was similarly in a symbolic and unconscious manner going to get the upper hand on death—control over it—by learning to be a funeral parlor director.

The tasks of therapy involved dealing with the rage surrounding the dependency issues within and outside the framework of the transference. The goal was to help the patient better handle her feelings and behavior in situations where it was appropriate for her to depend on others. Ideally, in this process a considerable amount of energy and resourcefulness could be constructively rechanneled. Over a period of two years the woman dealt with her anger and dependency conflict in therapy, and during that time she seemed to come to better terms with them. A turning point had clearly occurred when she finally agreed to visit her family.

This case example demonstrates several points. The impact of psychological health on the handling of physical disability can be seen. The converse can be seen as well—i.e., the impact of somatic change on thoughts, affect, and behavior. One can appreciate the difference between external dependency needs and internal dependency conflicts. Not the least that can be learned from this case is recognition that the capacity to deal with crisis and to grow psychologically continues throughout the life cycle.

With dementia the interplay of physical and mental factors affecting the severity of clinical course can be witnessed once more. So too can one witness the breadth of opportunties for psychotherapeutic interventions, where even in the case of Alzheimer's disease psychotherapy has a place. It is not uncommon in this regared for the Alzheimer patient to have a concomitant depression which in turn causes excess disabilty for the individual. Depression itself can cause difficulty in concentrating, thus adding to the dementia and making the Alzheimer patient even more impaired. Treating the depression can reduce overall disability and thereby improve quality of life for the Alzheimer patient at that stage of his or her illness, and likely ease the burden on others assisting the ill individual.

Of note is that psychodynamic phenomena continue to be relevant at an advanced stage of dementia as well. One illustration of this point is the double dilemma around one's own history experienced by the institutionalized older patient with severe dementia. The demented individual has not only lost touch with personal history, but has also lost the ability to convey his or her own history to others. In this sense we all have a compound history, a two-faceted history—a history of ourselves as we know it, and a history of ourselves as others know it. Not to be known by others, to be in effect without a history as a consequence of being unable to convey one's past, puts a person at a severe disadvantage in eliciting the understanding and empathy of others. The therapist can be enormously helpful here in conveying the individual's personal and dynamic history—his or her clinical biography, so to speak—to the various staff who will be working with the patient. The outcome is likely to be improved interpersonal exchange despite the patient's marked cognitive impairment. It might be said in this regard that how the Alzheimer patient is viewed late in dementia is as much a factor of biography as biology.

Effect of the Older Patient on the Therapist

It is common for a therapist working for the first time with older patients to be surprised in discovering how satisfying the experience can be. That older patients are often more realistic in their treatment objectives and more grateful for small changes in therapy is a pleasant realization. Victims themselves of negative stereotypes of old age, many elderly individuals may not initially expect much to happen in therapy, so when something does improve, a profound sense of satisfaction can be shared.

Therapsits also typically gain new information about themselves in providing psychotherapy to older patients. Whenever one works with any new age group—whether children, adolescents, young adults, the middle aged, or older adults—there is the opportunity to see oneself in a new light. New personal insights gained in this process clearly can benefit the therapist in his or her work with all age groups.

Work with those at an advanced age may, in addition, present the therapist with a unique opportunity to look back in time with the patient at the course of early life conflicts and problems across the life cycle, to examine in one person the interplay of development and disorder over a period of decades. It is as if one has a chance for a 60, 70, or 80 year follow-up of interactions among psychological, biological, and social changes in an individual. Psychotherapy with the elderly, in short, can add to one's general education; the therapist is allowed in this effort to have new glimpses in an attempt to further understand illness and the human condition (Cohen, 1979). The future of psychotherapy with the elderly should only add to these opportunities.

References

Abraham, K.: Applicability of psycho-analytic treatment to patients at an advanced age. In Selected Papers on Psychoanalysis. New York: Bruner/Mazel, 1979.

Berezin, M.A.: Some intrapsychic aspects of aging. In Zinberg, N.E., and Kaufman, I. (Eds.), Normal Psychology of the Aging Process. New York: International Universities Press, 1963.

Berezin, M.A.: Psychodynamic considerations of aging and the aged: An overview. *Am. J. Psychiatry 128*, 1483–1491 (1972).

Blum, J.E., and Tross, S.: Psychodynamic treatment of the elderly: A review of issues in theory and practice. In Eisdorfer, C. (Ed.), Annual Review of Gerontology and Geriatrics, pp. 204–234. New York: Springer-Verlag, 1980.

Butler, R.N.: The life review: An interpretation of reminiscence in the aged. *Psychiatry 26*, 65–76 (1963).

Cath, S.H.: Beyond depression—the depleted state; a study in ego psychology in the aged. *Can. Psychiatric Assn. J.* (Suppl.) *11*, 329–339 (1966).

Cohen, G.D.: Prospects for mental health and aging. In Birren, J.E., and Sloane, R.B. (Eds.), Handbook of Mental Health and Aging. Englewood Cliffs: NJ: Prentice-Hall, 1980.

Cohen, G.: Perspectives on psychotherapy with the elderly. *Am. J. Psychiatry 138*, 347–350 (1981).

Cohen, G.D.: The older person, the older patient, and the mental health system. *Hospital and Community Psychiatry 33*, 101–104 (1982a).

Cohen, G.D.: Geriatric psychiatry. In Oken, D., and Kakovics, M. (Eds.), A Clinical Manual of Psychiatry. New York: Elsevier/North Holland, 1982b.

Cohen, G.D.: Research on aging: A piece of the puzzle. *Gerontologist 19*, 503–508 (1979).

Comfort, A.: A Good Age. London: Mitchel Beazley, 1977.

Cumming, E., and Henry, W.: Growing Old: The Process of Disengagement. New York: Basic Books, 1961.

Foy, J.L.: Creative Psychiatry. New York: GEIGY Pharmaceuticals, 1979.

Freud, S.: On Psychotherapy (1905). In Complete Psychological Works, Vol. 7. Translated and edited by J. Strachey. London: Hogarth, 1978.

Granick, S., and Patterson, R.D. (Eds.): Human Aging—II: An Eleven-Year Followup Biomedical and Behavioral Study. Washington, D.C.: Dept. of H.E.W. publication HSM-71-9037, 1971.

Grotjahn, M.: Analytic psychotherapy with the elderly. I: The sociological background of aging in America. *Psychoanal. Rev. 42*, 419–427 (1955).

Hendricks, J., and Hendricks, C.D.: Aging In Mass Society. Cambridge, MA: Winthrop, 1977.

Jones, E.: The Life and Work of Sigmond Freud, Vol. 3, pp. 417–431. New York: Basic Books, 1957.

Myer, N.: The Seven Percent Solution. New York: Ballantine Books, 1976.

Pfeiffer, E.: Psychotherapy with elderly patients. In Bellak, L., and Karasu, T. (Eds.), Geriatric Psychiatry. New York: Grune & Stratton, 1976.

Rechtschaffen, A.: Psychotherapy with geriatric patients. A review of the literature. *J. Gerontol. 14*, 73–84 (1959).

Weinberg, J.: On adding insight to injury. *Gerontologist 16*, 4–10 (1976).

Part XI

A Look into the Future

Chapter 42

"Old Wine in New Bottles": Medical Care for the Elderly in the Year 2000

Roger J. Bulger

Summary

In this chapter an attempt is made to predict the characteristics and nature of medical care for the elderly 20 years hence. There is a discussion of the distinction between primary and secondary technologies and the implications of each kind of technology for improving health status and reducing the burden of disease.

There then follows a review of some of the promising new techniques and technologies which might have a particular bearing on the elderly. Next, an estimation is made of the possibilities for behavior modification and quantitative risk assessment for environmental hazards in health promotion and disease prevention in relationship to those maladies most detrimental to the aged population. Finally, some prognostications are presented regarding the way health care will be made available to our population in the year 2000.

I have wondered, repeatedly, why an administrator was asked to address this subject, and despite these efforts at understanding, my best guess remains that no biomedical scientist or practicing physician of distinction, wit, and common sense would have accepted the invitation! So it was out of necessity that they turned to an administrator . . . Obviously, there is no sense predicting anything with any certainty or confidence regarding the state of our world 17 years hence. Nevertheless, there may be some value in having someone make a stab at some prognostications for the year 2000 insofar as it may encourage more of us to do the same; the playing of the futurist game has the value of stimulating one to consider where he or she thinks we might be going and induces an implicit comparison with where one would like us to be going; and the latter step of course may lead more of us to be more active in working harder to bring about those outcomes we deem most desirable. In any case, it was on these terms that it seemed most appropriate for someone with my background to undertake this task and I therefore agreed to do so; I must confess that I have learned a lot in the process and very much appreciate the opportunity which has been offered me.

A few assumptions must be stated at the outset. First, it is assumed that there will be no nuclear holocaust, other major world conflagration, or widespread economic collapse, and that there will be relatively little change in the general directions of our nation in particular and western civilization in general. Second, it is assumed that other contributors will cover central nervous system and mental disorders and that their exclusion from this discussion is no reflection upon their relative importance, even primacy, in the scheme of things, when it comes to the health of the elderly. Finally, it is my own personal assumption that medical care, though obviously important, is less important than other social, psychological, and cultural factors in terms of the overall well-being of our aged population.

I have divided my approach to this subject into four sections as follows: First, a discussion of the implications of what Lewis Thomas has referred to as the distinction between primary and secondary technologies; second, a review of some of the promising new techniques and technologies which might have a particular bearing on the elderly; third, an estimation of the possibilities for behavior modification and quantitative risk assessment for environmental hazards in health promotion and disease prevention in relationship to those maladies which are most detrimental to the aged population; and fourth, a listing of some guesses about the way health care will be made available to our population in the year 2000.

In many ways, what has been referred to as the "creeping incrementalism" of social policy change in a democratic society may make the social and behavioral aspects easier to predict accurately than are the kinds of new technologies, either primary or secondary which will emerge in 20 years. Scientific breakthroughs are so unpredictable, technology transfer in many instances so rapid, and commercialization so effective that it is likely that many of the more important practical advances of the year 2000 cannot be imagined even by well-informed professionals in 1984. These caveats notwithstanding, my colleague Sue Feazel and I systematically interviewed 20 leading faculty in our Health Science Center and added their impressions on the subject to our own such that we share with them any of the credit for interesting insights or observations, but must take sole responsibility for errors or inept analysis.

Primary versus Secondary Technologies

It was about a decade ago, as part of his ongoing attempt to explain and advocate the value of basic science to the lay public and body politic, that Lewis Thomas introduced into the relevant rhetoric the distinction between a primary and a secondary technology. A prime example of a primary technology is the polio vaccine, which for relatively low unit cost effectively prevents the occurrence of a disastrous disease; the development of this primary technology required increased understanding of basic biological processes and followed hard upon the acquisition of the requisite core knowledge. (The Nobel Prizes went to the people who discovered the basic knowledge and not to Salk and Sabin). An example of the secondary technologies associated with the treatment of paralytic polio is the iron lung, used to sustain and improve the lives of severely stricken patients. The treatment of polio was and is enormously expensive and that expense has been virtually eliminated by the development of the primary technology.

Another, perhaps more relevant example to our discussion relates to chronic renal failure, the secondary technologies for which include dialysis and transplantation; the search for a vaccination or other primary technology goes on, but the prevention of chronic renal failure would save much misery and societal expense. Public health experts might argue that Dr. Thomas' definition of primary technology is too restrictive and that epidemiology, quantitative risk assessment for environmental hazards, and other disease prevention and health promotion devices can eliminate costly diseases even without understanding the basic biochemistry or possessing a vaccine. If these arguments prevail, then more money will be spent on basic research and development in the biological sciences and in those areas relating to behavior modification, multiple risk factor analysis, and disease prevention; and the citizens will benefit accordingly by the year 2000. But, of course, it requires a highly sophisticated form of political widsom and citizen unselfishness to vote more research dollars today to yield somewhat uncertain benefits in 5–10 years. In any case, these distinctions are useful to keep in mind as we explore what the experts tell us we may have in our armamentarium to treat the elderly two decades hence.

There is an interesting footnote to the chronic dialysis issue which may offer a lesson to us as we ponder how to control health costs and whether possibly just changing our system will offer more equitable distribution of care on the one hand or a more effective way to ration expensive care on the other. At the last International Congress on Nephrology, a comparative analysis was presented upon the utilization of chronic dialysis in various nations in the world. I found it interesting to note that the elderly had their greatest access to chronic dialysis in the United States, while Japan seemed to be catching up more quickly than were Germany, Sweden, and England. Second, for those who might argue that the rationing of these expensive technologies for the elderly while making them more fully available to the young is right and proper as seems to have occurred in England and Sweden, the upward trend in increasing accessibility for the elderly is clear even in those more centralized, socialized systems. It seems that, over time, no nation has been successful in preventing the widespread utilization of effective technologies throughout the population. If this experience and others offer us any lesson, it must be that we should assume that our society will be unable to selectively deny to the elderly those technologies that people are convinced are effective, no matter how expensive.

Aging—Primary Technologies

Lewis Thomas has expressed what, in my view, is perhaps the most realistic hope for optimal biological aging. Rather than denying our genetically programmed mortality and postulating an ever-increasing life span, he hopes for disease-free old age, with death occurring because of the inevitable winding down of the genetic and, therefore, the metabolic clock. One of the most exciting of the current research probes that bear upon this subject is being pursued by the immunologists. The complicated operation and modulation of our immune system is coming to light at last, and with these advances have come the so-called biological response modifiers, natural and synthetic agents able to influence the system at particular precise points and, in some cases, with a seemingly generalized action. The general significance of the host defense systems in the development of cancer, all infectious diseases, and the so-called autoimmune diseases is well known, but the descriptive details are pouring from the world's research laboratories in such profusion as to make it not unreasonable to predict access to immunomodulating agents by the year 2000, which will be capable of preserving the immune system intact, until the biological clock at last runs its course.

Our experience with immunosupressive agents has been extensive, but the leading primary technologies of the future in the field of aging may be stimulators of the immune system, such as Interleukin II, cyclosporine, isoprinosine, and a host of other agents currently under investigation. One way to view cancer is to consider it as an attempt at immortality on the part of a single cell cluster at the expense of the mortality built into the genomes of the entire organism, and one function of our host defences is to prevent such cancers from occurring. Fifty percent of men over 80 years of age have cancer cells in their prostate glands; other lines .of evidence point towards diminished immunologic competence as preconditions for many diseases. Thus, one can see the logic of seeking treatments to preserve immunologic competence before symptomatic disease occurs. It is in this regard that the current disturbing outbreaks of AIDS is offering us all some paradoxical benefits. It is a set of diseases which follow upon a basic dysfunction of the T-cells, a core component of the immune system; it seems that isopronisine, which restores T-cell function and the production of Interleukin II, can in fact restore the early AIDS patient to normal and prevent the serious sequelae of multiple bouts with serious infection and ultimately the development of Karposi's sarcoma. If the day may shortly come when we shall routinely screen for the early AIDS defect in populations at risk and make the proper intervention to restore the defect, then I believe the next fruitful exploration will be the screening of elderly people for immune system defects and population studies to determine the potential benefits of preventive correction of any recognized defects before an intercurrent illness becomes manifest. Such restorative therapies for a defective host defense system may be regarded as a kind of vaccination against a variety of illnesses. Thus, in increasing numbers, the elderly might conceivably be spared the nagging struggles with infections and neoplasia, which currently cut people down before their genetically predetermined time.

Although not a so-called primary technology, the monoclonal antibody technology offers some hope in the diagnosis and localization of neoplasia as well as in the treatment of some tumors, especially when the antineoplastic poison can be linked to the tumor-specific monoclonal antibody, and can thus be delivered directly to the tumor, minimizing undesirable side effects of the therapy.

There will be wonderful diagnostic advances, including, of course, the much heralded NMR and PET scanning and, by then, the matured role of the computer as an aid to diagnosis, choice of therapy, and advanced record keeping. It is the fond hope of all medical educators that these new technical aides will allow students to rediscover the most cost-effective diagnostic tool, i.e., the doctor's ears. If the available technology allow doctors more time to listen and therefore to take more effective histories, it is my belief that the patient interview and the physical examination will enjoy a return to popularity as more than an art form. The more accurate dissection of internal pathology made possible through NMR and PET scanning should bring a new era of comparisons of physical signs, devaluing some, but elevating others to new levels of utility in low-cost diagnosis. Hope springs eternal!

Aging—Secondary Technologies

Among the most promising "secondary" technologies will be refinement and expansion of successful transplantation procedures and an increase in useful artificial organs. Liver, kidney, heart, lung, bone, bowel, and pancreas must be listed among the former, while artificial joints may well become first among the latter, especially as regards the elderly. Surgery, in general, will be increasingly safe; anesthesiology will continue to improve, especially for the elderly; and the refinements in microsurgery will open new vistas for successful surgical intervention in a population of older people in generally better condition than their predecessors.

Laser treatments and surgical interventions will increase for the treatment of eye disease in the elderly, but early diagnosis of glaucoma and diabetes can be major elements which will be pursued more vigorously in the prevention of serious disease. Microcomputers seem likely to do wonderful things for the hard of hearing and those with speech impediments, and will certainly contribute importantly to the development of effective aids to independent locomotion.

Somewhere out there are the inventions which will allow for the dignified handling of incontinence such that otherwise intact patients will be able to pursue a meaningful existence. Advances in robotics will allow more people to live effectively outside of institutions for longer periods.

Diabetes will become more prevalent as more people live longer, but more effective therapies will make it a less burdensome disease. Hypertension should be less of a problem, but postmenopausal osteoporosis needs effective preventive measures not yet conceived. An effective treatment of the latter disorder is also much needed.

Advances in drug delivery systems and in the understanding of drug interactions in the elderly will enhance treatment markedly. The decreased and more appropriate use of psychotropic drugs should minimize therapy-induced poisonings. Refined radiation therapy should truly advance cancer therapy and minimize side effects.

Disease prevention and health promotion will have an impact on the elderly. Larry Green, the Director of our Center for Health Promotion Research and Development, points out that the elderly, surprisingly, seem better able than their younger colleagues at changing eating and smoking habits. On the other hand, the fact that as many women now smoke as men suggest that lung cancer will be supplanting breast cancer as the number one killer of women. By 2000, we may find that the number of men surviving into old age will equal the number of women. The high suicide rate of white males over 65 is a worrisome fact that warrants attention. Better nutrition, better mouth care, water flouridation, and improved dental restorative techniques all should lead to healthier mouths and, therefore, a better quality of life for the elderly in 2000.

Advances in epidemiology and in the capacity to make an accurate assessment of the multiple hazards in our world will allow for intelligent interventions in our environment and should do much to enhance the life of the elderly.

Old Wine in New Bottles

In closing, let me encapsulate my guesses about health care delivery in the year 2000, guesses based on the "creeping incrementalism" through which major national policies historically have emerged and evolved. In skeletal outline, it seems to me the projected surfeit of doctors and other health professionals will have become a reality and, to a larger extent than is now the case, health care will have become a buyer's market. Doctors and nurses will make house calls, and along with dentists will provide office hours on weekends and evenings; there will have been a shift away from compensation primarily for the execution of a technique and towards an upward valuation of the cognitive skills. Health promotion and preventative elements will be built into daily practice.

The overriding problem will be, of course, the economy of it all. How can we pay for all that it will be possible to provide? An aging population will be in better physical shape later and later in their lives, with more and more people at 70 and 75 having bodies doctors today are used to seeing in people 60 and 65. Thus, costly hospital-based secondary technologies will be potentially available to more and more people eligible for medicare . . . and by 2000 AD, the Medicare Trust Fund will have long been exhausted! Congress will have been politically unable to withold services to the elderly, all of whom will be voting; and the only viable approach to rationing of health care and keeping the cost below 15% of the GNP in a relatively affluent modern society will have been the establishment of some form of capitation or prepaid system. Instead of 10% of the population being covered this way, it will be 90% by 2000 AD, but the cost will be budgetable in advance.

Octagenarians with sufficient personal funds may be able to pay from their own pockets to have their heart, lung, and liver transplants, to acquire frequent face lifts, and to get braces for their teeth, but the level of health services made available to everyone as a matter of societal policy will be predetermined by the number of dollars made available on a capitation basis for health care for the elderly. Alternatively, those primary technologies deemed effective and efficient at preventing the common disorders of the elderly will be fully supported. For example, treatments which might prevent diabetes, postmenopausal osteoporosis, Alzheimer's disease, hearing loss, stroke, and tooth decay could easily prove cost effective to the society, much as certain immunizations and water flouridation have already proven.

There is one other related development currently evolving in the health care field which could have major implications for the provision of services for the elderly in 2000 AD. I refer to the emergence of the so-called "for-profit" chains of hospital and nursing homes, side by side with the growing trend among not-for-profit hospitals to link up with others to make the most of the management networks and cost-saving systems such as those associated with bulk purchasing, shared laundry, power and so forth. The "for-profit" chains now account for 7% of the hospital business in this country and Wall Street analysts believe their market share will grow to 20% in this decade. There are arguments about whether these efforts cut costs or do not; improve quality, diminish it, or do not affect it; and whether doctor and other health professional ownership is or is not in the public's and therefore the professions' best interest. One element of the for-profit trend, however, deserves the watchful consideration of all concerned parties' in the years ahead, and that element is the venturing into a far-reaching vertical integration of provider institutions, with home health care and primary services being connected to hospital care. Increasingly, linkages are occurring in management between and among nursing homes of all levels and hospitals; one of the big five for-profit corporations is building on a single campus, a primary care center, an acute-care hospital, a chronic care hospital, a nursing home, and a psychiatric hospital, literally offering care from cradle to grave.

When one recalls that the U.S. Veterans Administration operates the largest chain of hospitals in the world, including nursing home, dental, mental, and rehabilitative care, and appreciates further that by the year 2000 an enormous proportion of all those over 65 will be eligible for VA care, the potential for a publicly sponsored horizontally and vertically integrated system available to many people will be closer to reality than we suspect. In my mind, then, the VA, with its growing leadership in the field of geriatrics and the trend to vertical integration and nursing home and home care being fueled by the interest of the "for-profit" chains, deserves our continuing attention and, perhaps, support. Strange bedfellows indeed!

I know the prime character trait required of an administrator must be optimism—and my optimism lets me close on the hopeful note that the computerization of our own health care system and all the subsequent high technology will, in fact, encourage a new humanity in our system, a new appreciation of our ability to help one another through a renewed appreciation of the value of our capacity to listen, of our words as therapeutic tools, and of our spirit of helpfulness. The trust relationship between doctor and patient, between health professions and the public can be strengthened if we professionals make the most of the increasing patient time that will be made available to us by our new technologies and our increased numbers. If we cannot marry high technology and humanity more effectively in our sector of our national life, what hope can there be for the rest of society?

Chapter 43

Health Care in the 21st Century: The Social and Ethical Context

James E. Birren

Summary

Predictions about the health of the aged have not been noted for their accuracy. The current level of public interest in measures that promote well-being will influence the health of future older persons and the kind of care they will need. In the past, diagnosticians were taught to seek a single primary diagnosis for an illness. The chronic diseases of the aged are less the manifestations of invasions by foreign agents than manifestations of a changing host. In the phase of terminal decline, self-regulation breaks down, and energy and information must flow into the individual in order to reestablish an equilibrium. Studies of the physiology of aging must embrace the ecology of individuals. This is supported by the fact that there is a large increase in mortality rates associated with bereavement. A greater integration of our specialized disciplinary bodies of knowledge about aging will be required to develop new treatment methods for our future older population.

Historical Perspectives

The kind of predictions implied by the title of this chapter are not known to be very accurate. What disturbs our predictions is that they are made with implicit assumptions about many things being constant, and these constants may actually become variables at different times. In addition, inevitably there are those unanticipated scientific discoveries whose applications change the level of health. For example, the current wave of interest in not smoking, reduced caloric intake, moderate use of alcohol, regular exercise, and reduction of stress has greatly influenced individual well-being. These trends, coupled with the development of hypotensive drugs, have resulted in a dramatic reduction in the mortality rate from cardiovascular disease. This change would not have been predicted from trends evident during the period after World War II, when mortality rates in middle age were constant or increasing.

One way of improving our predictions for the future is to utilize our history. In an attempt to do this, one can explore the social roots of health care in our society; however, this does not always lead to improved predictions. For example, following World War II, I expected the United States to move toward a national health insurance system. This prediction was influenced by the fact that so many individuals in military service at the time were involved in a comprehensive health-care system. Thus, I expected that these millions of veterans would lean toward a centralized insurance system, if not toward a main federal health provider. That has not evolved. Of course, we have not yet seen the total impact of World War II veterans as they move into their later years with increasing health needs. One can foresee a major impact of the large numbers of older veterans on the health-care system in the United States, but how this impact will be expressed is still unknown.

Another belief of our American society is that science and technology will improve the quality of life. A major scientific institution which has had a profound influence on biomedical institutions in America is the National Institutes of Health (NIH). NIH has been effective in promoting basic biomedical research. This research is often carried out within the rubric of a "war on disease" and by institutes devoted to the study of categorical diseases. These orientations may not be those most suitable to the study of health in relationship to aging.

It is relevant to note that, prior to World War II, there existed at NIH an Institute of Experimental Biology and Medicine which in 1941 created a section for the study of gerontology. After World War II, however, categorically oriented disease institutes were promoted, and the National Institute of Experimental Biology and Medicine was incorporated into the National Heart Institute. In the spirit of the times, it was thought that the categorical disease institutes would fare better in competition for funds than would the more academically titled programs. The National Institutes of Health have been successful beyond anyone's dream in terms of creating a research enterprise, mobilizing congressional support, and creating in the public mind the image of waging war on specific diseases. This image is manifested in the public concept of disease as a takeover of the body by a foreign power.

Health and the Aging of Host Organisms

Robert Aldrich, the first director of the National Institute of Child Health and Human Development, once commented that we still suffer from a hangover of an earlier period of this century when our major battles were with infectious diseases. At that time, diagnosticians were taught to seek a single primary diagnosis. It has become apparent that, as infectious diseases were controlled and the population aged, there has been a dramatic increase in chronic diseases and these diseases have become the major killers. Chronic disease is usually less the manifestation of an invasion by a foreign agent than a characteristic disorder of the host. Therefore, a change in our approach is necessary.

T.B. Robertson (1923; cited in Lansing, 1959) once pointed out that "in actuality death is always in some measure accidental." This implies that the last small increment in a stimulus precipitates death in a vulnerable, aged organism. The important point here is the increasing vulnerability of the older organism. Early in the emerging field of gerontology there were many debates about whether there was anything that one might appropriately label "aging." At that time aging was considered to be merely an expression of disease. Today we regard these early debates as beside the point, and consider it more important to specify the energy and the information content of the stimuli that impinge on an organism, as well as its capability to adapt to perturbation. In order to be relevant to aging, the war on disease requires a translation in concept. I believe we are going to begin to look at the health of older individuals in terms of environmental interaction and disease–host interactions.

Over the life span there may be a change in the importance of environmental influences, both social and physical. Early in life, there are strong associations between mortality rates and a broad range of factors that can be clustered under the concept of socioeconomic status. Late in life, however, these influences may diminish. For example, the mortality rates of the nonwhite population, as compared to the white population, are higher in the early years through middle age; however, there is no appreciable difference after age 65. On the one hand, this may be expressing a survival of the biologically fittest in environments which are not necessary favorable (those who make it to the later years being unusually fit persons). A contrary point of view would hold that, with age, the individual's genetic constitution increasingly expresses itself. More dramatically said, "the genome will out" and, with increasing age, variations in mortality rates may be more controlled by genetic factors. Whether or not there is a decreasing contribution of socioenvironmental influences and an increasing influence of genetic factors in the health of aging populations can be a subject of research. I expect that by the year

2000 there will be marked advances in our concepts about aging and, indeed, about how we fit into an evolutionary pattern of aging.

George Sacher (1977) reviewed the evidence and concluded that there was a surprisingly high correlation between the brain size of a species and its length of life. More specifically, he believed that the extent of encephalization influenced prospects for longevity. If Sacher was right, mankind's long length of life may well be due to our comparatively enlarged nervous system relative to our body size. Another implication, however, is that for mammals with large nervous systems the aging of the nervous system becomes the major pacemaker of aging in general. This is not to suggest that we should initiate a quest for a single clock in the brain. The brain may, in fact, best be viewed as a clock shop.

Recently, Gary Lynch (1983) has suggested that there may be a difference in the way the avian brain and the mammalian brain age. He makes the point that the avian brain may show more neuronal replication, and the mammalian brain more dendritic development. Because the mammalian brain is programmed more on the basis of experience, aging may be expressed in reduced dendritic density. The mammalian nervous system, therefore, responds more to use than does the avian brain.

Evidence is accumulating that the structure of neural tissue in old animals depends on use. The density of receptor sites may well vary with the activities of the organism. In humans, functional differences are found between active and inactive men and women. Clearly, the physical activity of older persons influences the characteristics of the aging nervous system. We have need for a general physiological orientation to aging in contrast to a categorical disease approach.

Ecological Relations

One of the problems with extrapolating from laboratory research to real life is the question of the ecological validity of animal studies. In experimental studies it is customary to raise the question of whether a substance is within "a physiologic range." This implies that, in order to interpret an experiment, one needs to know the quantitative level of the experimental substance used in relation to the levels commonly found in the organism. Likewise, one should know whether the environmental conditions used are within a range to which the animals will be normally exposed during their lifetime. It is customary, for example, to house rodents singly in small cages over much of their life span; this is foreign to the way the animals would live in natural environments. In the wild state, rodents have a considerable amount of social contact and, ranging free, have the opportunity for ample physical activity. Experiments have shown that animals denied physical activity show altered brain morphology and behavior.

It is thus important, in establishing models for pathological aging, that we know the baselines for animals raised under ecologically valid conditions. In the same sense, it has been pointed out that the assessment of individuals' capacities for independent living should be done in their homes rather than in the artificial environment of a hospital or institution.

At the NATO conference on technological developments and aging societies, held at the University of Southern California (Robinson, Livingston, and Birren, in press), data were reported that indicate that disuse of function can mimic the changes that occur in aging. Shephard (in press) conducted a 10 year longitudinal study of Eskimos who moved into urban areas. Dramatic physiologic changes occurred, associated with the fact that the Eskimos' caloric expenditures were reduced by one-half as a result of their move from characteristic hunting and fishing areas into the city. The Eskimos showed an increase in body fat, lower maximum oxygen capacity, bone demineralization, and lower muscle strength.

Many of these characteristics sound like normal aging but, in fact, were in this case associated with altered ecological relationships. It is pertinent to point out that in our current urban environments more and more individuals add "physical loading" to their daily lives, replacing the physical effort lost by sedentary work. That is, we run and engage in other exercise to replace the lost physical effort since we apparently must maintain at least a minimal effort in order to remain in good health.

Perhaps we should enlarge our concept of added loading to include the use of cognitive functions. Perhaps we will lose our capacity for calculating if we excessively depend on computers; and gone may be the skills manifested by the market clerk who could keep a running tally of a series of individual purchases. It may also be desirable to speculate about affective loading, although here the principle of loading is less clear. Group therapy, however, may be a substitute or replacement for the broken affective bonds resulting from our highly mobile urban societies. My experience with the exchange of autobiographies by individuals leads me to suggest that it is a replacement for emotional exchanges that have been minimized by our technological society (Birren and Hateley, in press).

In the remainder of this chapter, I will touch upon five elements that would better equip us to improve the quality of life for older adults in the 21st century: (1) new concepts, (2) new data, (3) new research methods, (4) new methods for data analysis, and (5) new treatment methods. I will also discuss several implications that stem from new expectations that the future aged will have about their health care and their roles in society.

New Concepts

Some of the new concepts have already been pointed out, such as the idea that we should look at the human organism as a clock shop rather than as a single grandfather clock. However, at extreme conditions, this concept needs to be expanded because, with aging, the clocks begin to interact. The healthy and adaptive organism may be like a clock shop in which the subsystems show remarkable autonomy of function. In contrast, this autonomy of subsystem function may decline with age. Eugene Yates (1982) updated the concept of homeostasis as it is applied to aging. He observed that when the normal boundary conditions of biological systems are exceeded new relationships enter; and, as the systems interact, new nonlinear relationships appear.

This bears upon the issue that in the period of *terminal decline*, the organism appears to be in a qualitatively different state than previously existed during normal aging. In the phase of terminal decline, different principles operate and self-regulation breaks down. Therefore, energy and information must flow into the individual in order to reestablish an equilibrium. The phase of terminal decline should be viewed not only as being different from normal aging, but also as a phase of decompensation. Various domains of functioning in the organism that are usually autonomous early in life interact when boundary conditions are reached, and a phase of terminal decompensation begins. By the end of the century I suspect that we will have evolved a common language with which to describe such important phenomena.

As I alluded to earlier, I believe that the nervous system will be increasingly implicated in the process of aging. In the past, the nervous system tended to be regarded as a passive follower of changes beginning elsewhere in the aging organism, rather than as a primary factor in aging. The brain is the primary regulatory organ of the body and, because of its complexity, at least two kinds of language are needed to describe it. Many of the properties of the brain are reducible to biochemical and thermodynamic principles, as is true of any group of cells in the body. However, in addition to regulating the vegetative functions of the body, the brain has another role, the intrinsic character of which is not described by energy relations but by information. This reflects the principle that the brain is programmed not only by information in the DNA but also on the basis of experience. This raises the interesting question of how the thermodynamic systems and the information systems of the brain interact in the aging process.

New Data

One question that is often asked about aging is whether there can be symbolic or psychological events that are causal in the same sense that genetic predisposition is. The answer to this question is yes. A unique set of data gathered in Sweden on the effects of bereavement on the mortality of surviving spouses demonstrates this (Mellstrom, Nilsson, Oden, Rundren, and Svanborg, 1982). In these studies the effect of loss of a spouce was examined in relation to the mortality rates of the surviving partner. Outcomes following about 365,000 deaths were examined for a period of 5 years. It was found that the mortality rates went up 46% in the first 3 months following the death of a spouse for males and 22% for females. Admittedly there is some common variance due to the fact that individuals shared the same household and lifestyle as their spouse, but this would appear to be a small factor. In fact, one may question whether there is any biological factor that can raise the mortality rate so dramatically.

It is apparent that females have gained more from general improvements in the standard of living during this century, in terms of their life expectancy, than have males. The gap between female and male life expectancy has been widening, which may reflect the principle alluded to earlier that "the genome will out." Here we have an issue that will warrant new data; that is, what is the basis for the special vulnerability of the male organism?

New Research Methods

The fact that bereavement increases mortality rates would seem to defy explanation in the natural sciences. However, the paradigms or models developing in the neurosciences may provide some explanations. The power of the neuroscience approach lies not only in its experimental methods but in the fact that convergent evidence about phenomena is gathered from a variety of disciplines. Explanations of brain function are simultaneously undertaken from the points of view of morphology, neurochemistry, neurophysiology, and behavior. Although investigators are usually trained in one particular area, they utilize data from adjacent disciplines.

In a similar way, the issues of aging transcend the limits of any particular discipline and require integration of data from several methods of investigation. The causal relationships in issues of mortality and longevity involve interactions between individuals and environments. Presumably, they reflect ecological relationships which are broadly sociological in character, and invite a neuroscience orientation.

One breakthrough in the study of the nervous system has been Sokoloff's (1979) development of noninvasive techniques which permit the study of regional metabolic activity in the brain during normal functioning, as well as its orchestrated activities in the wakeful state. These methods promise to provide us with important distinctions between aging and pathological functioning, such as that which exists in Alzheimer's disease.

Our modern research methods may enable us to identify whom of the aged will be most at risk. Alternatively, they will also enable us to identify individuals who are least at risk and will survive to their late 90s, or even over 100 years of age, with their functional capacities intact in every sense of the word.

New Methods for Data Analysis

In addition to new methods of data collection, among the important research developments in recent years are new, powerful methods of data analysis. These developments make it possible to find and follow pathways in the organization of health changes with age. This is to say that one can develop hypotheses about causal pathways in a set of data, and test for those hypotheses by analytical programs such as those developed by Jöreskog and Sorbum (1979). These powerful analytical methods will enable us to describe patterns of change in normal and pathological aging for complex sets of data.

New Treatments

1983 saw the introduction of robots into nursing home care. The friendly little robot machine can do everything we can do—faster, more efficiently, and possibly better. However, the thought of introducing robots into nursing home care brings about some reservations. Human supporting contact or, if you will, an emotional element is not met by the machine; and this contact may be essential and life sustaining in the nursing home context. If culture is the DNA of society, then the *way* we do things is as important to the older individual as *what* we do. Perhaps we are faced with the fact that the decompensating older person is not only in need of energy and information, but also affect. If we wish to maximize function, we must take all three factors into account.

New Expectations

It has been pointed out in numerous contexts that there is a new group of elderly persons coming upon the scene who are better educated, more competent, and have higher expectations for care than past generations. These individuals have lived long and productive lives. I doubt that we will be able to tell them that they are not going to share equally in the new technology, such as the technological advances seen in renal and cardiovascular disease. For example, the largest membership group in the

United States is the American Association of Retired Persons, with about 15 million members. Their publication, *Modern Maturity*, has the third widest readership of any magazine in the country. Given this organization of articulate, informed individuals, it will not be easy to deny them equal access to new developments in health care.

It seems to me that there are two imperatives in the field we are discussing. One is the demographic imperative, namely, that the oldest portion of the population is increasing the fastest. The other is the technological imperative, in which our society has strong faith. I doubt if we can turn aside technological developments by adopting the approach of the Luddites in England, who tried to destroy the mechanically driven weaving looms that drove out handweaving. Because of the social organization of older persons who have lived constructive lives, have served society well, and are now informed about public policy issues, I believe that public policy dialogues are going to be increasingly open and intense. The recent discussions concerning social security serve as evidence of the fact that older persons are neither totally dependent nor passive in defining their needs. The old of tomorrow will be defining their needs more strongly in the face of pressure to reduce the proportion of the gross national product spent on health care for the elderly.

Discussions about the health and aging of the labor force are also relevant to this issue. Questions have been raised about whether we can afford to keep older workers in the labor force. The other side of this question is whether we can afford to keep older persons *out of* the labor force. Clearly we are living longer and working for a lesser number of years, and a large economic gap is being created.

The sequential longitudinal studies conducted in Gothenborg, Sweden (Mellstrom, Nillson, Oden, Rundren, and Svanborg, 1982) indicate that it is a small minority of persons who have severe health limitations in their 80s. In general terms, this means that individuals as old as 75–80 years of age have the capacity to work and to produce. Some individuals who live temperate lives, such as college teachers, have a much longer life expectancy than the population at large.

It is a strong temptation to link all aspects of personal productivity with being employed, as though nothing we do outside of an employed job is productive. This would mean that a worker employed in a cigarette factory is judged to be productive, but a grandparent who is retired and helping to rear a grandchild is not. Soon we are going to have to differentiate more carefully the concepts that relate to the productivity of a society. The concepts of productivity and profitability have been linked too closely. We need new concepts of productivity, concepts that can embrace the activities of older persons.

At the present time our state of knowledge about normal aging is very particulate; we have many islands of knowledge, but few bridges between them. The departmentalized knowledge of the various specialized disciplines and professions does not lend itself easily to research on aging, nor to an integrated approach to treating older persons. This leads me to suggest that educational institutions have a large responsibility to educate professionals and academics with regard to the issues of aging. In every future geriatrician there should be a little of the sociologist and psychologist, just as in every future social worker there should be a little of the geriatrician and biologist. Only then will we be able to address the issues of aging in their natural terms, and to bring about the introduction of new treatment methods in health care for the increasingly sophisticated older population that will be with us in the year 2000.

References

Birren, J.E., and Hateley, B.J.: Guided autobiography: A special method of life review. In Blum, R.H. (Ed.), The Art of Life and Family Writing. Portola Valley, CA: American Lives Endowment (in press).

Jöreskog, K.G., and Sorbum, D.: Advances in Factor Analysis and Structural Equation Models. Cambridge, MA: ABP Books, 1979.

Lansing, A.I.: General biology of senescence. In Birren, J.E. (Ed.), Handbook of Aging and the Individual, pp. 119–135. Chicago: University of Chicago Press, 1959.

Lynch, G.: Aging, synaptic plasticity, and neuronal stability. Invited address, 91st Annual Convention of the American Psychological Association, Anaheim, California, August 1983.

Mellstrom, D., Nilsson, A., Oden, A., Rundren, A., and Svanborg, A.: Mortality among the widowed in Sweden. *Scand. J. Soc. Med. 10*, 33–41 (1982).

Robertson, T.B.: The Chemical Basis of Growth and Senescence. Philadelphia: J.B. Lippincott, 1923.

Robinson, P., Livingston, J., and Birren, J. (Eds.): Aging and Technology. New York: Plenum (in press).

Sacher, G.: Life table modification and life prolongation. In Finch, C., Hayflick, L. (Eds.), Handbook of the Biology of Aging, pp. 582–638. New York: Van Nostrand Reinhold, 1977.

Shephard, R.: Technological changes and the aging of working capacity. In Robinson, P., Livingston, J., and Birren, J. (Eds.), Aging and Technology. New York: Plenum (in press).

Sokoloff, L.: Effects of normal aging on cerebral circulation and energy metabolism. In Hoffmeister, F., and Muller, C. (Eds.), Brain Function in Old Age, pp. 367–380. New York: Springer-Verlag, 1979.

Yates, F.: Outline of a physical theory of physiological systems. *Can. J. Physiol. Pharmacol. 60*, 217–248 (1982).

Chapter 44

Future Diagnostic and Therapeutic Strategies: A Realistic Forecast

Arvid Carlsson

Summary

The degenerative changes occurring in the aging brain appear to affect many different types of neurons in vast areas of the brain, leading to functional losses of varying type and severity. Senile dementia, depression, and Parkinson's disease may be looked upon as manifestations of severe imbalances between neuronal systems caused by degenerative processes. To combat the age-related losses of brain function will require a tremendous effort, involving the development of new diagnostic and therapeutic procedures. Recent progress in these areas offers promise that by the year 2000, some of these problems will be overcome.

Introduction

We are obviously facing a very serious problem. The "squaring off" of the human survival curve, repeatedly referred to in many of the chapters, will allow an increasing number of individuals to reach an age when their brains will no longer function properly. Epidemiological studies suggest that by the year 2000 a person who is now 60 years old—that would apply to myself—would run an almost 10% risk of being demented to a degree requiring care at an institution (see, for example, Adolfsson et al., 1981). With increasing age this risk rises dramatically to approach the 50% level at the age of 90–100 years. The risk of suffering from a cognitive defect of less severe degree, though still disturbing, should be substantially greater.

If we include other age-related brain disorders, such as depression (which is actually more common than dementia), Parkinson's disease, and other motor disturbances so frequently seen in the aged, we will obviously end up with alarming figures. We have good reasons for considering how to face this situation.

Diagnostic Strategies

The diagnostic problems in neurogeriatrics are by no means simple. To distinguish between dementia and depression, for example, may prove very difficult, especially since there is overlapping between them. How common is pseudodementia, where both depression and psychosocial factors may be involved?

Some workers in this field insist that the diagnosis Alzheimer's disease, or senile dementia of the Alzheimer type, can only be established by microscopic examination of the brain tissue. As a presumptive future patient I do not find such a diagnostic procedure very attractive, but I feel confident that by the year 2000 we are going to do a lot better than that. We are now witnessing a most spectacular development in the area of neuroimaging. Already at the present time the dopamine receptors of the basal ganglia can be visualized by means of positron emission tomography. By the turn of the century we can expect considerable advances along this line; it will no doubt be possible to visualize a large number of neurotransmitters and their receptors and to discover pathological changes in well-defined brain regions and transmitter systems.

However, these sophisticated techniques will probably continue to be very expensive, and it seems doubtful if they can be applied in routine diagnostic procedures. Hopefully serendipity will come in and indicate shortcuts, which will enable the clinician to recognize syndromes, previously defined and characterized by means of the imaging techniques, but later detectable by simpler methods.

In this context I would like to mention the neuroendocrinological research strategy, which has already given results of diagnostic interest in depression, as illustrated, for example, by the dexamethasone suppression test. This type of approach has not yet been much utilized in the diagnosis of senile brain disorders. Dr. Samorajski (Chapter 13) described some recent progress in this area, and a recent study at the University of Gothenburg shows that the dexamethasone test gives a positive result in many cases of dementia, even in the absence of clear-cut signs of depression (Balldin et al., 1983).

The neuroendocrinological approach permits us to look into the neurotransmitter machinery in a small but very important part of the brain: the hypothalamus. Admittedly it is a narrow keyhole, but it may provide us with a lot of useful information, based on blood samples, sometimes taken after relatively simple challenging procedures.

Therapeutic Strategies

Future therapeutic strategies will depend very much on new diagnostic procedures, and the two will thus to some extent have to be developed hand in hand. We can thus anticipate new subclassifications of some of the major senile brain disorders, such as depression and dementia, based on the actual biochemical disturbances in the brain. Possibly this will apply also to Parkinson's disease, but in this case we can rather anticipate improvement of the available drug therapy.

The present L-dopa therapy leaves much to be desired. The levels of L-dopa in the blood show tremendous fluctuations, which are probably harmful and may contribute to the "on–off" problems often observed after some years of treatment. Here we can expect considerable improvement by the advent of suitable pharmaceutical preparations.

In addition to L-dopa, direct dopamine-receptor agonists, such as bromocriptine and lisuride, have been found useful in the treatment of Parkinson's disease. They have, however, on the whole done less well than L-dopa. Nevertheless the principle of direct receptor agonist treatment may prove a lot more valuable in the future, with the advent of more efficacious and specific drugs.

In Parkinson's disease replacement of the missing neurons by grafting techniques would appear especially promising, since we are here dealing with a rather strictly localized lesion. The few attempts made thus far have not been successful, but we can foresee technical improvement of the grafting techniques, and thus a future successful outcome is by no means excluded. However, in more generalized brain disorders—and dementias may largely belong to these—grafting techniques will probably prove less useful. Drug therapy appears more promising in such cases, though still difficult.

In depression, especially senile depression, significant advances can be foreseen in the not too distant future. In particular, it will no doubt be possible to avoid the anticholinergic side effects characteristic of the now dominating tricyclic antidepressants. These side effects are particularly troublesome in the aged, not least because of their liability to cause delirious states. New antidepressants with more specific actions on serotonergic or adrenergic mechanisms are now being developed. They appear to be at least as efficacious as the tricyclic antidepressants, though with fewer side effects.

It remains to discuss further therapeutic strategies in dementia. They depend, of course, on the nature of the underlying disorder. At present there are two schools in this area (I am now discussing specifically Alzheimer's disease and senile dementia of the Alzheimer type). One school maintains that we are dealing with a strictly localized and specific disturbance, i.e., a degeneration of a cholinergic pathway originating in the nucleus basalis of Meynert and terminating in various parts of the cortex and in the hippocampus. The other school claims that these dementia disorders are more generalized and encompass cortical as well as subcortical areas of the brain, where many different neuronal systems and neurotransmitters are involved. I belong to the latter school. Thus I was most intrigued by the PET scan data presented by Dr. de Leon, (Chapter 17) which shows that glucose uptake is significantly reduced in the brains of Alzheimer patients, and that this disturbance occurs in vast areas of the brain. His observations thus support the notion of a generalized brain disorder. Another interesting observation by Dr. de Leon was that the biochemical disturbance, detected by PET scan as outlined above, correlated better with the clinical symptoms than did the structural abnormalities, detected by means of computer tomography. This was one of the most encouraging messages that has reached me recently, because it suggests that in dementia there is still enough brain tissue left; if only the biochemical disturbance can be corrected, the brain will then hopefully start to function properly again.

I was also interested in Dr. Bondareff's report (Chapter 19) showing that several subcortical neurotransmitter systems are deficient, as indicated by postmortem data from cases of Alzheimer's disease or senile dementia of the Alzheimer type. This is in line with the observations of our own research group, reported in Chapter 27.

The conclusion drawn from these studies will be that future therapeutic strategies in dementia must aim at alleviating multiple neurotransmitter deficiencies. A truly rational approach will probably have to await the development of refined diagnostic procedures, by means of which the profile of neurotransmitter deficiencies can be established in the individual patient. It will also have to await the advent of an arsenal of receptor agonists, substituting for the missing neurotransmitter molecules. These agonists will perhaps have to be given as cocktails, tailored for the particular deficiency profile of the individual patient.

Hydergine has a pharmacologic profile of some interest in this context. Dr. Markstein (Chapter 30) indicates that Hydergine is a partial agonist on dopamine and 5-HT receptors and an antagonist on alpha-adrenergic receptors. This seems to match the biochemical disturbances found in dementia of the Alzheimer type, i.e., a deficiency in dopamine and 5-HT systems with simultaneous evidence of a hyperactive noradrenergic system (see Chapter 27).

The moderate therapeutic activity of Hydergine in dementia may be related to this particular profile. It may thus serve as an interesting model substance in research aiming to develop more active therapeutic agents for dementia.

There is little doubt, however, that a deficiency in cholinergic systems forms an important aspect of senile dementia, and thus we must ask the pharmaceutical industry to develop more specific centrally active cholinergic agonists than those available today, and with less side effects. To this list will have to be added a number of other neurotransmitters. A couple of peptides are already known to be deficient in dementia.

Will Prophylaxis Be Possible?

Finally, a few words should be written about possible future preventive strategies. I restrict my discussion here to biomedical aspects, even though psychosocial measures, aiming, for example, to create a more stimulating environment, are probably of at least equal importance.

It seems doubtful if it will ever be possible to delay to any significant extent the fundamental aging process, which may reside in the genetic material. To do this might not even be desirable from our society's point of view. However, mechanisms may exist which are superimposed upon the basic aging process, causing some neurons to become more sensitive to aging than others. The imbalance thus arising between different neuronal systems may contribute more to functional disturbances than the aging process per se. A possible example will be briefly mentioned below.

There is both morphologic and biochemical evidence that the catecholaminergic neurons exhibit a more rapid age-related decay than many other types of neuron investigated so far. While it cannot be excluded that the catecholaminergic neurons are especially sensitive to the aging process per se, it is tempting to suggest that their sensitivity is somehow related to their specific biochemical products, i.e., the catecholamines. These compounds can undergo a nonenzymatic oxidative reaction, leading to the formation of cytotoxic semiquinones and quinones. The possibility may thus be considered that the catecholaminergic neurons are committing suicide slowly over the years by the formation of toxic compounds, and that this accounts for their apparently high sensitivity to the aging process. If this is so, it might be possible to prevent some of the functional loss occurring in the aging brain by interfering with the oxidative reactions leading to the toxic products. This might be achieved by raising the levels of protective antioxidants, such as vitamins C and E, or compounds possessing thiol groups (see Chapter 9).

Another possible approach would be to identify trophic factors which may be reduced during aging, leading to neuronal degeneration, and to try to stimulate their formation (see Chapter 7).

In conclusion, the degenerative changes occurring in the aging brain appear to affect many different types of neurons in vast areas of the brain, leading to functional losses of varying types and severity. Senile dementia, depression, and Parkinson's disease may be looked upon as manifestations of severe imbalances between neuronal systems, caused by degenerative processes. To combat the age-related losses of brain function will require a tremendous effort, involving the development of new diagnostic and therapeutic procedures. Recent progress in these areas offers promise that by the year 2000 some of these problems have been overcome.

References

Adolfsson, R., Gottfries, C.-G., Nyström, L., and Winblad, B.: Prevalence of dementia in institutionalized Swedish old people. *Acta Psychiat. Scand. 63*, 225–244 (1981).

Balldin, J., Gottfries, C.-G., Karlsson, I., Lindstedt, G., Långström, G., and Wålinder, J.: Dexamethasone suppression test and serum prolactin in dementia disorders. *Br. J. Psychiat. 143*, 277–281 (1983).

Epilogue

Our overview of conditions in 1984 has shown us that much can be done to help old people who have physical and mental impairments. What we know is still not universally applied, or even available in practice, however, and this gap can to some extent be explained by economic factors and disjointed dissemination of information. We hope, in the last years of the 20th century, to enable caregivers to help the aged in our population achieve a higher quality of life and to communicate what is available and attainable.

We are on the threshold of benefiting from technological advances that were little more than fantasy in the past. New knowledge in the neurosciences, for example, should help us unravel some of the relationships of brain function and disease. Progress in psychopharmacology, biology, and immunology, and knowledge gained from the new imaging techniques, positron emission tomography, and nuclear magnetic resonance, should give us a more rational basis for treatment. If we can relate this information with social and psychological parameters, which are equally important, we can look forward to a time when these advances, combined, will provide more opportunities for a meaningful existence late in life.

Those of us who are advocates for the aged—and implicitly for ourselves—must maintain our efforts to provide the elderly with their fair share of services. We must make it easier for them to have access to the best treatment available at the present time. Research in all fields must include, to an even greater extent than now, age as an important element for study. Specifically, of course, research has to be expanded to find answers to the problems of the elderly for which currently we have no answers.

Finally, we must be constantly aware that moral and ethical issues, and financial and economic factors even more than technical advances, determine the future of the elderly in our society. Such issues may transcend application of scientific advances. Perseverance, diligence, and vigilance by the advocates will be required to maintain the current initiative and interest in overcoming the handicaps of aging.

Index

MIX
Papier aus verantwortungsvollen Quellen
Paper from responsible sources
FSC® C105338

If you have any concerns about our products,
you can contact us on
ProductSafety@springernature.com

In case Publisher is established outside the EU,
the EU authorized representative is:
Springer Nature Customer Service Center GmbH
Europaplatz 3, 69115 Heidelberg, Germany

Printed by Libri Plureos GmbH
in Hamburg, Germany